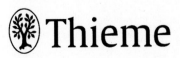

Oral Development and Histology

Third edition

James K. Avery, D.D.S., Ph.D.
Professor Emeritus, Dentistry and Anatomy
School of Dentistry and Medical School
University of Michigan
Ann Arbor, Michigan, USA

Editor
Pauline F. Steele, B.S., R.D.H., B.S. (Educ.), M.A.
Professor Emeritus and Director of Dental Hygiene
School of Dentistry
University of Michigan
Ann Arbor, Michigan, USA

Associate Editor
Nancy Avery, B.F.A.
Ann Arbor, Michigan, USA

850 illustrations, partly in color

Thieme
Stuttgart · New York

Library of Congress Cataloging-in-Publication Data

Oral development and histology / editor, James K. Avery; associate editor, Pauline F. Steele–3rd ed.
p.; cm.
Includes bibliographical references and index.
ISBN 3131001933 (GTV) – ISBN 1-58890-028-2 (TNY)
1. Mouth--Anatomy. 2. Teeth--Anatomy. 3. Mouth--Histology. 4. Teeth--Histology. 5. Embryology, Human. I. Avery, James K. II. Steele, Pauline F.
[DNLM: 1. Stomatognathic System--anatomy & histology. 2. Stomatognathic System--growth & development. WU 101 063 2001]
RK280 .0683 2001
611'.31--dc21
2001027523

2nd edition published 1994 by Thieme Medical Publishers, Inc., 333 Seventh Avenue, New York, NY 10001

© 2002 Georg Thieme Verlag,
Rüdigerstrasse 14,
D-70469 Stuttgart, Germany
Thieme New York, 333 Seventh Avenue,
New York, NY 10001, USA

Typesetting and reproductions by Menhir Produzione,
S. Egidio alla Vibrata (TE), Italy
Printed in Germany by Staudigl, Donauwörth

ISBN 3–13–100193–3 (GTV)
ISBN 1–58890–028–2 (TNY)   1 2 3 4 5

Preface

The aim of this text is to enable the student of dentistry to learn the fundamentals underlying clinical treatment of the patient. Oral structures are described in microscopic detail in this book. As in the past editions the book is divided into six sections. The first section describes developmental details of the head and neck and how these structures relate to the body as a whole. Also described is the relationship of cells to tissues, how tissues make up organs, and how organs relate to the total being. The developing body is followed postnatally through postadolescence. The second section describes the developing crowns and roots of the teeth and the tissues surrounding and supporting them. Tooth eruption and shedding is also included in this section. The third section is a description of the structure and function of the teeth in their mature form as well as a comparison of the primary and permanent dentitions. The fourth section describes the supporting tissues of the teeth including the gingiva and the periodontium, which consists of the cementum, alveolar bone, and periodontal ligament. These structures, including their innervation, are fully described. The fifth section describes the glands of the oral cavity and their products. The sixth and final section describes the perioral tissues, such as the bilateral nasal sinuses and the temporomandibular joints. Also considered in this section are tooth movement, tooth implantation, and healing of oral tissues. In comparison with the past edition, we believe this organizational pattern is more relevant to the teaching of these subjects.

This new edition is updated and expanded, bringing forth new information gained since production of the last edition. We have included more "Clinical Applications" to better relate basic and clinical information. The text contains a large number of illustrations that enhance understanding of the written descriptions. In this edition color has been added to further clarify the histologic photomicrographs and the diagrams. This should assist in gaining information about the structure of complex tissues. A glossary is again included to assist in defining terms that may be unfamiliar to the student. All of the authors wish to express their hope that the materials presented are clear and understandable. Please send any questions that arise to me or to the authors directly.

Fall 2001

James K Avery

Acknowledgements

The first edition of this text was developed with the assistance of a group of students of the oral histology class at the University of Michigan School of Dentistry. Dr. Donald Strachan, one of the instructors of the course, had encouraged development of a series of slide-tape sequences to stimulate interest in the subject. From this effort class manuals were developed, which then evolved into a textbook. Most of the students involved are now teaching at universities or are in dental practices. Some of them have written chapters of this book.

Again, the medical illustrations in this book were produced by students of dentistry. The first was Jeff Clark who produced much of the art throughout the book. The second was Alayne Evans, then a dental student, who listened to the needs of each of the authors and provided excellent illustrations. Both are practicing dentistry today. Much of the photography was also done by students such as Steve Olsen, Gary Bilyk, and Thomas Simmons, all of whom created the photography for yearbooks at the university and found it a challenge to produce the detailed illustrations required to publish this book.

I am also grateful to Drs. Daniel Chiego, Donald Strachan, and Charles Cox, who assisted in teaching this course and contributed in many ways to the evolution of this text. Guidance was also provided by Dr. Thomas Greene of the Department of Educational Resources who evaluated manuscripts and in many ways assisted in the production of class manuscripts and ultimately this text. Although many of these people were not on the scene for this edition, they helped immeasurably on earlier editions from which this edition was developed.

James K Avery

Contributors

James K. Avery, D.D.S., Ph.D.
Professor Emeritus, Dentistry and Anatomy
School of Dentistry and Medical School
University of Michigan
Ann Arbor, Michigan, USA

Sol Bernick, Ph.D.
Professor Emeritus of Anatomy
Department of Anatomy
University of Southern California
Los Angeles, California, USA

Daniel J. Chiego, Jr., M.S., Ph.D.
Associate Professor of Dentistry
Department of Cardiology, Restorative Sciences,
and Endodontics
School of Dentistry
University of Michigan
Ann Arbor, Michigan, USA

Marion J. Edge, D.M.D.
Chairperson and Associate Professor
Department of Diagnostic Sciences
Prosthodontics and Restorative Dentistry
School of Dentistry
University of Louisville
Louisville, Kentucky, USA

Carla A. Evans, D.D.S, D.M.Sc.
Professor of Dentistry
Chair of Orthodontics
University of Illinois
Chicago, Illinois, USA

David C. Johnsen, D.D.S., M.S.
Dean and Professor of Pediatric Dentistry
University of Iowa
College of Dentistry
Iowa City, Iowa, USA

Robert M. Klein, Ph.D.
Professor and Director of Medical Education
Department of Anatomy and Cell Biology
School of Medicine
University of Kansas Medical Center
Kansas City, Kansas, USA
rklein@kumc.edu

Robert B. O'Neal, D.M.D., M.S., M.ed.
Director Graduate Periodontics
University of Washington
Seattle, Washington, USA

Nicholas P. Piesco, Ph.D.
Associate Professor
Departments of Oral Medicine and Pathology and Restorative
Dental Sciences
School of Dental Medicine
University of Pittsburgh
Pittsburgh, Pennsylvania

Francisco Rivera-Hidalgó, B.S., D.M.D., M.S., F.I.C.D.
Associate Professor and Director of Research
Department of Periodontics
Baylor College of Dentistry
The Texas A & M University System, Health Science Center
Dallas, Texas, USA

James W. Simmelink, Ph.D.
Associate Professor of Restorative Dentistry
Director of Research
School of Dentistry
Case Western Reserve University
Cleveland, Ohio, USA

Geoffrey H. Sperber, B.Sc. Hons, B.D.S., M.S., Ph.D., F.I.C.D.
Professor Emeritus
Faculty of Medicine and Dentistry
University of Alberta
Edmonton, Canada

Donald S. Strachan, D.D.S., Ph.D.
Professor Emeritus of Dentistry
School of Dentistry
Associate Professor of Anatomy and Cell Biology
Medical School
University of Michigan
Ann Arbor, Michigan, USA

Dennis F. Turner, D.D.S., M.B.A.
Clinical Associate Professor of Dentistry
Department of Cardiology
Restorative Sciences and Endodontics
Assistant Dean for Patient Services
School of Dentistry
University of Michigan
Ann Arbor, Michigan, USA

Contents

Section VI
Related Functional Tissues of the Oral and Paraoral Areas

SECTION I
Development and Maturation of the Craniofacial Region

1 General Human Development

James K. Avery and Nagat M. ElNesr

Introduction

The purpose of this chapter is to describe many of the important developmental events that take place between conception and birth in the human. Early events leading up to and following conception are discussed, such as endometrial changes in preparation for implantation of the fertilized ovum. Changes in the endocrine level of estrogen and progesterone are noted and facilitate changes in the uterine wall and the fertilized ovum. Growth of the fertilized ovum into an embryoblast surrounded by a functioning and protective membrane system is next described. The embryo is then seen to undergo differentiation of various organ systems that will give rise to the brain, the spinal cord, and the gastrointestinal tube and its associated organs. Somites, a series of soft-tissue blocks located on either side of the neural tube, appear at 2.5 weeks. These somites enlarge to provide muscle and skeletal support of the body. Blood islands appear in the yolk sac and placenta. Blood vessels and cells of the vascular system develop and then prepare for the initiation of the first heartbeat. Blood circulates first from the yolk sac (vitelline circulation) to provide nutrition for the first few weeks of embryonic life. The vascular system then conducts oxygenated blood from the placenta. As the embryo continues to grow, a number of tissue types appear, enabling the embryo to develop many specialized functions. By 9 months the fetus has developed essential features and grown in size, enlarging sufficiently to be prepared for the changes associated with birth. Finally, a number of hereditary and environmental factors known to cause congenital defects are described.

Objectives

After reading this chapter, you should be able to discuss the important developmental events such as fertilization and further growth of the fertilized ovum. You should also be able to discuss the development of the organs and organ systems of the embryo and the fetus, some of the vital changes at birth, and finally, several of the important hereditary and environmental causes of abnormal development.

Origin of the Human Embryo

Human prenatal development begins with processes involved in the ovarian cycle and fertilization (Fig. 1.**1**). As the ovum develops, the uterine wall thickens and ducts and capillaries proliferate in the underlying endometrium. The uterus is thus preparing for the arrival of the fertilized ovum. The uterine changes from days 7 to 14 can be observed in Figure 1.1. Blood levels of the hormones estrogen and progesterone fluctuate cyclically; both function in uterine wall development (Fig.1.**1**). Progesterone also aids in the conversion of the empty ovarian follicles into the the "corpus luteum." The average menstrual cycle is 28 days, although this varies with the individual. If the cycle is defined from the first day of menstrual flow, ovulation will occur about 14 days later. By this time, a follicle ruptures on the surface of the ovary releasing a mature ovum. Note both ovarian and uterine changes in Figure 1.**1**.

Fertilization finally occurs in the distal one-third of the uterine tube (Fig. 1.**2**). It may occur elsewhere, leading to an ectopic pregnancy. It begins with the deposition of some 200 million spermatazoa in the vagina during coitus. The spermatazoa move 1.5 to 3 mm per minute toward and into the uterus and uterine tubes to the point of fertilization. However only 300 to 500 spermatazoa remain viable to surround the ovum. Finally, only one spermatazoon (generally) penetrates the ovum. The ovum is surrounded by the zona pellucida, which after fertilization becomes a fertilization membrane that prevents other spermatozoa from entering the ovum. Fusion of the male and female pronuclei then occurs, each pronucleus carrying 23 chromosomes. This process completes the fertilization process. The fertilized ovum is termed a "zygote," which then undergoes cleavage (cell division) and begins movement into the uterine tube where it passes toward the uterine cavity. Fluid in the oviduct assists the zygote in its movement to the uterine cavity. It takes 4 days for the changing zygote to reach the uterine cavity where it will implant into the wall of the uterus (Fig. 1.**2**). The zygote meanwhile has

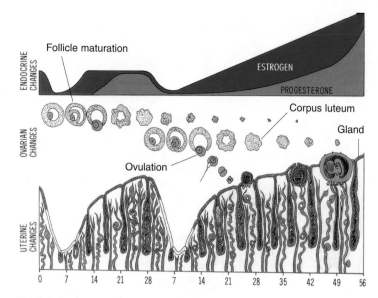

Fig. 1.**1**. Ovulation and fertilization.

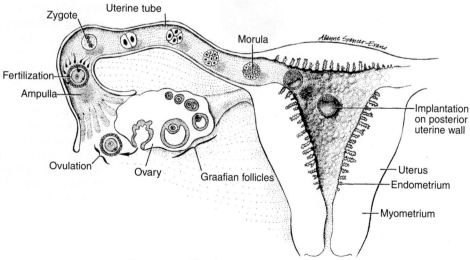

Fig. 1.**2** Site of fertilization.

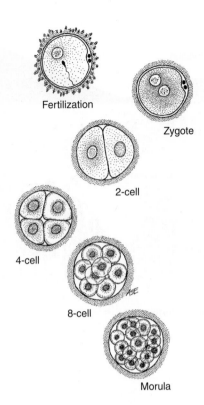

Fig. 1.**3** Cleavage stages

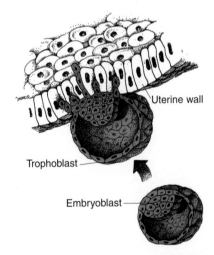

Fig. 1.**4** Implantation

changed into a multi-celled mass; this is termed the morula stage (Fig 1.**3**). As the cellular mass divides, it enlarges and gains a fluid-filled inner cavity termed the blastocele. The blastocele separates the cells into two parts: an outer cell layer, the trophoblast, and an inner cell mass, the embryoblast. This is called the blastocyst stage (Fig.1.**4**) and occurs at 4.5 days after conception and shortly before implantation.

On the sixth day, implantation takes place. The trophoblast at the embryonic end of the cell mass attaches to the sticky endometrial surface, usually on the posterior wall of the body of the uterus (Fig. 1.**2**). The uterine wall, in the meantime, has increased its vascularity in expectation of receiving the cell mass. The surface cells of the trophoblast produce hydrolytic enzymes that digest the endometrial cells, allowing a deeper penetration of the cell mass (Fig. 1.**4**). This event is termed "implantation."

Fundamentals of Development

In the past dozen years the molecular biology of vertebrate development has been the subject of intense study, yet today we are still not able to understand many of the processes vital to fundamental embryology. For example, a gene may have different functions at different periods of development. Also important, but not understood, is the role of mutant forms of developmentally important genes (**protoncogenes**), which convert normal cells to tumor cells. Rather than attempting discussion of this expansive subject, only examples of molecular control of developing structures will be used where appropriate in chapters in this text. Many of the molecules that guide embryonic development can be grouped into a small number of categories. Some molecules remain in the cells that produce them and act as **transcription factors**. Transcription factors are those proteins that possess domains and bind to DNA (deoxyribonucleic acid) in enhancer regions of genes. There are many kinds of transcription factors. Some act as intercellular effectors stimulating adjacent cells or those cells distant from the one from which they originated. However, each contain **signalling molecules** that affect growth. Signalling molecules are mediators of most interactions or inductions between two groups of embryonic cells. Transforming growth factor (TGF-B), fibroblast growth factor (FGF), and Hedgehog proteins are families of molecules that cause important inductive phenomena. **Nerve growth factor** is an example of one which stimulates the growth of sensory and sympathetic nerves and has been studied for many years. Other molecules function as receptors located on cell surfaces and can function from either an intercellular or extracellular location. Examples of some of these molecules will be described as their development is discussed.

Periods of Prenatal Development

Implantation and enlargement of the blastocyst, which contains the embryonic tissues, occurs within the first 2 weeks of development and is described as the "proliferative period." During this time, fertilization, implantation, and formation of the embryonic cell mass has taken place. After the second week the embryonic mass begins to take the shape of an embryo, so the period of 3 to 8 weeks is appropriately termed the "embryonic period." During this period the embryonic germ layers composed of ectoderm, mesoderm, and endoderm differentiate and form tissues, which then form organ systems within the embryo. At 4 weeks the heart forms and begins to beat, the neural tube forms, the gastrointestinal tract develops, and the face forms. At 8 weeks the embryo begins to look human, indicating the beginning of the fetal period that extends until birth (Fig. 1.**5**). Also an increase in body weight and size reflects the increase of tissues and organ systems during the fetal period.

Details of the Proliferation Period

In the second week blastocyst cells of the inner cell mass differentiate into two cell masses, each comprised of different cell types (Fig. 1.**6**). These are columnar ectodermal cells and cuboidal endodermal cells that lie side by side forming the embryonic disc (Fig. 1.**6**). A cavity, termed the amniotic cavity, develops between the ectodermal cells of the embryonic disc and the cells of the outer wall of the trophoblast (Fig. 1.**6**). Then a second internal cavity, the yolk sac, appears (Fig. 1.**7**). These cells give rise to yolk, or nutrition of the embryo, until blood vessels form and carry food from the mother's circulation to the embryo. Both cavities lie on either side of the embryonic disc (Fig. 1.**7**). The amniotic cavity, lined by a membrane, enlarges even more rapidly than the embryo and invests it in a membrane. The developing embryo is

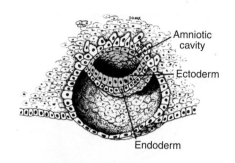

Fig. 1.**6** Differentiation of ectoderm and endoderm.

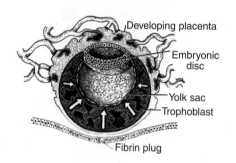

Fig. 1.**7** Formation of the embryonic disc.

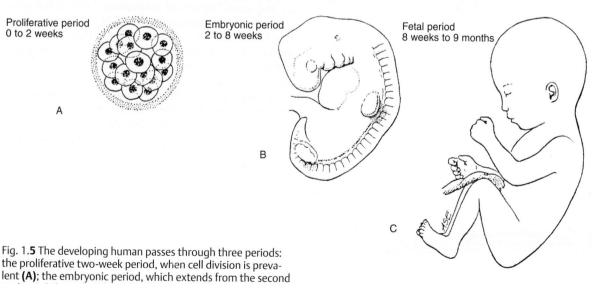

Fig. 1.**5** The developing human passes through three periods: the proliferative two-week period, when cell division is prevalent **(A)**; the embryonic period, which extends from the second to the eighth weeks **(B)**; the fetal period, from the eighth week to birth **(C)**.

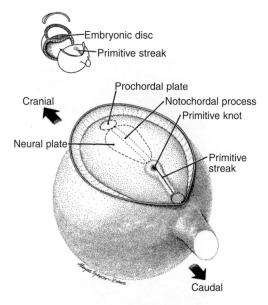

Fig. 1.**8** Primitive knot and streak on the embryonic disc.

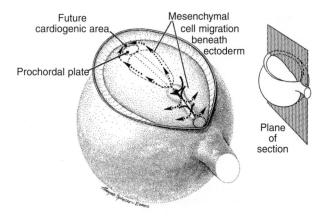

Fig. 1.**9** Formation of the mesoderm.

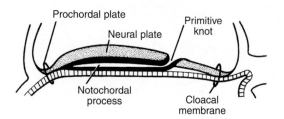

Fig. 1.**10** Sagittal view of the notocord.

provided with nutrition by cells of the oviduct and uterine glands until the heart begins to function at 4 weeks and nutrition is supplied via the umbilical blood supply.

During the second week, the blastocyst becomes embedded in the endometrium of the uterine wall. Fibrin plugs the endometrial implantation site. The placenta develops from the vascularized tissue that surrounds the enlarging blastocyst. The placenta is the zone of exchange of maternal oxygen and carbon dioxide from the embryo. From the surface of the blastocyst, cells grow as finger-like extensions from the surface of the trophoblast to invade the spongy vascular placenta. As these cells grow into villi, the placenta can begin to become functional during the third week (Fig 1.**7**).

Embryonic Period

The embryonic period ranges from 3 to 8 weeks and is the differentiation period for the three basic tissue types and their specialization into organs and organ systems. The embryonic disc is modified during the 15th day as a groove, called the "primitive streak," appears on its dorsal surface (Fig. 1.**8**). At the posterior end of the primitive streak a knot of cells appears, which is known as "Henson's node." From this node, cells producing the notochord grow anteriorly to provide the primitive axis of the embryo (Figs. 1.**8**–1.**10**). Mesodermal cells from the primitive streak and notochordal process grow laterally between the ectodermal and endodermal layers forming the embryonic shield or third germ layer, called the "mesodermal layer" (Fig. 1.**9**). During the third week, mesodermal cells grow anteriorly, posteriorly, and laterally from the midline, contributing to the forming embryo and uniting laterally with the extraembryonic mesoderm of the amniotic membrane and yolk sac wall. Mesoderm, however, fails to intervene between the ectoderm and endoderm at the rostral and caudal, giving rise to the prechordal and cloacal membranes of the oral cavity and anus. The neural tube arises distal to the notochord by the infolding of neural folds; from here these crests give rise to neural crest cells that behave like mesoderm, and are hence called ectomesenchyme. Anterior cranial derivatives of this tissue are the connective tissues and bones of the face.

The ectodermal cells contribute to the nervous system, the covering of the embryo and its appendages (nails, hair, sebaceous and sweat glands), the epithelium lining the oral and nasal cavities and sinuses, a part of the intraoral glands, and the enamel of the teeth. The embryonic endodermal cells form the lining of the gastrointestinal tract, the stomach, and associated organs such as lungs, pancreas, liver, gallbladder, and urinary bladder (Fig. 1.**11**).

During the next several weeks the pharyngeal arches appear as horizontally positioned tubular masses forming the mandible of the face and tissues of the neck. The mesodermal layer gives rise to the muscles, and structures derived from connective tissues such as the cartilages, bone, dentin, cementum, pulps of the teeth, and periodontal ligament are of neural crest tissue origin. The face takes form and develops during the fifth to seventh weeks. As these tissues begin to form, the embryonic period becomes the fetal period at the eighth week. This is marked by the first appearance of ossification centers that form bones.

Fetal Period

The embryonic period is the architect for the fetal period. All major and most of the minor organs begin development in the embryonic period, and then grow and specialize during the fetal period. This is the period of growth. It is said that if we continued to grow for the rest of our lives at this rate each of us would be larger than the world in which we exist. At the end of the fetal period, the head is proportionately larger compared to the less well-developed postcranial region (Fig.1.**5B**). If the embryonic period is the stage of organ differentiation, then the fetal period is the stage of organ growth and physiologic maturation. The remainder of this chapter is a description of the various organ systems that develop and mature during the fetal period. This period prepares the fetus for its entrance into life as an independent being.

Development of the Nervous System

The process by which the embryonic head and face are patterned is a continuum, beginning with specification of the anterior neural plate. The initially flat neural plate develops elevated folds at its lateral edges, where laterally located cells become located dorsally as the plate curls to form a tube. This tube is the forerunner of the brain and spinal cord (Figs. 1.**12** and 1.**13**). Cells located medially in the neural plate will be located ventrally in the developing tube. The SHH (Sonic hedgehog) proteins are essential to the patterning of the neural tube. The medially located notochord exerts a role in induction from its position underlying the neural plate (Fig. 1.**8**). The neural plate bends along its central axis to form a groove, and the raised margins form the neural tube. The neural folds gradually approach each other at the midline where they fuse. Contact of these folds begins in the central body region and proceeds in a cephalic (anterior) and caudal (posterior) direction. The folds remain temporarily open at the cranial and caudal ends forming the anterior and posterior neuropores. These close during

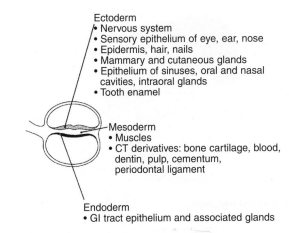

Ectoderm
• Nervous system
• Sensory epithelium of eye, ear, nose
• Epidermis, hair, nails
• Mammary and cutaneous glands
• Epithelium of sinuses, oral and nasal cavities, intraoral glands
• Tooth enamel

Mesoderm
• Muscles
• CT derivatives: bone cartilage, blood, dentin, pulp, cementum, periodontal ligament

Endoderm
• GI tract epithelium and associated glands

Fig. 1.**11** Derivatives of germ layers.

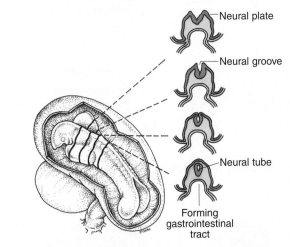

Neural plate

Neural groove

Neural tube

Forming gastrointestinal tract

Fig. 1.**12** Development of the neural tube.

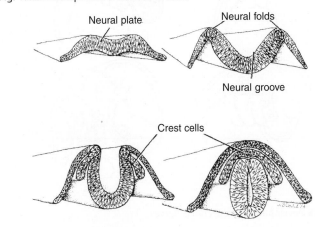

Neural plate

Neural folds

Neural groove

Crest cells

Fig. 1.**13** Development of the neural crest.

Clinical Application

The observation that wounds heal without scarring before birth has provided an ideal situation for correcting malformations such as a cleft lip and palate. Imaging devices have enabled surgeons to correct malformations prenatally in utero. Such operations are performed near the time of birth. Fetal wounds heal without any inflammation in the presence of cytokinins, which initiates epithelialization.

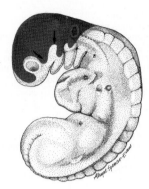

Fig. 1.**14** Neural crest migration.

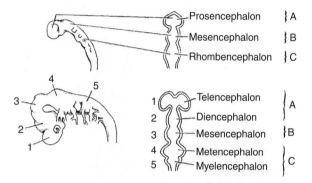

Fig. 1.**15** Development of the brain vesicles.

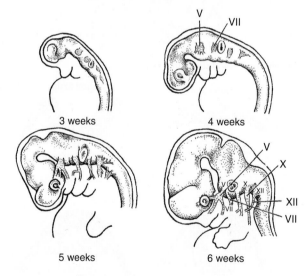

Fig. 1.**16** Development of the cranial nerves.

the fourth week, which signals the establishment of the nervous system. Upon closure of the neural tube, a unique population of cells known as "neural crest" cells separate from the crest of the folds (Fig. 1.**13**). These cells immediately begin to migrate ventrally along the lateral walls of the neural tube. This is especially apparent in the head and neck region (Fig. 1.**14**). Neural crest cells give rise to a variety of different cells that form components of many tissues, such as the sensory ganglia, sympathetic neurons, Schwann cells, pigment cells, leptomeninges, and cartilage of the pharyngeal arches. They also contribute to the embryonic connective tissue of the facial region, which includes dental tissues such as pulp, dentin, and cementum. Although the neural crest tissues arise from neural ectoderm, they exhibit properties of mesenchyme. As a result, the tissue they form is called "ectomesenchyme." Growth and differentiation of the neural tube begins anteriorly. By the fourth week the neural tube has formed three primary vesicles: forebrain, midbrain, and hindbrain or prosencephalon, mesencephalon, and rhombencephalon. Secondary vesicles rapidly develop from these primary vesicles (Fig. 1.**15**).

A lateral view of the developing brain is seen at the third, fourth, fifth, and sixth week (Fig. 1.**16**). The brain enlarges rapidly, bending anteriorly and expanding laterally. The cranial nerves grow downward from the lateral neural tube and floor of the brain, early enough to be included in the organization of the developing face, neck, and lower body tissues (Fig. 1.**17**). Growing evidence suggests that the molecular mechanism mediating craniofacial morphogenesis is the same as the molecules that regulate patterning and differentiation of other systems in the body.

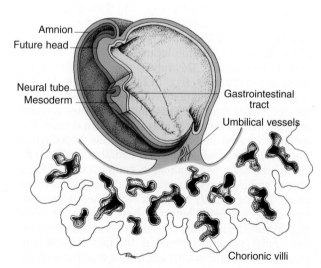

Fig. 1.**17** Development of the GI tract.

Development of the Gastrointestinal System

The developing neural tube and the gastrointestinal tube lie adjacent to each other. In the area between these two developing tubes, the somites form sheets of muscle from the mesoderm (Fig. 1.**19**). As the embryo grows in length, the alimentary canal lengthens as well. This canal extends from the prechordal plate to the cloacal plate, each of which will open to provide an entrance to and exit from the alimentary canal.

The next step in development is the appearance of several outpouchings throughout the gastrointestinal tube. Craniocaudally, the first and second pouches provide the parathyroid glands, the thyroid from the thyroglossal duct, the lungs, the enlarging area of the stomach, liver, gallbladder, and pancreas; more posteriorly the urinary bladder develops (Figs. 1.**18A** and **B**). The thyroid gland appears during the fourth week from the junction of the body and base of the tongue, and descends in the midline of the neck. Next the bilateral lung buds differentiate and enlarge, but since they are filled with fluid they remain nonfunctional until birth when they inflate with air. The stomach develops as a localized enlargement of the anterior gut and gradually develops as a mixing and digestive organ. The liver grows rapidly and by 6 weeks functions in red blood cell formation, the conversion of glucose to glycogen, and the storage of nutritional elements. The pancreas and its product, insulin, develop early and by 20 weeks are functional in the production of growth hormone, later becoming important in carbohydrate metabolism. The midgut rotates and pushes into the umbilical cord at 6 weeks, but by the 10th week the body has increased sufficiently in size to allow return of the gut. The midgut forms the duodenum, the remainder of the small intestine, and the ascending and transverse colon of the large intestine. The descending and terminal parts of the alimentary canal develop from the hindgut. The urinary bladder is the final outpouching of the alimentary canal and develops in conjunction with the genitourinary system (Fig. 1.**18**). The alimentary canal is filled with fetal meconium during the early prenatal life. Meconium is a combination of shed epithelial cells, lanugo hairs, and associated debris.

Development of the Muscular System

The muscular system is composed of specialized cells arising from the mesoderm, in which the property of contractility has been highly developed. On the basis of microscopic structure and function, three types of muscles are recognized (Fig. 1.**20**): 1) skeletal muscle, attached to and responsible for movement of the body skeleton; 2) smooth muscle found characteristically in the walls of the hollow viscera, ducts, and blood vessels; and 3) cardiac muscles, found only in the heart wall.

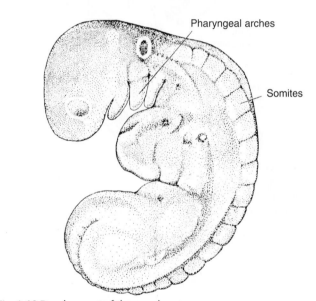

Fig. 1.**18** Derivatives of the GI tract at **(A)** 4.5 and **(B)** 5 weeks.

Fig. 1.**19** Development of the muscles.

Clinical Application

Ovulation is a monthly cyclic event controlled by the endocrine secretions estrogen and progesterone. The ovum matures and is expelled from the ovary and, if fertilized, will implant and be nourished in the uterine wall 7 days after fertilization. The function of the contraceptive "pill" is to maintain an increased level of progesterone and estrogen that will prevent follicle maturation (of the ovum) or ovulation. Without the ovum pregnancy will not occur.

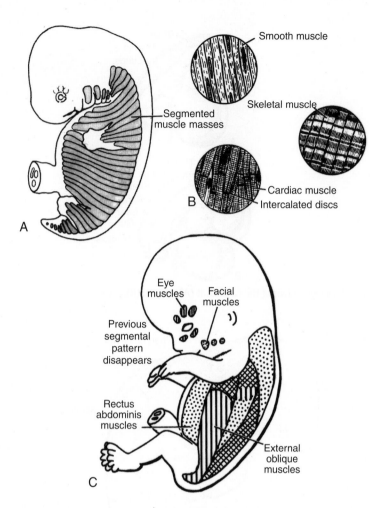

Fig. 1.**20 (A)**. Development of skeletal muscle **(B)**. Muscle types **(C)**. Differentiation of skeletal muscle

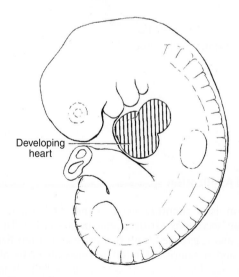

Fig. 1.**21** Cardiac muscle

Skeletal Muscle

At the end of 3 weeks the body has seven pairs of somites lying lateral to the neural tube. The somites are defined as segmented masses of tissue that contribute to the axial skeletal tissue, muscle, and connective tissue of the body wall. By the 35th day, 44 pairs of somites will have formed; four will be occipital, eight cervical, 12 thoracic, five lumbar, five sacral, and eight to ten coccygeal. Muscle masses following the same segmentation pattern grow from the somites along the body wall and appendages (Fig. 1.**20A**). The first occipital and the last five to seven coccygeal somites will later disappear. The somites contribute bone to the vertebral column, the dermis of the skin, muscles of the trunk and limbs, and some muscles of the orofacial region (Fig. 1.**20C**).

By 10 weeks, the myoblasts (muscle cells) have migrated and begin specializing into elongated, multinucleated muscle fibers (Figs. 1.**20A** and **B**). These fibers divide into groups: epimeres, which supply the dorsal surface of the limbs, and hypomeres which supply the ventral parts of the limbs. They also split into superficial and deep layers of muscle. In early development, the muscles follow the segmental pattern of the somites, but by the eighth week this pattern disappears (Fig.1.**20C**).

Smooth Muscle

At a very early stage of development, wandering mesenchymal cells concentrate around the epithelial linings of such structures as the gut tube, urogenital ducts, and the large vascular channels. These mesenchymal cells arrange themselves in zones where involuntary muscles (smooth) are destined to develop, and then lengthen in the direction their contractile power will be exerted. These developing smooth and cardiac muscle cells are both controlled by the autonomic nervous system (Fig. 1.**20B**).

Cardiac Muscle

In the early stages of differentiation, cardiac muscle cells are packed closely together around the developing heart tube and exhibit no definite plan or arrangement (Fig. 1.**21**). As the developing tissue is pulled into spiral bands about the chambers of the heart, the strands become more regular in arrangement until they appear to continue in a general parallel fashion. The last characteristic feature to appear in the development of cardiac muscle are the intercalated discs (Fig. 1.**20B**). Electron microscope studies have shown these transverse markings to be highly modified cell boundaries. Myofibrils on either side of the disc are attached in such a manner that their contractile power can function through the interaction of many cells.

Development of the Heart and Blood–Vascular System

The developing embryo or fetus is attached to the placenta by a connective-tissue stalk that elongates during development to become the umbilical cord. Both arterial and venous blood vessels form in this cord and carry carbon dioxide away from the embryo to the placenta and oxygen and nutrition to the embryo or fetus (Fig. 1.**22**). Blood flows to the embryo during the first 2 weeks through the vitelline circulatory system, which carries nutrition from the yolk sac to the heart. During the third week, the umbilical circulation takes over carrying oxygen and nutrition to the fetus. Yolk-sac-derived nutrition is much more prevalent in lower animals than in the human. At the end of the first month, the embryonic heart begins to beat. Oxygen is then transported from the maternal capillaries of the placenta across a membrane separating the two systems. The fetal red blood cells are developed in the embryo. Both vascular systems are shown in Figure 1.**22**. In the umbilical cord, a vein rather than an artery carries oxygenated blood to the fetal heart. After this blood circulates throughout the fetus, it is then carried by two umbilical arteries to the placenta (Fig. 1.**22**). At birth the lungs replace the placenta, and the pulmonary arteries will then conduct oxygenated blood to the newborn's heart.

The placenta functions as a nutritional link between mother and fetus (Fig. 1.**23**) and serves as a storage bank of nutrition and a site of exchange of oxygen and carbon dioxide. However, there is no direct contact of the blood elements in the placenta as both systems are separated by a membrane. The maternal blood flow effectively removes the waste products that cross the placental membranes.

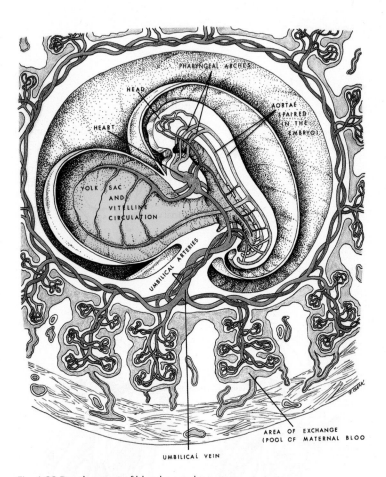

Fig. 1.**22** Development of blood–vascular system.

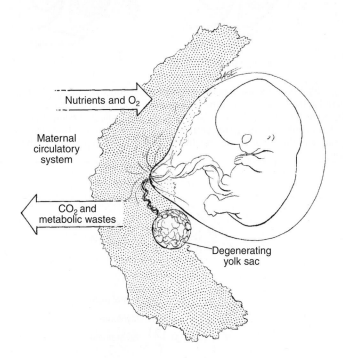

Fig. 1.**23** Placenta and exchange.

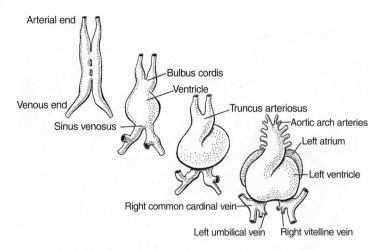

Fig. 1.**24** Development of the heart.

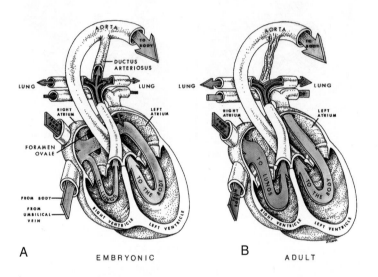

Fig. 1.**25 A** Prenatal heart. Both oxygenated and nonoxygenated blood collected in the right atrium to the right ventricle and mixed blood pumped to the body. **B** Postnatal heart. At birth the foramen ovale (between atria) closes, forcing blood to the right ventricle, then to the lungs. It returns oxygenated to the left atria and then the left ventricle and is pumped to the body.

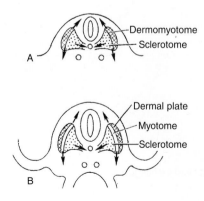

Fig. 1.**26** Differentiation of bone, cartilage, ligaments, and muscle.

Heart

The embryonic heart initially develops by fusion of two vessels into a single blood vessel forming the endothelial heart tube. In a series of steps (Fig. 1.**24**), this vessel enlarges and bends on itself, and its tissue differentiates. Then a septum divides the heart into right and left chambers. Septa and valves develop which separate the atria from the ventricles. In the embryonic heart, blood collects in the right atrium where most of the blood passes into the left atrium through the foramen ovale. Blood then passes to the left ventricle where it is pumped throughout the body by the aorta (Fig. 1.**25A**). Very little blood passes from the right atrium to the right ventricle, where it is pumped to the developing lungs. Blood bypasses the lungs, passing through the ductus arteriosus to the aorta (Fig. 1.**25A**). The fetal heart is relatively larger and beats more rapidly than the postnatal heart, since it carries blood to the body and the placenta.

At birth, several major changes occur to the heart (Fig 1.**25B**). When the infant takes its first breath the lungs inflate and a small slip of muscle slides over the foramen ovale, which is the opening between the right and left atria. This closure forces all the blood in the right atrium into the right ventricle and to the lungs. The blood is then returned to the left atrium from the lungs by the pulmonary veins. After birth, the ductus arteriosus begins to close, which prevents blood from passing directly from the pulmonary arteries to the aorta (Fig. 1.**25B**). These changes at birth are vital to prevent a "blue baby" (oxygen deficient). As a result, postnatally all the blood is oxygenated before being circulated to the entire body.

Skeletal Development

The skeletal and articular systems develop from the mesodermal somites, which differentiate into sclerotomes and dermomyotomes. The sclerotomes will form cartilage, bone, and ligaments (Fig. 1.**26**). Several types of

Clinical Application

One dramatic change at birth is the transformation from the closed system of the heart to an open one. Before birth this is accomplished by utilizing blood flow from the placenta and conducting it to and through the heart, then circulating it to the rest of the body. At birth the heart forces the blood into the lungs, where it is oxygenated. The blood is then returned to the heart and pumped throughout the body.

cartilage develop to supply the body's needs. Hyaline cartilage forms throughout the embryonic and fetal body and is the most prominent type. However, elastic cartilage forms to the ears and fibrous cartilage forms in the axial skeleton. Bone later develops by two types of connective-tissue formation, either endochondral or intramembranous (Figs. 1.27 and 1.28).

Cartilage

The first skeleton to develop in the embryo is composed of cartilage; it develops in a segmental pattern. Cartilage appears throughout the body: in the axial skeleton, the base of the cranium, and the appendages (Fig. 1.27). Cartilage cells first appear during the fourth and fifth week, and cartilage matrix soon appears throughout the body. Cartilage provides the skeletal strength and forms a matrix where bone cells will later form bone. Later nutrient blood vessels enter the cartilages, and bone forms initially in the shafts and later in the proximal and distal heads of the bones (Fig. 1.28B). By the 20th week, bone has replaced most of the cartilage in the body. Cartilage will ultimately be limited to the covering of the heads of long bones, the nasal septum, the trachea, and specialized cartilages will provide support for the ears (elastic) and the spinal column, (fibrous).

Bone

Bone may develop through replacement of cartilage by endochondral means, or transformation of connective tissue to bone by the intramembranous route (Fig.1.28). Regardless of the means by which bone forms, the resultant skeleton will have the same appearance and function whether compact (dense bone) or spongy (cancellous bone). The external portion of bones is usually compact and the internal part surrounding the marrow space is cancellous or spongy. The developing skull is a classic example as it contains both membranous bone, which covers the brain and face, and cartilage-developed components that support the base of the brain. They function in synchrony to support and protect the brain and face. This will be described in detail in Chapter 4. Figure 1.28 shows the initial formation of membranous bone (flat bones), which forms in connective tissue, as well as a representative area of cartilage that is modified by endochondral bone formation.

Morphologic Changes during Prenatal Development

Embryos increase in size first by cell multiplication, second by growth in intercellular deposition, and third through a modification of same cell size. From the fertilized ovum stage until birth, the human increases in length from 140 μm to more than 50 cm, and in weight

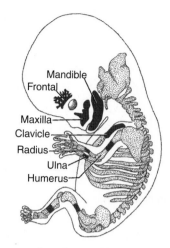

Fig. 1.**27** Development of cartilage and bone. ■bone; ▨cartilage.

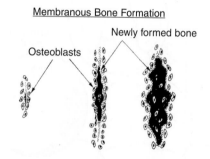

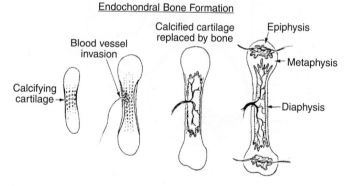

Fig. 1.**28** Types of bone formation.

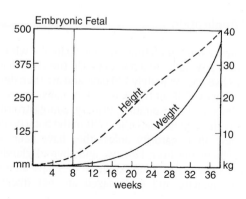

Fig. 1.**29** Increase in weight and length of body.

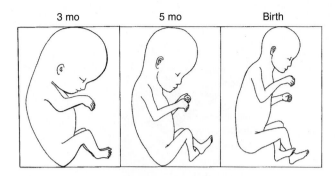

Fig. 1.**30** Changes in body proportion.

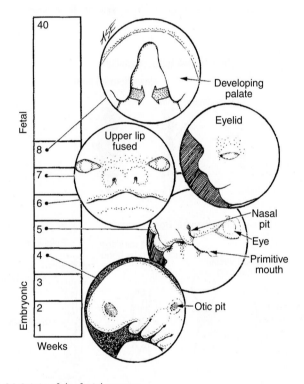

Fig. 1.**31** Origin of the facial process.

from a few milligrams to more than 3000 g in approximately 266 days (Fig. 1.**29**) Thus, from fertilization to birth the body increases in size about a million times. The embryonic period is one of rapid growth and differentiation of cells, organs, and organ systems. All major features are established during this time. Growth may be interstitial, involving an increase in bulk within a tissue or organ, or appositional, involving enlargement by surface deposition of tissue. Interstitial growth is a characteristic of soft tissue, whereas appositional growth is a characteristic of mineralized tissue, such as bone and dental hard tissues. An exception is cartilage, a hard tissue that increases in size by both interstitial and appositional growth. Much of the interstitial growth occurs during development when this tissue is soft or in a less-mineralized stage. At that time each cell or cell group deposits a matrix around the cell.

Differential growth is essential to produce changes in size and shape of different body parts. An example would be the change in proportion of head size by the end of the embryonic period at 8 weeks. During the fetal period from eight weeks to birth the body increases in size at a rate greater than the head. The head represents one-half of the total body at 3 months, one-third at 5 months, and one-fourth at birth (Fig. 1.**30**).

During the first 2 prenatal months the heart develops, blood begins to circulate, the body elongates, and the human face develops (Fig. 1.**31**). At the end of the third month the upper limbs reach a length proportionate to the rest of the body. By the end of the fourth month, ossification centers have made their appearance in most of the bones and individual differences become apparent. At the end of the fifth month the fetus is about the length of a full-term fetus; however it weighs about 500 g, which is one-sixth its birth weight. By the end of the sixth month the face is infant-like, although the skin is wrinkled because of its rapid growth and lack of developing adipose tissue. By the end of the seventh month, however, the fetus has developed subcutaneous fat, eliminating the skin wrinkles. At this time, the eyelids are no longer fused together. Body movements now become progressively more noticeable. Movement of the lower jaw begins as early as the eighth week, but such a minor movement is not felt by the mother. Arm and leg flexing begins as joints mature, and these movements are quite noticeable to the mother. During the eighth and ninth months, hair and fingernails increase in length and the body becomes more plump. In the late prenatal months the body increases in weight until the fetus reaches about 3.2 kg, the average weight of an infant at birth.

Birth

Parturition or labor begins with muscular contractions when the fetus has attained the proper position deep in the pelvis. The amniotic fluid is squeezed into the thin part of the chorion that overlies the uterine cervix. This acts as the preliminary dilator of the cervical canal. As contractions become more powerful and frequent, the investing membranes rupture and the infant is freed from the fetal envelope. The amniotic fluid starts to flow from the mother, which lubricates the birth canal (Fig. 1.**32**). Because the process of birth usually lasts several hours, it is important that the placenta remains attached to the uterus. If the fetus were cut off prematurely from its maternal associations, it could not survive the prolonged interruption of its oxygen supply.

Combined contractions of smooth muscle in the uterus, aided by contractions of the skeletal muscles in the abdomen, literally squeeze the fetus into the slowly dilating cervical canal. When dilation is sufficient, the fetus is pushed out of the uterus. This is the first phase of labor. The second phase is much more brief than the first. The fetus passing through the cervical canal moves promptly through the vagina and "presents" itself. The vulval orifice dilates rapidly, and when the head passes the outlet the rest of the body emerges quickly. With delivery and the tying and cutting of the umbilical cord, maternal connections are terminated and, for the first time, the newborn subsists independently of another individual.

Approximately 15 to 20 minutes after the birth of the baby, the uterus begins another series of contractions which serve to loosen and expel the placenta and amniotic remnant. This entire mass is referred to as the "afterbirth." This abrupt shedding of tissue from the uterus involves some hemorrhage, but the continued contractions of the uterus minimize blood loss by compressing the ruptured vessels, which thereby facilitates coagulation. Following parturition, there is a period of repair of the uterine lining similar to the one that occurs after menstruation.

The process of birth occurs about 9 to 9.5 months after conception. A complete environmental transformation takes place at that time. The infant is catapulted from a warm, dark, and relatively quiet environment, having been submerged in fluid at a body temperature of 37°C, into a lighted, noisy environment approximately 7°C cooler, in which it must support itself by breathing air through its own lungs and live independently. Thus, at birth the infant must survive a number of physiologic changes, such as the inspiration of air through its lungs, changes in the circulatory pathways, shunting of blood through the lungs, oral feeding, use of the gastrointestinal tract, utilizing sense organs of sight, sound, and smell—all of which create new and complex feelings.

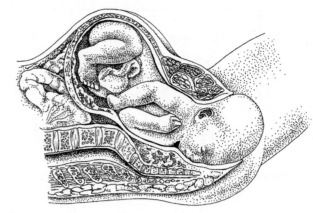

Fig. 1.**32** Birth

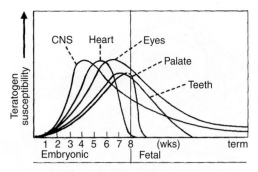

Fig. 1.**33** Decrease in susceptibility to teratogens with prenatal age.

Abnormal Development

The causes of congenital malformations may be hereditary and/or environmental (genetic and epigenetic). The majority of congenital defects are the result of interaction between hereditary and environmental factors occurring at a specific time of development. It was recently reported that SHH protein presence is necessary for growth of the frontonasal prominence (stage 23 chick). Signaling from this protein is critical to normal development of the mid and upper face.

Beyond prenatal examinations and parental counseling, not much can be done to reduce hereditary hazards in humans. Recent experiments are being directed toward altering the effects of abnormal genetic endowment through changes in the environment, such as stress reduction and dietary changes.

Our increased knowledge of noxious environmental agents (teratogens) and the time of their maximum effects on fetal development is of great importance in the understanding and prevention of such malformations. The developing human is least susceptible to teratogens during the proliferation period (first 2 or 3 weeks). At that time damage may be compensated for by the remaining cells that have not yet become committed or differentiated. The embryonic period (third through the eighth week) is the most critical time period because it is the period of differentiation of tissues and organs. At this time, teratogenic agents may be highly effective and result in numerous malformations. During the fetal period (end of eighth week until birth) susceptibility to teratogens rapidly declines and may cause only minor defects (Fig. 1.**33**).

Hereditary Causes of Congenital Malformations

Hereditary causes of congenital malformations can be attributed to either chromosomal or genetic abnormalities.

Chromosomal Abnormalities

Many congenital defects are now known to be the result of an abnormal number of chromosomes. The abnormality in number is expressed as either a decrease or increase in the normal number of chromosomes (46 in humans), euploidy. A decrease in one chromosome, monosomy (45 chromosomes), is usually lethal. Turner syndrome (XO) is not lethal. An increase in one or more chromosomes is teratogenic and results in congenital malformations. The extra chromosome may be an auto-some or a sex chromosome. If an extra chromosome member is present, a condition known as trisomy devel-ops. The best known example is trisomy 21 or Down's syndrome (Figs. 1.**34** and 1.**35**). In this condition three members of chromosome 21 are present in the somatic cells of the affected individual, which results in the cells containing 47 chromosomes each. The malformation is characterized by mental retardation, upward slanting of the palpebral fissures, a flat nasal bridge, and a fissured protruding tongue (macroglossia). Another example of chromosomal abnormality is Kleinfelter syndrome. There are several types, one is the XXY indicating an increase in the female sex chromosome . The male is tall of stature, has deficient testes development, and requires additional testosterone to function normally. Other more serious and severe forms of this condition are the XXXY and XXXXY syndromes.

Genetic Abnormalities

Genes are segments of the DNA chain for stored infor-mation that can perpetuate from one generation to another. Abnormal development may be the result of expression of defective genes, which may be dominant or recessive. A dominant gene expresses itself whether it is present on one member of the pair of homologous chromosomes (heterozygous) or on both pairs (homozy-gous). A recessive gene expresses itself only when it is present on both members of the homozygous pair of chromosomes. (Fig. 1.**36**). The following abnormalities are examples of autosomal dominant genes: acro-cephalosyndactyly (Fig. 1.**37**), achondroplasia, cleidocra-nial dysostosis, mandibulofacial dysostosis, and dentino-genesis imperfecta. Achondroplasia is a defective devel-opmental condition of bones ossified in cartilage (partic-

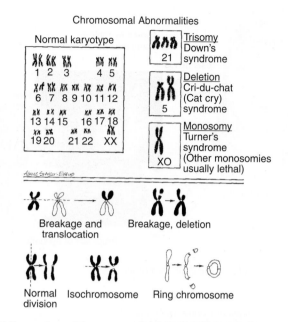

Fig. 1.**34** Comparison of three types of chromosomal abnormalities.

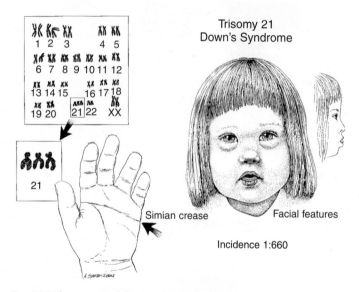

Fig. 1.**35** Chromosomal abnormalities

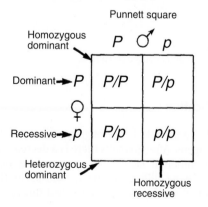

Fig. 1.**36** Gene expression

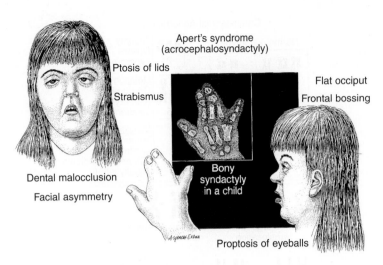

Apert's syndrome
(acrocephalosyndactyly)

Ptosis of lids

Strabismus

Flat occiput

Frontal bossing

Bony
syndactyly
in a child

Dental malocclusion

Facial asymmetry

Proptosis of eyeballs

Fig. 1.**37** Craniofacial and digit syndrome.

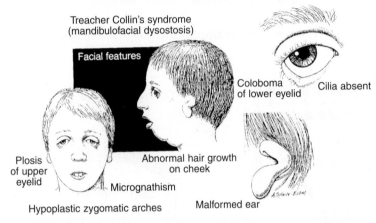

Treacher Collin's syndrome
(mandibulofacial dysostosis)

Facial features

Coloboma
of lower eyelid   Cilia absent

Plosis
of upper
eyelid

Abnormal hair growth
on cheek

Micrognathism

Hypoplastic zygomatic arches

Malformed ear

Fig. 1.**38** Lack of neural crest cell migration resulting in multiple facial abnormalities.

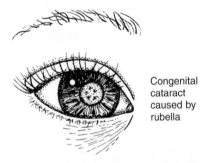

Congenital
cataract
caused by
rubella

Fig. 1.**39** Congenital cataract caused by rubella.

Clinical Application

The period of 3 to 8 weeks is one of greatest sensitivity to the action of teratogens. After 8 weeks there is a decreasing sensitivity to environmental factors. The tissues are no longer undergoing as many differentiating factors as in the early weeks. The risk of malformations is greatest during embryogenesis.

ularly long bones). On the other hand, cleidocranial dysostosis is a condition of defective development of bone ossified in membrane (cranial vault, face, and clavicles). Some of the defects are facial and dental malformations. Mandibulofacial dysostosis, also called Treacher Collins' syndrome, results from a defective gene that seems to cause a disturbance in the migration of neural crest cells. This is expressed as an underdeveloped face (Fig. 1.**38**). Dentinogenesis imperfecta, a hereditary condition, results in defective dentin formation.

Environmental Causes of Congenital Malformations

Environmental causes of congenital malformations may be classified as infectious agents; radiation, drugs, hormones, nutritional disorders, and teratogenic habits such as smoking or consuming caffeine-containing substances or excessive alcohol, especially during pregnancy.

Infectious Agents

Viral infections affecting the mother during early pregnancy can cause congenital malformations. A well-known example is rubella virus, which causes German measles. When a pregnant woman is infected with rubella, many defects in the child can result, including cleft palate, central nervous system anomalies, and cataracts (Fig. 1.**39**).

Radiation

The direct teratogenic effects of X-rays on the embryo result in specific congenital malformations, including cleft palate. The indirect effect of irradiation causes gene mutation (alteration) in the germ cells. This leads to the occurrence of congenital malformations in succeeding generations. To alleviate the dangerous effects of radiation, all personnel dealing with X-rays should use proper protective measures for both themselves and their patients. They should also protect women of reproductive age as though these women were pregnant.

Drugs

Although specific drugs used during pregnancy have not been implicated as causing teratogenic effects, drugs should be avoided unless necessary during early pregnancy. Remember the tragic effects of thalidomide, a drug once considered to be a safe hypnotic and antinauseant. It caused partial and total absence of the limbs (Fig. 1.**40**). Aminopterin is another dangerous drug used to induce an abortion, when necessary. Tetracycline administered as a useful antibiotic, taken during tooth and bone calcification during the second and third trimesters, causes permanent brownish discoloration of dentin and hypoplasia of the enamel of deciduous teeth. Although widely used some few years ago, these drugs are used to a lesser extent today. To date little is known about the teratogenesis of the interactive effects of drugs.

Hormones

The action of hormones such as teratogens has not clearly been demonstrated in humans. Cortisone, however, has been shown to cause cleft lip and palate in some experimental animals. These effects have not been shown in humans. The use of steroids by some athletes may cause side effects, although to date there is inadequate information.

Nutritional Disorders

Nutritional disorders have been reported in case histories of humans. However, these reports are few and most relate to the effects of nutritional disorders on developing teeth. Vitamin deficiencies and hypervitaminosis A, C, and D have been reported as teratogenic in some animals. Hypervitaminosis A is implicated in effects in early pregnancy in humans. Treatment with vitamin A for skin disorders is now avoided in women of child-bearing years. Folic acid deficiency has been implicated in neural tube defects leading to spina bifida and rachischisis (fissure in spinal column). Folic acid is now recommended during early pregnancy.

Teratogenic Habits: Smoking, Alcohol, and Caffeine

Infants of heavy-smoking mothers were shown to have offspring with higher incidence of cleft lip and palate. In many cases, the birth weight was decreased. Alcohol abuse during early pregnancy may also produce congenital defects such as mental retardation, growth deficiency, and facial defects. This is known as fetal alcohol syndrome. Maxillary hypoplasia has also been reported. Even excessive caffeine consumption has been implicated in some developmental defects.

In general, to reduce teratogenic hazards, all women of reproductive age should avoid drugs and questionable habits at the time of the first missed menstrual period and for at least 12 weeks thereafter. This will protect the developing human embryo during the time when it is most susceptible to teratogenic effects.

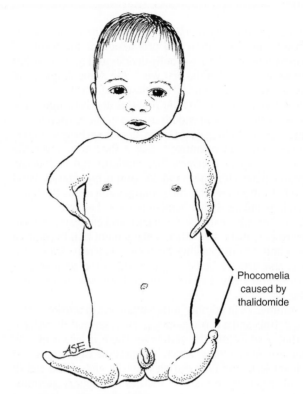

Phocomelia caused by thalidomide

Fig. 1.**40** Effects of thalidomide.

Summary

The contact of the sperm and the ovum in the distal uterine tube results in fertilization and production of the fertilized ovum or zygote, which then rapidly divides as it moves toward the uterus. At the end of the first week, the zygote implants in the uterine wall and the resulting blastocyst, with an embryonic disc developing within it. At first this disc is composed of two layers, ectoderm and endoderm. A notochord then develops and the disc elongates. On its dorsal surface a groove appears, which is the primitive streak. A third germ layer, the mesoderm, develops between the ectoderm and endoderm. The neural plate elongates, and its lateral boundaries bend upward to form a tube. This tube enlarges and forms the bilateral cerebral and cerebellar hemispheres of the brain.

A yolk sac forms beneath the notochord and elongates to form the gastrointestinal tube with an enlargement that becomes a stomach and an outpouching for lungs, pancreas, liver, gallbladder, and urinary bladder. Above this tube segments or somites extend along the body wall on both sides of the neural tube.

These somites, 38 in number, differentiate into a portion forming the dermis and a cartilaginous portion termed the sclerotome that ossifies into the vertebrae. There is also a muscle portion termed myotome, which supports the gastrointestinal tract, body wall, and limb muscles. By the end of the eighth week, all major organ systems such as the neural, gastrointestinal with associated organs, reproductive, and urinary, and systems such as the vascular have developed. The face appears human by the beginning of the ninth week, at the start of the fetal period.

There is a general increase in body length, and then an increase in weight occurs. At this time, specialization takes place as the body prepares for birth. At birth, a number of very rapid and important changes take place. One is the shift from placental oxygen and carbon dioxide exchange to that of the lungs. This shift is associated with dramatic changes in the heart and circulatory pathways. At birth the lungs inflate and the baby goes through a change of environment, from fluid to air, the new environment being some 7°C cooler than that in which it has existed for 9 months.

Self-Evaluation Review

1. Define the terms: ovulation, fertilization, and implantation.
2. Describe the two vascular systems of the embryo and the contribution of each.
3. What do somites contribute to embryonic development?
4. From what does the gastrointestinal tract develop? Which organs develop from it?
5. What is the common feature of muscle tissue? Name the three types that develop and the functions of each.
6. Compare the prenatal and postnatal heart and describe the important changes that occur at birth.
7. What is the origin and function of neural crest cells, and what is derived from them?
8. Name the three germ layers and the derivatives of each.
9. Describe the development of each type of cartilage and bone.
10. What may develop from genetic and chromosomal aberrations?
11. Discuss the various environmental agents that can act teratogenically on the human.
12. Describe the birth process.

Acknowledgements

Dr. Alphonse R Burdi provided Figures 1.**35**, 1.**37**, and 1.**38**.

Suggested Readings

Avery JK. Development and structure of cells and tissues. In: Steele PF ed. Essentials of Oral Histology and Development. St. Louis: Mosby Inc.; 1999:1–16.

Carlson BM. Human Embryology and Developmental Biology. St. Louis; Mosby Inc.; 1999.

England M. Color Atlas of Life Before Birth. Chicago, Ill: Year Book Medical Publishers; 1993.

Guggenheim B, Shapiro S. Oral Biology at the Turn of the Century. Basel: Kaarger; 1998.

Moore KL. Essentials of Human Embryology. Toronto: BC Decker Inc.; 1988.

Moore KL. The Developing Human. 4th ed. Philadelphia, Pa: WB Saunders; 1993.

Nishmura H, Okanoto N. Sequential Atlas of Human Congenital Malformations. Baltimore, Md: University Park Press; 1976.

Poswillo D. The Pathogenesis of the first and second branchial arch syndrome. Oral Surg. 1973;35;302–328.

Sadler T ed. Langman's Medical Embryology. 6th Ed. Baltimore, Md: Williams & Wilkins; 1990.

Sperber GH. Craniofacial Embryology. 4th ed. London: Butterworth; 1989.

Sperber GH. Craniofacial Development. Toronto: BC Decker Inc.; 2000.

Tortora GJ. Principles of Human Anatomy. 8th ed. Menlo Park, CA: Addison Wesley Longman Inc.; 1999.

2 Development of the Pharyngeal Arches and Face

James K. Avery

Introduction

Initiation of the oral cavity occurs in the third prenatal week as a pit or invagination of the tissues underlying the forebrain. The pit increases in length as the forebrain expands anteriorly at this time. This pit will later develop into the oral cavity, and the tissues surrounding it will form the face. The lower part of the face and neck are formed by the pharyngeal arches that surround the oral pit on both sides of the neck. The pharyngeal arches contribute much of the face and neck. In the third week the first pharyngeal arch forms the mandibular arch and cheeks. Grooves separate the pharyngeal arches initially. Gradually, however, the components of the face unify as they grow, allowing them to merge into the cheeks, mandible, and neck structures. Facial development is fairly rapid, spanning only a 2-week period from the fifth to the seventh prenatal week. Initially, there are four primary tissue masses, termed the frontal or frontonasal prominence, that lie above the oral pit, two maxillary masses on the right and left sides of the oral pit, and the mandibular mass or first pharyngeal arch below it (Fig. 2.1). In addition to these primary processes, small thickenings appear in the epithelium of the two placodes that form lenses of the eye. Bilateral nasal placodes also develop. The latter are located above the developing upper lip. Placodes also appear bilaterally; these form our organs of hearing. The nasal thickenings gradually develop into pits, termed nasal pits, which deepen to become our organs of smell. Other endothelial thickenings appear internally in the oropharyngeal area, forming the glands: pituitary, parathyroids, thyroids, and thymus.

The focus in this chapter is on the second month of prenatal life, when the tissues of the face and oral cavity are first differentiated and begin to form.

Objectives

After reading this chapter, you should be able to describe the formative process of the primitive oral cavity, the appearance and modification of the pharyngeal arches

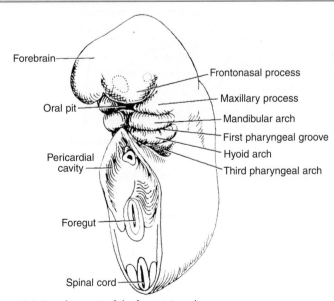

Figure 2.**1**. Development of the face at 4 weeks.

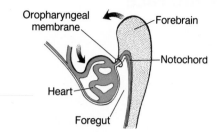

Figure 2.**2**. Anterior growth of brain vesicles at 2.5 weeks.

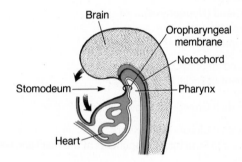

Fig. 2.**3** Further growth of the brain anteriorly at 3 weeks.

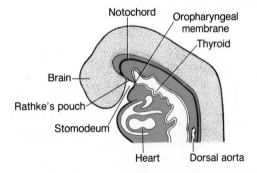

Fig. 2.**4** Development of the stomodeum at 3.5 weeks.

and their contribution to the face. You should also be able to define the pharyngeal pouches and their contribution to oral development and describe the development of the tongue and palatine shelves. Finally, you should be able to describe various malformations of the face and discuss how these malformations occur.

Development of the Primitive Cranium and Oronasal Cavity

The primitive oral pit, or stomodeum, is an invagination of the surface epithelium positioned anteriorly between the forebrain and the adjacent ventrally developing heart (Fig. 2.**1**). This invagination appears as a result of the forebrain's anterior growth and enlargement of the developing heart. The oral cavity is positioned in a space under the forebrain (Figs. 2.**2**–2.**4**). During the third prenatal week the deep end of the oral pit is lined with ectoderm, which is in close contact with the endoderm of the foregut (Fig. 2.**1**). The area of contact of the two epithelia is termed the "oropharyngeal membrane" since it forms part of the oral and pharyngeal cavities and separates them. The oropharyngeal membrane then disintegrates to create an anterior external opening of the gastrointestinal tract in the fourth week of life (Figs. 2.**5** and 2.**6**). The origin of the head and face is the flat neural plate that lies in the anterior area of the embryonic disc at 18 days. The neural plate then bends into a tube to form the brain. The lateral margins of the neural plate then assume a dorsal position, and neural crest cells arise from the dorsal neural tube. These cells then begin their migration down the outside of the neural tube and give rise to the cells that form the tissues of the head and face. The developmental pattern of these structures is thought to be a continuum from the initiation of these cells to their ceasing to grow. SHH (sonic hedgehog) protein is essential for mediolateral patterning of the neural plate, and later dorsoventral patterning of the neural tube.

Pharyngeal Arch Development

The tissues bordering the oral pit inferiorly and laterally develop into five or six pairs of bars that form the lower part of the face or neck. These bars are termed "pharyngeal arches." The first four pharyngeal arches (numbered I to IV craniocaudially) are well developed in humans. Only the first and second arches extend to the midline, and each arch is progressively smaller from the first to the last. The mandibular pharyngeal arch is the first to develop (Figs. 2.**5** and 2.**6**) and the hyoid is the second. Thus there is an anteroposterior growth gradient (Fig. 2.**7**).

The third, fourth, and fifth arches also consist of paired bars of epithelial-covered mesoderm, which are divided in the midline by a cleft in which the heart is positioned (Fig. 2.**4**). Each arch lies horizontally in the neck and is separated from adjacent arches by shallow grooves externally (Fig. 2.**1**) and by deep pharyngeal pouches internally (Figs. 2.**5** and 2.**6**). The outer surface of pharyngeal arches is covered by ectoderm and the inner (pharyngeal) surface by endoderm, except for the first arch which is lined by ectoderm of the oral mucosa. Within each pharyngeal arch are neural crest cells, which lie around a core of mesodermal cells. In each arch there will be differentiation of muscles, cartilages, bones, blood vessels, and nerves.

Figures 2.**5** and 2.**6** are illustrations of the external as well as the pharyngeal views of the arch system. The pharyngeal arches are denoted by Roman numerals I to V; the pharyngeal grooves and the corresponding internal pharyngeal pouches are designated by Arabic numerals 1 to 5.

The first pharyngeal groove deepens to form the external acoustic meatus, or ear canal. The ectodermal membrane in the depth of the groove persists and forms the tympanic membrane together with mesoderm and endoderm from the adjacent first pharyngeal pouch (Fig. 2.**6**). The external features of the second, third, and fourth pharyngeal grooves are obliterated by the overgrowth of the second pharyngeal arch anteriorly, which

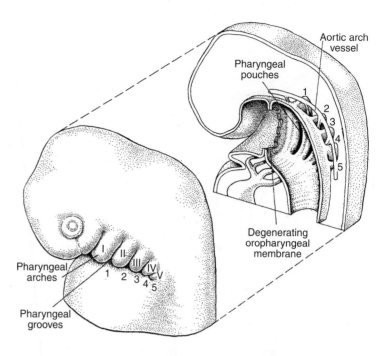

Fig. 2.**5** Sagittal view of the branchial region at 4 weeks. Observe the blood vessels that arise from the heart below and pass through each pharyngeal arch.

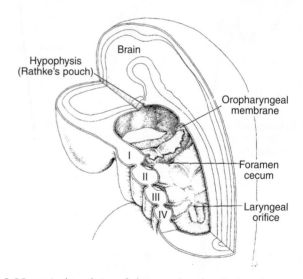

Fig. 2.**6** Posterior lateral view of pharyngeal–oral cavity loss of oropharyngeal membrane.

Clinical Application

The lack of normal growth changes in the pharyngeal arches can cause defects to appear in the lateral aspects of the neck. These defects may develop into cysts, causing localized swellings or fistulas that drain mucous secretions on the neck.

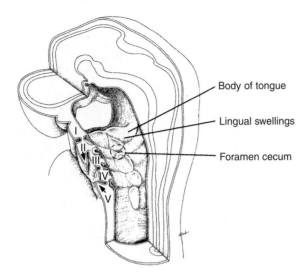

Fig. 2.**7** Pharyngeal arches I to V.

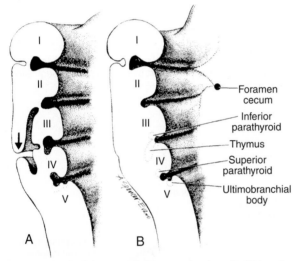

Fig. 2.**8 A** Overgrowth of the second pharyngeal arch to the fifth arch on the external surface. **B** Development of the pharyngeal pouches and their derivatives in the pharynx.

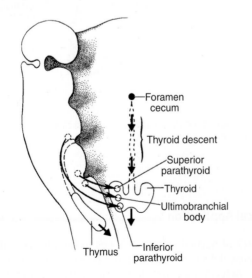

Fig. 2.**9** Site of endocrine glands in the pharyngeal pouches in the oropharynx.

after fusion with the fifth arch provides a smooth surface for the neck (Figs. 2.**7** and 2.**8**).

Endodermal epithelium, which lines the pharyngeal pouches, develops into a variety of organs. The middle ear and eustachian tube develop from the first pouch, the palatine tonsils from the second, and the inferior parathyroid and thymus from the third. From the fourth pouch, the superior parathyroid glands develop, and from the fifth the ultimobranchial body (Figs. 2.**8B** and 2.**9**).

The thymus is relatively large at birth and continues to grow until puberty. Thereafter it gradually atrophies, disappearing later in life. The ultimobranchial body fuses with the thyroid and contributes parafollicular cells to this gland. The parathyroid glands function throughout life in calcium regulation; the tonsils function in lymphocyte development and immunologic response factors.

Thyroid Gland

In the fourth week the thyroid gland appears as an epithelial primordia in the floor of the mouth; it is located in a depression at the junction of the body and base of the dorsal surface of the tongue (Fig. 2.**7**). This area becomes a blind duct, the "foramen cecum," from which the thyroid primordia will develop. This small mass then lengthens to descend in the midline of the neck as a bilobed diverticulum, reaching its final destination in front of the trachea in the seventh week (Fig. 2.**9**). During this migration, the gland remains connected to the floor of the mouth by an epithelial cord that later develops a lumen and becomes the thyroglossal duct. This duct later becomes a solid cord of epithelial cells that subsequently disintegrates and disappears. The thyroid gland begins to function by the end of the third prenatal month, when colloid-containing follicles begin to appear. Its secretions will later have an effect on the body's metabolism.

Pituitary Gland (Hypophysis)

As the oral cavity enlarges, a second important endocrine gland develops in the roof of the oral cavity as an ectodermal-lined pouch, termed Rathke's pouch. The pouch grows dorsally in the connective tissue toward the ventral surface of the brain (Fig. 2.**6**), where the middle and posterior lobes of the anterior pituitary develop. Both the middle and posterior lobes of this gland develop from oral epithelium. The posterior lobe—the neurohypophysis—develops from the infundibulum, which in turn develops from the brain. The pituitary gland is the master endocrine gland and interacts with all the other endocrine glands of the body.

Facial Development

The face develops during the fifth to seventh week of uterine life from four primordia that surround a central depression, the primitive oral pit. The facial primordia are: the frontal process, a single process located above the oral pit; two maxillary processes located lateral to the oral pit; and the mandibular arch or prominence, located below the oral pit. The two maxillary processes arise from the first pharyngeal arch (Fig. 2.**10**). These primordia arise because of centers of neural crest derived from mesodermal cell proliferation and differentiation. Any interruptions in timing or interaction at this early stage can result in malformation. The mandibular process appears initially as a partially divided structure, but soon merges at the midline to form a single structure (Figs. 2.**10** and 2.**11**). This process or arch gives rise to the mandible, the lower part of the face and the body of the tongue. The upper face arises from the frontal process that overlies the forebrain. The two maxillary processes are inconspicuous at 4 weeks, but later will form the cheeks and most of the upper lip.

By the late fourth week, nasal placodes develop bilaterally at the lower margin of the frontal process. These placodes quickly become recessed as the tissue around them grows, causing them to appear depressed. These depressions are now termed the nasal pits, and the area in which they appear the "frontonasal process." As the nasal pits deepen, they form the nostrils; the tissue around the pits enlarges, developing into horseshoe-shaped elevations with their open ends in contact with the oral pit below (Fig. 2.**11**). The medial nasal process is the tissue medial to the nasal pit. The lateral process, lateral to the pit, is in close contact with the maxillary process (Fig. 2.**12**). The contact zone of the epithelial-covered medial nasal and maxillary processes becomes the fusion site of the upper lip. A lack of fusion at this site results in a cleft lip. As the epithelial coverings of the

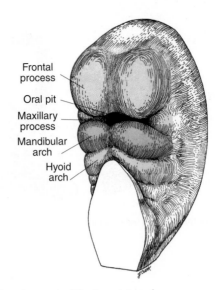

Fig. 2.**10** Development of the face at 4 weeks.

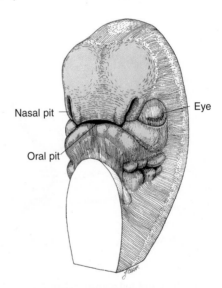

Fig. 2.**11** Development of face at 5 weeks.

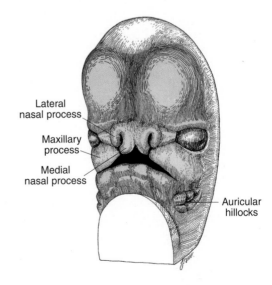

Fig. 2.**12** Development of face at 6 weeks.

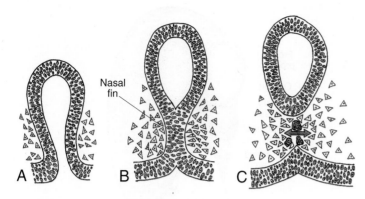

Fig. 2.**13** Breakdown of the nasal fin. Arrows indicate zone of intermingling.

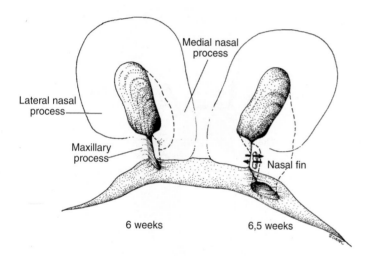

Fig. 2.**14** Formation of the nostril and primary palate. Arrows indicate zone of penetration.

maxillary and medial nasal processes come into contact, they normally fuse to form a "nasal fin" (Fig. 2.**13**). This vertically positioned sheet of epithelial cells is in the process of growing and also disintegrating. As these tissue masses expand, the epithelial sheets allow connective-tissue cells to penetrate the sheets, and bands of connective tissue then bind the lip contact area together.

A number of factors can interfere with the fusion process, such as genetic predisposition and/or a lack of blood supply, poor nutrition, chemical agents, physical interference, and timing. Fusion of the epithelial-covered processes occurs anteriorly, but not posteriorly where the floor of the nostril remains open. However, when fusion of the lip occurs, connective tissue and muscle cells grow through the nasal fin (barrier) to form tissue bands that strengthen the lip fusion site (Fig. 2.**14**). Normally the nasal fin will disappear in a few days and the lip will proceed to form.

During the sixth week, the two medial nasal processes merge in the midline to form the intermaxillary segment of the lip (Fig. 2.**12**). This removes the midline notch and allows the primary palate, immediately posterior to the lip, the opportunity to develop and also provides a site for the four maxillary incisor teeth to develop. Later, the segment of tissue in the center of the lip forms the philtrum. The philtrum is limited laterally by the two vertical ridges of tissue under the nostrils (Fig. 2.**12**). Initially, at the lateral boundary of the medial segment (the philtrum), there is a fissure where the line of fusion of the maxillary and medial nasal process meet (Fig. 2.**13**). This is the vulnerable area of the lip; disintegration of the fusion site will result in a cleft lip (Fig. 2.**12**). The upper lip is thus composed of three parts: the two maxillary processes grow inwardly from the sides, and the medial maxillary segment grows in a downward direction from above to interdigitate between the maxillary processes. These events occur during the sixth week of intrauterine life.

The floor of the nostril then fuses in an anteroposterior direction, and at its most posterior point there is an opening into the roof of the oral cavity (Fig. 2.**14**). Thus, the nostrils open on the front of the developing face and terminate in an opening in the roof of the mouth. This will soon change when the palatine shelves, which arise from the maxillary processes (cheek tissues), grow to meet in the midline of the palate. The palatine shelves fuse, separating the nasal and oral cavities.

The eyes develop during the fifth week of prenatal life. A localized thickening of the epithelium develops on the sides of the head, from which lens placodes form. These are positioned between the maxillary processes and the frontonasal processes (Fig. 2.**11**). Growth of the lateral forebrain causes lateral expansion of the face. The broadening of the face during the sixth week causes the eyes to be positioned more anteriorly on the front of the face and the nasal pits to appear more central in the face (Fig. 2.**12**). The distance between the nasal pits does not decrease, although it appears to do so, as seen in Figures

2.**11** and 2.**12**. Instead the width of the lateral face increases by lateral expansion of the brain, which causes the eyes to move to the front of the face. This widening of the face occurs during the sixth prenatal week (Fig. 2.**15**).

Ear Development

External ear. During the sixth week, the external ear (auricle) develops from six mesenchymal swellings or hillocks: three from the first pharyngeal arch and three from the second or hyoid arch (Fig. 2.**15**). These six hillocks appear in the upper and lower part of the cheek that surrounds the first branchial cleft. This cleft will develop into the external auditory canal. The hillocks will grow and merge to form the external ear (Fig. 2.**16A**). As the face grows forward and downward, the ears will maintain their position on the lateral face (Fig. 2.**17**).

Middle and inner ear. The middle ear is bounded externally by the tympanic membrane (eardrum) and internally by a thin, bony partition that contains two small membrane-bound openings. The middle ear contains three small bones: the malleus (hammer), which is attached to the tympanic membrane; the incus (anvil), which is the second bone; and the stapes (stirrup), which is attached to the oval window and opens into the inner ear (Fig. 2.**16B**). The three hearing bones are attached by minute (new) ligaments. The function of these three bones is to amplify and conduct sound to the inner ear, where nerve endings carry impulses to the brain. The inner ear or labyrinth consists of a complicated series of canals. The second part of the inner ear is the vestibule, which is concerned with balance. (Fig. 2.**16B**).

Development of Facial Features

The continued development of facial features is the result of differential growth brought about by the increase in breadth of the medial and lateral nasal processes and by the increased growth of the maxillary processes. By the seventh week, the face has acquired a

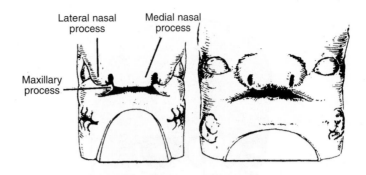

Fig. 2.**15** Development of the face at weeks 6 and 7.

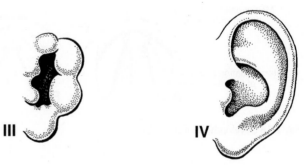

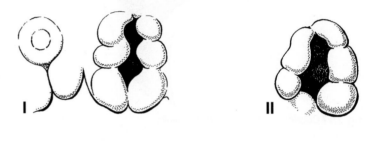

Fig. 2.**16 A** Development of the external ear.

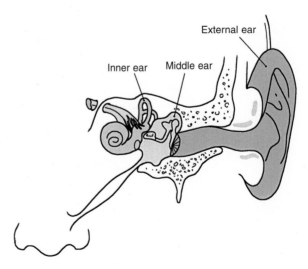

Fig. 2.**16 B** Anatomy of the inner, middle, and external ear.

Clinical Application

Alterations in the developmental timing of a structure can result in a developmental defect. In the vascular supply of the face, for example, a defect may result if the normal shift from internal to external carotid artery occurs, causing a vascular deficiency, at the time of organization and differentiation of the facial structure. Vascular and nutritional balance is critical during the seventh week.

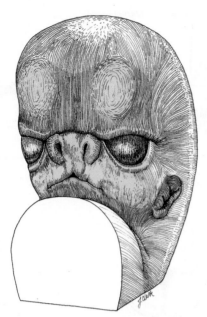

Fig. 2.**17** Development of the face at 7 weeks.

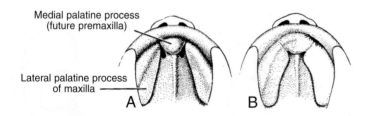

Medial palatine process
(future premaxilla)

Lateral palatine process
of maxilla

A   B

Fig. 2.**18** Development of the palate.

more human appearance (Fig. 2.**17**). At this time the medial part of the face increases in an anterior direction. As vertical height increases the bridge of the nose will develop, so that the nostrils and eyes will not be on the same horizontal plane. The mouth is very large at the fifth week, but merges at the angles to limit the size by the seventh week.

In the newborn, the nose is not yet fully developed and does not acquire its inherited size and shape until puberty. The eyes have moved from the lateral aspect of the face to the front, and as the orbits develop the eyes do not protrude as in the seventh and eighth weeks. In normal development, the distance separating the eyes greatly influences the appearance of the face. A narrow interocular distance (hypotelorism) confers a sharp fox-like appearance. An increased interocular distance (hypertelorism) causes the face to appear broad. The orbital cavities attain their adult dimensions when a child is about 7 years of age.

During early development, the mandible is at first small in comparison to the upper part of the face. It then grows at a more rapid pace in the eighth to twelfth weeks. Growth of the mandible then lags behind that of the maxilla, so the fetus displays a small lower jaw (micrognathia). In 2 weeks, the fifth to seventh, a recognizable human face takes shape. The face is formed from five unassociated masses: the frontonasal, maxillary, and mandibular processes. The development of the face is a marvel, the primordia growing, fusing, merging, and enlarging to become a recognizably human face with all the acquired hereditary features.

Palate

Palatine Shelf Growth and Elevation

The term "palate" refers to the tissue interposed between the oral and nasal cavities. The palate develops from three parts: one medial and two lateral palatine processes (Fig. 2.**18**). The medial palatine process is also called the "primary palate" because it appears before the secondary palate, at the beginning of the sixth week. As with the lip, the primary palate develops as an intermaxillary segment (a wedge-shaped mass) between the maxillary processes of the developing jaw (Fig. 2.**18**). The premaxillary bones, which support the four maxillary teeth, develop in the primary palate.

At the end of the sixth week, the lateral palatine processes that form the secondary palate develop from the medial edges of the maxillary processes that bound the stomodeum. The lateral palatine processes (shelves) first grow medially (Fig. 2.**18**), then grow downward or ventrally on either side of the tongue (Fig. 2.**19**). At this stage of development, the tongue is narrow and tall (Fig. 2.**20**), almost completely filling the oronasal cavity, and reaches the nasal septum. Elevation of the palatine shelves occurs after descent of the tongue, which allows for their meeting in the midline and fusion.

Tongue

Because the tongue is believed to take part in palatine shelf closure, it is appropriate to discuss its development at this time. The tongue is a muscular organ composed of an anterior movable part, termed the body, and the posterior firmly attached base or branchial part. The tongue originates from the first, second, and third pharyngeal arches and from a migration of muscles from the occipital myotomes (Fig. 2.**21**). The anterior part arising from the first arch is formed from three masses, the two lateral lingual swellings and the tuberculum impar (Fig. 2.**21**). These lateral lingual swellings rapidly enlarge, merge with each other, and overgrow the tuberculum impar to form the oral part of the tongue. A U-shaped sulcus develops in front of and on both sides of this oral part, which allows it to be free and highly mobile, except at the region of the lingual frenulum where it remains attached to the floor of the mouth.

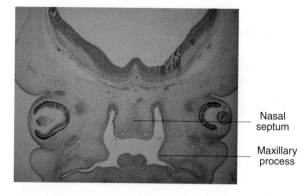

Nasal septum

Maxillary process

Fig. 2.**19** Palate at 6 weeks, prenatally.

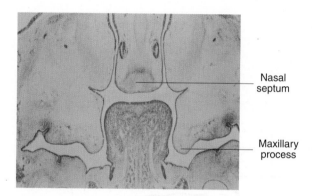

Nasal septum

Maxillary process

Fig. 2.**20** Palate at 7 weeks, prenatally.

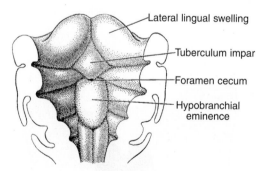

Lateral lingual swelling

Tuberculum impar

Foramen cecum

Hypobranchial eminence

Fig. 2.**21** Tongue development from three primary masses: two lateral lingual swellings and one tuberculum impar.

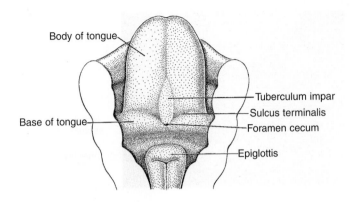

Fig. 2.**22** Fully formed body and base of tongue.

The base of the tongue develops mainly from the third pharyngeal arches (Fig. 2.**22**). Initially it is indicated by a midline elevation that appears behind the tuberculum impar, which is a large branchial eminence of the third and fourth arches. Later this eminence overgrows the second pharyngeal arch, to become continuous with the body of the tongue. The site of union between the base and the body of the tongue is delineated by a V-shaped groove called the "sulcus terminalis" (Fig. 2.**22**). Muscle cells from the occipital myotomes migrate anteriorly into the tongue during the fifth to seventh weeks, a diagram of which will be seen later in this chapter. In later stages of development, various types of papillae will differentiate on the dorsal mucosa that covers the body of the tongue, whereas lymphatic tissues develop on the branchial part of the tongue.

Palatine Shelf Closure and Fusion

At about 8 to 8.5 weeks of intrauterine life, the lateral palatine shelves slide or roll over the body of the tongue (Figs. 2.**23** and 2.**24**). The process of shelf elevation occurs when the shelves are capable of sliding over the tongue. This process usually occurs from the combined action of both shelf and tongue movement. (Fig. 2.**24**).

Step 1: The posterior parts of the palatine shelves are above the tongue because the posterior part of the tongue is attached to the floor of the mouth. Step 2: Palatine shelf action begins in this posterior area by rolling forward, which depresses the tongue and pushes it forward so that the tongue tip extends out of the mouth. Step 3: This forward rolling action releases the shelves from beside and under the tongue. Step 4: The shelves then assume a position overlying the tongue and gradually move together and fuse (Fig. 2.**25**). It is believed that the tongue and shelves function together in a combined action. Shelf elevation occurs as rapidly as swallowing and is therefore difficult to observe. The important consideration is that the shelves move over the tongue, and that the tongue then broadens and uti-

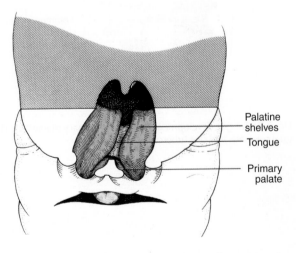

Fig. 2.**23** Palatine shelves positioned beside the tongue anteriorly and above it posteriorly.

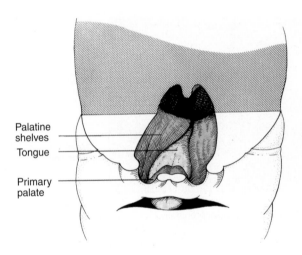

Fig. 2.**24** Palatine shelf elevation over the tongue. Observe the position of the tongue as the palatine shelves move it anteriorly during their elevation process.

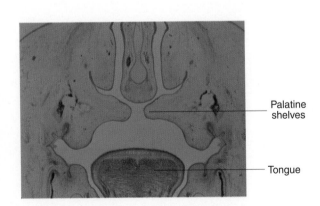

Fig. 2.**25** Palatine shelves positioned above the tongue.

lizes the space originally occupied by the shelves (Fig. 2.**26**). Step 5: Because the muscles of the tongue are well differentiated (Fig. 2.**26**), it is possible for the tongue to make a final action in this process and press against the shelves, aiding in the closure process.

After the shelves are positioned horizontally, there is a final growth spurt causing the shelves to make contact in the midline (Fig. 2.**27**). Initial closure or fusion of the lateral palatine shelves first occurs immediately posterior to the median palatine process (Fig. 2.**28**). Palatine closure involves the process of both fusion and merging (Fig. 2.**28**). When the shelves come into initial contact, the intervening epithelium breaks down and the shelves are then united by an intermingling of cells across the midline (Fig. 2.**28A–C**, Fusion). From the point of initial contact in the anterior palate, the lateral palatine processes fuse with the medial palatine process anteriorly (Fig. 2.**28**). Posteriorly, closure then takes place gradually over the next several weeks by the merging of the two lateral palatine processes. In merging, the depth of a groove separating the processes is diminished by growth underlying the groove (Fig. 2.**28A–C**, Merging). Fusion of the lateral palatine processes also occurs with the overlying medial nasal septum (Fig. 2.**26**), except posteriorly where the soft palate and uvula are unattached dorsally. In the initial stages palatine fusion involves fusion of soft tissues, but later at 12 weeks bone appears in the palate from the ossification centers (Fig. 2.**28**).

Development of Structural Components of the Head and Neck

Vasculature

The pharyngeal arches or aortic arch vessels supply blood to the face and neck. The vessels arise from the dorsal aorta, carrying blood from the ventral area through the arches dorsally, and return blood to the heart by a series of branchial veins. These arches are said to be vestigial remnants of fish and amphibians that oxygenate their blood by means of gills and gill slits which circulate the surrounding water. Not all of these paired arches are present at the same time. The anterior right and left arches develop first during the fourth week, and

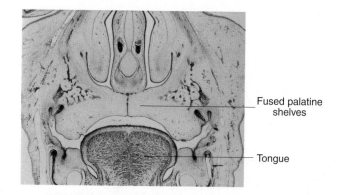

Fig. 2.**26** Histology of palatine fusion.

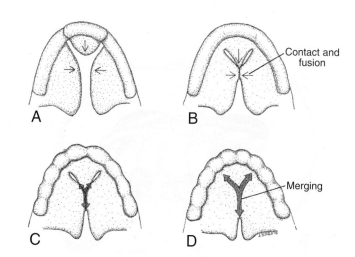

Fig. 2.**27** Fusion and merging of the palatine shelves. Arrows indicate the direction of growth.

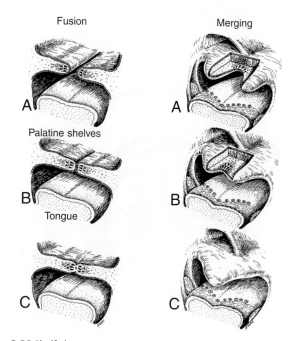

Fig. 2.**28** Shelf closure

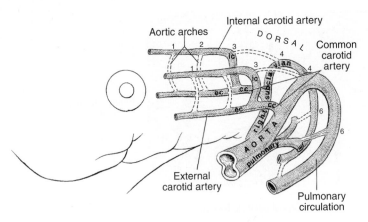

Fig. 2.**29** Aortic arch vascular development; ec, external carotid; ic, internal carotid.

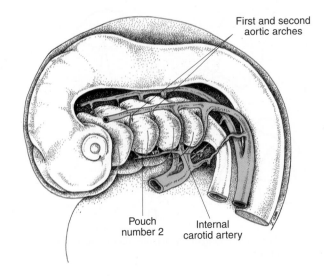

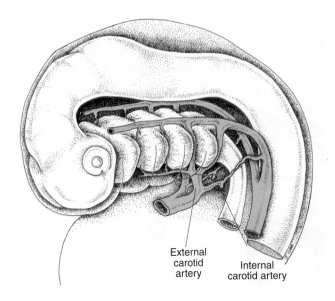

Fig. 2.**30** Aortic arch vessels at 4 weeks.

begin to degenerate as more posterior arches enlarge and begin to function (Fig. 2.**29**). As the second arch vessel begins to dwindle, the third arch vessel enlarges and begins to function. This third vessel will maintain its function and forms the common carotid (Figs.2.**30** and 2.**31**). The fourth and fifth arch vessels appear next, the fourth arch vessels forming the dorsal aorta supplying blood to the entire body. The fifth arch vessel then disappears and the sixth arises, forming the pulmonary artery supplying blood to the lungs. Therefore, of the six pairs of branchial vessels that develop, only the third, fourth, and sixth continue to function throughout life (Fig. 2.**29**).

Figure 2.**30** illustrates the embryo at 4 weeks; the paired branchial blood vessels are shown passing through the pharyngeal-arch tissue. The heart is located ventral to the arches, and blood passes dorsally through the arches to the face, brain, and rest of the body. By the fifth week (Fig. 2.**31**), the first and second arches have disappeared; blood to the face, brain, and body passes through the carotid circulation, which is the third pharyngeal arch. The common carotid then divides into the external and internal carotid artery. The external carotid artery supplies blood to the face (lower part) and the internal carotid artery supplies blood to the brain (Fig. 2.**32**). In the region of the ear, the internal carotid artery gives rise to a small vessel, the stapedial artery, which supplies blood to the upper part of the face and palate (Fig. 2.**33**). Blood supply to the face by the internal carotid artery is a characteristic of the embryo at the sixth and seventh weeks.

An important change in the vascular supply to the human face and palate takes place in the seventh prenatal week. At that time, the stapedial artery suddenly occludes and separates from the internal carotid artery. The vascular supply to the upper face and palate is immediately terminated. A strange development then occurs: the terminal portions of the stapedial artery

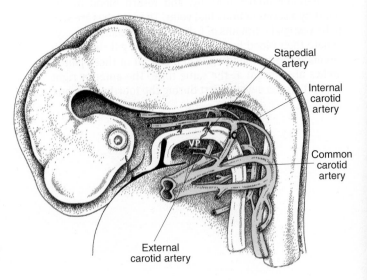

Fig. 2.**31** Aortic arch vessels at 5 weeks.

Fig. 2.**32** Aortic arch vessels at 6 weeks.

attach themselves to the terminal branches of the external carotid artery and blood begins flowing in the opposite direction through the stapedial vessels. The area of the upper face and palate then have a renewed blood supply (Fig. 2.**34**). The interesting aspect of this is that blood flowing through the stapedial artery to its terminal capillaries then reverses itself, starting in the fused capillaries and flowing to the artery. If this event occurs too late or too early, or if the vessels do not fuse properly, this can result in facial malformations such as cleft palate or facial cleft. The seventh week is important for facial growth and fusions, and also for facial vascular shift. The shift in blood supply from the internal to external carotid artery is shown in Figures 2.**33** and 2.**34**.

Skeletal Elements

The initial skeleton of the pharyngeal arches and face develops from the mesenchymal tissue within the arch. In the first arch these cartilage bars are termed Meckel's cartilage, after the man who first described and named them. The right and left Meckel's cartilage bars persist for the first few weeks of embryonic and fetal life, but later they are replaced by the bony mandible. The cartilage bars gradually disintegrate, leaving part of the perichondrium as the sphenomalleolar ligament (anterior ligament of the malleus) and part as the sphenomandibular ligament (Fig. 2.**35**). The posterior terminal parts of Meckel's cartilage are the malleus and incus, small cartilages that ossify and then function as middle ear bones.

In the second arch, Reichert's cartilage develops sup-

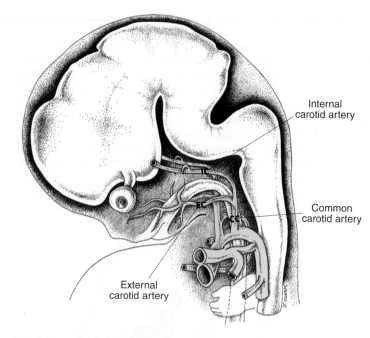

Fig. 2.**34** Shift carotid facial blood supply from internal to external carotid artery.

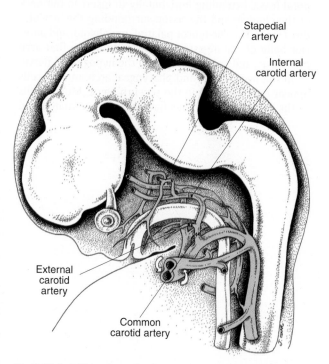

Fig. 2.**33** Facial blood supply of internal carotid artery by strapedial artery. Note relations of common and external carotid arteries at 7 weeks.

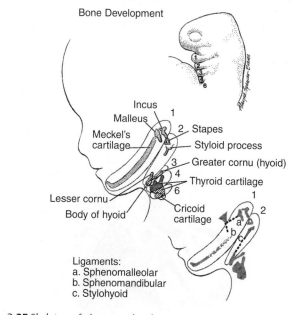

Fig. 2.**35** Skeleton of pharyngeal arches.

Clinical Application

Syndromes associated with the pharyngeal arches are frequently seen clinically as a group of defects. They can include: a malformed ear or mandible, small mouth, enlarged tongue or unequal growth of the sides of the tongue, malocclusion of teeth, cleft palate, and swelling caused by a cyst or clefts on the sides of the neck. Usually several or more defects appear, which leads to the classification as a syndrome. These include Treacher Collins' syndrome (mandibulofacial dysostosis), Goldenhar's syndrome (hemifacial microsomia), and the otocephalic first arch syndrome.

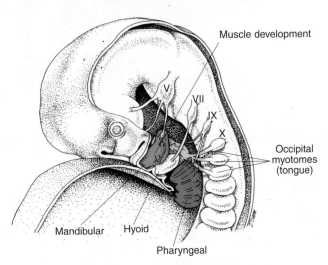

Fig. 2.**36** Development of nerves and muscles to pharyngeal arches, 5 weeks.

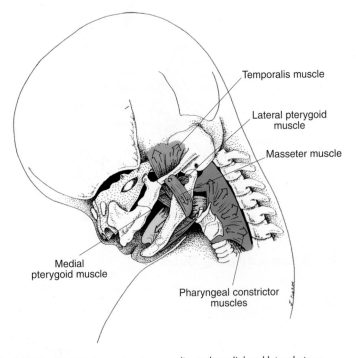

Fig. 2.**37** Masticatory (masseter, temporalis, and medial and lateral pterygoid) muscles at 10 weeks.

porting the function of the pharyngeal bar. This cartilage later breaks down, giving rise to the third middle-ear bone, stapes, styloid process, lesser horn, and the upper part of the hyoid body. The stylohyoid ligament is formed by the perichondrium at the site of disappearance of this second arch cartilage.

The third pharyngeal-arch cartilage forms the greater horn and lower part of the body of the thyroid (Fig. 2.**35**). The fourth arch cartilage forms the thyroid cartilage; the fifth has no adult derivatives; and the sixth arch cartilages form the laryngeal cartilages. Further skeletal structures are discussed in Chapter 3.

Facial Muscles

During the fifth and sixth weeks, myoblasts within the first arch begin proliferation (Fig. 2.**36**). The muscle cells become oriented to the sites of origin, carrying their initially established nerve supply (mandibular division of trigeminal). The myoblasts will then initiate insertion of these muscles of mastication, which will continue to develop. By 10 weeks, the masseter, medial and lateral pterygoid, and temporal muscles of mastication have emerged (Fig. 2.**37**). Muscle cell migration occurs before the skeletal ossification centers form bone in the mandible. The muscle cells of the masseter and medial pterygoid now form a vertical sling, inserting into the site that will form the angle of the mandible. The temporalis muscle differentiates in the infratemporal fossa and inserts into the developing coronoid process. The lateral pterygoid muscle fibers also arise in the infratemporal fossa, extending horizontally to insert in the neck of the condyle and the tissue surrounding the articular disc (Fig. 2.**37**). The tensor palatini, mylohyoid, and anterior belly of the digastric also arise from the first arch myoblasts, and are innervated by the hypoglossal nerve.

In the hyoid or second pharyngeal arch, muscle cells appear differentiated in the seventh week. Muscle cells in the occipital myotomes have also differentiated and are undergoing anterior migration, forming muscles of the tongue. This anterior migration will follow the path of development of the tongue (Fig. 2.**37**). By 10 weeks, muscle cells of the hyoid arch continue migration over the first arch muscle masses and extend upward over the face. One group of muscle cells grows upward anterior to the ear, and one group posterior to the ear. This is shown by arrows in Figure 2.**38**. These facial muscle cells follow a path not unlike that of the platysma muscle, up the side of the neck and over the mandible. The facial muscles arising from the hyoid arch extend upward over the face. They further develop a superficial and deep group of fibers that attach themselves to skeletal elements of the face (Fig. 2.**38**).

At the same time, muscle cells of the third and fourth arches form the branchial muscles: stylobranchial, cricothyroid, levator palatini, and constrictor muscles of the pharynx (Fig. 2.**38**). These muscles then enclose; their function is constriction of the pharynx (Fig. 2.**37**). All muscles of the throat as well as the face will continue developing to meet the increasing functional demands.

Innervation

By the seventh week, the fifth nerve has entered the mandibular muscle mass and the seventh nerve the second arch muscle mass. This means that the nerves are incorporated in these muscle masses early and lead or follow the muscle cells as they migrate and differentiate. The trigeminal (V) nerve innervates the muscles of mastication and the facial (VII) nerve innervates the muscles of facial expression (Fig. 2.**39**).

The fifth nerve supplies sensory fibers to the mandible and maxilla, and motor fibers to the four mus-

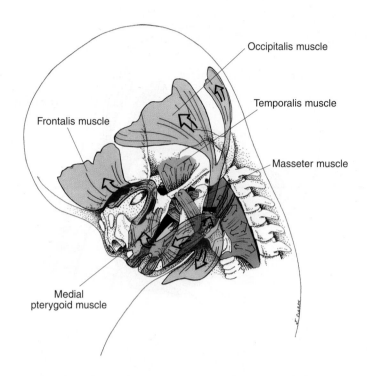

Fig. 2.**38** Facial muscles overlying masticatory muscles at 10 weeks.

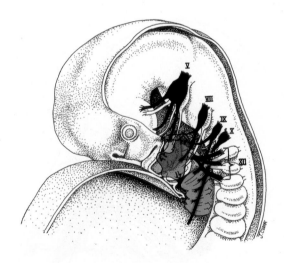

Fig. 2.**39** Cranial nerve and muscle relations at 7 weeks.

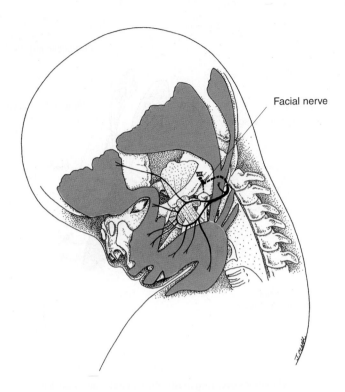

Facial nerve

Fig. 2.**40** Facial nerve distribution at 10 weeks.

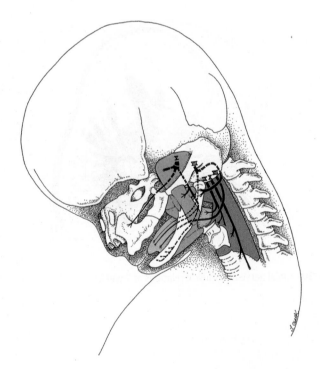

Fig. 2.**41** Face and tongue innervation pattern, 10 weeks.

cles of mastication and to the mylohyoid, tensor palatini, tensor tympani, and anterior belly of the digastric muscles. The seventh nerve follows the migration of the facial muscle mass from the neck to the face, where at 10 weeks this loop of motor nerves can be seen distributed to these muscles (Fig. 2.**40**). The seventh nerve also supplies the stylohyoid and stapedius muscles and the posterior belly of the digastric muscles (Fig. 2.**40**). The ninth or glossobranchial nerve supplies the stylobranchial and upper branchial muscles; the tenth cranial nerve, or vagus, supplies the branchial constrictor and branchial muscles.

As the occipital muscle masses migrate anteriorly, the ninth and twelfth nerves are carried along in the migrating tongue muscle mass. This muscle mass migrates anteriorly and acquires the seventh and fifth nerves as it reaches the oral cavity. The fifth nerve supplies the sensory nerves and the seventh nerve the taste fibers to the anterior two thirds of the tongue (Fig. 2.**41**). The ninth nerve supplies sensory taste fibers to the posterior third of the tongue, and the 12th nerve supplies the intrinsic muscles (longitudinal, vertical, and transverse) as well as the extrinsic muscles (styloglossus, hyoglossus, and genioglossus) of the tongue.

Clinical Application

The embryonic period is from the third to the eighth week. This is a high defect time when environmental agents are most likely to cause facial malformations. Facial malformations relate to timing because the face develops during the fifth to seventh weeks and the body tissues are also concurrently differentiating during the third to eighth week. The adverse effects are likely to alter closure and differentiation of the neural tissue, alimentary canal and its associated organs, and vascular, glandular, skeletal, and muscular formation.

Developmental Anomalies

Facial malformations are usually due to environmental and hereditary factors that may affect the timing of proliferation, migration, or even the death of tissue. Failure of growth, merging, or fusion of the various embryonic units of the face results in the persistence of developmental grooves and the formation of clefts. These defects are most common in the lip and palate. Most developmental anomalies of the neck arise from transformation of the branchial system into the adult derivatives. In recent experiments on chick and mouse, the introduction of excess SHH protein to the frontonasal processes led to the expression of other proteins (gli and bmp2). This expression leads to expansion of the midface and a cleft of the secondary palate.

Cervical Cysts and Fistulas

Caudal overgrowth of the second arch gradually covers the second, third, and fourth cervical grooves. These grooves lose contact with the surface of the neck and temporarily form an ectoderm-lined cavity, the cervical sinus, which would normally disappear (Fig. 2.**42**). Failure of complete obliteration of the cervical sinus results in a cervical cyst. If the cyst opens to the surface of the neck, a cervical fistula develops. Cervical cysts or fistulas are found anywhere on the side of the neck along the anterior border of the sternocleidomastoid muscle (Fig. 2.**43**).

Another cause of a cervical cyst or fistula is incomplete caudal overgrowth of the second arch, which leaves an opening on the surface of the neck (Fig. 2.**44**). A rarer condition is an internal pharyngeal fistula, in which the cervical cyst is connected to the pharynx by a small canal that usually opens in the tonsillar region (Fig. 2.**42**).

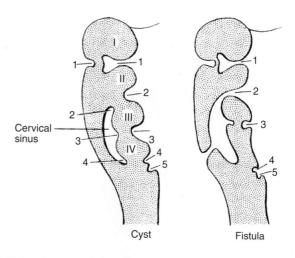

Fig. 2.**42** Development of pharyngeal cyst and fistula.

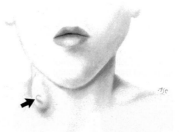

Fig. 2.**43** Location of potential branches cysts of fistulas.

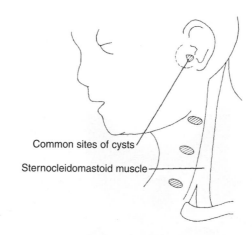

Fig. 2.**44** Clinical view of site (arrow) of cervical cyst and fistulas.

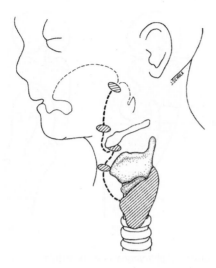

Fig. 2.**45** Sites of thyroglossal cysts and fistulas along descent path of thyroid gland.

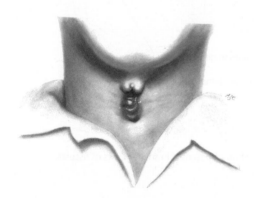

Fig. 2.**46** Clinical view of midline thyroglossal duct cyst.

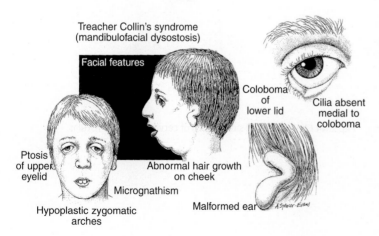

Fig. 2.**47** First pharyngeal arch defects.

Thyroglossal Cysts and Fistulas

Cysts and fistulas found along the midline of the neck usually develop from remnants of the thyroglossal duct. Generally, thyroglossal cysts may be found at any point along the course of the thyroglossal duct as it descends in the neck. The most common sites of these cysts are the areas of the hyoid bone and thyroid cartilage (Fig. 2.**45**). A thyroglossal cyst is a blind swelling commonly located in the region of the hyoid bone. A thyroglossal fistula is a swelling that opens to the surface of the neck by a small canal (Fig. 2.**46**). It usually results from a ruptured cyst.

Mandibulofacial Dysostosis or Treacher Collins' Syndrome

Mandibulofacial dysostosis, or Treacher Collins' Syndrome, results from failure of complete migration of the neural crest cells to the facial region. As its name implies, it is characterized by underdevelopment of the mandible and other facial bones. The zygomatic bone is severely hypoplastic. The face appears to be drooping, and the ears appear to be malformed. The lower border of the mandible appears concave, and cleft palate is occasionally seen (Fig. 2.**47**).

Cleft Lip

Cleft lip is a malformation of the maxillary lip. It may be unilateral or bilateral. The cleft varies from a notch in the vermilion border to a cleft extending into the floor of the nostril.

Unilateral cleft lip results from a failure of the maxillary process on one side to meet and fuse with the medial nasal process, which results in a division of the lip into medial and lateral parts. Unilateral clefting results in nasal distortion as lip and nasal tissues are pulled toward the attached side (Fig. 2.**48**).

Bilateral cleft lip occurs in much the same way on both sides. The defects may be symmetric or asymmetric. In bilateral cleft lip, the medial mass interposed between the two maxillary processes grows downward following a path of migration of neural crest cells from the closing forebrain. The timing of the proliferation, migration, positioning, and fusion is of vital importance for normal lip development. In some cases, the medial nasal process has not descended into proper position and a bilateral cleft lip occurs (Fig. 2.**49**). Recently, fibroblast growth factor (FGF) has been noted in the tips of ectoderm, comprising the medial nasal and maxillary processes, and can act as an organizer in these facial primordia. If the maxillary processes are widely separated, a unilateral or bilateral cleft lip can be associated with a cleft palate. In some cases, however, a cleft lip will not be associated with a cleft of the palate.

A median cleft lip is extremely rare and results from partial or complete failure of the medial nasal process to merge in the sixth week (Figs. 2.**12** and 2.**50**). This has been compared incorrectly to a "hare lip" of rabbits, as their maxillary processes meet in the midline leaving a notch in the upper lip. In the human, the median nasal process interposes between the two maxillary processes, forming the upperlip. Human clefts are sometimes incorrectly regarded as "hare lips": this term should be left with the rabbits.

A median cleft of the mandible is a rare condition that results from failure of the mesenchymal masses of the mandibular processes to merge together at 5 weeks of prenatal life. The mandible can then develop with no hard-tissue union in the midline (Fig. 2.**51**). A dimple in the chin is the slightest form of incomplete merging of the two mandibular processes.

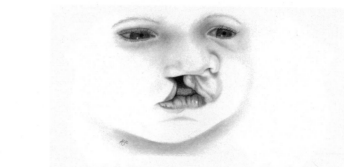

Fig. 2.**48** Unilateral complete lip cleft.

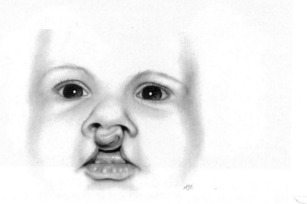

Fig. 2.**49** Bilateral complete lip cleft.

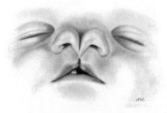

Fig. 2.**50** Midline cleft of maxilla

Clinical Application

Cleft lips and palates are two of the most common congenital malformations in the human population today. They appear in 700 live Caucasian births and one in 2000 in the Afro-American population in the United States today. Such defects are even more common in the Oriental population. They appear in one in 500 births in Chinese, Japanese, and native Americans, suggesting a strong hereditary factor.

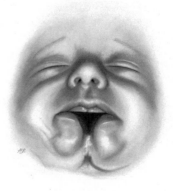

Fig. 2.**51** Midline cleft of mandible.

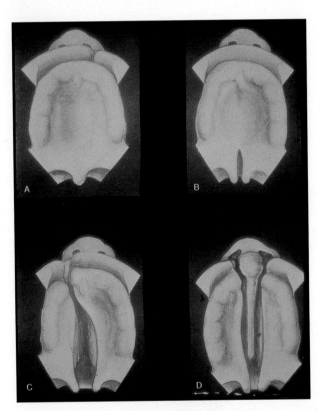

Fig. 2.**52** Examples of cleft lip and palate. **(A)**. Cleft lip.
(B). cleft of soft palate, **(C)**. Unilateral cleft lip and palate, **(D)**. Bilateral cleft lip and palate.

Cleft Palate

Cleft palate is less common than cleft lip. It can result as lack of growth or failure of fusion between the medial and lateral palatine processes and the nasal septum. Other causes are initial fusion with interruption of growth at any point along its course and interference in elevation of the palatine shelves. Clefts of the palate can be unilateral or bilateral (Fig. 2.**52**) and are classified as clefts of the primary palate, secondary palate, or both. Clefts of the primary palate, that is, clefts anterior to the incisive foramen, result from failure of the lateral palatine processes to meet and fuse with the median palatine processes or primary palate. The four maxillary incisors develop in the anterior median palatine segment; canines and molars develop in the lateral palatine segment. Clefts of the primary palate are usually associated with missing or malformed teeth adjacent to the clefts, such as lateral incisors and canines.

Because fusion of the secondary palate begins in the anterior region and progresses posteriorly, the degree of cleft can vary from the simplest form of bifid uvula to a complete cleft involving both the hard and soft palates. Therefore clefts of the secondary palate, that is clefts posterior to the incisive foramen, are the result of partial or incomplete failure of the lateral palatine processes to meet, fuse, and merge with each other and with the nasal septum (Figs. 2.**52B–D**).

Clefts of the primary and secondary palates are the result of failure of growth or lack of fusion of the three palatine processes with each other and with the overlying nasal septum (Figs. 2.**53** and 2.**54**). Clefts of the palate create many problems, the severity varying according to their extent. Although a bifid uvula causes practically no discomfort and is usually accidentally discovered, a cleft of the soft palate causes varying degrees of speech difficulty and swallowing problems. Clefts of both the hard and soft palates usually produce a severe feeding problem, as food can be aspirated into the lungs. Early correction of this problem should be sought.

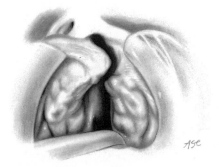

Fig. 2.**53** Clinical view of unilateral cleft.

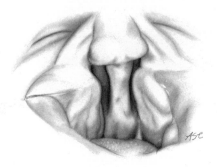

Fig. 2.**54** Clinical view of bilateral cleft.

Summary

The primitive oral cavity appears during the fourth prenatal week, initially as a pit located between the growing forebrain cranially and the growing heart ventrally. The pharyngeal arches develop as five or six pairs of horizontally positioned mesenchymal bars, located lateral and ventral to the oral pit and surrounding the oropharynx. The first pharyngeal arch gives rise to the mandible, which in turn forms the maxillary processes. From the mandibular arch, the bony mandible and the masticatory muscles develop. The mid upper face is formed from the frontal and nasal processes, from which the forehead, nose, and mid upper lip (philtrum) develop. The expansive growth of the second, or hyoid, arch gives rise to both the superficial and deep muscles of the face and scalp. The ectodermal lining of the oral cavity provides two endocrine glands, the thyroid gland from the tongue and the anterior pituitary gland from the roof of the mouth. Each pharyngeal arch gives rise to specific blood vessels, muscles, skeletal components, and neural elements. Contributions of each arch are shown in the summary diagram (Table 2.1). Other contributions of the pharyngeal pouches are pharyngeal tonsils from the second pouch, the parathyroid glands from the third and fourth pouch, and thymus gland from the third and fourth arches.

The roof of the mouth develops from three tissue areas: the anterior central portion, from the median palatine process, and the two lateral posterior parts from the palatine processes arising from the maxillary processes. The palatine processes "elevate" from beside the tongue to position themselves above it. This action is believed to begin with the tongue sliding forward, allowing the shelves to move over the tongue. The palatine shelves then make contact and fuse with the medial palatine process anteriorly; the right and left shelves fuse posteriorly in the midline.

Malformations can arise from the pharyngeal arches, where defective development results in clefts or fistulas between the arches. These defects are located along the anterior margin of the sternocleidomastoid muscle in the lateral neck. They can occur as a result of abnormal overgrowth of the second arch in the fifth prenatal week. Defects that appear in the anterior neck are usually due to thyroglossal duct cysts or fistulas. Clefts may appear, unilaterally or bilaterally, in the maxillary lip. This is due to lack of contact and fusion of the maxillary and medial nasal tissues during the sixth prenatal week. Midline clefts of the maxilla or mandible are rare and occur due to a lack of merging of tissues in that specific area. Palate clefts occur between the medial palatine process and the lateral palatine processes and can be isolated to that area or extend along the palatine margins to the back of the throat. Any variation in the length of the cleft can occur.

Table. **2.1** Contributions of brachial arches

BRANCHIAL GROOVES	BRANCHIAL ARCH STRUCTURES					PHARYNGEAL POUCHES
Adult derivative	**Arch no.**	**Cranial nerve**	**Branchiomeric muscles**	**Skeletal derivative**	**Aortic arch**	**Adult derivative**
Ext. auditory meatus	**I** Mandibular	**V** Trigeminal	Muscles of mastication, anterior belly digastric, mylohyoid, tensor tympani, tensor palatini.	Malleus, incus, sphenomandibular ligament, sphenomalleolar ligament (Meckel's cartilage)	**I**	Middle ear Eustachian tube
	II Hyoid	**VII** Facial	Muscles of facial expression, stapedius, stylohyoid, posterior belly digastric	Stapes, styloid process, stylohyoid ligament, lesser cornu hyoid, upper part body hyoid	**II**	Palatine tonsil
Cervical fistula	**III**	**IX** Glossopharyngeal	Stylopharyngeus	Greater cornu hyoid, lower part body hyoid	**III**	Thymus, inferior parathyroid
	IV	**X** Vagus	Laryngeal musculature, pharyngeal constrictors	Laryngeal cartilages	**IV**	Superior parathyroid / Ultimobranchial body
	V	**XI** Spinal accessory	Sternocleidomastoid Trapezius		**VI**	

Structures formed from the first pharyngeal groove, the pharyngeal pouches, and pharyngeal arches.

Self-Evaluation Review

1. Describe the process of the eyes migrating from the side to the front of the face.
2. Describe the origin of the thyroid gland and its descent in the neck to its location in the newborn.
3. Of the five vascular aortic arches that develop in the embryo, which ones disappear and which continue to function? What is their function in adults?
4. Describe the relative timing, function, and importance of the shift from the internal to the external carotid artery in the face.
5. What muscles develop from the second pharyngeal arch and what are their functions?
6. Name the four initial masses from which the face is formed. What does each of these contribute?
7. Describe the development of the maxillary lip.
8. Describe the process of palatine shelf elevation and fusion.
9. What cartilage elements arise from the first pharyngeal arch. Do they make any contributions in the adult?
10. Describe the contribution of the structures that arise from the pharyngeal pouches.
11. Describe the origin of the tongue musculature and its innervation.

Acknowledgements

The author acknowledges the original suggestions of Dr. ElNesr to this chapter. Dr Alfonse Burdi kindly provided Figure 2.47 from research in his laboratory.

Suggested Readings

Diewert VM. Course of the palatine arteries during secondary palate development in the rat. J. Dent. Res. 1973;52:273–280.

Gasser RF. The early development of the parotid gland around the facial nerves and its branches in man. Anat. Rec. 1970;167;63–78.

Maher WP, Swindle, PF. Submucosal blood vessels of the palate. Dental Progr. 1962;2:167–180.

Millard RD, Williams S. Median cleft lips of the upper lip. Plastic and Reconstr. Surg. 1968;42:4–14.

Padget DH. The cranial venous system in man in reference to development of adult configuration and relation to the arteries. Am J. Anat. 1956;98:307–356.

Poswillo D. The pathogenesis of the first and second pharyngeal arch syndrome. Oral Surg. 1973;25:302–328.

Sadler T, ed. Langman's Medical Embryology. 7th ed. Baltimore, Md.: Williams and Willkins; 1995.

Sperber GH.Craniofacial Embryology. 4th ed. London UK: Butterworth; 1989.

Sperber GH. Craniofacial Development and Growth. Toronto: B Decker Inc.; 2000.

Sulik KK. Craniofacial defects from genetic and ter atogen induced deficiencies in presomite embryos. Birth Defects. 1984;20:79–98.

Sulik KK, Johnson MC. Embryonic origin of holopros encephaly. Interrelationship of the developing brain and face. Scan Elem. Microsc. 1982;309–323.

Sulik KK, Lauder JM, Dehort DB. Brain malformation in prenatal mice following acute maternal ethanol administration. Int. J. Dev. Neurosci. 1984;2:203–214.

Sulik KK, Johnson MC, Smiley SJ, Speight HS, Jarvis BE. Mandibulofacial Dysostosis (Treacher Collins' Syndrome), a new proposal for its pathogenesis. Am. J. Med. Genet. 1987;27:354–372.

Ten Cate AR. Oral Histology, Development, Structure and Function. 5th ed. St Louis: Mosby Inc.; 1998

Van der Meulen JC, Mazzola R, Vermey-Keers C, Stricher M, Raphaie B. A morphogenetic classification of craniofacial malformations. Plastic Reconstr. Surg. 1983;71:560–572.

3 Development of Cartilage and Bones of the Craniofacial Skeleton

James K. Avery

Introduction

The facial skeleton is derived from both cartilage and bony elements. Centers of hyaline cartilage forming the base of the skull appear above and medial to the forming maxilla to support the developing brain. As the brain enlarges to form the bilateral cerebral and the cerebellar hemispheres, the cartilage centers grow laterally to underlie and support the brain. Anteriorly, the nasal capsule surrounds the olfactory sense organ, and laterally the otic capsule cartilage supports the hearing sense organ. The greater and lesser wings develop from the sphenoid midline cartilage and support the base of the brain. The three cartilages—nasal capsule, sphenoid, and basioccipital—are joined in the midine as a single unit, extending from the nasal septum to the foramen magnum. By the seventh week ossification centers surround the medial cartilages, as bone replaces them with endochondral bone formation. Ossification centers next appear in the connective tissue overlying the brain, forming bones for protection. These are the frontal, parietal, temporal, and occipital bones. The facial bones—nasal, premaxilla, maxilla, and zygomatic—then appear, which support the orbits and the cheeks. As these bones grow larger and come into closer contact, syndesmotic sutures form between them. Below in the mandibular arch, bilateral cartilage bars support the first pharyngeal arch. In addition to support, they provide the mandibular articulation of the malleus and incus, limited to a hinge action—the primary jaw joint. Bone then appears lateral to Meckel's cartilages forming the body of the mandible. A cartilage condyle next forms and soon fuses with the body of the mandible, resulting in a single unit. The temporal bone forms a fossa for articulation of the condylar heads. This is the secondary mandubular joint that begins functioning in the 16th prenatal week, as the malleus and incus cartilages transform into bone. These bones then function as hearing bones in the middle ear. There is further bone formation in the condyle, but cartilage continues forming on the condylar head throughout postnatal life and until the 22nd to 25th postnatal year. Examples of unilateral and bilateral clefts of the palate demonstrate lack of bone development where the soft tissue processes fail to form.

Objectives

After reading this chapter, you should be able to describe the skeletal components that form the skull and developing face. You should have acquired information regarding the cartilages and bones of the cranial base, maxilla, mandible, and primary and secondary mandibular joints. Also, you should be able to define the various articulations of the face and palate. Finally, you should be able to describe abnormal development resulting from a unilateral or bilateral cleft palate.

Early Skull Development

Those cartilages and bones developing around the brain are termed "neurocranial" elements and those supporting the face are termed "viscerocranial" elements. The cranial skeleton differs from the axial and appendicular skeleton in that the latter are composed of two major tissue types and are derived from one single mesodermal cell lineage, whereas the skull is derived from four different tissue types and two cell types. The mesoderm provides a minor source while the major contribution comes from ectomesenchyme originating from the lateral neural plate.

Cartilaginous Neurocranium

The first cartilages to form in the skull are those that support the base of the brain and develop initially in the midline as a continuous cartilaginous bar extending posteriorly from the nasal septum to the foramen magnum (Fig. 3.**1**). Attached to the midline bar anteriorly are the lateral wings of the nasal capsule, the sphenoid cartilage, and the lateral otic capsule, and posteriorly the supraoccipital and parachordal plate (Fig. 3.**2**). The nasal and otic capsules form around the nasal and auditory nerve endings. All of these cartilages underlie and support the developing brain and are termed cartilaginous neurocranial elements (Fig. 3.**3**). Gradually, ossification centers appear within these cartilages and they ossify to form the ethmoid and sphenoid bones. Lateral extensions of the sphenoid bone become the lesser and greater wings. Part of the otic capsule (squamous) and basiocciput also become the petrous portion of the temporal bone(Fig. 3.**4**).

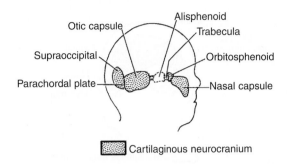

Fig. 3.1 Early cartilage formation.

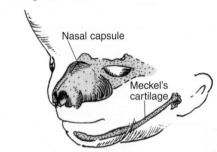

Fig. 3.2 Cartilages of the face at 6 weeks.

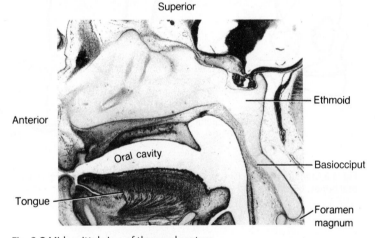

Fig. 3.3 Midsagittal view of the nasal septum.

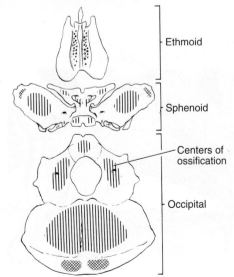

Fig. 3.4 Development of the cranial base.

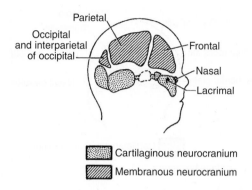

Fig. 3.5 Development of the membrane bones of the cranium.

Membranous Neurocranium

Intramembranous ossification sites appear in the mesenchyme covering the brain and are termed membranous neurocranium (Fig. 3.**5**). These sites first appear at 8 weeks, the beginning of the fetal period, as ossification centers. This membranous tissue will develop into flat bones of the skull and form the nasal, frontal, lacrimal, parietal, and part of the occipital bones. These bones are each separated by serrated connective-tissue sutures. In the sixth month bone-free spaces, covered by connective tissue, appear in the skull between bones. These spaces are known as "fontanelles"; they enable the skull to undergo alterations in shape or molding at birth (Fig.3.**6**).

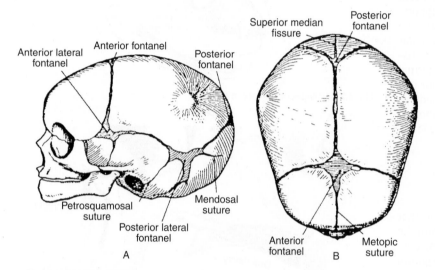

Fig. 3.**6** Cranium at birth. Observe the fontanelles at the corners of the parietal bones.

Cranial Base Development

In the 18th week, the cranial base cartilages begin to ossify by endochondral bone formation. This process will continue throughout prenatal and early postnatal life. In addition, the cranial base cartilages transform into bone, and membrane bone centers develop at the periphery of these cartilages. These bone centers produce membrane bone expansions of the cranial base to support the developing and enlarging brain (Fig. 3.**5**). Sutures then appear between the ethmoid and sphenoid and the sphenoid and occipital bones. These cartilage sutures, the ethmospenoid and sphenooccipital, are classified as synchondroid. They are named after the bones with which they articulate (Fig. 3.**7**). These cartilage sutures

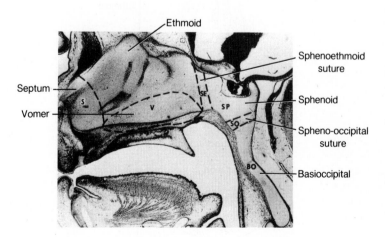

Fig. 3.**7** Location and identity of sutures in the cranial base.

continue to function, and are a site of new bone formation at the periphery of the cartilage sutures (Fig. 3.**8**).

The cranial base forms a 135° angle very early in life (Fig. 3.**9**). This angle is maintained until early childhood, when major changes in the face and cranial base occur.

Early Skeletal Development of the Upper Face

Cartilaginous Viscerocranium

The cartilaginous viscerocranium (facial) originates from the first and second pharyngeal arches, comprising the cartilaginous nasal capsule in the maxilla and, right and left, Meckel's cartilage bars in the mandible (Fig. 3.**10**). These mandibular cartilages extend from an anterior location near the midline to a posterior location in the middle ear, where they form an articulation between the malleus and incus cartilages (Fig. 3.**11A**). Meckel's cartilage terminates in the malleus, which is a rounded ball with a flat articulating face in contact with the incus cartilage. During the 8th to the 16th prenatal week these cartilages, known as the "primary temporomandibular joint" (1st TMJ) function as a simple hinge joint. The malleus then separates from Meckel's cartilage and ossifies into bone, forming the hearing bones of the middle ear.

In the second arch, a parallel cartilage to Meckel's cartilage forms. It is termed "Reichert's cartilage" and forms the lesser cornu and the upper part of the hyoid body, the stapes, and the styloid process (Fig. 3.**11A**). This diagram shows the third pharyngeal arch that gives rise to the body of the hyoid cartilage; the cricoid and thyroid cartilage arise from the fourth and fifth arches (Fig.3.**11B**).

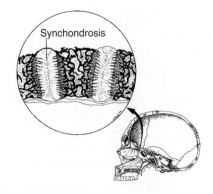

Fig. 3.**8** Diagram of cartilage suture development.

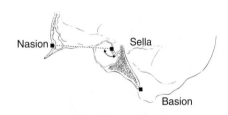

Fig. 3.**9** Diagram of landmarks to determine the cranial base angle.

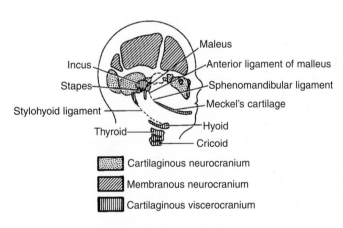

Fig. 3.**10** Diagram of facial cartilage development.

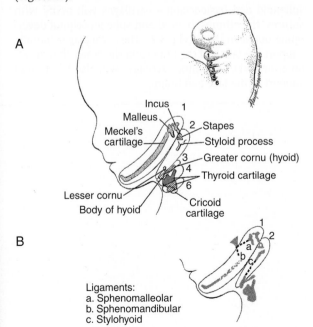

Fig. 3.**11** Diagram of pharyngeal-arch skeletal differentiation.

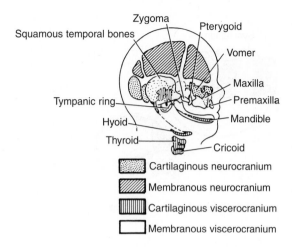

Fig. 3.**12** Diagram of craniofacial bony skeletal development.

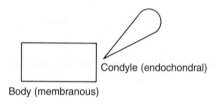

Fig. 3.**13** Diagram of mandibular development: body and condyle.

Membranous Viscerocranium

Membranous bone formation in the face occurs in the maxillary process of the first pharyngeal arch to form the premaxillary, maxillary, zygomatic, and temporal (squamous portion) bones (Fig. 3.**12**). The premaxilla may or may not form a separate ossification center. In some cases a single center develops and in others bilateral centers appear that soon fuse on the facial surface as an anterior extension of the maxilla. For the sake of discussion the premaxilla will be described as separate bilateral bones as they later form a suture on the lingual palatine surface with the maxilla. Mesenchyme in the mandibular arch tissue, lateral to Meckel's cartilage, also undergoes membranous ossiffication to form the body of the mandible. The body of the mandible appears as a small rectangular piece of bone. It attaches anteriorly to Meckel's cartilage and posteriorly develops a carrot-shaped piece of cartilage that will later form the mandibular condyle (Fig. 3.**13**). This is an example of the cooperation of the two types of bone formation producing a single bone. Therefore, the mandible is initially formed from membrane bone with a cartilaginous condyle. Then they fuse together, and the cartilage is transformed into bone.

Later Skeletal Development of the Upper Face

Medial Cartilage Contributions

The cartilage that develops in the upper face, noted earlier as the nasal capsule, comprises the medially positioned nasal septum and two lateral wings, which form the ethmoid. Posterior to this cranial base cartilage, the sphenoid and basioccipital cartilages will ossify with sutures, the ethmosphenoid and sphenooccipital developing between them (Fig. 3.**7**). These cartilages initially support the face and the brain, and the bones that develop around these midline cartilages will also function in support of the face and brain.

Peripheral Bony Centers

Bony ossification centers first appear representing the nasal (also considered a cranial bone), the premaxillary, maxillary, and more posteriorly the zygomatic and temporal (squamous) bones. These sites then enlarge in the face. The premaxilla grows cranially upward toward the nasal area, and the maxilla also grows upward around the nose to support the orbits. As seen in Figure 3.**14**, at 8 weeks the frontal bone covers the forebrain, forming the forehead: 1) Nasal bones appear on the surface of the nasal capsule; 2) Premaxillary sites may appear separately or united with (3) the maxillary, (4) the zygomatic, (5) sphenoid-cartilage center of the face; 6) The temporal sites appear posterior to the maxillary centers; 7) in the mandibular arch this bone appears lateral to Meckel's cartilage and forms the body and appears fused to the condyle forming a single unit (Fig. 3.**14**). The bony mandible is derived from the membrane body and the cartilage condyle. The head of the condyle maintains a cap of cartilage throughout prenatal life.

A human specimen, with the bones stained and the soft tissue cleared, is shown at 10 weeks (Fig. 3.**15**). Above the orbits the temporal bones are well developed, and the premaxillary and maxillary bones are near fusion. By 12 weeks, the premaxillary and maxillary centers are fused but the cranial base cartilages are still in evidence (Fig. 3.**16**). During the 10th week, a midline bony site appears below the nasal septum. The vomer forms a "V"-shaped bone, as seen anteroposteriorly, growing up either side of the nasal septum. As the face increases in height, the vomer becomes more prominent (Fig. 3.**17**). This is also evident in a cross-section of this area as the bone below and on either side of the septum

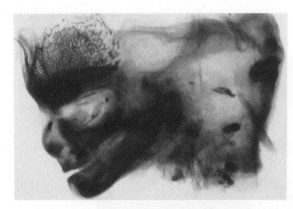

Fig. 3.**14** Relation of cartilages and bones of the face at 9 weeks.

1. Nasal
2. Premaxilla
3. Maxilla
4. Zygomatic
5. Sphenoid
6. Temporal
7. Mandible

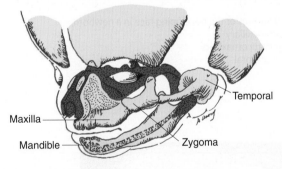

Fig. 3.**15** Human skeleton at 10 weeks. Note the extent of facial bone development.

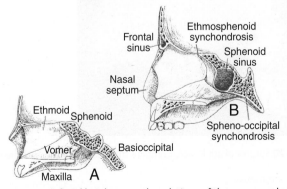

Fig. 3.**16** Illustration of bones of the face at 10-12 weeks.

Maxilla

Mandible

Temporal

Zygoma

Clinical Application

The face has a parallel suture system that provides for growth and projection of the face in a downward and forward direction. The sutures are situated between the maxillary, zygomatic, and temporal bones and all have a very similar inclination. These bilateral sutures are part of a network contributing to facial growth that occurs in the midline of the cranium, palate, and mandible, as well as the external surface of the facial bones.

Frontal sinus

Ethmosphenoid synchondrosis

Sphenoid sinus

Nasal septum

Ethmoid

Sphenoid

Vomer

Basioccipital

Maxilla **A**

B

Spheno-occipital synchondrosis

Fig. 3.**17** Increase in facial height: note the relations of the vomer and ethmoid bones at birth (**A**) and in the adult (**B**).

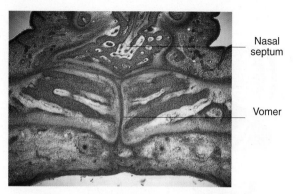

Nasal
septum

Vomer

Fig. 3.**18** Cross-section of the face. Note the midpalatine suture
(arrow) and overlying vomer.

(Fig. 3.**18**). Note that the palatine bones are immediately
beneath the vomer and contact the vomer in the midline. The relationship of the septum, vomer, and sphenoid can be seen during the fetal period and in a young
adult in Figure 3.**17**. The disproportionately large eye
sockets displaced inferiorly by the brain throughout this
period by its increased relative size during later prenatal
life. Bone resorbs on the superior (nasal) side of the
palate, but forms on the oral palatine side during the
prenatal period.

Facial Articulations

The bones of the nasomaxillary complex continue to
enlarge and maintain sutural contact at the frontomaxillary, zygomaticomaxillary, zygomaticotemporal, and
pterygopalatine sites. A comparison can be seen in the
appearance of these bones and sutures at birth in Figure
3.**19**, and in the adult in Figure 3.**20**. Note the general
increase in the height of the face and cranial skeleton.
The sutures have remained relatively in the same position, although the face has grown in height and length.

Simple sutures are those in which the bones meet
end to end with connective tissue between them (Fig.
3.**21**). Serrated sutures are characterized by interdigitating opposing bone fronts, such as the calvarial bones
(Fig. 3.**22**). They exhibit cells and fibers between the

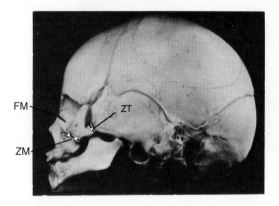

FM

ZT

ZM

Fig. 3.**19** Sutures of the developing face in a newborn.
FM: frontomaxillary
ZM: zygomaticomaxillary
ZT: zygotemporal

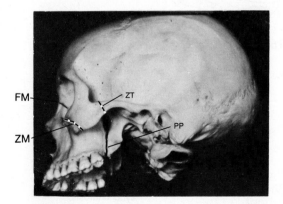

FM

ZT

ZM

PP

Fig. 3.**20** Sutures of adult face. Compare the location to those of the new-
born.
FM: frontomaxillary
ZM: zygomaticomaxillary
ZT: zygomaticotemporal

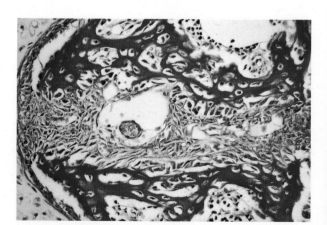

Fig. 3.**21** Simple syndesmosis suture. Observe the connective
tissue between two bony interfaces.

bones in a relationship similar to the simple sutures, except that they consist of dense fibrous bands extending across them. Squamous sutures, such as the temporoparietal one, are characterized by overlap. Growth of the opposing bones is at an angle to each other (Fig. 3.**23**).

In addition to fibrous connective-tissue syndesmotic sutures, there are cartilage junctions between two bones. These were described previously as sutures found between the midline ethmoid, sphenoid, and occipital bones. It is interesting that areas of cartilage that ossify develop cartilage sutures between them, whereas areas of forming bone develop connective-tissue sutures between them. Such cartilage junctions are termed synchrondroses (Fig. 2.**24**). These sutures have the appearance of an epiphyseal plate or "line" in an X-ray. At the center of each suture, new cartilage cells differentiate in the "resting zone." As these new cells differentiate in the center of the cartilaginous suture, the cells that previously occupied this zone move peripherally to multiply and develop new cartilage matrix. The peripheral cartilage then calcifies and degenerates as new bone forms. Growth of the opposing bones takes place in the periphery of these cartilage sutures (Fig. 3.**25**).

The prevalent theory of cranial sutural expansion is growth of the underlying structure, such as the brain, which causes the bones to separate (Fig. 3.**25A**). Therefore, sutural expansion compensates for the intrinsic growth process. The growth of the four facial sutures could be a response to the force of the facial-tissue growth downward and forward. Another theory of sutural growth is that the force resides within a suture, and that growth of the face results from this sutural force (Fig. 3.**25B**).

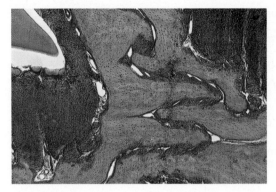

Fig. 3.**22** Serrated suture of the cranium. Observe the intedigitating bony extensions.

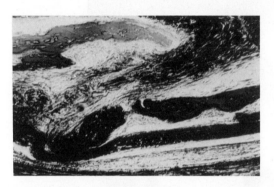

Fig. 3.**23** Squamous suture. Observe the overlapping bony fronts.

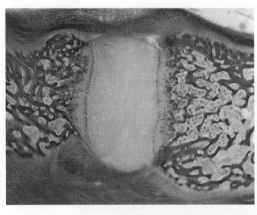

Fig. 3.**24** Cartilage suture. Synchondrosis with new cartilage cells in the center and bone forming along the lateral boundries.

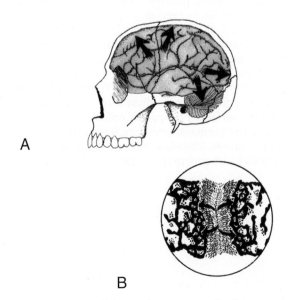

A

B

Fig. 3.**25 A** Diagram of the cartilage suture and its location in the cranial base. **B** Growth of cartilage ion suture between adjacent bones.

Clinical Application

Sutures are sites of growth but also provide a hinge–like action of the cartilage or bony interfaces, and may be strengthened with fibrous bands or interdigitating or overlapping projections formed to fulfil the needs of a particular location. The ability to judge the amount and timing of growth in a particular site is of considerable clinical importance in planning orthodontic and surgical procedures.

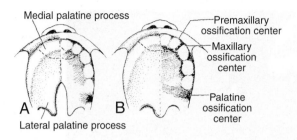

Fig. 3.**26** Palate formation. Observe the ossification centers. **A** Palatine shelves. **B** Location of the ossification centers.

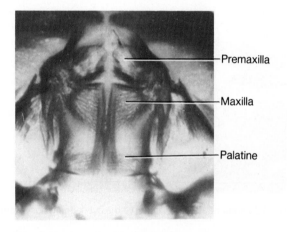

Fig. 3.**27** Ossification centers in the palate at 13 weeks. Observe the location of the premaxillary, maxillary, and palatine centers.

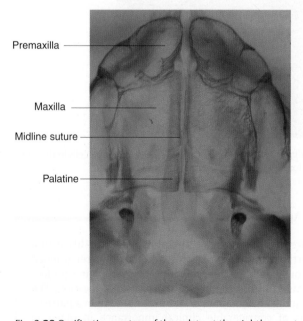

Fig. 3.**28** Ossification centers of the palate at the eighth prenatal month. Note the location of the palatine sutures.

Palatine Ossification

Medial Palatine Centers

In Chapter 2 we learned that the roof of the oral cavity develops from one medial and two lateral palatine processes (Fig. 3.**26A**). Six tiny ossification centers appear within these three processes. Two centers, the premaxillary and maxillary, appear adjacent at the junction of the medial and lateral palatine processes (Figs. 3.**26A** and **B**). The bone from these centers grows medially and then a midline palatine suture forms at this site (Figs. 3.**26** and 3.**27**). The two premaxillary centers develop in the medial palatine process. The premaxillary bone has both lingual and labial plates of bone that surround the four developing incisor teeth. After palatine bone growth occurs in the lateral palatine processes, the midline suture extends between the right and left sides of the palate (Fig. 3.**27**). A suture is then positioned between the more posterior palatine and maxillary bones (Fig. 3.**27**). This suture and the anterior premaxillary–maxillary suture provide for anterior growth of the palate, and the midline suture provides for lateral growth. These sutures can be more clearly seen in the eighth prenatal month (Fig. 3.**28**).

Lateral Palatatine Centers

From the lateral palatine ossification centers, the right and left maxillary and palatine ossification sites grow medially to support the soft tissues of the palate. A prenatal palate of 13 weeks is seen in Figure 3.**27**. This stained fetal skull shows many fine trabeculae of bone extending medially in the palate. At this time there is a white space between the maxillary and palatine centers, indicating that bone has not formed there but will later fill in this area. The palatine center then forms a suture with the maxilla, as seen in a specimen at 8 prenatal months (Fig. 3. **28**). The maxillary bones will support the primary maxillary cuspids and molars and later provide alveolar bone support for the permanent cuspids, premolars, and molar teeth. Crypts for the primary cuspids and molar teeth can be seen in Figure 3.**28**. Lateral growth will occur at the midline suture as well as laterally on the surface of the palate. Anterior growth is provided at the premaxillary–maxillary and maxillary–palatine sutures. Therefore, growth in the palate keeps pace with facial growth (Fig. 3.**28**).

Mandibular Development

Meckel's Cartilage Contributions

As the nasal capsule becomes the prominent cartilage skeleton of the upper face, Meckel's cartilage is established as bilateral support in the mandibular arch during the seventh and eighth weeks (Fig. 3.**29**). The posterior part of each Meckel's cartilage bar enlarges to form the malleus and articulates with the incus, which is the second cartilage. These two minute cartilages become enclosed in bilateral otic capsules and later develop later into the middle-ear bones. This joint is known as the "malleoincudal" or primary mandibular joint. It is important as the mouth is opening and closing at this early time (Figs. 3.**29**–3.**31**). The primary joint functions until the 16th week when the "secondary temporomandibular joint" (2nd TMJ) assumes the function. During the 14th to 15th week the malleus and incus begin to calcify and ossify. Throughout this period the malleus and incus are transformed into bone. Their function of articulation changes as they develop into hearing bones. The stapes, arising from the second-arch (Reichert's) cartilage will also function as a hearing bone. The remainder of Meckel's cartilage will then degenerate as the bony mandible enlarges. The TMJ begins to develop anterior to the otic capsule and will assume a more complex function of the bony mandible than the primary joint (Figs. 3.**32** and 3.**33**).

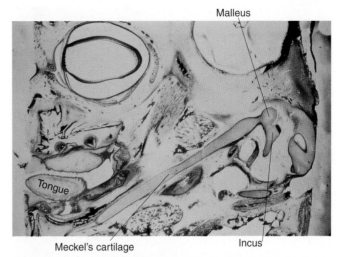

Fig. 3.**29** Lateral views of Meckel's cartilage and the articulation between the malleus and incus.

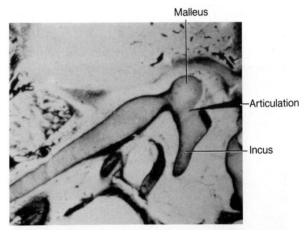

Fig. 3.**30** Lateral view of the malleus attached to the posterior end of Meckel's cartilage. Observe its articulation with the incus cartilage.

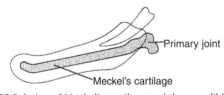

Fig. 3.**32** Relation of Meckel's cartilage and the mandible.

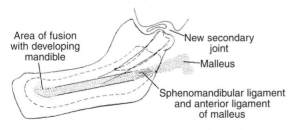

Fig. 3.**33** Relation of the mandible and Meckel's cartilage at 20 weeks. Note the developing temporomandibular (TMJ) joint.

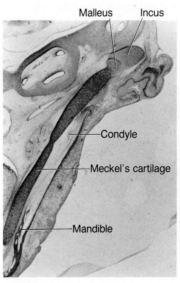

Fig. 3.**31** Frontal view of Meckel's cartilage and the articulation of the malleus and incus.

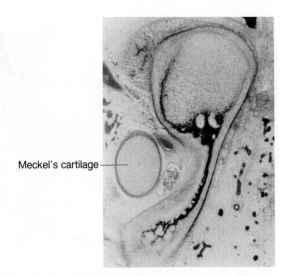

Fig. 3.**34** Coronal view of the mandibular condyle and its relation to the medially located Meckel's cartilage at 11-12 weeks.

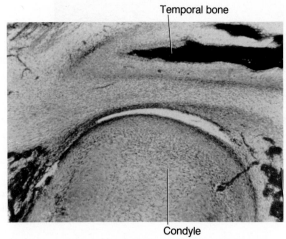

Fig. 3.**35** Lateral view of the condylar head and appearance of the cleft outlining it.

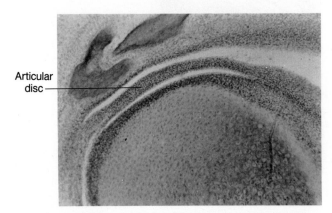

Fig. 3.**36** Lateral view of the condylar head and appearance of the second cleft outlining the articular disk overlying the condylar head.

Formation of the Body and Ramus

The body of the mandible forms as a rectangular piece of membrane bone developing lateral to Meckel's cartilage (Figs. 3.**32** and 3.**33**). The condyles develop posterior to the body as carrot-shaped cartilages in the 8th to 12th weeks. Initially these cartilages develop independently, but by the 13th week they fuse with the body to form a single mandibular unit. The condyle develops in the area anterior to the ear and posterior to the body of the mandible. The condyles develop first in cartilage before ossifying; as they enlarge, the condylar heads are formed (Fig. 3.**34**). The first appearance of a TMJ cavity appears in the fetus of 12 weeks (Fig. 3.**35**). The first of the compartments to develop is the inferior or mandibular compartment. A split appears in the mesenchyme overlying the cartilage condyle, and develops into a small cleft (Fig. 3.**35**). Within another week, the superior or temporal compartment is formed by a second split in the connective tissue, parallel to the first (Fig. 3.**36**). The synovial cavity outlines the condylar head. The precise mechanism of tissue cavitation remains unknown. The process is probably due to programmed cell death (apoptosis), which occurs along the path of condylar movement with the adjacent connective tissue. Then a spicule of the temporal bone develops superior to the forming articular disk (Figs.3.**35** and 3.**36**).

With continued bone formation, the small segments soon coalesce to form the glenoid fossa (Fig. 3.**37**).

By the 16th week bone has formed around the cartilages by endochondral bone formation, which then fuses with the body of the mandible. The condyles and the body of the mandible initially form an angle of 135°, which is maintained during the remainder of prenatal life. Later in prenatal life, near birth, bone is deposited near the angle of the mandible where the masseter and medial pterygoid muscles attach. This action serves to strengthen the union of the attachment of the mandibular body and condyle. Growth of the condylar head increases the height of the condyle. However, most enlargement of the mandible occurs postnatally. The coronoid process becomes a prominent part of the mandible and continues to develop until near the time of birth (Fig. 3.**38**). The two halves of the mandible become united at the anterior midline, which is termed the mental symphysis. This suture continues to grow almost until the end of the first postnatal year when it ossifies.

Fate of Meckel's Cartilage

The anterior aspect of Meckel's cartilage fuses to the medial wall of the bony mandible during the 10th prenatal week. This process occurs by endochondral bone formation. Therefore, some endochondral bone is formed on a membrane body of the mandible. As the mandible enlarges, remnants of Meckel's cartilage become smaller in relation to the mandible, as seen in Figure 3.**37**. By the 15th prenatal week, the malleus and incus have begun transformation into bone by endochondral bone formation. (Fig.3.**37**). As Meckel's cartilage then degenerates in the area anterior to the ear, the anterior malleolar and the sphenomandibular ligaments develop in its path (Fig. 3.**33**). When the TMJ begins functioning in the 16th prenatal week, Meckel's cartilage loses its function and almost disappears. The structure that supported the mandibular arch and functioned in articulation as the primary jaw joint, is replaced by a jaw bone with an advanced articulation capable of anterior, posterior, and bilateral motion.

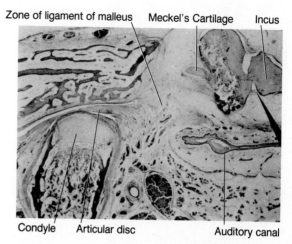

Fig. 3.**37** Lateral view of the condyle and fossa on the left. Upper right: the malleus and incus are seen undergoing transformation into bone. The arrow indicates the articulation point of the malleoincudal joint.

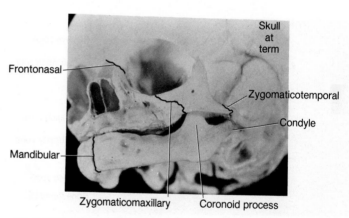

Fig. 3.**38** The skull at birth. Observe location of the facial sutures.

Clinical Application

Two growth centers are found in each of the condyles and account for their rapid growth and increase in size. First, new cartilage cells differentiate in the cartilage underlying the perichondrium, which lies on the surface of the condylar head. These cells proliferate and deposit a new cartilage matrix at this site. A second center lies deeper in the condyle where new bone replaces the mature cartilage by endochondral bone deposition. This bone-forming center also adds to the volume of the condyles.

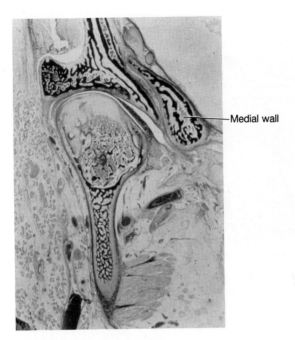

Fig. 3.**39** Frontal view of the TMJ joint at 22 prenatal weeks.

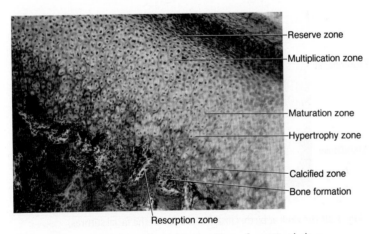

Fig. 3.**40** Condylar head. Cartilage above and bone formation below.

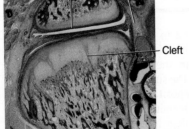

Fig.3.**41** Frontal view of the TMJ at 26 prenatal weeks. Observe the clefts of connective tissue in the condylar cartilage.

Development of the Secondary Mandibular Joint

Once the component parts of the TMJ have been established by the 12th prenatal week, no major changes occur other than further differentation of the joint tissues and a general increase in size of the glenoid fossa and condylar head. Note the appositional growth of cartilage on the surface of the condyle in Figure 3.**37**. Cartilage is deposited interstitially around the cells in the matrix (Fig. 3.**39**). This condition develops since there is enlargement of the cartilage cells and then deposition of cartilage matrix around these cells (Fig.3.**40**). Below the cartilage mass of the condyle, bone can be observed which replaces the cartilage beneath the cartilage cap. New cartilage cells can be seen arising from the reserve zone (top of figure) and passing into the multiplication zone (middle of figure), where cell division occurs. Below that is the Maturation zone where cells mature and enlarge. The cartilage cells enlarge further into the Hypertrophy zone. Below this zone, the matrix surrounding the cells begins to calcify. In the bottom of Figure 3.**40**, bone cells invade the cells of the calcified zone and deposit bone on the cartilage. Bone also increases in the neck, as well as the head, of the condyle. Again, there is an increase of bone in the superior medial wall of the glenoid fossa by 22 prenatal weeks (Fig. 3.**39**). The primary joint begins to function in the 16th week as a TMJ.

The major change in structure of the TMJ is an increase in the size and density of the condyle. This bone changes in shape and size as the mandible becomes associated with differentiation and function of masticatory muscles. One noteworthy feature of the TMJ cartilage occurs in late prenatal life, as connective-tissue clefts extend into the cartilage front from the overlying fibrous perichondrium (Figs. 3.**41** and 3. **42**). The function of these clefts is to bring blood vessels into close contact with the rapidly growing area of cartilage. Cartilage is considered avascular, but the mandibular condyle is an exception to this rule. Another change in the condyle is the thinning of the cartilage cap, which occurs in the late prenatal period. During the eighth and ninth prenatal months, the endochondral bone replacement of the cartilage is more rapid than the cartilage deposition on the condylar surface. At this time, all clefts have disappeared, indicating that the cartilage is no longer in a rapid growth phase. The narrow band of cartilage seen on the condylar head persists until the 25th postnatal year.

Maturation of the Mandibular Body

Although the body of the mandible develops from membrane, fusion of Meckel's cartilage to the anterior medial aspect of the mandible is by endochondral bone formation. There are several other cartilage growth centers known as secondary growth cartilages of the mandible. These are: the coronoid cartilages, cartilage around the tooth germs, and the symphyseal cartilage in the anterior midline (Fig. 3.**43**). The cartilage in the coronoid area appears in the 14th to 16th week, and signals formation of the coronoid process. This cartilage disappears by the 16th week, when function begins. Bone replacement of this cartilage then occurs as the temporalis muscle differentiates and originates at this site. During this time bone formation is rapid, creating a bone comparable to the condyle at birth.

Tiny sites of cartilage surround most of the forming tooth buds, especially on the buccal. These are soon transformed into thin plates of bone protecting the tooth germs. Only the symphyseal cartilage between the growing halves of the mandible persists until birth or later. These two cartilages wrap over the anterior bodies of the right and left mandibles. They are covered by perichondrium and are united at the midline. The symphyseal cartilages undergo endochondral bone formation throughout prenatal life, and contribute to anterior growth of the mandible. Since these cartilages are positioned between the anterior ends of the mandible, this cartilage provides an increase in a width as well. Growth cessation of these cartilages occurs in the early postnatal months, although the suture contributes to an increase in mandibular width during early postnatal life.

Abnormal Development

Unilateral and bilateral clefts of the palate produce defects in the nasomaxillary skeleton and bones of the palate. Figure 3.**44** shows a cleared human palate at 11 prenatal weeks. In this figure, a near vertical white line is seen extending through the alveolar ridge and palate. Note the absence of premaxillary bone formation on the left side. Compare the size of the right and left maxillary bones. Bone formation on the left side is deficient. In the case of a unilateral cleft palate, the bone forms on the normal side and there is bone deficiency where the cleft occurs (Fig. 3.**44**). A lack of palatine bone, as well as the absence of the bony alveolar ridge, and tooth buds in the region of the cuspid and lateral incisor can be observed

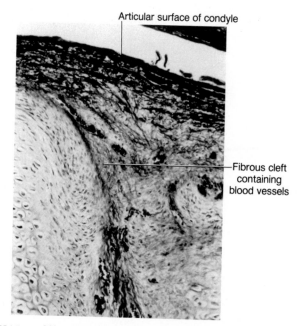

Fig. 3.**42** View of fibrous cleft with blood vessels in the condylar cartilage.

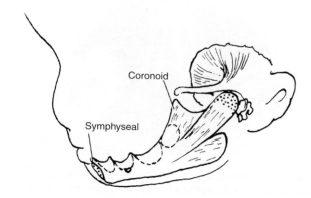

Fig. 3.**43** Diagram of the mandible and TMJ at 20 prenatal weeks. Observe the areas of secondary cartilages around the tooth germs, coronoid process, and symphysis.

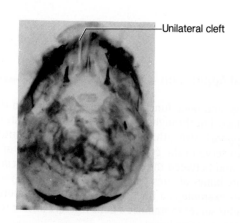

Fig. 3.**44** Unilateral cleft palate in a human fetus at 11 prenatal weeks.

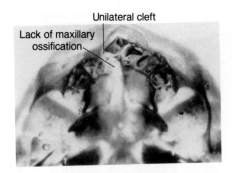

Fig. 3.**45** Unilateral cleft palate in a human fetus at 20 prenatal weeks.

in this specimen. Alveolar ridge deficiency occurs where the premaxilla and maxilla join developmentally (Fig. 3.**45**).

A bilateral cleft illustrates a bony deficiency on both the left and right sides (Fig. 3.**46**). In this palate there is an absence of bone at the junction of the premaxilla and maxilla, as both of these bones are much smaller than they would be normally. The lateral incisors, cuspids, and primary molar teeth are missing, along with their bony crypts. Prior to bone formation, a soft-tissue deficiency would have occured in the 5th or 6th prenatal week. In Figure 3.**45** it can be noted that the lateral incisors and cuspids are missing, since they are adjacent to the cleft.

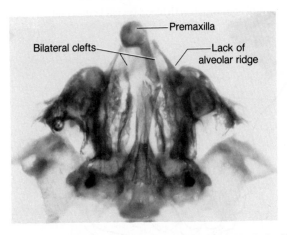

Fig. 3.**46** Bilateral cleft palate in human at term. Observe the lack of bone formation anteriorly isolating the premaxilla that bears two tooth buds.

Summary

The initial skeleton of the face is cartilaginous and composed of the nasal capsule in the upper face and Meckel's cartilage in the mandibular arch (Fig. 3.**47**). Later the nasal, premaxillary, maxillary, zygomatic, and temporal bones appear in the upper face; bone of the mandible appears in the lower face (Fig. 3.**48**).

The connective-tissue sutures between the bones of the face are termed "syndesmoses" (Figs. 3.**19** and 3.**20**). Syndesmoses may be further classified as simple, serrated, or squamous and are located between the frontal and maxillary, the maxillary and zygomatic, the zygomatic and temporal, and the palatine and pterygoid lamina of the sphenoid bones. Other sutures in the midface appear between the ethmoid, sphenoid, and occipital bones. Cartilage is present between these latter midline bones, and these sutures are termed "synchondroses" (Fig. 3.**24**).

Palatine ossification appears at the junction of the medial and lateral palatine processes. Bone trabeculae grow medially to the midline from both premaxillary and maxillary centers. Posteriorly, palatine ossification centers appear on the periphery of the palate and grow toward the midline. By the 8th month of intrauterine life, bone covers the palate. Premaxillary–maxillary and maxillary–palatine sutures, as well as a midline suture extending the entire length of the hard palate, provide for palatine growth. Further growth of the palate occurs on the periphery by appositional growth. Compare the size relationship of the face at birth with the adult face (Figs. 3.**49** and 3.**50**). It is also helpful to compare the position of sutures in the face at birth with those in the adult face (Figs. 3.**19** and 3.**20**).

Meckel's cartilage is the primary cartilage of the mandibular arch and provides support, allowing jaw movement for the first 4.5 months of intrauterine life. At the superior posterior surface, the

Clinical Application

Cartilage and bone function in concert not only in the developing face, but throughout the human skeletal system to provide support, strength, and flexibility. Cartilage sutures continue to serve in the cranial base, ears, epiphysis of the long bones, and between the vertebrae. They work in conjunction with the bones at sites where growth and motion is needed. Another example is a fracture site, where a temporary cartilage callus serves to stabilize a bone fracture until it is replaced by slower growing bone.

malleoincudal cartilages serve as articulators for the lower jaw at 8 weeks (Fig. 3.**47**). The TMJ becomes functional at 16 weeks. Then Meckel's cartilage resorbs and disappears. Its most posterior elements, the malleus and incus, transform into bone, developing into hearing bones of the middle ear along with the stapes of the second arch. The condyle of the mandible begins as a cone-shaped cartilage, at the posterior superior surface of the bony mandible. The temporal bone forms the socket for the TMJ by intramembranous bone formation, although the socket soon becomes lined with cartilage. This cartilage gradually transforms into bone. There are several differences in the growth of cartilages in the mandibular condyles and the growth of long bones. Long bones develop primary bone fronts, and then produce secondary bone fronts in their epiphysis. These bone fronts face each other with a cartilage band between them and are termed epiphyseal lines (Fig. 3.**40**). Only a primary ossification center develops in the condyle, therefore no epiphyseal line develops. Also, cartilage cells are scattered rather than formed in rows as they appear in long bones. In early months of prenatal life, perichondrium covers the condylar head and vascular tracts extend into the condylar cartilage, which is unlike cartilage at other sites.

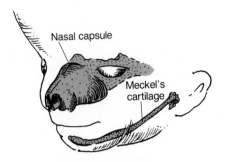

Fig. 3.**47** Cartilages of the face at 8 prenatal weeks.

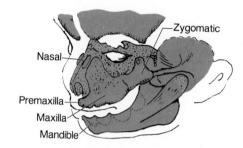

Fig.3.**48** Facial skeleton at 4.5 prenatal months.

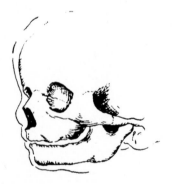

Fig.3.**49** Cranium and facial skeleton at birth.

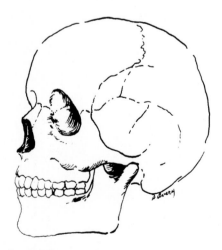

Fig. 3.**50** Adult craniofacial skeleton.

Self-Evaluation Review

1. Name the components of the primary mandibular jaw articulation.
2. Name the components of the secondary mandibular jaw articulation.
3. Compare the function of the primary and secondary TMJs.
4. Define and give examples of a syndesmosis and synchondrosis suture.
5. Describe the function of Meckel's cartilage and its final contributions.
6. Name the early developed cartilages of the cranial base and describe their functions.
7. Name and locate the bones of the facial skeleton.
8. Describe the histology of a simple, serrated, and squamous suture.
9. Name and locate the ossification centers of the palate.
10. Describe how the palate grows, and name the important sutures.

Suggested Readings

Carlson BM. Human Embryology and Developmental Biology. St Louis: Mosby Inc.; 1999;166–170.

Dixon AD and Sarnat BG, eds. Normal and Abnormal Bone Growth. New York, NY: Alan Liss Inc.; 1985.

DuBrul EL. The craniomandibular articulation. In: Sicher's Oral Anatomy. 7th Ed. St Louis: The CV Mosby Co.;1980; 74–210, 527–535.

Enlow DH. Introductory concepts of the growth process: Handbook of Facial Growth. Philadelphia Pa: WB Saunders Co.; 1982:24–66.

Griffin CJ, Hawthorne R, Harris R. Anatomy and histology of the human temporomandibular joint. Monogr. Oral Sci. 1975;4:1.

Jaxobson A. Embrylogical evidence of the nonexistence of the premaxilla in man. Journal Of the Dental Association of South Africa. 1955;10:189–210.

Mikie MC. The role of the condyle in the postnatal growth of the mandible. Am. J. Orthop. 1973;64:50–62.

Moore KL. Articular and skeletal systems: Essentials of human embryology. Toronto, Canada: BC Decker Inc.; 1988: 137–145.

Ross RB, Johnson MC. Facial development from cleft formation to birth. In: Cleft Lip and Palate. New York, NY: Robert Kreiger Pub.; 1978:68–87.

Sarnat BG; Laskinm DM. Temporomandibular Joint: Biological Basis for Clinical Practice. Springfield, Ill: Charles C Thomas; 1979.

Sadler TW. Skeletal System. In: Langman's Medical Embryology. 5th Ed. Baltimore, Md: Williams and Wilkins; 1985:133–147.

Sperber GH. Craniofacial Embryology. 4th Ed. London: Wright; 1989.

Sperber GH. Craniofacial Development and Growth. Toronto, Canada: BC Decker Inc.; 2000.

Thjorgood P, Sarker S, More R. Skeletogenesis in the Head. In: Oral Biology at the Turn of the Century. Guggenheim B and Shapiro. Basel: Karger; 1998:93.

Wood NK, Wragg LE, Stuttreville, OH. The premaxilla: Embryological evidence that it does not exist in man. Anat. Rec. 1967; 158: 485–390.

4 Postnatal Facial Growth, Birth through Postadolescence

Carla A. Evans

Introduction

The basic organization of the head is established early in the developing embryo through a series of critical steps involving differentiation of tissues, migration of cell masses, and fusion of facial processes. Throughout the remainder of the prenatal period and after birth, growth phenomena continue until the attainment of an adult appearance (Fig. **4.1**). This chapter explains important concepts of postnatal facial growth that emphasize various biologic processes and their timing in the developmental sequence, growth-control mechanisms, specific growth sites in the facial skeleton, and variations in abnormal development.

The maturation of an infant's face into its adult form results from growth, which means an increase in size, and development, which means progressive evolution toward the final state. Important changes occur in the size, shape, position, and composition of all cranial tissues, including bones, muscles, nerves, and sense organs. Bones enlarge and change shape; muscles lengthen and alter their attachments; innervation matures; skin proliferates to cover the growing face. The oral cavity and nasal spaces, eyes, and brain increase in size but at different rates. Sinuses form within the facial structures, the teeth erupt and emerge, and the dentition changes. The adult face differs markedly from the fetal or infant face in size, proportions, structure, and function.
Aging further alters appearance as minor skeletal modifications continue, skin loses elasticity and wrinkles, and fat deposits produce jowls under the lower jaw and bags around the eyes. The differences between the newborn and adult skulls are striking (Fig. **4.2**). The calvaria, or skull vault, is much more prominent in infancy than later. The membranous bones of the vault are separated by areas of fibrous tissue known as "sutures" and "fontanelles," or soft spots. At birth, the endochondral bones at the base of the skull are separated by bars of cartilage; these synchondroses are gradually replaced by bone. The anterior portion of the nasal septum, another remnant of the embryonic cartilaginous skull, retains its cartilaginous composition in the adult. Most of Meckel's cartilage is resorbed before birth, but secondary cartilages that develop independently of the primary cartilaginous skull can be observed in the newborn mandible.

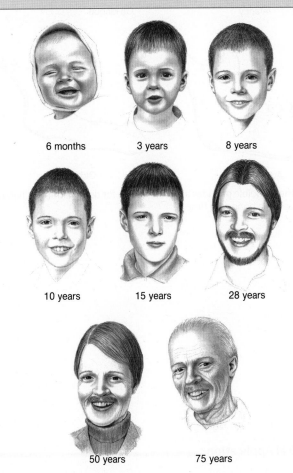

6 months   3 years   8 years

10 years   15 years   28 years

50 years   75 years

Fig. **4.1** Growth and maturation of the face from birth to old age.

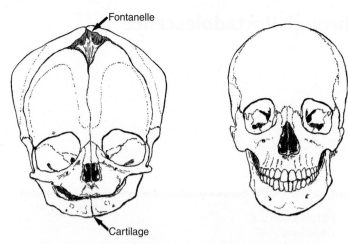

Fig. 4.**2** The adult human skull differs markedly from the infant skull in its proportions.

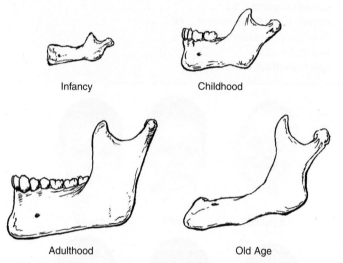

Fig. 4.**3** The mandible provides a good example for demonstrating changes in the shape of a bone with time.

These secondary cartilages are the mandibular condyle and the soon-ossified coronoid process and mandibular symphysis.

Proportionally, far more facial than calvarial growth occurs after birth. The newborn head has attained 55 to 60% of adult breadth, 40 to 50% of adult height, and 30 to 35% of adult depth. In the postnatal period, the mandible grows proportionally more than the early developing cranial base and brain. Quantification of skull growth is based on measurements of standardized skull radiographs, called "cephalograms" or "cephalometric radiographs."

Generally, all skull bones change throughout life. For example, in the newborn, the mandible has a wide gonial angle, no chin, small ramus, and very immature joint and, relative to the rest of the face, is retruded (Fig. 4.**3**). A compatible relation between maxilla and mandible is achieved, however, by rapid growth within the first year. During infancy and childhood, relations and proportions in the mandible continue to change: teeth erupt and emerge, the gonial angle decreases, the mandibular plane become less steep, and a chin develops. In adolescence, the alveolar region becomes less prominent as the upper face and chin project forward. These changes decrease the convexity of the profile, if the highly variable nose is not included. Skeletal modifications that emphasize individual features of the facial contours continue in adults. The adolescent and post-adolescent changes continue for a longer time in males. In old age, teeth may be lost, the mandible loses mass, and the gonial angle widens.

Objectives

After reading this chapter, you should be able to explain the important concepts of postnatal facial growth, emphasizing various biologic processes and their timing in the developmental sequence. You should be able to describe growth control mechanisms, specific growth sites in the facial skeleton, and variations in abnormal development.

Clinical Application

Relapse of lower anterior dental crowding after orthodontic treatment is a controversial issue in orthodontics. Both late adolescent mandibular growth and third molar eruptive pressures have been blamed.

Timing of Growth

Individual children differ not only in the amount of growth and their ultimate size, but also in the timing of different phases of their growth.

Growth of the face follows the general timetable of the skeleton, the abdominal and thoracic organs, and the musculature. Periods of rapid growth (dependent on the systemic control of hormones) occur after birth, in mid-childhood, and during adolescence. Other tissues have their own timetables: neural tissues (e.g., brain) develop early, the reproductive tissues (e.g., genital organs) develop late, and the lymphoid tissues are variable (e.g., the thymus hypertrophies in childhood and subsequently shrinks). The face is considered to be intermediate in timing, as it follows the somatic growth of the child.

Within a person, considerable variation between growth rates of different body parts occurs. For example, during the adolescent growth spurt in height, the sequence of growth acceleration is foot, calf, thigh, trunk, and finally, weight. The head also demonstrates considerable variation in the growth of its parts. The upper nasal cavities nears adult size by 1 year of age, the anterior cranial base is essentially complete in size by 7 years of age, the maxilla finishes growing between 14 and 16 years of age, and the mandible finishes growth at an older age. The maximum growth rate of the face in adolescence is believed to take place a little later than does maximal change in body height.

The adolescent growth maxima for the maxilla and mandible occur simultaneously, but growth slows and stops at different times (Fig. 4.**4**). The mandible continues to increase in length for approximately 2 years after the facial sutures become inactive. The extended period of mandibular growth makes it difficult to predict the final size for surgical correction of mandibular overgrowth and may be responsible for the crowding of lower incisors that is often observed in late adolescence.

The specific growth pattern of the head is influenced by many variables such as gender, ethnic or racial characteristics, physique, illness, and nutritional level. Boys grow "later, longer, and larger" than girls. Consequently, girls mature earlier and pass through the adolescent growth spurt more rapidly than boys (Fig. 4.**5**). Although African American babies generally weigh less than caucasian babies at birth and during childhood, they achieve their developmental milestones earlier. Asian children tend to be smaller than both African American and Caucasian children. Physique or body build also influences the timing of growth and development. For example, the extremely tall, thin person usually has later, more prolonged periods of growth during adolescence than the shorter, highly muscular individual. The nonmuscular, obese adolescent usually lacks an intense spurt and, instead, gradually increases in size over a long time. Illness or poor nutrition may delay or prevent proper growth. Another factor influencing timing of growth is the so-called "secular trend." Some surveys suggest that in the developed areas of the world, children are maturing at increasingly early ages.

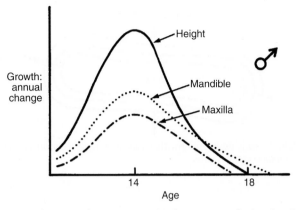

Fig. 4.**4** Growth curves show average growth increments for height of the maxilla and the mandible in young men. The peak growth rate for the face is believed to occur shortly after the maximum increment in height. Growth ceases at different times, however.

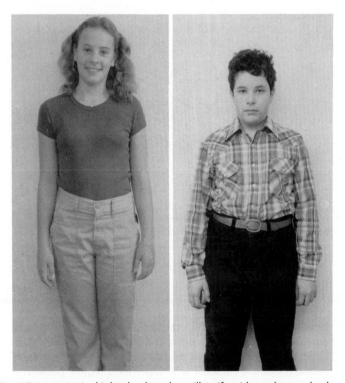

Fig. 4.**5** As any junior high school teacher will verify, girls tend to reach adolescence earlier than boys. A 13-year-old girl may be taller and developmentally more mature than a 13-year-old boy.

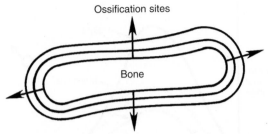

Fig. 4.6 In the early period of growth, ossification may occur on all surfaces of a developing cranial bone.

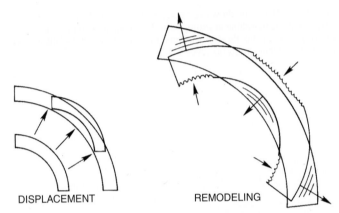

Fig. 4.7 Later cranial bone growth occurs as a combination of remodeling and sutural growth.

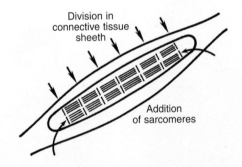

Fig. 4.8 Muscle fibers grow by addition of sarcomeres at the end of the myofibrils. The cells in the connective-tissue sheath, however, divide throughout the length of the muscle.

Clinical Application

Gender differences for skeletal age may be greater than for dental age. Because girls attain skeletal maturity earlier than boys, some girls may have mature facial bones but still have primary teeth. A clinician who waits for a female patient to have a full permanent dentition may miss the opportunity to correct a skeletal disharmony with dentofacial orthopedic appliances.

However, recent data indicates a leveling-off tendency as good nutrition and preventative health measures become widespread.

The marked variations in growth timing have led to the concept of biologic age, which is determined from the level of maturity rather than chronologic or calendar age. Typically, biologic age is based on developmental milestones in development of the long bones of the skeleton (skeletal age) or in the formation or emergence of the teeth (dental age). Assessments of skeletal maturity are commonly made from hand-wrist radiographs, and dental maturity is best determined from radiographs of the jaws. Readiness for treatment is based on biologic maturity rather than chronologic age.

Growth Processes

Bones of the head grow on surfaces, at synchondroses, and at sutures, but do not grow by internal expansion. Some basic biologic processes involved in skeletal growth and development are most clearly illustrated by examining the growth of the bones of the cranial vault. In the early period of growth, bone is deposited incrementally on all surfaces of the enlarging bones (Fig. 4.6). This type of growth continues only for a short time. Later growth of a calvarial bone is a complex response to the outward displacement of the bones by the expanding brain (Fig. 4.7). Their enlargement and flattened contour result from both remodeling of the bone as it is displaced and sutural growth at the edges. Remodeling modifies bone structure by the process of bone deposition and resorption on the bone surface.

Bones also change their position in the growing face by displacement and drift. Displacement involves a change in position of an entire bone as the result of growth at its border or the movement of an adjacent bone. Drift results from apposition on one side and resorption on another. Changes in proportion as well as size are achieved through differential growth, or variations in relative rates and amounts of growth. For example, the mandible grows proportionately more after birth than do other skull bones, and some bone edges on either side of a suture may grow at different rates.

With growth, the changes in the facial soft tissue are not as clearly delineated as are the bony changes. It is known that muscles increase in bulk by an increase in the size of individul muscle cells, not by an increase in the number of cells. Sarcomeres are added to the myofibril at its end (Fig. 4.8). The sheath covering the muscle, however, grows as a result of cell division throughout the length of the muscle. The fact that the muscular pattern of the face is determined very early probably has important consequences in facial development.

Specific Areas of Growth

In the mandible, three areas of activity account for the growth changes observed: 1) remodelling of the ramus and coronoid process (Fig. 4.**9**); 2) growth at the condyle (Fig. 4.**10**); and 3) alveolar growth and slight growth at the inferior border. Remodeling of the ramus in a growing child provides space for the second and third molars (Fig. 4.**11**). The condyle grows by proliferation of cartilage in the condylar head and endochondral bone formation. The formed bone is remodelled as it becomes part of the ramus, and the cartilage proliferation continues (Fig. 4.**10**). Relatively stable areas are located at the inner border of the symphysis, along the mandibular canal, on the chin, and on the contour of tooth germs before root formation. Chin growth is deceptive because the chin "grows" as a result of resorption of bone above the chin rather than deposition of bone at the chin itself (Fig. 4.**12**). The maxilla changes position in the growing face as a result of both drifting by remodeling, and displace-

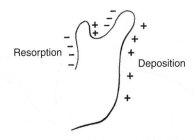

Fig. 4.**9** Remodeling of the mandibular ramus and coronoid process.

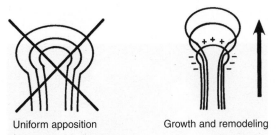

Fig. 4.**10** The condyle does not grow by the process of uniform apposition but by a complex process of growth and remodeling. +, deposition of bone. -, resorption of bone.

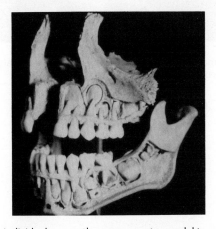

Fig. 4.**11** As an individual grows, the ramus must remodel to provide adequate room for eruption of the second and third molars.

Clinical Application

That dental arches display only minor changes in transverse and anteroposterior dimensions during childhood is remarkable, especially considering that the teeth erupt several millimeters to maintain dental occlusion as the face grows in height. This allows the clinician to make reasonable predictions about the need for treatment even in young children.

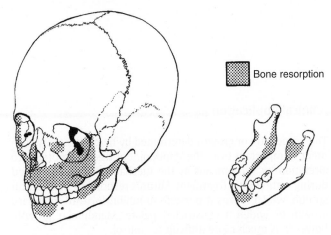

Fig. 4.**12** Areas of bone resorption in the growing human face.

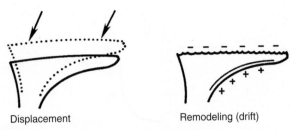

Fig. 4.**13** In the growing face, the maxilla relative to the cranial base changes as a result of both displacement and remodeling (drift).

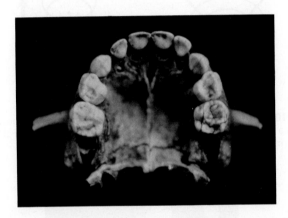

Fig. 4.**14** The maxillary tuberosity increases in length to create space for the developing second and third molars.

ment due to growth at the maxillary sutures (Fig. 4.**13**). The tuberosity increases in length to create space for the molar teeth (Fig. 4.**14**). The increased height of the palate with maturation is due to the eruption of teeth carrying the alveolar process along. The area of least change is around the nasopalatine foramen. As the maxilla moves forward and downward, the anterior surface is resorbed (Fig. 4.**12**).

Dental arch relations are usually maintained during the increase in facial height. As the face enlarges, teeth compensate by erupting further. Eruption of teeth continues throughout life to maintain occlusion. An ankylosed primary molar serves as a good marker of eruptive changes because it is fused to the alveolar bone and does not keep pace with the active movements of other teeth. Both cartilaginous and sutural growth contribute to the growth of the nasal region and upper face. The nasal septum is a cartilaginous remnant of the chondrocranium that ossifies posteriorly as the vomer bone. The anterior part remains as cartilage and continues growing later than most of the rest of the face. The gains in nose length and width are unrelated to other facial measurements. The forward growth of the forehead is due to the development of brow ridges and frontal sinuses. These sinuses are present at birth but are not aerated. Although the sutures of the upper face are nearly parallel in arrangement, the upper face does not grow in a particular downward and forward direction away from the cranial base. Individual sutures may grow in a vertical, horizontal, or anterior–posterior direction, or permit sliding of bones along the suture line. Moreover, the overall vector of sutural growth is not consistent over time. Changes in direction are fairly common.

Growth Control

Even more important than descriptions of specific growth changes in individual bones and relations of bones is information related to the questions of how and why growth occurs. It is necessary to define the factors controlling growth and to understand growth mechanisms to promote normal facial development and alter deviant growth patterns.

Heredity and Environment

Heredity and environment jointly determine the facial growth pattern. The close resemblance of identical twins shows that the heredity component is important. However, environmental influences are also active. For example, Inuits developed a much higher prevalence of malocclusion within a generation of the arrival of modern civilization. Also, human traditions and animal experiments have shown that growth of bone can be altered. Bound Chinese feet and deformed Indian skulls demonstrate the adaptability of skeletal growth to environmental influences.

Clinical Application

The proportion of growth determined by heredity or environment is important from the standpoint of tissue receptivity to alteration by such means as the mechanical appliance used during orthodontic treatment. Sutures respond to mechanical stimuli, which makes it possible to inhibit forward maxillary growth or widen a constricted palate. Mandibular growth, however, is much more difficult to control.

Abnormal Development

The biologic concepts developed in this chapter can be applied to individuals who have abnormal growth patterns. Knowledge of normal growth processes can be helpful in recognizing aberrant growth and in planning treatment. The gaps in our understanding of deviant growth processes and causes of facial deformity, however, are major and limit preventative and corrective efforts.

Some perplexing growth problems are seen in the genetic syndromes. For example, a patient with Apert syndrome has a peculiarly shaped cranial vault; a retruded midface with the maxilla sometimes fused to the sphenoid bone; abnormalities of the cranial base and upper spine; intraoral abnormalities including bulbous alveolar processes in the maxilla and crowding of teeth; and fusion of the digits of the hands and feet (Fig. 4.**15**). Premature fusion of the cranial sutures produces an unusual skull form by preventing skull growth at the fused suture lines. Because the increased pressure produced by the growing brain may lead to severe mental and neurologic handicaps, early release of the fused sutures is a critical step in optimizing brain development. Treatment methods now in use are not effective, however, because osseous bridges between cranial bones soon recur. It is not known whether the sutures are themselves defective or whether the cells function through normal mechanisms but respond to an abnormal environment. Growth abnormalities are not limited to congenital malformations or inherited metabolic defects. Injury to the temporomandibular joint in a child can cause ankylosis or joint damage that leads to asymmetry and underdevelopment of the mandible on the traumatized side (Fig. 4.**16**). Mobility of the joint should be restored as soon as possible to maximize normal function and growth.

Mandible prognathism is one of the most common facial deformities (Fig. 4.**17A**). Unlike many congenital deformities, malocclusions become apparent during postnatal development. Many explanations regarding the etiology of mandibular prognathism have been advanced, but no single explanation has proved to be adequate. Although some families seem to have more

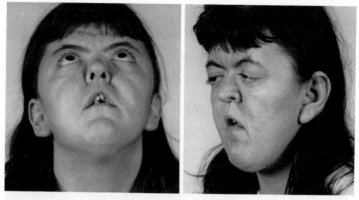

Fig. 4.**15** An example of Apert syndrome.

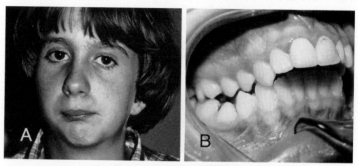

Fig. 4.**16** Injury to this child's temporomandibular joint has impaired growth, which has resulted in both facial **(A)** and dental **(B)** asymmetries.

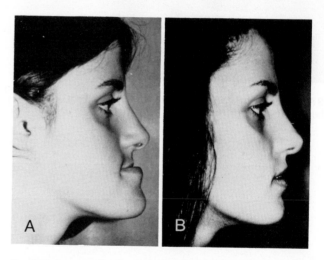

Fig. 4.**17** An example of mandibular prognathism before **(A)** and after **(B)** surgical correction.

Clinical Application

Only about half of young people in the United States have normal jaw and dental relations. The proportion of very severe malocclusions is the same in African Americans and Caucasians, approximately 15%. The types of disharmonies, however, differ with race; African Americans are more likely than caucasions to have anterior open bite malocclusions, and caucasions are more likely than African Americans to have severe crowding of teeth.

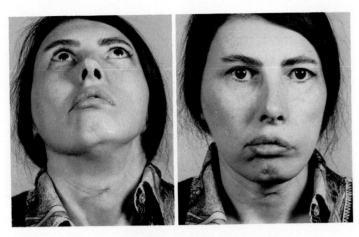

Fig. 4.**18** Facial asymmetry following partial facial nerve palsy.

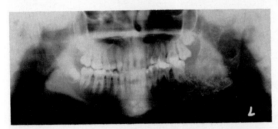

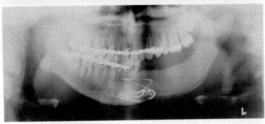

Fig. 4.**19** A mandible before (upper) and after (lower) placement of a successful bone graft.

individuals affected than do other families, the pattern of genetic transmission has been unclear, and in many cases it is found to occur sporadically. The mechanisms of mandibular growth have been explored in animal experiments, but these studies have not progressed to the point of providing a basis for altering human growth. Consequently, the most effective treatment has been surgical reduction of mandibular length (Fig. 4.**17B**). Growth is a factor that must be considered in planning treatment of facial deformities. For example, early surgical treatment of mandibular prognathism is often unsuccessful because the mandible continues to grow abnormally. In areas in which growth mechanisms are better understood, however, growth can be used advantageously. One argument in favor of early treatment holds that a primary defect causes secondary deformities in adjacent tissues. For example, lack of appropriate muscle function followed a partial facial nerve palsy and resulted in asymmetries in facial form, including underdevelopment of the mandible on the paralyzed side and deviation of the nasal tip (Fig. 4.**18**).

In more severe deformities, tissues that are initially normal can be distorted even more than those shown in Figure 4.**18**. If proper relations are achieved at an early age, growth is more likely to proceed along a normal vector. In the development of normal dental relations, normal function of the lips, lip seal, and nasal breathing are thought to be important. Function is also important during remodeling of bone grafts into normal bone structure after surgical reconstruction. A successful mandibular bone graft can be difficult to detect on a radiograph, except to the stabilizing wires that remain (Fig. 4.**19**). A piece of iliac crest bone from the patient's hip was used to replace the diseased half of the mandible that included the condyle. After remodeling had occurred, not only did the graft assume an appropriate shape, but the bone trabiculations had the appearance of mandibular rather than iliac crest bone.

Some attempts to modify abnormal facial structures in children may actually inhibit growth. Surgical repair of clefts of the lip and palate have resulted in extensive scarring that retards forward development of the maxilla, especially when older techniques have been used (Fig. 4.**20A**). With use of these techniques, a different type of midface deformity is produced that necessitates other operations to advance the midface. If oral clefts are not treated, as has occurred in remote villages in India, even the severe bilateral clefts seen in adults are not accompanied by marked anterior–posterior discrepancies (Fig. 4.**20B** and **C**). Despite the devastating functional and cosmetic effects of the untreated oral cleft in the individual seen in Figure 4.**20B** and **C**, jaw relations are quite good.

Although many questions regarding growth mechanisms remain, some basic points that recognize the importance of growth can be stated. A program aimed at achieving or maintaining normal facial structure and function should: 1) remove inhibitions of normal growth; 2) promote normal function; 3) reduce iatrogenic damage to tissues, such as surgical scars; and 4) consider the effect of growth on the final result when intervention during the growth period is necessary.

Summary

The principles of facial growth and development discussed in this chapter include specific biologic processes, sites of growth, timing, hereditary factors, receptivity of environmental cues, and variations found in abnormal development. Changes in the dental arches and alveolar processes are coordinated with facial growth. Postnatal growth of the face is complex and varies considerably among children.

Growth processes and their timing must be assessed carefully for individual patients to achieve optimal results from clinical treatment. Knowledge of growth concepts is important because, in some instances, growth improves the treatment outcome, whereas in other situations, growth interferes with attainment of a successful result.

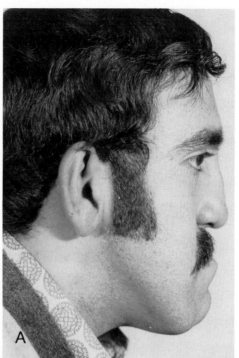

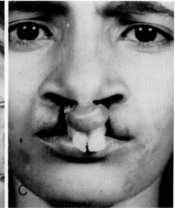

Fig. 4.**20 A** Example of midface underdevelopment resulting from restriction of maxillary growth by excessive scarring after early surgical repair of cleft lip and palate. **B, C** Untreated bilateral cleft of lip and palate in an adult. Growth of the jaws has not been retarded, and jaw relations are quite good.

Self-Evaluation Review

1. When does the face grow with respect to other parts of the body? During the postnatal period, which areas of the face grow proportionately more than other areas?
2. What factors may influence an individual's specific growth pattern?
3. Distinguish between biologic age and chronologic age. Why is maturity so important in determining timing of treatment?
4. How do growing bones change position in relation to other bones?
5. Name areas of the maxilla and mandible that change relatively little during growth.
6. Describe remodeling changes in the growing mandible that create space for the permanent molars.
7. List the cartilaginous structures of the face and identify whether they are primary or secondary in origin.
8. How does scarring affect maxillary growth in patients with cleft lip or palate?
9. Why is growth significant in the treatment of facial deformities?
10. How is the shape of bones influenced by function?

Acknowledgements

Figures 4.**15**, 4.**18**, and 4.**20** were provided courtesy of Dr. Joseph Murra. Figures 4.**16** and 4.**17** were provided courtesy of Dr. Walter Guralnick.

Suggested Readings

Bjork A. The Face in profile. Lund: Berlingska Boktryckeriet; 1947.

Enlow DH. Facial Growth. Philadelphia, PA: WB Saunders Co; 1990.

Horowitz SL, Hixon EH. The Nature of Orthodontic Diagnosis. St. Louis, MO: CV Mosby; 1966.

Lundstrom A. Dental genetics. In: Dahlberg AA, Graber TM, eds. Orofacial Growth and Development. The Hague: Mouton Publishers; 1977.

Marshall WA, Tanner JM. Puberty. In: Davis JA, Dobbing J, eds. Scientific Foundations of Paediatrics. Philadelphia, PA: WB Sauders; 1974.

Moore WJ, Lavelle CLB. Growth of the Facial Skeleton in the Hominoidea. London: Academic Press; 1974.

Moorees CFA, Gron AM, Lebret LML, Yen PKJ, Frolich FJ. Growth studies on the dentition: a review. Am J Orthod. 1969;44:600.

Tanner JM. Growth at Adolescence. Oxford: Blackwell Scientific Publications; 1962.

SECTION II
Development of the Teeth and Supporting Structures

5 Development Of Teeth: Crown Formation

Nicholas P. Piesco and James K. Avery

Introduction

Overview of Dental Tissues

As an aid in establishing developmental relationships during tooth development (odontogenesis), it is important to briefly review the structure of a fully developed tooth (Fig. 5.**1**). Detailed descriptions of tooth anatomy are found in texts on dental anatomy and will not be considered here. Under gross inspection the tooth consists of two parts, the crown and root(s). The crown provides the chewing or biting (occlusal or incisal) surface of the tooth while the root provides the necessary supporting functions. The anatomic crown is the part of the tooth covered with enamel, and the clinical crown is the part of the tooth exposed to the oral cavity. In young individuals the clinical crown may be smaller than the anatomic crown (especially true during eruption). In older individuals with gingival recession, part of the anatomic root may be exposed to the oral cavity. Then the clinical crown will be larger than the anatomic crown, since it would include some anatomic root structure. For simplicity, the term "crown" as used hereafter will refer to the anatomic crown. Unlike the crown that needs a durable covering, the roots of teeth are covered with cementum that functions instead as an attachment surface. The junction between cementum and enamel, the cementoenamel junction, lies at the cervix (or neck) of the tooth and is an important developmental landmark worth noting.

By examining a ground histologic section of an erupted tooth, one can see that the enamel covering the crown consists of tightly packed enamel rods or prisms. One can also observe that the bulk of the mineralized tissue that underlies the enamel consists of dentin. Dentin is tubular in nature. Unlike enamel, dentin is permeable and contains tissue fluid and cell processes. Enamel and dentin contain microscopically visible landmarks that indicate the incremental nature of matrix deposition (appositional growth). These are the incremental lines, Retzius' striae in enamel and incremental lines of von Ebner in dentin (described in detail in Chapters 9 and 10). The junction between the enamel and dentin (dentinoenamel junction [DEJ]) is another important developmental landmark.

Cementum covering the root encases the ends of collagen fibers (Sharpey's fibers) and therefore provides firm anchorage points (dental attachment) for fibers of the periodontal ligament. Additionally, the roots of the teeth remain in sockets or alveoli. The alveolar surfaces provide bony attachment sites for periodontal ligament fibers (also Sharpey's fibers). That part of the mandible and maxilla containing the tooth sockets is called the alveolar process and consists of alveolar bone. Between the root and alveolar bone is the periodontal space. It contains blood vessels, nerves, fibers, cells, and ground substance. Details of its structure and development will be considered in Chapters 6 and 7.

The dentin of the tooth encloses a mass of soft tissue, the dental pulp. In the crown the dental pulp resides in the pulp chamber, and in the root it exists as extensions of the pulp chamber termed root (radicular) canals. Odontoblasts are the outermost cells of the pulp and are responsible for forming the protein matrix of dentin (mostly type I collagen) and its eventual mineralization. Between the odontoblasts and the calcified dentin is a layer of predentin matrix that has not yet been mineralized. The junction between the dentin and predentin is the dentin mineralization front or dentin–predentin junction. At the apex of the root there is an opening, the apical foramen, which allows the passage of blood vessels, lymphatics, and nerves through the root canal to and from the pulp chamber.

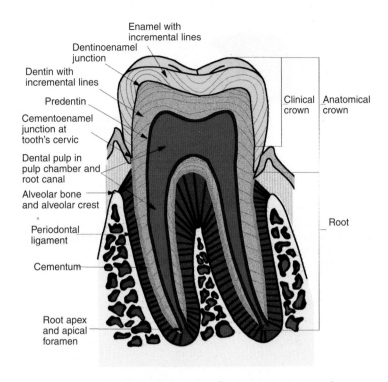

Fig. 5.**1** Diagram of a longitudinal section of an incisor in situ. Note the anatomic boundaries between the mineralized tissues. DEJ: dentinoenamel junction. CEJ: cementoenamel junction.

Introduction to Tooth Development

Teeth and other organs develop as a result of a complex series of interactions between epithelium and underlying mesenchymal tissue. In the tooth 20 primary tooth germs develop initially, with 32 additional tooth germs differentiating to form the permanent dentition. Although each tooth germ develops as an anatomically distinct unit, the fundamental developmental process is similar for all teeth. Each tooth develops through successive bud, cap, and bell stages (Figs. 5.**2A–C**). During the early stages, the tooth germs grow and expand, and the cells that will form the mineralized components of the teeth differentiate. Once the formative cells of the tooth germ differentiate, formation and mineralization of the dentin and enamel matrices take place (Figs. 5.**2D–F**). Subsequently, the completed tooth erupts into the oral cavity (Fig. 5.**2G**). As eruption occurs, the tooth roots surrounded by periodontal ligament and supporting alveolar bone develop (Figs. 5.**2G** and **H**). Root formation proceeds until a functional tooth and its supporting apparatus are fully developed (Fig. 5.**2H**).

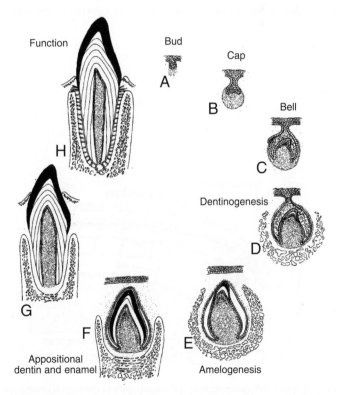

Fig. 5.**2 A–H** Diagram depicting the stages of tooth development beginning with the bud stage **(A)**.

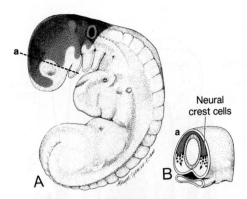

Fig. 5.**3 A** Map of neural crest cell migration in a 4-week-old embryo. **B** Frontal section representing the plane of section "a" in **A** and illustrating neural crest migration.

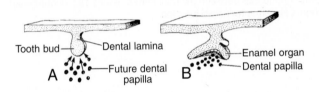

Fig. 5.**4 A** Induction of tooth primordia. **B** Further induction of the enamel organ.

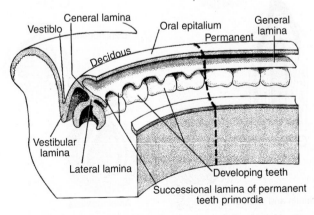

Fig. 5.**5** Stylized diagram depicting the continuity of the dental lamina system for deciduous and permanent teeth. Note that the permanent molars arise from the general and not the successional lamina.

Objectives

The overall objectives of this chapter are to enable the student to: 1) Describe, in detail, the origin of the formative cells of the tooth. 2) Describe the role of induction in tooth formation. 3) Describe the stages of tooth formation. 4) Describe the process of mineralization and how it differs in enamel and dentin. 5) Describe the formation of the tissues that surround each tooth.

Origin of Dental Tissues

Neural crest cells constitute much of the mesenchyme of the head and neck. Since these cells are originally derived from the ectodermal germ layer that forms the nervous system, they are also termed ectomesenchyme or neuroectoderm. These cells form all of the connective tissues of the face, including the dental structures (Figs. 5.**3A** and **B**). The role of the neural crest in the development of teeth and their supporting structure is not completely understood. These cells arise from the neural folds. As these folds close, neural crest cells migrate down the sides of the head along pathways underlying the ectoderm (Figs. 5.**3A** and **B**). It is interesting to note that in the cephalic region of the embryo the cells of the neural crest begin their migration before the closure of the neural tube, while in the trunk these cells leave at a slightly later developmental stage. Because of their extensive migrations and propensity to differentiate along many different developmental pathways, some investigators consider neural crest cells to be a fourth germ layer. Others consider these to be a merging of two cell types, ectodermal and mesodermal, which in turn form cells that resemble both types.

During the sixth week in utero the ectoderm covering the oral cavity is composed of an epithelial layer, two to three cells thick. In the region of the future alveolar processes, the oral epithelium proliferates and forms the dental laminae (Fig. 5.**4**). These are horseshoe-shaped bands that traverse the perimeters of the lower and upper jaws and give rise to the ectodermally-derived portions of the teeth (Fig. 5.**5**). The dental laminae undergo further proliferation at sites corresponding to the positions of the 20 primary teeth. This results in the formation of rounded or ovoid structures (placodes) that protrude into the mesenchyme (primitive embryonic connective tissue). These placodes later develop into tooth buds or tooth germs (Fig. 5.**4**). The maxillary and mandibular dental laminae eventually give rise to 52 such buds, 20 for the primary teeth, which arise between the sixth and eighth prenatal week, and 32 for the permanent teeth, which appear at later prenatal periods (Figs. 5.**5** and 5.**6**). Successional tooth buds of the permanent dentition develop lingually to the tooth buds of their deciduous predecessors (Fig. 5.**4** and 5.**5**). This occurs in utero at 5 months of age for the central incisors and 10 months of age for the premolars. The lingual extension of the dental lamina that gives rise to the successional teeth is therefore called the successional lamina (Fig. 5.**5**).

Permanent molars develop posteriorly to the deciduous molars. Posterior growth of the dental lamina gives rise to the first permanent molar buds during the fourth prenatal month and the second permanent molars at 4 years of age. A second lamina, the vestibular lamina, develops simultaneously and in association with the dental lamina. The vestibular lamina first forms a wedge of epithelial cells facial or buccal to the dental lamina (Fig. 5.**5**). It will form the oral vestibule or the space between the teeth and cheeks or lips (Fig. 5.**6**). Teeth develop anteroposteriorly, which means that the anterior teeth develop slightly ahead, temporally speaking, of the posterior ones. Again, each tooth is of a different type (Fig. 5.**5**). It is interesting that most all organ systems such as the digestive system, cardiovascular system, urinary systems, etc. are functionally completed within 9 months (at birth), but the development of teeth continues long after birth. This prolonged development period means that the developmental processes (cell differentiation, matrix production, mineralization, etc.) are susceptible to many different environmental stimuli (diseases, diet, drugs, etc., Chapter 8).

Bud, Cap, and Bell Stages

Tooth formation is a continuous process that may be characterized by a series of distinguishable stages. The stages are classified according to the shape of the epithelial component of the tooth and are named accordingly. Four different stages are recognized, for example the lamina, bud, cap, or bell stage (Figs. 5.**2** and 5.**7**–5.**9**).

The dental lamina stage is characterized by a thickening of the oral epithelium. At this stage there are no distinguishable tooth sites. The bud stage is the initial stage of definitive tooth development. The bud stage designates a rounded, localized growth of the epithelial cells of the dental lamina (Figs. 5.**7A** and **B**). It is also defined as the initiation or proliferative stage because it is the stage in which the initial proliferation of oral epithelial cells and adjacent mesenchymal cells occurs. Proliferation of oral epithelial cells results in the formation of a bud-shaped epithelial (enamel) organ. Proliferating mesenchymal cells surround the bud and form an ectomesenchymal condensation. Gradually, the epithelial bud gains a concave surface, and the enamel organ is then considered to be in the cap stage (Figs. 5.**8A** and **B**). Dental mesenchyme that is partially surrounded by the cap-shaped enamel organ is called the dental

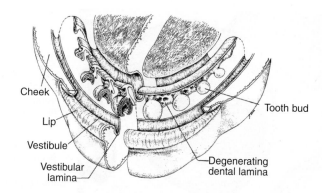

Fig. 5.**6** Development of tooth buds in developing alveolar processes.

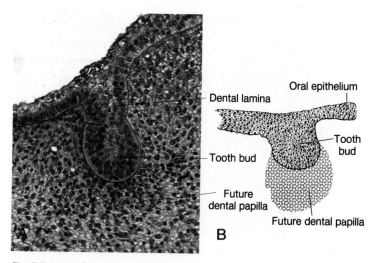

Fig. 5.**7 A** Histology of tooth development at the bud stage. **B** Diagram of tooth development at the bud stage.

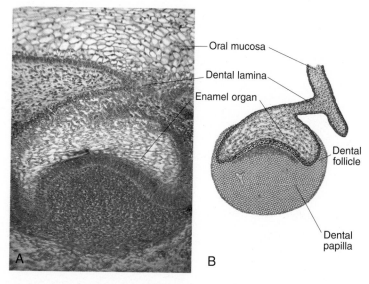

Fig. 5.**8 A** Histology of tooth development at the cap stage. **B** Diagram of tooth development at the cap stage.

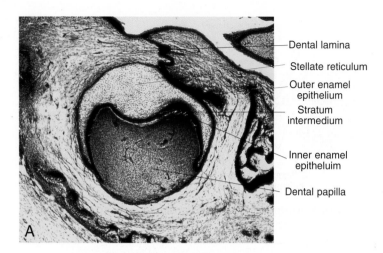

Dental lamina

Stellate reticulum

Outer enamel epithelium

Stratum intermedium

Inner enamel epitheluim

Dental papilla

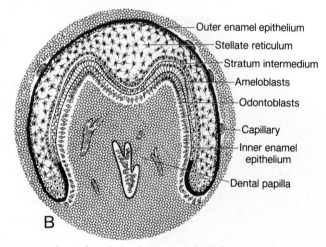

Outer enamel epithelium

Stellate reticulum

Stratum intermedium

Ameloblasts

Odontoblasts

Capillary

Inner enamel epithelium

Dental papilla

Fig. 5.**9 A** Histology of tooth development at the bell stage. **B** Diagram of tooth development at the bell stage.

papilla or embryonic dental pulp. Cells adjacent to the dental papilla and those that lie outside the enamel organ divide and grow around the enamel organ to form the dental follicle or sac.

All three structures, the enamel organ, dental papilla, and dental follicle, are seen in the cap stage. These three structures constitute the tooth germ and give rise to the tooth and its supporting structures (Figs. 5.**8A** and **B**). The epithelial component, the enamel organ, forms enamel. The dental papilla forms the dentin and pulp. The dental follicle forms the cementum, periodontal ligament, and adjacent alveolar bone. Note that the collagenous matrices (dentin, cementum, periodontal ligament, and bone) are formed from the neural crest mesenchyme and the noncollagenous matrix (enamel) is formed by the epithelium.

After the enamel organ and adjacent dental papilla increase further in size, the tooth germ proceeds from the cap stage to the bell or differentiation stage. This stage has two characteristics: 1) The shape of the future tooth crown is defined and outlined by the junction between the inner enamel epithelium and dental papilla. This process, a change from an undifferentiated cap-stage tooth germ to a more differentiated adult-looking bell-stage tooth germ, is called morphodifferentiation. 2) The inner enamel epithelial cells (those cells closest to the papilla) elongate and differentiate into ameloblasts, the future enamel-forming cells. Adjacent to the ameloblasts, the stratum intermedium is formed from a layer of spindle-shaped cells that lie in an axis perpendicular to that of the differentiating ameloblasts. The stratum intermedium cells are thought to function with ameloblasts in the mineralization of the enamel. The outer enamel epithelial cells become associated with a capillary plexus, which will function to bring nutritional substances and oxygen to ameloblasts and other enamel organ cells (Fig. 5.**9**). The stellate (star-shaped) cells lying between the stratum intermedium and outer enamel epithelium comprise the stellate reticulum.

The enamel organ in the bell stage consists of four different types of cells: 1) Those that cover the convex surface, which are the outer enamel epithelial cells. 2) Those that line the concavity of the enamel organ, which are the inner enamel epithelial cells. 3) Those forming a layer adjacent to the inner enamel epithelium, referred to as the stratum intermedium; 4) Those that fill the remainder of the enamel organ, which are termed the stellate reticulum. The stellate reticulum is sometimes called the enamel pulp. The area of the enamel organ where the inner and outer enamel epithelial cells join one another is called the cervical loop. The cervical loop is an area of active cell proliferation and lies in a region that will become the cervix of the tooth. Following the formation of the crown, the cells in the cervical loop will give rise to the epithelial root sheath and epithelial diaphragm (discussed in Chapter 6). During the bell stage, the cells in the periphery of the dental papilla differentiate into odontoblasts. As they differentiate, they elongate and will function in the formation of dentin. The process of differentiation of the various cells of the enamel organ and dental papilla is called cytodifferentiation. Differentiation of the various dental tissues during these stages is called histodifferentiation. At this time, the general and lateral dental laminae begin to degenerate. The tooth bud has differentiated and is independent of the oral epithelium. In this process, the epithelial cells of the dental lamina undergo lysis until the lamina disappears (Figs. 5.**6** and 5.**11**). The general lamina is maintained more posteriorly in the mouth, however, where other teeth are less advanced in development (Figs. 5.**10** and 5.**11**).

Development of the Dental Pulp

The young dental papilla is more densely packed with cells than the tissues surrounding the teeth (Figs. 5.**8**, 5.**9**, and 5.**12**). In Figure 5.**12**, two primary maxillary tooth buds are seen above two mandibular molars in the lower jaw. Both are in the bell or dentinogenesis stage. The high cell density in the papillae is an indication of cell division in the papilla, which will keep pace with growth of the enamel organ.

As peripheral dental papilla cells transform into columnar-shaped odontoblasts they develop cell

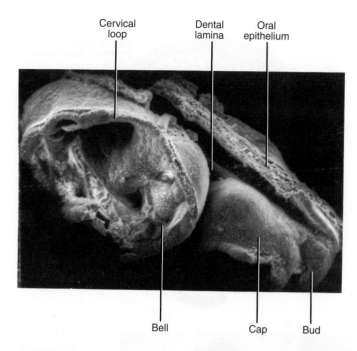

Fig. 5.**10** Scanning electron micrograph of the dental lamina with attached enamel organs at the bud cap and bell stage of development. Epithelium was separated from dental mesenchyme by enzyme treatment and gentle mechanical force.

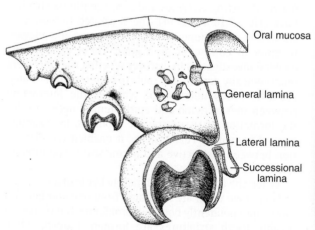

Fig. 5.**11** Diagram depicting the general and lateral lamina as well as the beginning of the dissolution of the dental lamina.

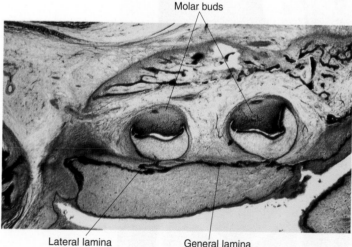

Fig. 5.**12** Sagittal section of the jaws of an embryo illustrating developing teeth.

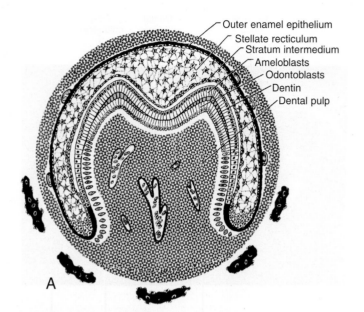

Outer enamel epithelium
Stellate recticulum
Stratum intermedium
Ameloblasts
Odontoblasts
Dentin
Dental pulp

A

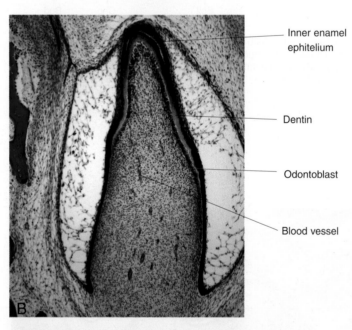

Inner enamel ephitelium

Dentin

Odontoblast

Blood vessel

B

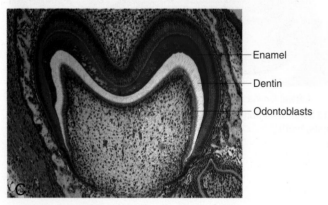

Enamel

Dentin

Odontoblasts

C

Fig. 5.**13 A** Diagram of tooth development and initial dentinogenesis.
B Light micrograph demonstrating the histology of initial dentinogenesis and the beginning of the appositional stage. **C** Light micrograph demonstrating the stage when apposition is near completition.

processes (Fig. 5.**13**). Odontoblasts then begin the process of dentin formation, which is termed dentinogenesis (Fig. 5.**9** and 5.**13**). During dentinogenesis, the dental papilla becomes surrounded (except at the apical area) by dentin and it is then termed the dental pulp. The dental pulp and dentin are closely related forming the dentin–pulp complex. Dentin-forming odontoblasts reside in the periphery of the pulp and recede as they form the dentin matrix. These cells maintain cell processes in dentinal tubules.

On close examination, most of the cells of the dental pulp are seen to be fibroblasts and appear as a delicate reticulum (Fig. 5.**13**). A few larger blood vessels traverse the central area of the pulp; smaller ones are seen in its periphery. Although large nerve trunks are located near the developing young teeth, only a few small nerves associated with blood vessels enter developing young pulps. Later as the teeth erupt and come into function, the larger myelinated nerves become more abundant throughout the pulp organ.

Induction in Tooth Development

Role of the Epithelium and Mesenchyme in Tooth Development at the Tissue Level

Initial experiments designed to determine the role of epithelium and mesenchyme in the initiation of tooth development and cell differentiation made use of epithelial-mesenchymal recombinations. In these experiments the epithelium and mesenchyme of developing teeth are experimentally separated (with the aid of matrix-digesting enzymes and some gentle mechanical force (Figs. 5.**10** and 5.**14**). The separated tissues were allowed to grow alone or were recombined and allowed to grow in culture or as a graft. These experiments enabled investigators to discover whether the cells were embryonically determined (able to secrete differentiated products independently) or whether the interaction between mesenchyme and epithelium is necessary for the formation of tissue-specific products, for example enamel or dentin. Furthermore, it enabled the distinction between instructive and permissive tissue interactions.

When the epithelium and mesenchyme of a bud, cap, or later stage tooth are separated from one another and grown independently both will proliferate, but no recognizable tooth structures are formed. Indeed, when grown independently, these tissues loose their shape (cap or bell) as well as their ability to form dentin or enamel. At best, the epithelium may keratinize and the papilla may form a mineralized tissue resembling bone. This demonstrates that the interaction of the two dental tissues is necessary for tooth formation, and that neither tissue can continue along a path of differentiation independently.

Since these two dental tissues must cooperate to form a tooth, one would like to know which tissue is providing the instructions and which tissue is responding to inductive cues. This question is answered by separating the dental tissues, recombining them with dental tissues from different teeth or nondental tissues (heterotypic recombinations), and putting them in an environment in which they can interact (usually as a graft). When cap-derived dental mesenchyme from a molar tooth is recombined with epithelium from an incisor, a molar tooth will result. Furthermore, when papilla mesenchyme is recombined with epithelium from the diastema (a toothless region in the jaw) or even non-oral epithelium, the result is the formation of a complete tooth that has its morphology dictated by the dental mesenchyme. Recombination of cap-stage dental epithelium (enamel organ) with non-dental mesenchyme does not result in the formation of tooth structures (Fig. 5.**14**). These experiments show that the mesenchyme, at the bud stage of development and beyond, determines tooth type (shape) and can induce dental development (secretion of enamel) from nondental epithelium. In this case the mesenchyme is said to exert an instructive influence on the epithelium because it carries "instructions" that can change the fate of the epithelium (from the original stratified squamous keratinizing or non-keratinizing epithelium to an enamel organ that secrets enamel). On the other hand, the epithelium exerts a permissive influence on the dental mesenchyme because only its presence is necessary for dental development. The mesenchyme is determined since its fate is not changed by the epithelium.

The above recombination experiments are true for interactions occurring during the morphogenesis and proliferative stages of tooth development. A different picture emerges when examining similar experiments performed during the period in which the patterning or positioning of teeth occurs, that is, prior to the bud stage of development, the lamina stage in which epithelial thickenings are beginning to become apparent. Recombinations have been made between premigratory neural crest and early oral epithelium. Furthermore, recombinations between first-arch (maxillary) and second-arch (hyoid) mesenchyme and epithelium have also been made at a stage prior to the formation of tooth buds. In these circumstances tooth development would only proceed if oral (first-arch) epithelium was included in the recombination. This indicates that the epithelium plays an instructional role during the earliest stage of tooth formation and that the fate of the neural crest cells is not predetermined. It appears that these reciprocal cell interactions occur in two stages. In the first stage, the epithelium specifies the "dental nature" of the mesenchyme, and in the second stage the mesenchyme specifies the tooth type and the nature of products produced by the epithelium. By the late-bud or early-cap stage and beyond, mesenchymal dominance over the epithelium is established.

To determine the mechanism of induction during the differentiation of dental tissues, dental papilla and

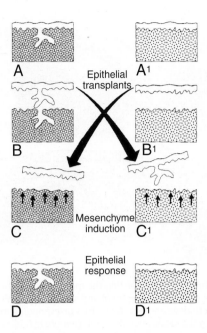

Fig. 5.**14** Induction of tooth primordia by neural crest cells in mesenchyme.
A Transplantation of enamel organ from the site of the alveolar process to the lip or cheek mesenchyme. The result is a lack of continued induction of tooth primordia.
B Transplantation of enamel organ from the lip or cheek mesenchyme to the dental alveolar process. The result is the induction of tooth primordia.

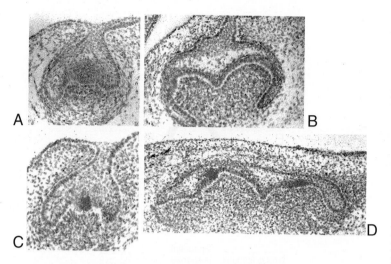

Fig. 5.**15** Light micrographs depicting the morphology of the enamel knot at the cap stage of tooth development and secondary enamel knots at the bell stage of tooth development (**A** and **B**). Corresponding micrographs (**C** and **D**) depicting the localization of FGF-4 by *in situ* hybridization.

enamel organ have been cultured on opposite sides of a porous membrane. These transfilter experiments test the hypothesis of whether cell–cell contact or diffusible molecules are involved in the signaling process. Close cell–cell contact, without the formation of specialized junctions, between preamelobalsts and preodontoblasts has been seen with the electron microscope in the differentiation stage of amelogenesis (see description of amelogenesis below). During this period the basal lamina, between preodontoblasts and preameloblasts, is penetrated by epithelial processes. It becomes discontinuous and is eventually eliminated allowing the formation of heterotypic contacts between epithelium and mesenchyme. Filters that had pore sizes less than 0.2 mm prevented differentiation. Pores of this size do not prevent the diffusion of molecules but do prevent cell processes from either the mesenchyme or epithelium from reaching one another. This rules out the existence of a diffusible molecule as the signal. Since inhibitors of matrix synthesis inhibit tooth development and processes of dental mesenchyme have been seen reaching the epithelial basement membrane, it has been concluded that contact with the basal lamina and its associated matrix is the trigger for odontoblastic differentiation. This would be an example of a short-range, matrix-mediated interaction. (Matrix-mediated reactions are discussed below.)

Molecular Control of Tooth Development

The sequential and reciprocal interactions governing tooth development and patterning are complex. Molecules and signaling pathways responsible for providing "instructions" that regulate initiation, patterning, and morphogenesis are intricate and have not been fully elucidated. However, there are some fundamental principles that can be used to facilitate the understanding of mechanisms involved with dental development. In so doing, one must keep in mind that the final product (human dentition) is a culmination of a series of processes or extracellular signaling events involving morphogenic movements, as well as short, mid, and long-range cell–cell and cell–tissue interactions. The response of cells to short, mid, and long-range signals depends upon their developmental history or lineage. Previous encounters with other cells, the exposure to signaling molecules (or morphogens), and the number of prior cell divisions are some of the other criteria influencing cell competence (the ability to respond to positive and negative signals) and ultimately cell differentiation.

Short-range signaling involves direct cell–cell contact. Such interactions are mediated by cell surface molecules. Although this type of interaction has not been shown to be involved in the induction of epithelial and mesenchymal tissues of the tooth, intercellular junctions are certainly important for cell–cell communication and formation of differentiated tissue layers within the developing enamel organ and dental papilla. Mid-range interactions involve the diffusion of signaling molecules to responding cells in the immediate vicinity. Such interactions have been shown to be crucial during dental development. The role of the extracellular matrix in mid-range signaling cannot be overlooked. Gradients of morphogens contained within the extracellular matrix can direct cell migration and influence cell differentiation. The interaction of morphogens with the extracellular matrix may even be essential for morphogenic activity. In contrast to short and mid-range interactions, long-range interactions have a more generalized influence on the development of body plan. These interactions coordinate development of teeth, bones, and muscle into a functional architecture. They are also involved in regulating the symmetry between the left and right sides of the body (or dentition).

The patterning of the dental arches (positioning of teeth and tooth types) is dependent upon local concentrations of signaling molecules and positional signals that may influence the rate of cell division, the plane of division, the tendency of cells to migrate, the direction of migration, the differentiation of cells, and cell death (apoptosis). It is important to remember that the behavior or fate of a cell is determined by the summation of received intercellular signals. During the processes of induction and differentiation certain combinations of gene activity may be switched on or off. The response of a cell to inductive stimuli (its competence) is not only dependent upon the response to presently perceived signals, but also upon its developmental history (number of previous cell divisions, encounter with previous inductive stimuli, etc.).

Although there is still much to be learned concerning dental development, a general picture is emerging concerning the identity of the mid-range signaling molecules and genes expressed at the various stages of development (summarized in Table 5.**1**). Recently, the importance of the sequential expression of certain homeobox transcription factors and signaling molecules has been highlighted in tooth development. Transcription factors bind to specific sites on DNA to facilitate gene expression. A single transcription factor may activate the expression of a cascade of genes. Concerted gene expression is important for many biologic processes including embryonic development, activation of the immune system, and hormonal responsiveness. Additionally, signaling molecules (and their receptors) and transcription factors may be expressed alternately in the epithelium or mesenchyme at various times during tooth development. This accentuates the observation that the reciprocal interactions first observed at the tissue level are now being substantiated at the molecular level. Our understanding of histologic tissue interactions occurring during tooth development and the molecular mechanisms described here come from studies of the murine dentition. Although the human dentition differs in number (16 teeth per arch vs. eight for the mouse; no lateral inci-

Table. 5.**1** Molecular and tissue interaction in tooth development

STAGE	MORPHOLOGY	TISSUE INTERACTIONS	MOLECULES INVOLVED
Undetermined		Migration of neural crest	Wnt has been implicated in neural tube formation and neural crest migration.
Initation		Initiation of tooth development	FGF-8 from the epithelium induces the mesenchyme to establish an undetermined tooth bud. Msx-Dlx-Barx expression (pre-patterning of tooth type) may be established in the mesenchyme (initiation to bud stage).
Bud		Epithelial mesenchymal interactions establish tooth shape. Appearance of the enamel knot.	Pax 9 expression in mesenchyme initiates tooth bud. Induction of the enamel knot by BMP-4 produced by the mesenchyme late in the bud stage.
Cap		Beginning of morphogenesis. The dental papilla is formed and mesenchymal dominance is established.	The primary enamel knot acts as a putative signaling center inducing cusp formation through the production of signaling molecules like SHH, BMP-2, BMP-7, and FGF-4. The shape of the tooth is determined by mesenchyme.
Bell		Definitive shape of the tooth is established. The primary enamel knot disappears and secondary enamel knots appear over the tips of developing cusps. Histodifferentiation of components of the dental papilla and enamel organ occur.	The secondary enamel knots produce many of the same signaling molecules as the primary enamel knot; The most important appear to be the members of the FGF and BMP family. Extracellular matrix molecules, especially sulfated proteoglycans found in the basement membrane, may be important in facilitating growth factor activity (at this and other stages of development).
Apposition		Secondary enamel knots elaborate many of the signalling molecules expressed by primary enamel knots. A signal beginning at the cusptips initiates wave of differentiation that progresses in an apical direction (toward the cervical loop). Differentiation of ameloblasts and odontoblasts and elaboration of their respective matrices proceeds similarly.	Final differentiation of odontoblasts and ameloblasts. Secretion of dentin and enamel matrix proteins.

sors, canines, or premolars in the mouse), and in dental morphology (shape and size of teeth), many of the conclusions drawn from these studies can most likely be applied also to the human dentition. The process as described here is condensed and simplified. The references cited in the bibliography offer a detailed description and more complete discussion of the processes outlined here.

As expected, many potential signaling molecules (inductive or morphogenic stimuli) have been found to be expressed during tooth development. The most prominent of these include sonic hedgehog (SHH) as well as members of the Wnt (vertebrate homolog of Drosophila wingless), fibroblast growth factor (FGF), and transforming growth factor beta (TGF-β) families. The latter also include the bone morphogenetic proteins (BMPs) which, in addition to their role in dental development, are important regulators of bone growth and regeneration postnatally. These signaling molecules interact with specific receptors to set up intracellular signals that result in specific gene expression. Among the genes activated during early tooth development are also those coding for transcription factors. Homeobox transcription factors are highly conserved genes that are important in controlling the patterning of a variety of developing structures, including teeth. The transcription factors implicated in controlling the initiation of tooth development, tooth morphogenesis (tooth type), and dental patterning (placement of tooth types at specific sites) are Lef1, Pitx2 (Otlx2), Barx1, Lhx6, Lhx7, and Pax9 as well as members of the Msx and Dlx groups (note that by convention genes are italicized and their products are cited in conventional font). Although the location and timing of the expression of these transcription factors have been documented, the number and identity of the genes they are responsible for activating have not been fully elucidated.

Members of the Wnt family of signaling molecules have been linked indirectly to two early embryonic processes, neural tube formation and morphogenetic movement. This suggests an involvement for Wnt in the early events of craniofacial development, including neural crest migration and those functions leading to the establishment of facial processes comprising the dental arches. Following the establishment of the first branchial arch, Pitx2, an early homeobox transcription factor is expressed in oral epithelium during the initiation stage (before the appearance of any recognizable tooth structure). Its expression extends broadly into non-dental areas as well. Its expression may be controlled by mesenchymal positional signals. Failure to express this factor results in Reiger syndrome, a condition associated with dental hypoplasia and even the absence of teeth. Following the establishment of epithelial dental thickenings (or placodes) the signaling molecule, FGF-8, is expressed widely in oral epithelium. Experimental data suggests that expression of FGF-8 is responsible for the initiation of budding. FGF-8 may induce budding by stimulating proliferation (mesenchymal condensation) and the expression of the transcription factor, Pax9, in the mesenchyme. Animals failing to express Pax9 lack teeth entirely. Actually tooth formation is arrested in the early bud stage indicating that expression of Pax9 is necessary for the tooth anlage to develop further. Interestingly, Pax9 expression in certain areas is inhibited by epithelially-produced BMP-4. At this early stage of development BMP-4 is expressed in areas of the dental arch where teeth will not form. Therefore, it has been speculated that production of this signaling molecule may restrict Pax9-expression and tooth development to specific sites in the dental arch. Although this may be an over simplification, it does suggest how expression of several different factors might regulate site-specific odontogenesis.

At the bud stage, FGF-8 induces the expression of Lhx6 and Lhx7 in dental mesenchyme. During development expression of these transcription factors occurs only in the forebrain and the first pharyngeal arch. At slightly later stages, their expressions are restricted to sites of tooth formation, indicating a close correlation with dental development. Furthermore, in addition to FGF-8 the transcription factor Lef1 is expressed first in the epithelium and later in the mesenchyme. As a transcription factor, Lef1 does not work alone. It activates genes in collaboration with other DNA-binding proteins and may be working in concert with one or several of the signaling pathways during this and subsequent stages of tooth development. Curiously, Lef is also a component of the Wnt signaling pathway. Recombination experiments using tissues from Lef1-deficient and normal mice have shown that failure of the epithelium to express Lef1 results in total absence of teeth. Again, these teeth are arrested at the bud stage. Once Lef1 is expressed by the epithelium normal development will occur even if the mesenchyme is incapable of Lef1 synthesis. Expressions of genes activated by Lef1 and Pax9 are needed for progression to the cap stage of development.

While the epithelial component appears to initiate the process of odontogenesis (most likely by FGF-8 signaling), the "instructions" providing the pattern (placement of specific tooth morphologies at distinct sites) probably lie in the mesenchyme. In the developing mouse dentition it is interesting to note that there appears to be a pattern of homeobox genes expressed along the dental arch prior to the initiation of tooth development. Among these are Msx1, Msx2, Dlx2, and Barx1. Of these, one transcription factor, Barx1, is restricted to the molar field of tooth development. Additionally coexpression of Dlx1 and Dlx2 appears to be restricted to the presumptive molar region. Double knockout mice (lacking both Dlx1 and Dlx2 genes) lack maxillary molar teeth. However, lower molars are normal, indicating that the mechanism for patterning differs in the upper and lower dentitions. Given the developmental histories of these two arches this observation is not surprising. Remember that the lower arch is formed by fusion of left and right mandibular processes and each process carries both incisor and molar fields. In the upper arch the right and left maxillary processes must fuse with the incisor-bearing median nasal process. While Dlx1 and Dlx2 and Barx1 appear to be important in molar patterning, Msx1 is expressed in the incisor fields. Its expression may be linked to the formation of incisors. However, transgenic mice lacking Msx1 develop no teeth. This suggests a more general role for this gene in dental development. Other Msx genes have been shown to be expressed in the mesenchyme, and all may be involved in some way in patterning of the dentition.

SHH, a morphogenic signaling molecule, is expressed early. In fact, it is expressed in the prechordal plate and has been proposed to act as a midline patterning molecule. In this regard, SHH may be an early patterning molecule for the incisor fields by acting prior to the establishment of the epithelial thickenings. It may work by regulating the expression of Pax transcription factors in early facial processes. Mutations in the SHH gene result in lethality early in development. Therefore, it is not possible to determine directly the role of SHH using gene deletion. However, the expression of SHH, its receptor (patched), and some of the genes activated by SHH (Gli 1, 2, and 3) have been determined and demonstrate that SHH has important roles during the initiation and morphogenic stages of dental development.

Interestingly, the specification of dental patterning is apparent in early mandibular epithelium. BMP-4, expressed in epithelium overlying incisor fields, induces Msx1 while FGF-8 is expressed over molar fields and induces Barx1. Removal or inhibition of the epithelial BMP-4 signal over the incisor field at the appropriate time results in the expression of Barx1 instead of Msx1 in the mesenchyme and the eventual formation of a molar in the place of an incisor. Additionally, in these experiments a tooth with intermediate characteristics (of a molar and incisor) was also formed. It is tempting to speculate that this may suggest that morphogenic fields play a role in determining the expression of canine and premolar teeth. These experiments also indicate the importance of early epithelial signals in specification of tooth type, and that specification of tooth shape is not predetermined prior to neural crest migration.

During the process of morphogenesis (acquisition of tooth morphology, i.e., size, number, and location of cusps), the enamel knot plays a central role as a developmental regulator (Fig. 15.**5**). The enamel knot has been likened to other well-known signaling centers such as the neural tube and notochord during early development, and the apical ectodermal ridge and zone of polarizing activity during limb development. As previously mentioned, the enamel knot is a transitory structure making its appearance during the early cap stage of development. Its initiation and differentiation are thought to be triggered by signaling molecules in the mesenchyme. The most likely candidate is BMP-4, although other signaling molecules are likely to be needed. This is consistent with tissue recombination experiments, showing that at this stage of development the mesenchyme asserts its dominance over the epithelium and provides "instructions" for the determination of tooth shape.

Expression of p21 (also cyclin-dependent kinase inhibitor or CKI) by cells within the enamel knot is correlated with their withdrawal from the cell cycle and subsequent differentiation. Cells within the enamel knot are unresponsive to the potential autocrine proliferative signaling because they lack appropriate receptors. Among the signaling molecules produced by the enamel knot are SHH, BMPs 1, 2, 4, and 7, FGFs 4 and 9, and Wnt 10a and 10b (Fig. 5.**15**). The proliferative signals affect both epithelium and mesenchyme, causing growth of future cusps. Cells of the enamel knot then undergo programmed cell death (apoptosis) and the enamel knot disappears. Later secondary enamel knots appear over the tips of cusps of multicuspid teeth. These secondary enamel knots also control the cell proliferation and differentiation occurring around the forming cusps, by producing many of the same signaling molecules found in the primary enamel knot. A gradient of signaling molecules produced from the occlusal or incisal region to the apical region is responsible for the gradient of cell differentiation seen along the developing cusps, during the appositional stage of tooth development.

As signaling molecules, retinoids are essential powerful modulators of growth and development. However, their role as signaling molecules in tooth development is not well understood. Excessive application of retinoids affects both limb and tooth development. Studies in animal models demonstrate that retinoids can induce multiple limb segments. Similarly, *in vitro* application of retinoids induces multiple dental lamina formation, indicating that they may play a role in initiation of teeth. Excessive application or ingestion of retinoids can adversely affect almost any stage of tooth development, including the processes of proliferation, matrix formation, and mineralization. However, the mechanism of retinoid action in dental development remains unclear, in that studies of animals possessing mutant retinoic acid receptors have failed to reveal significant dental defects.

In addition to signaling molecules, receptors, and transcription factors, the extracellular matrix plays an important role in development. The basement membrane is a unique extracellular matrix lying between the two interacting tissues. Molecules contained within it or which diffuse through it are likely to play important roles in regulating developmental processes. This is especially true for members of the FGF family. FGFs have been shown to be sequestered by heparan sulfate containing proteoglycans found in basement membranes. Additionally, an association of FGFs with heparan sulfate actually appears to be required for signal transduction. In addition to FGF signaling, sulfated proteoglycans are important in Wnt signaling. It has been proposed that they may serve either to cross link Wnt molecules and induce clustering of receptors or act as low affinity co-receptors that serve to increase the local concentration of Wnt available for binding to high-affinity cell surface receptors. Although not required, the interaction of the extracellular matrix molecule tenascin with a cell surface molecule, syndecan, seems to facilitate mesenchymal condensation at the bud stage of development. In later stages of development the extracellular matrix molecules, especially collagens, play an important role in maintaining tooth shape and dental development. Loss of collagen synthesis (*in vitro* application of lathyrogens or tetracycline to tooth organ cultures) or inhibition of glycosylation of matrix proteins profoundly disrupts tooth structure and subsequent development. Therefore, the extracellular matrix is required for the facilitation of epithelial–mesenchymal signaling and the stabilization of dental morphology. Interactions and events during the stages of tooth development are briefly summarized in Table 5.**1**.

Dentinogenesis

Odontoblast Differentiation

Odontoblasts and ameloblasts differentiate in a tempo-ral spatial pattern. This means that the cells derived from proliferating cells near the cervical loop are the youngest cells developmentally. As one moves in an occlusal or cuspal direction, away from the cervical loop, these developmentally older cells cease dividing and begin the process of differentiation and matrix secretion. Accordingly, the cells near the tips of the cusps of devel-oping teeth in the late bell or appositional stages are developmentally older than those nearer the cervical loop. Therefore, in a developing tooth the sequential stages of development and matrix secretion can be visu-alized along the side of a developing cusp.

Odontoblast differentiation begins with the oval or polygonal cells located near the basal lamina, separating the enamel organ from the dental papilla. These cells are the preodontoblasts. Following a finite number of divi-sions they cease dividing, elongate, and become young differentiating odontoblasts. With further elongation comes the establishment of cell polarity and the forma-tion of an apical process (odontoblastic process). Observe the first-formed predentinal matrix in Figures 5.**16D** and **E**. As the odontoblasts elongate, their nuclei occupy a basal position in the cell and their organelles become more evident toward the apical ends of the cells (Fig. 5.**16D**). Occasionally a single cilium or flagellum may arise from the cell body of the odontoblast. The function of the cilium is unknown. However, the appear-ance of such organelles in other cells is often related to a sensory function. It is also likely that this is a rudimen-tary structure related to the developmental origin of these cells from neuroepithelium and that it has no real function.

Odontoblasts secrete matrix proteins externally, via transport vesicles, at the apical part of the cell and along

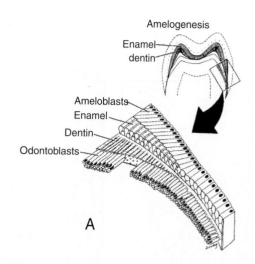

Fig. 5.**16** Diagram of histodifferentiation within the developing tooth. **A** Sites of initial dentin and enamel formation.

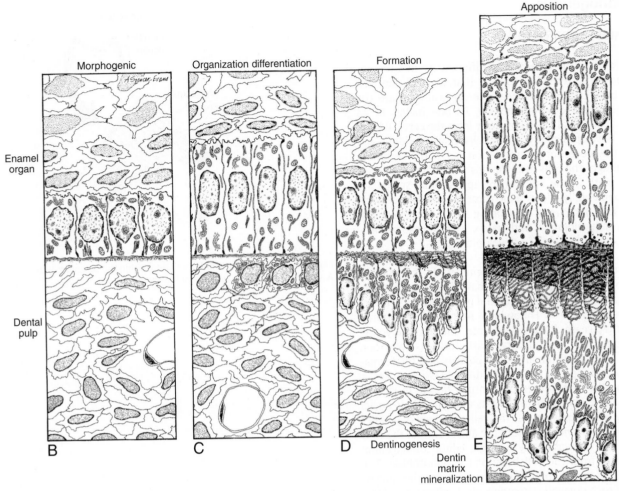

Morphogenic   Organization differentiation   Formation   Apposition

Enamel organ

Dental pulp

B   C   D   E

Dentinogenesis

Dentin matrix mineralization

Fig. 5.**16 B–D** Represent the early stages of odontoblastic differentiation and dentin formation. **B–I** Represent the important stages of ameloblastic differentiation and the formation of enamel. Note in panels **G** and **H** that the ameloblasts modulate, alternating these forms during amelogenesis.

its process (Figs. 5.**17** and 5.**18**). The collagenous dentinal matrix is not mineralized when it is first deposited and is thus termed predentin. When full polarity and final differentiation have been achieved these cells are termed odontoblasts. As the odontoblasts secrete predentin matrix materials, consisting of collagen fibrils and other organic materials, they migrate inwardly (toward the center of the pulp) and away from the basal lamina (Figs. 5.**16A** and **D**). It can also be observed that the DEJ lies at the former junction between the inner enamel epithelium and dental mesenchyme or site of the basement membrane.

The degree of polarization distinguishes odontoblasts from other collagen-producing cells. Odontoblasts are the most polarized connective-tissue producing cells in the body. Unlike osteoblasts or chondrocytes, odontoblasts are never surrounded by a dense matrix (except during pathologic situations) and are always found at the pulpal surface of the dentin. Unlike fibroblasts they only release their secretory products at their apical end. In these respects odontoblasts resemble secretory epithelial cells more than mesenchymal matrix-producing cells. Another indication of their polarity is the acquisition of specialized junctions. The apical terminal bar apparatus, consisting of a zonula adherens and zonula occludens, becomes apparent at the apical end of the

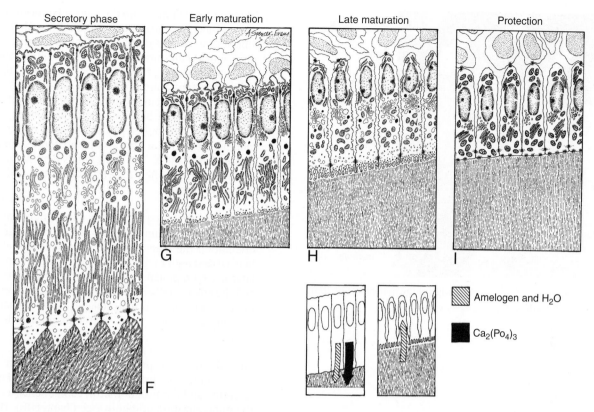

Fig. 5.**16**

cell. The fact that some nerve fibers and von Korff fibers (see next section) run between odontoblasts to enter the predentin matrix suggests that the occluding junctions are not completely tight. Experiments using low-molecular-weight tracer molecules demonstrate that the odontoblastic layer is slightly permeable. Gap junctions are also formed. These communicating junctions allow cells within the odontoblastic layer to share cytoplasmic components such as ions and low-molecular-weight secondary messenger molecules. This allows the odontoblastic layer to function as a unit and groups of odontoblasts to respond to physiologic stimuli.

Matrix Secretion

The appearance of the granular endoplasmic reticulum, Golgi complex, and mitochondria indicates the protein-synthesizing nature of these cells (Figs. 5.**16D** and **E**). Odontoblasts immediately begin forming the precursors of collagen on the ribosomes of the granular endoplasmic reticulum, and the protein is concentrated in the Golgi complex. However, during differentiation and with the initiation of matrix secretion some of the first-formed collagen fibers have been found to pass between the differentiating odontoblasts and extend toward the basal lamina where they end in a fan-like arrangement. These fibers, Korff's fibers, (or von Korff fibers) stain with silver salts (they are argyrophilic) and have been shown with the electron microscope to consist of both collagenous and proteoglycan or glycoprotein components. Since these fibers run between odontoblasts, and

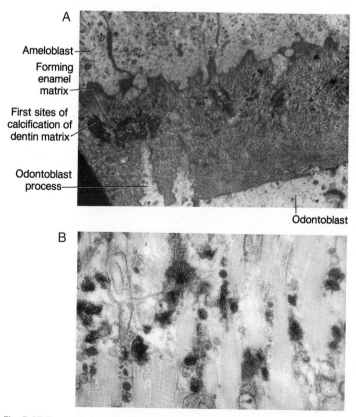

Fig. 5.**17** Transmission electron micrograph of initial mineralization sites of dentin, which appear in small vesicles.

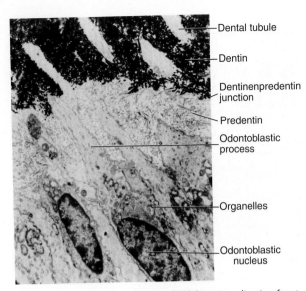

Dental tubule

Dentin

Dentinenpredentin junction

Predentin

Odontoblastic process

Organelles

Odontoblastic nucleus

Fig. 5.18 Transmission electron micrograph of the mineralization front, dentin–predentin junction.

from the basal lamina into the pulp, it has been concluded that they must originate from cells beneath the odontoblast layer or cells that have migrated there during the time when cell junctions are not well established. Additionally, during the stage of odontoblastic differentiation and formation of the early dentinal matrix, the cells secrete type III in addition to type I collagen. In time the type I collagen becomes the predominant collagen type (possibly the only type) produced by mature odontoblasts. Observe the first-formed predentinal matrix in Figures 5.16D and E. The collagenous dentinal matrix is not mineralized when it is first deposited and is thus termed predentin.

The fibers of the first-formed or mantle dentinal matrix are oriented perpendicularly to the DEJ. Because of this orientation the mantle dentin is positively birefringent in polarized light in the mature tooth. The dentin formed later is circumpulpal. It lies beneath the mantle dentin, and the collagen fibers have a more random orientation. In the root the first-formed collagen fibers are parallel to the long axis of the tooth. Therefore, no mantle dentin exists there.

The odontoblastic process plays an important role in maintaining the distribution of matrix proteins, the secretion and removal of matrix components, as well as the mineralization of dentin (see Chapter 10). The ends of the processes maintain their positions (Figs. 5.16D and E) near the DEJ and the odontoblastic process lengthens as the odontoblast retreats. During the lengthening process, the odontoblastic process exhibits many terminal branches as well as numerous lateral branches. These branches in the mature tooth are recognized as numerous canaliculi extending from the primary dentinal tubule. The extent of the odontoblastic process within the dentinal tubule is still somewhat controversial. It is interesting to note that the release of many matrix components, including collagen from the odontoblast, occurs at the base of the process or from the apical portion of the cell body. However, the release of phosphoproteins seems to occur at the junction of mineralized dentin and predentin. These phosphoproteins must travel from the Golgi area through the odontoblast processes to be released at the mineralization front (dentin–predentin junction Therefore, is not entirely correct to state that predentin is merely unmineralized dentinal matrix since it lacks some of the organic components found in mineralized dentin. The preferential location of phosphoproteins at the mineralization front indicates that they may play a role in matrix mineralization. The matrix that forms around the elongated cell processes eventually mineralizes and the odontoblastic process will lie within a dentinal tubule.

Mineralization of Dentin

The mineralization of the first-formed predentin is thought to occur in one of two ways: 1) Small mineral crystals appear in extracellular vesicles, matrix vesicles, (Fig. 5.**17B**; see Chapter 10). Mineralization spreads from these sites throughout the first-formed predentin; 2) Small mineral crystals are nucleated in spaces that exist within the collagen fibrils (due to the staggered arrangement of tropocollagen molecules). Dentinogenesis takes place in a two-phase sequence. The first is the formation of the organic collagen matrix. The second is the deposition of calcium phosphate (hydroxyapatite) crystals. After the initial calcification, all crystals are associated within or on the surface of the collagen fibrils. Crystals are oriented along the long axis of these fibrils. These minute crystals grow and spread throughout the predentin until only the newly formed band of collagen along the pulp is uncalcified. The average crystal attains a size of 100 nm in length and 3 nm in width. Processes of matrix formation and mineralization, therefore, are closely related. Mineralization proceeds by a gradual increase in mineral density of the dentin. As each daily increment of predentin (the amount laid down on the preexisting surface each day, i.e., incremental growth) forms along the pulpal boundary, the more peripheral adjacent predentin, which formed during the previous day, mineralizes and becomes dentin (Fig. 5.**19**). As the predentin calcifies and becomes dentin the mineralization front or dentin–predentin junction becomes established. Following the establishment of the dentin–predentin junction, the dental papilla becomes the dental pulp. Predentin is continuously formed along the pulpal border during crown formation and following eruption, and is calcified along the predentin–dentin junction (Fig. 5.**17**). This results in a decrease in the volume of the pulp organ.

During the period of crown development and during eruption, approximately 4 μm of dentin is laid down in each 24-hour period (Fig. 5.**18**). After the teeth reach occlusion the rate decreases to a level of less than 1 μm per day. Incremental lines (Fig. 5.**1** and 5.**19**: see also Chapter 10) in dentin are believed to result from hesitation in matrix formation and subsequently altered mineralization. This may occur when the basal metabolism is lowest each day. Dramatic changes in metabolism, such as occur at birth or during illness, result in an enhancement of these lines, for example the neonatal line (see Chapter 10). Incremental deposition and mineralization of dentin begins at the tips of the pulp horns at the DEJ and proceeds by the rhythmic deposition of conical layers in the cusps until the crowns are completely formed (Fig. 5.**19**). Dentinogenesis is continued until the entire crown is complete and long after the tooth begins to erupt (Figs. 5.**1** and 5.**2**). Root development continues during and after tooth eruption These details are described in detail in Chapter 6. Details of dentinal structure and composition will be covered in Chapter 10.

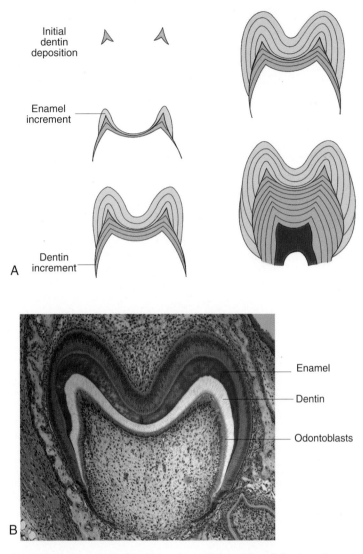

Fig. 5.**19** Diagram depicting the incremental deposition of dentin and enamel.

Organization of Other Components of the Pulp

The organization of structural components within the pulp chamber is a continuing process. The pulp of the erupted tooth is described as having a cell-free and cell-rich zone beneath the odontoblastic layer. These layers only become apparent following eruption and their importance will be considered in Chapter 10. Pioneering nerve fibers enter the tooth at an early stage of development and seem to retreat. The establishment of a mature pattern of innervation occurs late in dental development. The arrangement of nerve fibers within the pulp is also described in Chapter 10. The vascular pattern also evolves as the tooth erupts.

Histologic Events during Amelogenesis

Differentiation stage of amelogenesis. As the preameloblast differentiates to become a secretory ameloblast it also polarizes (Figs. 5.**16D–F**). Intracellular changes involve a lengthening of the cell, proliferation of endoplastic reticulum (ER), and redistribution of cellular organelles (basal migration of the nucleus and apical migration of the Golgi apparatus, i.e., repolarization). Prior to secretion of the enamel matrix the preameloblasts begin the process of eliminating the basal lamina that lies between them and the preodontoblasts. In the initial phase of basal lamina elimination many ameloblastic processes are sent through the basal lamina. Additionally, processes from the odontoblasts are now able to enter epithelial territory and some may insinuate themselves between the differentiating ameloblasts. The heterotypic contacts (differentiation of ameloblasts and odontoblasts) have been thought to play a role in inductive processes during differentiation. However, this is not the case because the inductive process begins prior to the elimination of the basal lamina (with the formation of the dental lamina and epithelial cap). While enamel matrix is deposited, the ameloblast migrates in an outward direction. As enamel matrix synthesis continues, the tips of the odontoblastic processes that entered epithelial territory become surrounded by enamel matrix. The result is the formation of an enamel spindle. During the differentiation process, ameloblasts acquire a set of apical and basal terminal bars as well as a specialized apical process, Tomes' process. Tomes' process can be defined as that part of the ameloblast apical (or distal) to the apical terminal bars. It contains numerous secretion granules and is usually devoid of endoplasmic reticulum and mitochondria. Tomes' process can be divided into two portions, a proximal and distal part. The proximal part of Tomes' process contacts adjacent ameloblasts. The distal part, also called the interdigitating part, is surrounded by (or interdigitates with) enamel (Figs. 5.**20A** and **B**). Acquisition of Tomes' process signals the beginning of the secretory stage of amelogenesis.

The supranuclear cytoplasm of the ameloblast contains a cylindrical Golgi apparatus. The trans (maturing)

Fig. 5.**20 A** Diagram depicting enamel rods. The arcades represent the rod ▶ sheaths, and a line connecting the open ends encloses an enamel rod; the rest is interrod enamel. The hexagonal profile represents the secretory territory of one ameloblast. Note that it takes four ameloblasts to form the outlined keyhole structure, but only one forms an enamel rod. **B** Diagram of the Tomes' process of a secretory ameloblast. The distal part projects into the enamel (see also Fig. 5.24) and forms the enamel rod. The proximal part rests on the enamel surface forming interrod enamel.
C Diagram depicting a longitudinal section through Tomes' process. Note that there are two growth sites, one for the rod and one for interrod enamel. The smooth face of the distal Tomes' process slides along the enamel matrix as the ameloblast retreats. Lines represent the orientation of enamel crystallites, which grow perpendicular to the forming membrane. Note the abrupt change in direction at the tip of the Tomes' process (see Fig 5.21). **D** Electron micrograph of the distal portion of Tomes' process. Note the secretion granules and the rod sheaths in the enamel.

face is more centrally located. Mitochondria are scattered throughout the cytoplasm. Laterally, ameloblasts are connected to one another by gap junctions, tight junctions, and desmosomes. The part of the ameloblast that lies basal to the basal terminal web is called the basal bulge. Numerous blunt processes extend from it to contact neighboring stratum intermedium cells. Ameloblasts and cells of the stratum intermedium are connected to one another by desmosomes and gap junctions. Gap junctions between ameloblasts and ameloblasts and the cells of the stratum intermedium provide the basis for cell–cell communication and coordination of cellular activities.

Secretion Stage of Amelogenesis

Secretory ameloblasts, like the odontoblasts, are polarized cells with a secretory or apical end and a non-secretory or basal end. They migrate in an outward direction away from the DEJ and secrete enamel. The production and secretion of enamel matrix proteins follow the traditional cellular pathway (mRNA → rER → Golgi → secretion granules → liberation at the apical cell surface) as revealed by radioautographic and immunohistochemical procedures. The accumulation of newly liberated enamel-matrix proteins can be visualized by electron microscopy as "stippled material." The initial or first-formed enamel is aprismatic. As the ameloblast develops and acquires a Tomes' process, enamel rods (prisms) are formed.

Concept of the Enamel Rod

The structure of fully developed enamel will be explained in Chapter 9. However, a general understanding of the enamel rod provides an important foundation for the understanding of its development. Mature enamel, when sectioned perpendicularly to its free (external) surface is seen to consist of arch–like structures, rod sheaths or arcades that serve as the boundaries of the enamel rod. The alternate arrangement of these arcades in rows roughly outlines a keyhole or paddle–like pattern (Fig. 5.**20A**). This pattern is seen neither near the DEJ nor near the enamel surface. These areas represent areas of prismless enamel. The formation of enamel into rods or prisms is due to the staggered secretory front created by the orientation of the distal end of the secretory ameloblast (Tomes' processes, Figs. 5.**20B** and **D**). When enamel secretion occurs along a flat secretory front, during the initial and final secretion of enamel (see below), there are no prisms in the enamel. When enamel secretion occurs by fully developed secretory ameloblasts in the presence of a Tomes' process, enamel rods are formed.

There are two different concepts of an enamel rod. One definition holds that the keyhole–like or paddle–like structures referred to above represent the enamel rod. If the secretory territory of an ameloblast is

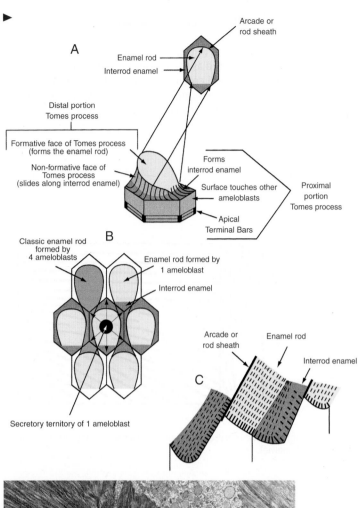

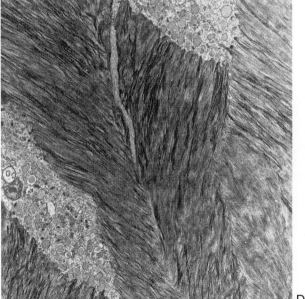

Fig. 5.**20** Legend see opposite page.

Clinical Application

During enamel secretion in the intercuspal areas, ameloblasts may become strangulated as their bases become apposed (Fig. 5.**21**). In the fully formed crown these areas become pits and fissures. They are extremely difficult to clean. Pit and fissure sealants are used to keep bacteria out of these areas.

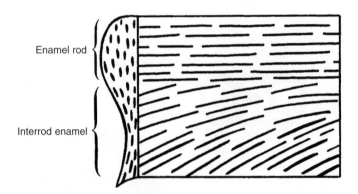

Fig. 5.**21** Diagrammatic representation of the orientation of crystals in rod and interrod enamel.

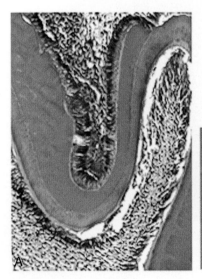
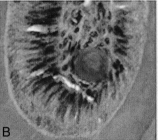

Fig. 5.**22 A** Development of an enamel pit in the intercuspal area of the tooth. **B** Higher magnification showing the lack of vasculature and an epithelial pearl in the developing pit.

projected over these keyhole-shaped rods we can see that four different ameloblasts contribute to the synthesis of one enamel rod or keyhole (Figs. 5.**20A**, **B**, and **D**). With this view there can be no interrod enamel.

Other investigators hold the view "one enamel rod, one ameloblast." With this view an enamel rod is defined as the enamel bounded by the rod sheaths (arcades) and a line connecting the two ends of the arcades. This corresponds to the head of the fish or keyhole and it is made by one ameloblast. The "tail" would then represent interrod enamel, enamel that lies between the enamel rods (Fig. 5.**20B**). The difference between rod and interrod enamel is not a chemical one but is based on the orientation of the hydroxyapatite crystals (Figs. 5.**20B** and 5.**22**–5.**24**). The initial enamel is formed when the basal lamina is being eliminated and is secreted prior to the formation of a fully developed Tomes' process. Therefore, it lacks enamel rods and is aprismatic. The final enamel is produced when the Tomes' processes are regressing and the ameloblasts are in the stage of postsecretory transition and maturation. One may also hold the view that during the formation of the initial and final enamel layers that only the proximal, or the non-interdigitating portion of Tomes' process is present. Since this is the portion of Tomes' process responsible for forming interrod enamel, the initial and final enamel layers would resemble one another because of their similar origin. With the "one ameloblast, one rod" view, the enamel rods can be thought of as bounded by interrod enamel on their sides and capped by aprismatic initial and final enamel. The initial and final enamel would be continuous with interrod enamel, and could be considered interrod enamel. Whilst neither of these views is "wrong," the "one ameloblast, one rod" concept allows better correlation of the formation of the enamel rod during development and with other species that have a very different prismatic arrangement.

Relationship of Tomes' Process to the Enamel Rod

Figure 5.**19** (**B** and **C**) is a diagrammatic representation of a Tomes' process that might be seen in human enamel. The interdigitating (distal) portion of Tomes' process is surrounded by enamel. It has a sloping surface that faces the newly forming enamel rod (the formative face) and an opposing (non-formative) face lying adjacent to interrod enamel. As can also be seen in the diagram, Tomes' process has a "trough"at its base. The interrod enamel is formed in this area. The trough representing the face of the proximal portion of Tomes' process can also be thought of as a formative face. However, it forms the interrod enamel while the formative face of the interdigitating portion of Tomes' process forms the enamel rod.

When the Tomes' processes are removed from developing enamel, the exposed enamel surface consists of "pits" in which the Tomes' processes resided (Fig. 5.**25**). These pits have three relatively steep "walls" and one gently sloping "floor." The "floor" of the pit represents the enamel rod (and its blending with the wall), and is formed by the sloping formative face of the interdigitating or distal portion of Tomes' process. The walls of the pit represent interrod enamel formed by the formative face of the proximal portion of Tomes' process. Since the floor is sloped, the enamel of the floor blends with the wall or interrod enamel. It should also be obvious that the enamel formed at the "deeper regions" of the floor of the pit, the enamel rod, is developmentally younger than the adjacent walls or interrod enamel.

When examined in section triangular profiles of the ameloblasts are seen in the surrounding enamel (Fig. 5.**20C**). This appearance is somewhat deceiving in that the outline of the Tomes' process is not triangular but really consists of the apex of the triangle, one side being the formative and the other the non-formative face of Tomes' process, and an extension from the side of an adjacent triangle.

The crystals in enamel tend to grow with their long axis perpendicular to the membrane that produces the matrix. It can be observed that the orientation of the crystals changes in conjunction with that of the membrane. Sharp changes in crystal direction can be seen at the boundary of the rod sheaths, and more subtle changes occur from the "open end" (the line joining the ends of the arcade or sheath) of the rod to interrod enamel (Figs. 5.**20B** and **D** and 5.**24**).

Postsecretory Transitional Stage of Amelogenesis

The stage of postsecretory transition occurs toward the end of enamel secretion and is marked by two developmental events, a change in the ameloblast's morphology and programmed cell death. Following the deposition of the majority of the enamel matrix, ameloblasts loose their Tomes' process; they become shorter and many (up to 25%) of the ameloblasts die. A basal lamina and associated hemidesmosomes, which provide attachment to the enamel surface, is formed between the enamel and ameloblasts.

There are also noticeable changes in the stellate reticulum. These cells that were once stellate and separated by extracellular spaces are now compact. With the stratum intermedium and outer enamel epithelium these cells will form a papillary layer of cells beneath the ameloblasts.

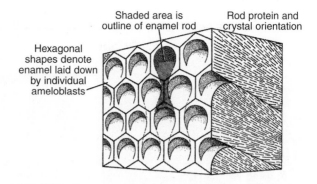

Fig. 5.**23** Diagram of the ameloblast–enamel rod interface.

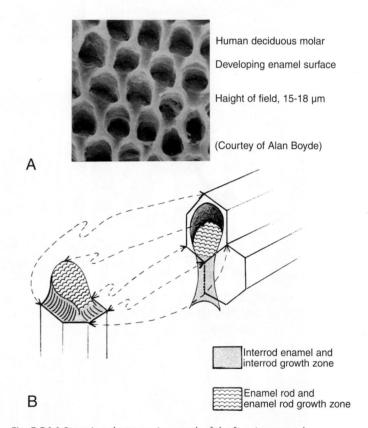

Human deciduous molar

Developing enamel surface

Haight of field, 15–18 μm

(Courtesy of Alan Boyde)

Interrod enamel and interrod growth zone

Enamel rod and enamel rod growth zone

Fig. 5.**24 A** Scanning electron micrograph of the forming enamel rod–ameloblast interface. **B** Diagram of the relationship of the Tomes' process to the interface in A. Note that the edge of the Tomes' process corresponds to the rod sheath.

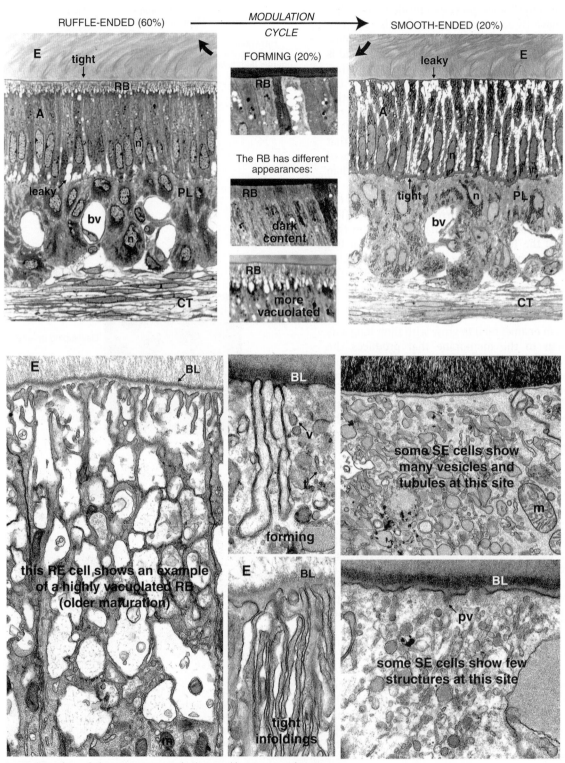

Fig. 5.**25** Light and electron micrographs (top and bottom panels, respectively) illustrating the morphologic appearance of ameloblasts in the rat incisor enamel organ (A) as they modulate rhythmically between the ruffle-ended (left side and middle) and smooth-ended (right side) morphologies during the maturation stage of amelogenesis. Top: right and left panels x 700; middle panels x l000. Bottom: left and top right panel x l7 500; two middle panels and bottom right panel x 28 750. Connective tissue of the dental sac (CT); ameloblast (A); basal lamina (BL); enamel (E); ruffled border (RB); mitochondria (m); nucleus (n); papillary layer (PL); pinocytotic vesicles (pv); tubules (t); vesicles (v); and blood vessel (bv). For a complete description see text.

Maturation Stage of Amelogenesis

During the process of maturation enamel becomes fully mineralized. The organic and water content of enamel becomes reduced and the inorganic component (principally hydroxyapatite) increases. The process of maturation is really an ongoing process that begins early in the secretion stage. Enamel matrix becomes mineralized as soon as it is formed and it continues to mature. This feature distinguishes it from dentin and bone. Unlike dentin and bone there is no "preenamel" whereas predentin or osteoid exists as unmineralized matrices in dentin and bone, respectively. During the secretion stage, enamel nearest the DEJ, being developmentally older, is more mineralized or mature. The maturation process is continuous, but acquisition of full mineralization, with loss of almost all the water and protein, occurs during the stage of maturation. This stage is first recognized by the formation of a ruffled apical border in ameloblasts (Figs. 5.**16** and 5.**25**).

During the stage of maturation, ameloblasts have been found to modulate. Modulation is a reversible change in cell activity and morphology. Two types of ameloblasts, as well as transitional forms, have been seen in this stage. They are the ruffle-ended (RE) and smooth-ended (SE) ameloblasts. Ruffle-ended ameloblasts, as their name suggests, possess a ruffled distal border. Ruffle-ended ameloblasts predominate during this stage. In the rodent incisor, a rapidly growing and continuously erupting tooth often used as a model for studying amelogenesis, approximately 60% of the ameloblasts are ruffle-ended. Only 20% of the ameloblasts are smooth-ended and the other 20% are in various stages of transition between the two types (Fig. 5.**25**). The apical specialization of ruffle-ended ameloblasts resembles that of intestinal villi epithelium, but is more irregular (thus the term ruffled instead of striated). Because of their superficial resemblance to resorptive cells, these cells may be responsible for the uptake of peptides and amino acids from the matrix. The ruffle border also varies in appearance during maturation. It initially appears loaded with dark/dense staining material during early maturation and then becomes more vacuolated and dilated as the enamel matures (Fig. 5.**25**). The pH of the extracellular fluid in enamel related to ruffle-ended ameloblasts is characteristically mildly acidic (as low as pH 5.8). Ameloblasts periodically lose their ruffle borders (modulate) to become smooth-ended. This occurs very rapidly, usually resulting in large spaces appearing between the cells and their apical junctions becoming more leaky or disappearing while their basal junctions become more tightly sealed. The apical area of these cells sometimes shows few structures or it can appear to be loaded with vesicles and tubules (Fig. 5.**25**). These smooth-ended ameloblasts also show numerous pinocytotic vesicles (Fig. 5.**25**). The pH of the extracellular fluid in enamel related to these smooth-ended ameloblasts is nearly neutral (pH 7.2). In the rodent incisor enamel organ ameloblasts remain smooth-ended for a short

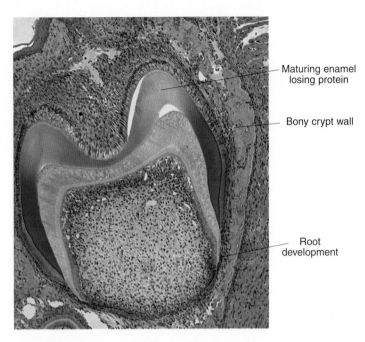

Maturing enamel losing protein

Bony crypt wall

Root development

Fig. 5.**26** Developing tooth with a nearly completed crown residing in a bony crypt.

duration (20% of cycle) and then they begin the process of recreating the ruffle border which takes time to form (20% of cycle time). Ameloblasts from the teeth of other mammals undergo as many as three full modulation cycles per day as the enamel matures (RE → SE → RE every 8 hours). The timing of the modulation cycle in human teeth is presently unknown. Ruffle-ended ameloblasts have well-developed distal junctional complexes but lack proximal junctions (Fig. 5.**25**). Interestingly, during maturation ameloblasts continue to produce low levels of enamel matrix proteins.

The net result of the activity of maturation ameloblasts is a gain in the mineral content (mostly calcium and phosphate) of the enamel and a loss of protein and water. Loss of protein from the matrix and a gain in mineral is easily visualized in decalcified histologic sections. The tips of the cusps have less matrix and more mineral content and exhibit poor staining or complete lack of staining (enamel space). In contrast, the cervical areas that have a higher protein content stain intensely (Fig. 5.**26**). Spaces between enamel crystals diminish in size with the addition of more mineral to the matrix. The crystals of young enamel are long and slender. During maturation the crystals get thicker and wider. The enamel rod core or head of the rod appears to be most mineralized during maturation. The rod periphery or rod tails (interrod enamel) still contain sufficient material to be seen. A Grenz X-ray illustrates spaces between rods, which indicates a lower mineral content (Figs. 5.**27A** and **B**). Measurements of these rods indicate that they are less than the 5 x 9 μm mature rod size. Therefore, the final mineral (96%+) is probably added to the rod periphery. This final process of mineralization may occur shortly before eruption.

Final enamel thickness (from 2 mm to 2.5 mm over the cusps) is attained following completion of enamel formation. The cervical regions of the crown and the central grooves are the last zones to mineralize and rarely reach the extent of the cusps. The ameloblasts in these regions may loose functional capacity before mineralization is complete. Lack of complete mineralization at sites, such as in pits and at the bases of cusps, is believed to be a reason for the prevalence of caries in these areas.

In summary, enamel mineralization follows the pattern of matrix formation from the DEJ peripherally (Fig. 5.**28**). The extent of mineralization is indicated by the dark-to-light shaded zones proceeding from the DEJ peripherally. The very dark zones are the most highly mineralized and the white areas the least mineralized. The final stage of mineralization of the enamel rod may be in its periphery, and at a time just prior to eruption of the crown into the oral cavity.

Physical and Biochemical Events during Amelogenesis

Proteins of the Enamel Matrix

From the above description of the morphologic events that occur in the cells of the enamel organ and the enamel matrix itself, we can conclude that the morphologic alterations reflect changes in cell function and that these alterations lead to differing molecular and biochemical events. Since the process of secretion occurs during differentiation, secretion, postsecretory transition, and maturation stages of amelogenesis, it is appropriate to view changes in matrix organization and cellular function in a molecular, biochemical, and physiologic context.

During the process of amelogenesis, ameloblasts secrete several classes of matrix proteins and enzymes. The exact role of these proteins in crystal nucleation, crystal orientation, crystal growth, and maturation is not fully understood. However, it is interesting to note that some matrix proteins appear to be spatially distributed in the enamel. Additionally, the secretion of certain classes of enzymes appears to be stage-related. Purification and identification of enamel-matrix proteins have been difficult, because they are degraded soon after they are released. Furthermore, "contaminating" proteins from the serum (especially albumin) also find their way into the enamel. The enamel matrix is a complex mixture of proteins. Tissue-specific proteins (produced by ameloblasts) and cellular activities of ameloblasts during maturation are central to the development of this unique mineralized tissue. The proteins of the enamel matrix are classified as belonging to one of two major groups, amelogenins or non-amelogenins. Amelogenins, as a class, are predominant enamel-matrix proteins and comprise about 80% of the young enamel matrix. Due to alternative splicing of RNA, a number of amelogenin isoforms have been found in enamel. They have been detected in secretory ameloblasts by immunocytochemical staining and are ameloblast-specific secretory products. Amelogenins are generally hydrophobic proteins with a hydrophilic sequence at their carboxy terminal (anionic) end. Additionally they contain high levels of the amino acids proline, glutamine, histidine, and leucine. They have a tendency to aggregate in solution and to form supramolecular structures 20 nm in diame-

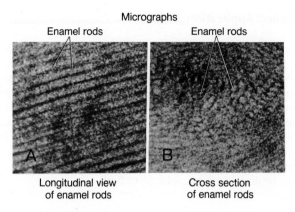

Fig. 5.**27** High-magnification view of microradiographs of forming enamel with rods cut in longitudinal **A** and cross section **B**.

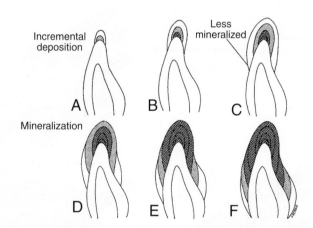

Fig. 5.**28** Summary of the stages of enamel mineralization. Initial enamel is formed in **A** and becomes more mature (more calcified) in **B** as further matrix is formed. **C** Further increments are formed. **D** Mineralization and matrix deposition increases. **E** Enamel matrix is formed on the side of the cusps. F Final matrix is formed and progresses cervically.

Clinical Application

The replacement of the hydroxyl anion with fluoride in hydroxyapatite during the secretion and maturation stages of amelogenesis decreases the solubility of the mineral phase making enamel more "caries resistant." This substitution, which occurs during enamel formation and maturation, produces a fluorapatite throughout the thickness of the enamel. During fluoride treatments on erupted teeth exchange of fluoride for hydroxyl ions occurs in surface layers only. Excessive fluoride results in a condition known as fluorosis. The enamel may be discolored, hypoplastic, or both.

ter, known as enamel nanospheres (Fig. 5.**29**). Each nanosphere consists of an aggregated mass of approximately 100 amelogenin molecules. "Stippled material" resembling the nanospheres is produced by secretory ameloblasts and is found at enamel growth fronts (Fig. 5.**30**).

The crystals of mature enamel are by far the largest crystals found in mineralizing tissues of the body. Their growth in length, thickness, and width is controlled by their interaction with amelogenins during development. In developing enamel, amelogenin nanospheres electrostatically adhere to the developing enamel crystals. The initially thin hexagonal shape of the crystals is maintained by adherent amleogenin nanospheres. Crystal growth occurs along the c-axis (longitudinal axis) of the crystal by preferential deposition of mineral at the end of the crystal. Growth of enamel crystals, in width and thickness, is prevented or controlled by the presence of

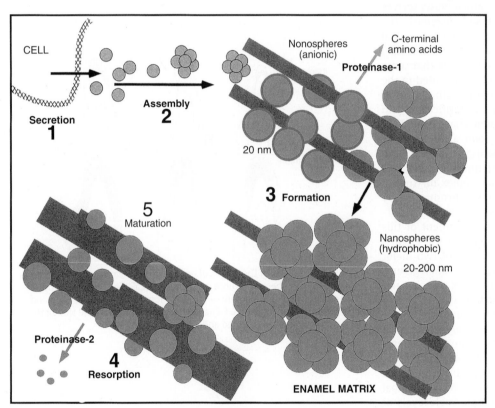

Fig. 5.**29** Summary of the role of the proposed role of amelogenins in enamel mineralization:
1. Amelogenins are synthesized by the ameloblasts and secreted extracellularly.
2. Amelogenin monomers assemble to generate nanospheres (~20 nm diameter) with hydrophilic (anionic) carboxy terminals externalized.
3. Anionic nanospheres initially interact electrostatically with the crystal faces parallel to the c-axis (long axis), preventing crystal–crystal fusions and acting as 20 nm spacers. Enamelysin (proteinase 1) processes the exposed carboxy terminals and progressively reduces their anionic character. Hydrophobic nanospheres assemble and stabilize the matrix containing the initial crystallites, which continue to grow by ion accretion at their exposed ends.
4. Enamel serine protease action degrades the hydrophobic nanospheres (amelogenins), generating smaller amelogenin fragments. Amelogenin fragments and other peptide fragments are resorbed by ameloblasts.
5. Removal of amelogenin nanospheres from the crystal leaves the surface "unprotected" (see point 3). This allows the crystals to grow in thickness, interlock, and possibly fuse.

amelogenins and perhaps enamelins on these surfaces. Besides directing growth, amelogenins have been proposed to serve as "20 nm spacers" to prevent premature fusion of crystals (Fig. 5.**28**).

The role of non-amelogenins in crystal growth is less well understood. The major matrix proteins in this group are tuftelin, sheathlin (also termed ameloblastin or amelin), and enamelin. Tuftelin appears to be restricted to an area near the DEJ (in enamel tufts; see Chapter 9) and appears to be a product of both young ameloblasts and preodontoblasts. Due to its restricted location it has been proposed to play a role in induction, the initiation of mineralization, and/or as a junctional material linking enamel and dentin. Sheathlin, when initially secreted, is found throughout rod and interrod enamel. However, as its name suggests it is preferentially located in the rod sheaths or arcades in deeper enamel layers. In developing enamel the rod sheath area is poorly mineralized. Enamelin is an acidic, phosphorylated, and glycosolated protein. It is the largest enamel-matrix protein and is preferentially restricted to the enamel-rod area. Its phosphorylated nature and initial accumulation near the growing ends of crystals suggests that enamelin may play a role in crystal growth or nucleation. Similar to amelogenin, enamelin has also been proposed as a factor in limiting crystal growth.

Role of Proteolytic Enzymes in Enamel Development

In addition to matrix proteins, hydrolytic enzymes have been found in the enamel matrix. Enamelysin is a matrix metalloprotease. As such, its activity in the enamel matrix can be regulated by tissue inhibitors of metalloproteases. Enamelysin is secreted with matrix proteins during the secretory stage of amelogenesis. It is probably responsible for the limited proteolysis that occurs at this time. Matrix alterations occurring during secretion include cleavage of the carboxy terminus of the amelogenins, initial processing of enamelin, and processing of sheathlin resulting in its mobilization to sheath areas. During postsecretory transition, production of enamelysin becomes reduced; the production of more aggressive serine proteases begins and continues throughout the maturation stage of amelogenesis. Serine proteases remove amelogenins from the intercrystal areas, allowing growth in crystal width and thickness.

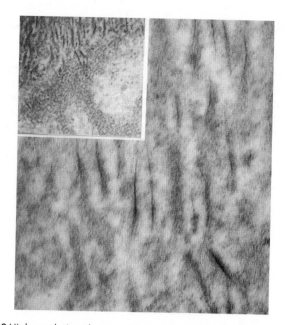

Fig. 5.**30** High-resolution electron micrograph showing developing enamel crystals. Electron micrograph showing the accumulation of "stippled material" at the enamel growth front (inset).

Clinical Application

Amelogenesis imperfecta is a genetic disease in which the enamel is poorly formed or mineralized. Such genetic disturbances can be the result of defective enamel-matrix synthesis, defective protease formation (enamelysin or serine proteases), or defects in other cellular functions.

Clinical Application

Certain antibiotics, like tetracyclines, have an affinity for calcified tissues. They may become incorporated within the mineral phase during maturation and cause discoloration of enamel and underlying dentin. Additionally, during earlier development, tetracyclines may interfere with the differentiation of a cohort of ameloblasts and cause hypoplastic areas of enamel on the crowns of teeth.

Mineral Phase and Mechanisms of Enamel Maturation

The mineral phase of enamel is considered to be carbonated hydroxyapatite. However, the smallest repeating unit, the unit cell, is calcium hydroxyapatite having the formula $Ca_{10}(PO_4)_6(OH)_2$. Generation of H+ ions during maturation results in increased acidity within the matrix (Figs. 5.**25** and 5.**31**). This increased acidity, if allowed to continue, could result in crystal dissolution. During the secretory phase of amelogenesis, the zwitterions provided by enamel matrix proteins or peptide degradation products could provide the buffering effect needed to prevent a large drop in pH. However, during maturation the protein content of the matrix decreases significantly and another buffering system must take over. The generation of bicarbonate anions by carbonic anhydrase has been proposed as a buffering mechanism during enamel maturation. High concentrations of carbonic anhydrase occur in the cytoplasm of all maturation ameloblasts.

Hydroxyapatite Unite Cell

$$10Ca^{2+} + 6\ HPO_4^{2-} + 2\ H_2O \leftrightarrow Ca_{10}(PO_4)_6(OH)_2 + 8H^+$$

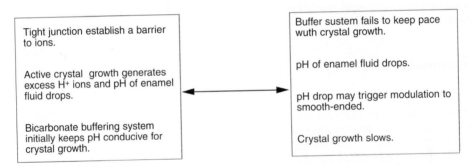

Tight junction establish a barrier to ions.

Active crystal growth generates excess H+ ions and pH of enamel fluid drops.

Bicarbonate buffering system initially keeps pH conducive for crystal growth.

Buffer sustem fails to keep pace wuth crystal growth.

pH of enamel fluid drops.

pH drop may trigger modulation to smooth-ended.

Crystal growth slows.

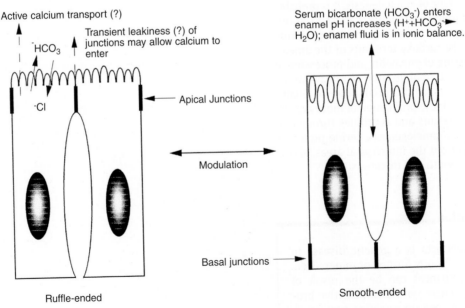

Active calcium transport (?)

-HCO3

Transient leakiness (?) of junctions may allow calcium to enter

-Cl

Apical Junctions

Modulation

Serum bicarbonate (HCO3-) enters enamel pH increases (H++HCO3- H2O); enamel fluid is in ionic balance.

Basal junctions

Ruffle-ended

Smooth-ended

Fig. 5.**31** Summary of the events which occur during the maturation of enamel (cf. Fig. 5.**25**).

Carbonic anhydrase is especially abundant in the apical cytoplasm of ruffle-ended ameloblasts. Measurements of enamel matrix pH during maturation demonstrate that the pH steadily declines beneath ruffle-ended ameloblasts as maturation progresses, indicating that as these cells actively pump calcium into the matrix (remember their apical junctions are tight) the buffering mechanism fails to keep pace with the generation of H+ ions. Although the exact mechanism triggering a change from ruffle-ended to smooth-ended ameloblasts is not known, it has been suggested to be related to the drop of pH (below a critical level) occurring beneath ruffle-ended ameloblasts during active crystal growth. Following the transition from ruffle-ended to smooth-ended, there is an abrupt rise in pH. The leaky apical junctions over smooth-ended ameloblasts allow for rapid influx of fluids and buffering components (carbonate and serum proteins) into the enamel. Re-establishment of a "pH balance" may be part of the triggering mechanism that signals the modulation from smooth-ended to ruffle-ended ameloblasts. Additionally, the increase in crystal dimensions (thickness and width) occurring during maturation allows for interlocking of crystals.

Crown Growth and Completion

Crowns of the teeth increase in size by incremental deposition of enamel matrix (Figs. 5.**28** and 5.**32**). The first area of the crown to completely form is the cusp tip, and the last is the cervical region. Crowns increase in height or length by differentiation of new ameloblasts. This is followed by enamel formation at the cervical aspects of the enamel organ (Figs. 5.**28**, 5.**32**, and 5.**33**). Crowns also increase in size by cell division of the inner enamel epithelial cells between the cusps. This results in a slight separation of the cusps with a resultant slight increase in crown size. From the inception of dentinogenesis to the completion of amelogenesis, the crowns increase in size about four times. This is primarily due to cell division at the cervical region and the deposition of enamel to the thickness of 2.5 mm. When the ameloblasts differentiate (in any area), they can no longer divide. The last areas to differentiate, therefore, are the intercuspal and cervical areas. Therefore, after cell differentiation, crown size is dependent upon incremental growth (enamel deposition).

Enamel completion is signaled not only by attainment of crown size, but also by mineral content. At the final stage of mineralization, the flattened ameloblasts and their basement membrane along with the remainder of the cells of the enamel organ (reduced enamel epithelium) form a membrane on the surface of the enamel (Figs. 5.**33** and 5.**34**). This is termed Nasmyth's membrane or the primary cuticle.

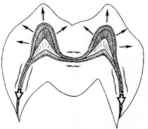

Growth of cusps to predetermined point of completion

{Zones of cell division}

Fig. 5.**32** Diagram depicting the growth of the developing crown at cuspal, intercuspal, and cervical sites.

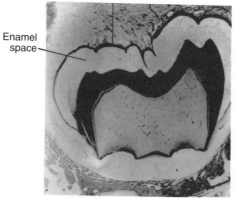

Enamel space

Fig. 5.**33** Enamel formation is near completion. Mineralization is not complete at the cervical region. The enamel organ is now in the form of a reduced enamel epithelium.

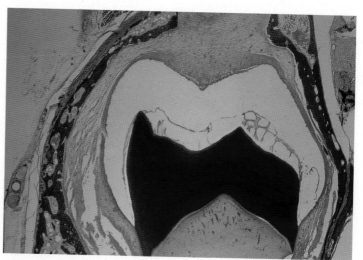

Fig. 5.**34** Completed crown residing in a crypt with a cuticle formed on the surface of the enamel.

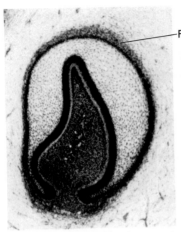

Follicle cells migrate away from the enamel organ to initiate periodontal development

Fig. 5.**35** Cells near the surface of the outer dental epithelium at the bell stage migrate outward to induce the formation of surrounding periodontal structures.

Clinical Application

The enamel cuticle may remain adherent to the tooth after eruption, appearing as a reddish or brown spot on the crown. This may cause undue concern for parents. However, this layer is soon shed or easily removed with a toothbrush.

Crown and Surrounding Tooth Crypt

The mesenchymal cells immediately surrounding the crown appear as a capsule known as the dental follicle (Fig. 5.**35**). Those follicular cells of ectomesenchymal origin that are adjacent to the young enamel organ in the cap and bell stages (Figs. 5.**9A** and **B**) migrate away from their origin into the follicle, and induce the formation of the surrounding alveolar bone and periodontal ligament. The future periodontal ligament is a connective-tissue zone that surrounds the tooth and is positioned between the protective thin shell of alveolar bone and the developing tooth. Later, as the tooth erupts, root formation takes place and the periodontal ligament matures.

Summary

Tooth development is the result of the inductive interactions that occur between the oral epithelium and the cells of the neural crest. The oral epithelium develops a dental laminar system from which 20 primary and 32 permanent enamel organs develop. All enamel organs pass through the same bud, cap, and bell stages. The proliferating cells differentiate into the tooth formative cells during the bell stage. Ameloblasts arise from the inner enamel epithelial cells and induce the adjacent cells of the dental papilla to differentiate into odontoblasts, which form dentin. The formation of enamel and dentin matrices occurs nearly simultaneously. Following the deposition of a layer of aprismatic enamel, ameloblasts deposit enamel in the form of rods or prisms that become highly mineralized. During enamel maturation, ameloblasts function to resorb much of the water and organic matrix from enamel to provide space for the growing enamel crystals. Enamel and dentinal matrices form by the incremental deposition of about 4 μm of matrix daily.

Odontoblasts first form an increment of collagenous matrix, called predentin, that is later mineralized. As daily increments of predentin form, the adjacent earlier-formed increment mineralizes as dentin. The odontoblastic process grows in length as more matrix is deposited, and is instrumental in controlling the environment at the mineralization front between dentin and predentin. Dentin consists of 70% mineral, 18% organic material, and 12% water.

Hydroxyapatite crystals in enamel increase in size, which results in enamel being 96% mineral and 4% organic material and water. The arrangement of ameloblasts with their Tomes' process results in the formation of enamel rods. The process of amel-

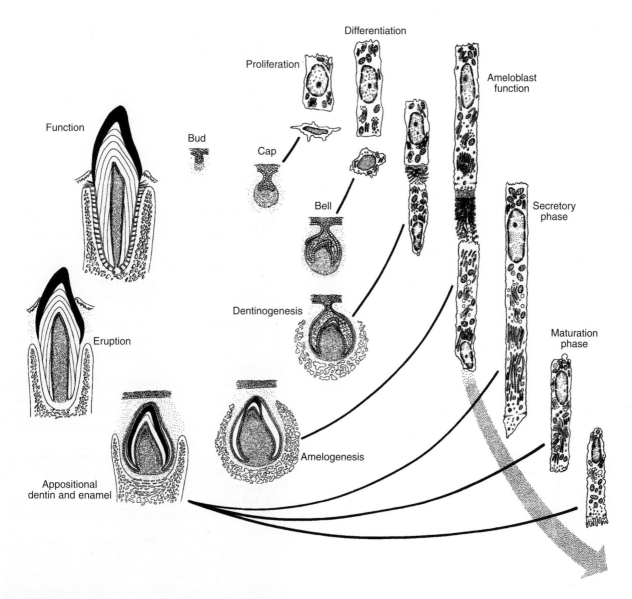

Fig. 5.**36** Summary of cell activity correlated to early stages of tooth formation that are important to the development, eruption, and function of teeth. Ameloblastic and odontoblastic differentiation and function are seen on the right and tooth development stages on the left.

ogenesis is a series of successive stages of proliferation, differentiation, secretion, and maturation (diagramed in Fig. 5.**36**). A four-fold increase in the size of the crowns occurs from initiation until the completion of hard-tissue deposition. This increase is accomplished by cell division and incremental deposition. The tooth follicle develops around the tooth and eventually gives rise to supporting structures.

Self-Evaluation Review

1. From what tissue does the mesenchyme of the tooth originate? When does this tissue gain its specificity?
2. What are the stages of tooth development (morphologic and physiologic)?
3. What three components make up the tooth germ? What structures do they form?
4. What cell types comprise the bell-stage enamel organ?
5. Define the terms morphodifferentiation and cytodifferentiation as they relate to tooth development.
6. What are the roles of the oral epithelium and mesenchyme in the induction of odontogenesis prior to and following the bud stage? What is meant by the terms instructive and permissive as they relate to epithelial–mesenchymal interactions?
7. What role does the enamel knot provide in the development of the crown's shape?
8. What causes the induction of dentin-forming cells?
9. Describe the changes that occur during odontoblastic differentiation.
10. Compare and contrast the role of the extracellular matrix in the mineralization of enamel and dentin.
11. Describe the changes in the inner enamel epithelium during the process of ameloblastic differentiation. What is Tomes' process?
12. Describe the distribution of prismatic and aprismatic enamel in the crown. What accounts for the arrangement of enamel into prisms?
13. What are the two definitions of an enamel rod? How many ameloblasts form an enamel rod according to each definition?
14. Describe the relationship between Tomes' process and the developing enamel rod.
15. What is meant by the term "modulation"? At which stage in amelogenesis do ameloblasts modulate? What is happening to the enamel matrix during this stage? What are the roles of proteolytic enzymes in this process?
16. How much does the crown increase in size between early development and completion?
17. Is the cervical region usually as highly mineralized as the cusp tip?

Acknowledgements

The authors would like to thank Dr. Irma Thesleff for her suggestions and the following persons who provided figures for this chapter: Dr. Paivi Kettunen, Department of Anatomy and Cell Biology, University of Bergen, Bergen, Norway for Figure 5.**15**; Dr.Thomas Diekwisch, Texas A&M University System, Baylor College of Dentistry, for Figures 5.**20D** and 5.**30**; Alan Boyde for Figure 5.**24A**; Dr. Charles E Smith, McGill University, and Antonio Nanci, University of Montreal, for Figure 5.**25**; and Alan Fincham, University of Southern California, for Figure 5.**29** (with permission of Academic Press).

Suggested Readings

Aoba T. Recent observations on enamel crystal formation during mammalian amelogenesis. Anat. Rec. 1996;245:208–218.

Bhaskar SN, ed. Orban's Oral Histology and Embrylogy. St. Louis: CV Mosby; 1986.

Boyde A. The development of enamel structure. Proc. R. Soc. Med. 1967;60(9):923.

Diekwisch TGH. Subunit compartments of secretory stage enamel matrix. Connect. Tiss. Res. 38:101–111.

Fincham AG, Simmer JP. Amelogenin proteins of developing dental enamel. Ciba Found. Symp. 1997;205:118–130.

Fincham AG, Moradain-Oldak J, Simmer JP The structural biology of the developing dental enamel matrix. J. Struct. Biol. 1999;126.

Jernvall J, Aberg T, Kettunen P, Keranen S, Thesleff I. The life history of an embryonic signaling center: BMP-4 induces p21 and is associated with apoptosis in the mouse tooth enamel knot. Dev. 1998;125(2):161–169.

Kollar EJ. Odontogenesis: A retrospective. Eur. J. Oral Sci. 1999;106:(S1):2–6.

Kratochwil K, Dull M, Fariñas I, Grosschedl R. Lef1 expression is activated by BMP-4 and regulates inductive tissue inter actions in tooth and hair development. Genes Dev. 1996;10:1382–1394.

Neubuser A, Peters H, Balling R, Martin GR. Antagonistic inter actions between FGF and BMP signalling pathways: A mechanism for positioning the sites of tooth formation. Cell. 1997;90:247–255.

Robinson C, Kirkham J, Shore R, eds. Dental enamel: Formation to destruction. Boca Raton: CRC Press; 1995.

Robinson C, Brookes SJ, Bonass WA, Shore RC, Kirkham J. Enamel maturation. Ciba Found. Symp. 1997;205:156–170.

Robinson C, Brookes SJ, Shore RC, Kirkham J. The developing enamel matrix: nature and function. Eur. J. Oral Sci. 1997;106(suppl 1):282–291.

Sasaki T, Takagi M, Yanagisawa T. Structure and function of secretory ameloblasts in enamel formation. Ciba Found. Symp. 1997;205:32–46.

Simmer JP, Fincham AG. Molecular mechanisms of dental enamel formation. Crit. Rev. Oral Biol. Med. 1995;6:84–108.

Smith CE. Cellular and chemical events during enamel maturation. Crit Rev.Oral Biol. Med. 1998;9:128–161.

Smith CE, Nanci A. Overview of morphological changes in enamel organ cells associated with major events in amelogenesis. Internat. J. Dev. Biol. 1995;39:153–161.

Ten Cate, AR. Oral Histology Development, Structure, and Function. 4th ed. St. Louis: CV Mosby; 1998.

Thesleff I, Sharpe P. Signalling networks regulating dental development. Mech. Dev. 1997;67(2):111–123.

Tucker AS, Sharpe P. Molecular genetics of tooth morphogenesis and patterning: The right shape in the right place. J. Dent. Res. 1999;78:827–834.

Weiss K, Stock D, Zhao Z. Dynamic interactions and the evolutionary genetics of dental patterning. Crit. Rev. Oral Biol. Med. 1998;9:369–398.

Weiss K, Stock D, Zhao Z, Buchanan A, Ruddle F, Shashikant C. Perspectives on genetic aspects of dental patterning. Eur. J. Oral Sci. 1998;106:(S1):55–63.

6 Development of the Teeth: Root and Supporting Structures

Nagat M. ElNesr and James K. Avery

Introduction

Root development is initiated through the contributions of the cells originating from the enamel organ, dental papilla, and dental follicle. The cells of the outer enamel epithelium contact the inner enamel epithelium at the base of the enamel organ, the cervical loop (Figs. 6.1 and 6.2A). Later, with crown completion, the cells of the cervical loop continue to grow away from the crown and become root sheath cells (Figs. 6.2B and 6.3). The inner root sheath cells cause root formation by inducing the adjacent cells of the dental papilla to become odontoblasts, which in turn will form root dentin. The root sheath will further dictate whether the tooth will have single or multiple roots.

The remainder of the cells of the dental papilla will then become the cells of the root pulp. The third component in root formation, the dental follicle, is the tissue that surrounds the enamel organ, the dental papilla, and the root. It will give rise to cells that form the supporting structures of the tooth—that is, the cementum that forms on the surface of the root, the periodontal ligament, and the surface layer of the alveolar bone. This bone initially encloses the developing crown of the tooth and later surrounds the roots (Fig. 6.3). It attaches to the periodontal ligament fibers, which also attach to the root by means of the cementum.

Objectives

After studying this chapter, details of the following topics should be understood: root formation including origin; functions of the root sheath in the initiation of root dentin and intermediate cementum formation; development of cementum and periodontal ligament; formation of alveolar bone.

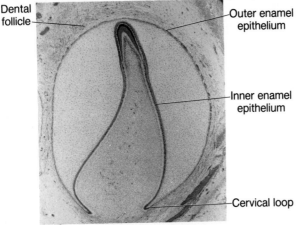

Fig. 6.1 Formation of cervical loop.

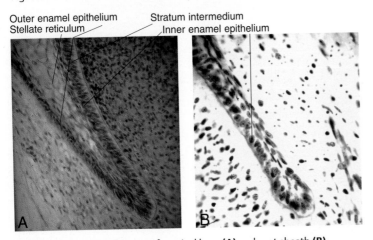

Fig. 6.2 Higher magnification of cervical loop (A) and root sheath (B).

Root Sheath Development

After the crown is completed, the inner and outer enamel epithelium at the base of the cervical loop (Fig. 6.**2A**) proliferate to form a bilayer of epithelial cells called the (Hertwig's) root sheath. The first formed part of the epithelial root sheath bends upward at a 45° angle to form a disc–like structure. This part is called the epithelial diaphragm (Fig. 6.**3**) because it reduces the size of the primary apical opening, which finally becomes the apical foramen. The epithelial diaphragm maintains a constant size during root development because the continuity of the root sheath grows in length at the angle of the diaphragm (Fig. 6.**4A**) and not at its tip. The newly formed vertically disposed part of the epithelial sheath (Fig. 6.**4B**) induces the adjacent cells of the dental papilla to differentiate into odontoblasts, which will form the root dentin (Fig. 6.**4C**). With increased root length, the crown begins to move away from the base of the crypt. This uplifting of the tooth provides space needed for continued root growth. As a result, the epithelial diaphragm maintains its position in relation to the base of the crypt. The root therefore lengthens at the same rate as the tooth moves occlusally (Figs. 6.**5A** and **B**).

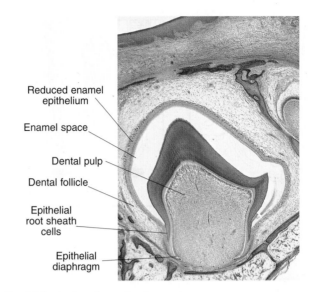

Fig. 6.**3** Beginning of root development.

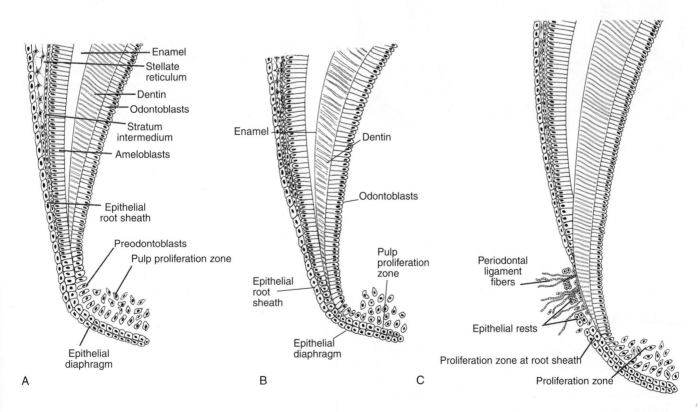

Fig. 6.**4** Formation of epithelial diaphragm. **A** Early epithelial diaphragm formation. **B** Later epithelial diaphragm formation. **C** Later root development.

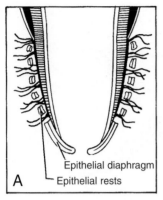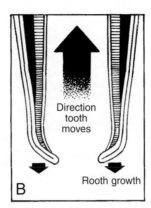

Fig. 6.**5** Root elongation **(A)** and tooth eruption **(B)**.

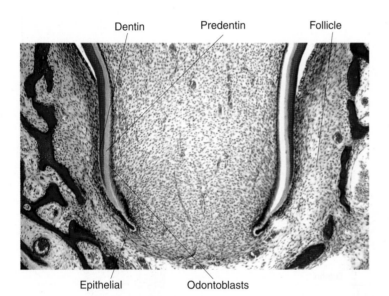

Fig. 6.**6** Root sheath and epithelial diaphragm.

Single-Root Formation

Formation of single-rooted teeth occurs through the growth of the root sheath, like a cuff or tube, around the cells of the dental pulp (Fig. 6.**4B**), followed by development of the root dentin (Fig. 6.**5A**). Cells of the inner layer of the root sheath induce adjacent cells of the dental papilla to differentiate into odontoblasts, which in turn form dentin. The odontoblasts secrete the dentinal matrix in consecutive layers or increments. As the first layer of dentinal matrix mineralizes, the epithelial root sheath cells separate from the surface of the root dentin and breaks occur in its continuity (Fig. 6.**5A**). The breaks are due to the degeneration of some epithelial cells. The separated root sheath cells then begin to migrate away from the root surface, deeper into the follicular area. Mesenchymal or ectomesenchymal cells of the dental follicle then migrate between the remaining epithelial cell groups to contact the root surface. At this surface, they differentiate into cementoblasts and secrete cementum matrix (cementoid), which subsequently mineralizes to form cementum. As root cementum forms, the remaining cells of the root sheath in that area migrate farther away from the root surface. They persist in the developing periodontal ligament as (Malassez's) epithelial rests (Fig. 6.**5A**). Root elongation continues progressively, with proliferation of the remaining root sheath cells at the base of the angle of the epithelial diaphragm. This is accompanied by proliferation of the adjacent cells of the dental papilla and dental follicle (Fig. 6.**6**). As the root lengthens the compensatory movement of eruption provides space for further root development (Fig. 6.**5B**).

The root sheath is never seen as a continuous layer because it breaks down rapidly once root dentin begins to form. The zone of the epithelial diaphragm, however, remains constant and is the last part of the root sheath to degenerate after root completion. The process of root development continues after the tooth has erupted into the oral cavity.

Clinical Application

The presence of the root sheath initiates development of the root and determines the size and shape of the root, its length, and whether the root will be curved or straight. Before root formation occurs, the root sheath must be present. Its interruption may result in root deformities.

Multiple-Root Formation

Human multirooted teeth have in common a root trunk, which is the area of common root base located between the cervical enamel and the area at which root division occurs (Figs. 6.**7** and 6.**10**). Development of multirooted teeth proceeds in much the some manner as development of single-rooted teeth, until the furcation zone is complete (Figs. 6.**7** and 6.**10**). Division of the root takes place through differential growth of the root sheath. In the region of the epithelial diaphragm, tongue–like extensions develop (Fig. 6.**7**) and grow until contact is made with one or two opposing extensions that fuse with each other. This divides the original single opening of the root trunk into two or three openings. The epithelium then continues to proliferate at an equal rate at the perimeter of each of the openings and forms epithelial diaphragms and cuffs to map the individual roots as they elongate. The areas of contact of the tongue–like extensions form epithelial bridges at the furcation zone (Fig. 6.**8**). A view of a section through the future bifurcation zone at a higher magnification is seen in Figure 6.**9**. At

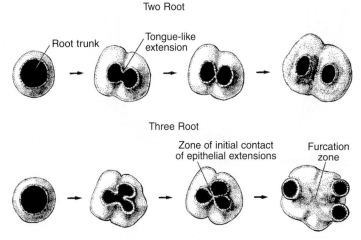

Fig. 6.**7** Multiple-root development. Note that the number of tongue–like extensions dividing the single root on the left is equal to the number of roots to be formed on the right.

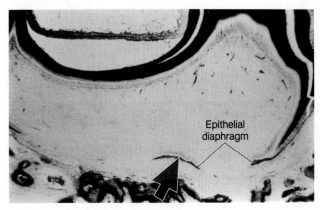

Fig. 6.**8** Development of furcation zone. Bifurcation bridge (arrow).

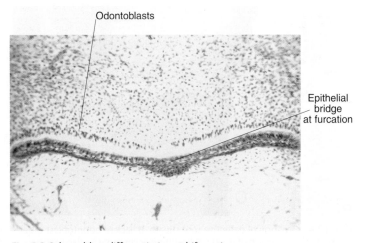

Fig. 6.**9** Odontoblast differentiation at bifurcation zone.

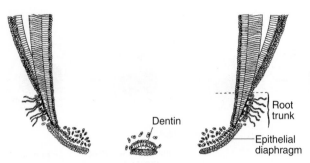

Fig. 6.**10** Formation of root trunk.

each bridge, the inner cells of the epithelial root sheath induce formation of odontoblasts, which in turn will produce a "span" of dentin between and around each root (Fig. 6.**10**). Odontoblasts continue to differentiate along the coronal pulpal floor. Dentin formation will then follow the root sheath and produce multiple roots (Fig. 6.**11**). Some root sheath cells will then degenerate in the same manner as in single-root formation (Fig. 6.**11**), which will provide space for cementoblasts to deposit cementum on the root surface.

Root Formation Anomalies

The continuity of the epithelial root sheath and the timing of its proliferation and degeneration are believed to be essential to normal root formation. If the continuity of the root sheath were broken before dentin formation, the result could be missing or defective epithelial cells. Odontoblasts would then not differentiate, and dentin would not form opposite the defect in the root sheath (Fig. 6.**12A**). The result would be a small lateral canal connecting the periodontal ligament with the main root canal. This supplemental canal is called an accessory root canal and may occur anywhere along the root, particularly in the apical third (Figs. 6.**12B** and **C**). Defects also are seen in the furcation area of multirooted teeth. These are due to incomplete fusion of the tongue–like extensions of the epithelial diaphragm dividing the root trunk. Accessory root canals are therefore seen at this site.

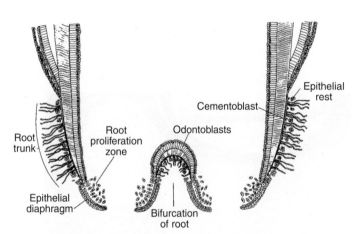

Fig. 6.**11** Development of individual root.

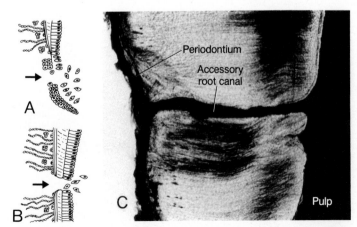

Fig. 6.**12 A** Formation of defective root sheath. **B** Lack of odontoblast differentiation and formation of dentin. **C** Resulting accessory canal in mature tooth.

If, on the other hand, the epithelial root sheath does not degenerate at the proper time and remains adherent to the surface of the root dentin (Fig. 6.**13A**), mesenchymal cells of the dental follicle will not come into contact with the dentin. There would then be no differentiation into cementoblasts and no cementum formation, resulting in areas of the root being devoid of cementum (Fig. 6.**13B**). Areas of exposed root dentin may be found in any area of the root surface, particularly in the cervical zone (Fig. 6.**13B**), and may be the cause of cervical sensitivity later in life when gingival recession takes place.

The epithelial root sheath may also remain adherent to the dentin in the cervical area near the furcation zone. In this case, the inner cells of the root sheath may differentiate into functional ameloblasts and produce enamel droplets known as enamel pearls. Enamel pearls often are found lodged between the roots of the permanent molars (Fig. 6.**14**).

If the epithelial root sheath becomes dislocated after partial root mineralization, the remaining portion of the root may eventually be bent or twisted resulting in a condition called dilaceration or root distortion. This condition is seen more in the permanent dentition. Usually it is caused by a blow on a deciduous predecessor resulting in displacement of the underlying, partly mineralized permanent tooth. A dilacerated root may prevent tooth eruption and also causes orthodontic and extraction problems.

Fate of the Epithelial Root Sheath (Hertwig's Sheath)

After dentin formation the epithelial root sheath breaks down, and its remnants migrate away from the dentinal surface. These remnants come to lie some distance from the root, in the periodontal ligament, and become known as the epithelial rests of Malassez. These cells persist in the periodontal ligaments throughout life. They are often found near the apical zone in young individuals up to 20 years of age. Later these cells tend to be seen more in the cervical areas of the tooth. This could be because the epithelial cells have an inherent characteristic of moving toward the surface and exfoliating. In humans, some of the epithelial cell remnants of the root sheath may become trapped in bay–like depressions between the dentin and cellular cementum, forming what is known as enameloid or intermediate cementum.

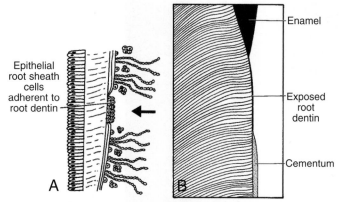

Fig. 6.**13 A** Root sheath cells fused to dentin. **B** Area of exposed dentin.

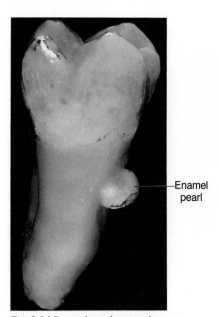

Fig. 6.**14** Enamel pearl on tooth root.

Clinical Application

Accessory root canals can spread infection from one site to another. Infection may occur initially in the tooth pulp and be transmitted to the periodontal space, or it may start from infection in the periodontium and pass to the pulp tissue.

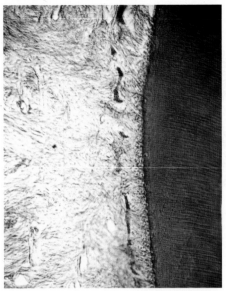

Fig. 6.**15** Development of epithelial rests.

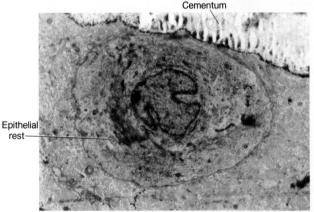

Fig. 6.**16** Electron micrograph shows the ultrastructure of an epithelial rest, with desmosomes between adjacent cells.

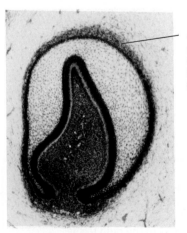

Fig. 6.**17** Dental follicle in developing tooth.

Microscopically, epithelial rests appear either as a network of epithelial strands along the root surface, as isolated islands of cells surrounded by connective tissue (Fig. 6.**15**), or as isolated cells in close contact with the cementum. Three types of epithelial rests develop: proliferating, resting, and degenerating. This description is dependent on whether the epithelial rests are in the process of dividing, inactive, or undergoing cell lysis.

Ultrastructurally, the epithelial cells are surrounded by basal lamina and hemidesmosomes. Each cluster is composed of a few irregularly shaped cells with ovoid, oblong, or indented nuclei (Fig. 6.**16**). The cytoplasm is rather dense with mitochondria, ribosomes, and tonofilaments appearing singly or in bundles. These are seen anchored to attachment plaques at sites of desmosomes and hemidesmosomes. Dense granules are also seen in the cytoplasm. When singly present, the epithelial cell has a uniform shape surrounded by a basal lamina with a smooth and round nucleus outline. When chronic inflammation or other pathologic conditions occur, the epithelial rests may proliferate into cysts or tumors. Degenerated epithelial cells, however, may form a nidus for calcified bodies contributing to the formation of a cementicle in the periodontal ligament.

Currently, the physiologic role of epithelial rests is unknown. The behavior of these cells is said to be species dependent. In teeth of persistent growth, such as a rat incisor, where collagen turnover is rapid, the epithelial rests are reported to degrade collagen by phagocytosis. In vitro studies have also shown procine epithelial rests to phagocytose collagen.

Dental Follicle

The dental follicle (sac) is the ectomesenchymal condensation that initially surrounds the enamel organ and the enclosed dental papilla (Fig. 6.**17**). Later, it surrounds the crown and eventually the tooth root. Cells of the dental sac initiate the development of the supporting tissues of the tooth (Fig. 6.**17**). They arise from the area near the outer enamel epithelium and migrate peripherally. Cells of the sac will therefore give rise to cells that produce cementum, the periodontal ligament, and the alveolar bone (crypt or alveolus). Dental follicular cells thus control the formation of future periodontal structures and are first apparent in very early developmental stages.

At all stages of development, teeth are protected and stabilized by follicular tissue. When the tooth germs of the permanent (successional) teeth first appear, they are in the same dental sac as their deciduous predecessors (Fig. 6.**18A**). This relationship is maintained until the deciduous teeth begin to erupt. The permanent tooth germs then develop separate sacs within separate crypts (Fig. 6.**18B**). A crypt is the bony cavity enclosing a developing tooth and is formed by the dental sac. Each crypt has an opening in its roof through which dental sac fibers extend for communication with the oral mucosa. The fibrous extension of the dental sac, which connects the permanent tooth germ to the oral mucosa, is called the gubernacular cords (Figs. 6.**19** and 6.**20**). Some authorities believe that after the eruption of the deciduous teeth the gubernacular cords lie in bony canals known as gubernacular canals, which are extensions of the bony crypts of the successional teeth. Although the gubernacular cord is formed of fibrous tissue (extension of the tooth sac), it may contain epithelial cells, possibly remnants of the dental lamina (Fig. 6.**20**). Some of these remnants proliferate and form small epithelial masses composed of keratinized material and known as epithelial pearls, epithelial cell nests, or cysts. The dental sac (follicle) initially surrounds the young tooth (Fig. 6.**21**). As the root forms and the tooth erupts, the follicular tissue becomes the supportive tissue of the teeth: the cementum, the periodontal ligament, and the supporting alveolar bone. Therefore, the functions of the dental sac are: to protect and stabilize the tooth during formation and later eruption; to provide nutrition and nerve supply to the developing tooth; and to give rise to the cells that form the cementum, the periodontal ligament, and the inner wall of the bony crypt or alveolus.

It has been proven that the function of the follicular cells is regulated by many autocrine and paracrine actions of local factors such as prostaglandins, epidermal growth factor, transforming growth factor, etc.

Also, it is now known that the dental follicle plays a key role in tooth eruption, as its removal causes complete cessation of eruption (see Chapter 7).

Fig. 6.**18** Development of bony crypt. **A** Relationship of primary and permanent tooth buds in early development. **B** Relationship of primary and permanent tooth buds in later development.

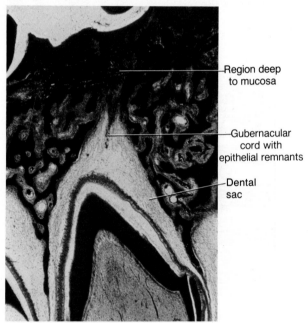

Fig. 6.**19** Eruption pathway

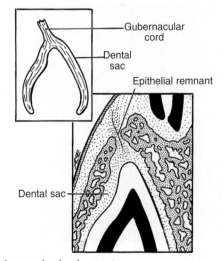

Fig. 6.**20** Gubernacular development.

Clinical Application

The dental follicle is important because it contributes to each of the supporting tissues of the tooth root, the periodontal ligament, cementum, and alveolar bone. The formative cells of these structures are important in the initiation, formation, and maintenance of these tissues.

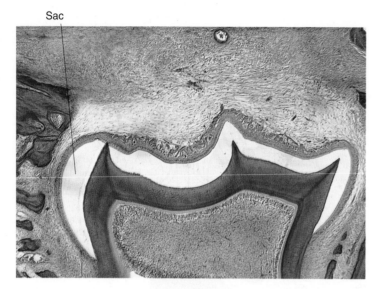

Sac

Fig. 6.**21** Tooth in crypt.

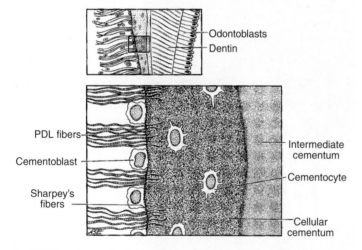

Odontoblasts
Dentin

PDL fibers
Cementoblast
Sharpey's fibers

Intermediate cementum
Cementocyte
Cellular cementum

Fig. 6.**22** Development of intermediate cementum. PDL: periodontal ligament.

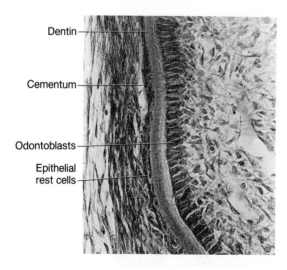

Dentin
Cementum
Odontoblasts
Epithelial rest cells

Fig. 6.**23** Histology of early cementum and dentin formation.

Development of (Intermediate) Cementum

Just before the degeneration of the epithelial root sheath, root dentin is deposited adjacent to it as a thin, amorphous, structureless, and highly mineralized secretion appears on the surface of the root dentin. This substance is devoid of collagen but contains tryptophan, an amino acid, also found in the enamel matrix. Its consistency is similar to that of the thin layer of peripheral enamel, aprismatic enamel. This secretion is more evident in the apical region of the root and averages some 10 to 20 μm in thickness. The deposit is believed to be formed by the root sheath cells, just before they break up and begin migration from the root surface. This cementum is deposited on the root surface and functions to attach the secondary cementum to its surface (Fig. 6.**22**). Recently, it has been reported that this substance may contain occasional epithelial cells. The root sheath cells have an odontoblast-stimulating ability as well as possible secretory functions in producing the intermediate cementum.

Cellular and Acellular Cementum

After root sheath cells begin migration, the ectomesenchyme cells from the dental follicle then contact the surface of the intermediate cementum and begin the formation of cementum. Cementum then covers the roots and functions to attach the periodontal ligament fiber bundles.

Cementogenesis proceeds at a slower pace than that of the development of adjacent root dentin (Figs. 6.**23** and 6.**24**). The cementoblasts exhibit features characteristic of cells capable of protein synthesis and secretion. They have a well-developed, rough-surfaced endoplasmic reticulum, a notable Golgi apparatus, numerous mitochondria, a large nucleus that contains prominent nucle-

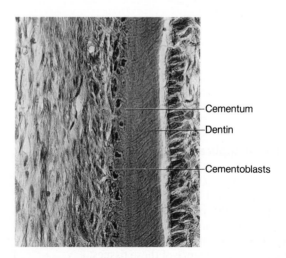

Cementum
Dentin
Cementoblasts

Fig. 6.**24** Development of cellular cementum.

oli, and abundant cytoplasm (Fig. 6.**25**). The newly differentiated cementoblasts first elaborate the organic matrix or cementoid. This matrix consists of collagen fibers and a ground substance with two components. The first is proleaglycans, consisting of glycosaminoglycans with predominance of the sulfated type attached to a core of protein. The second is glycoproteins. The collagen fibers produced by the cementoblasts are called the intrinsic fibers. They run parallel to the cementum surface in an irregular manner. Next, the organic matrix is mineralized and cementum is laid down in successive layers or increments until a predetermined thickness is reached. Thereafter, the cementoblasts enter a quiescent state near the cementum front, ready to function according to need, whether for further growth or repair. Adjacent fibroblasts elaborate collagen fibers, which become embedded in the cementum matrix, to provide attachment of the tooth to the surrounding bone. The embedded portions of the periodontal ligament fibers in the cementum are known as perforating fibers or Sharpey's fibers (Fig. 6.**22**). These are the extrinsic fibers of the cementum and run at right angles to the root surface (Fig. 6.**28**).

Cementum is described as either cellular or acellular, depending on whether it contains cells in its matrix. The behavior of cementoblasts during matrix formation determines the type of cementum to be formed. Cellular cementum develops when some of the cementoblasts elaborating the matrix become embedded in it as cementocytes (Fig. 6.**28**). Acellular cementum, on the other hand, develops when all the cementoblasts retreat into the periodontal ligament, leaving no trapped cells behind. Generally, acellular cementum covers the cervical half of the root dentin whereas cellular cementum is found on the apical half. However, layers of acellular and cellular cementum may alternate at any site (Fig. 6.**26**). In cellular cementum, trapped cementoblasts develop cytoplasmic processes (Fig. 6.**25**) and reside in the cementum matrix to become cementocytes.

Development of the Periodontal Ligament

The periodontal ligament originates from the dental follicle and is the specialized, soft, connective-tissue ligament that provides the attachment for the teeth to the adjacent alveolar bone. Its fibers are embedded in the cementum on the tooth's surface and in the alveolar bone at the other end.

Some delicate fiber bundles of the forming periodontal ligament first appear as root formation begins. At this time, the follicular cells show increased proliferative activity. The innermost cells near the forming root differentiate into cementoblasts and lay down cementum. The outermost cells differentiate into osteoblasts and furnish the lining of the bony socket (Fig. 6.**27**). The more centrally located cells in the ligament differentiate into fibroblasts. These produce collagen fibers that will

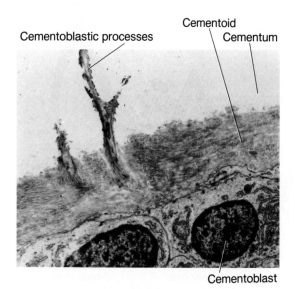

Fig. 6.**25** Ultrastructure of early cementum.

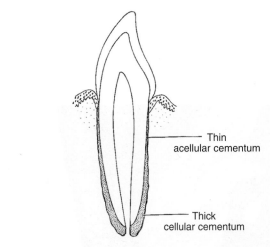

Fig. 6.**26** Cemental deposition pattern.

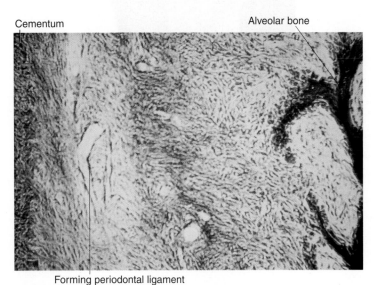

Fig. 6.**27** Differentiation of periodontal ligament.

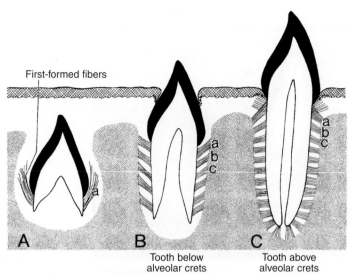

First-formed fibers

A   B   C

Tooth below
alveolar crets

Tooth above
alveolar crets

Fig. 6.**28** Formation of periodontal ligament. **A** Relation of periodontal fibers on unerupted crown. **B** Relation of periodontal fibers during intraoral eruption. **C** Relation of fibers in the adult tooth. Note the orientation of the first-formed fibers in **A**, **B**, and **C**.

become embedded in both forming cementum and bone. At first, all the developing fibers of the periodontal ligament run obliquely in a coronal direction, from tooth to bone (Fig.6.**28A**). The apical fibroblasts are the stem cells that proliferate and migrate cervically to form the first group of collagen fibers. As tooth eruption proceeds, the obliquity of the fibers gradually decreases and the position of the cementoenamel junction, which was originally apical to the crest of the crypt (Fig. 6.**28A**), becomes level and then coronal to the alveolar crest (Fig. 6.**28B** and **C**). This change between the cementoenamel junction and alveolar crest may relate to their functional role during tooth eruption. It also brings about the final arrangement of the principal fiber groups of the mature periodontal ligament (Figs. 6.**28A–C**).

The periodontal ligament is in a continuous state of remodeling, both during development and throughout the life-span of the tooth. The ligament persistently maintains support of an erupting or functioning tooth (Fig. 6.**29**). Remodeling is achieved by fibroblasts that rapidly synthesize and secrete collagen. Rapid turnover of collagen takes place throughout the whole thickness of the ligament, from bone to cementum. Turnover is not restricted to the metabolically active middle zone, which is sometimes referred to as the intermediate plexus. There is a differential rate of collagen turnover in the ligament, in an apicocervical direction. The highest turnover is in the apical region, and the lowest in the cervical region of the ligament. Maturation and thickening of the fiber bundles of the periodontal ligament occur as the teeth reach functional occlusion.

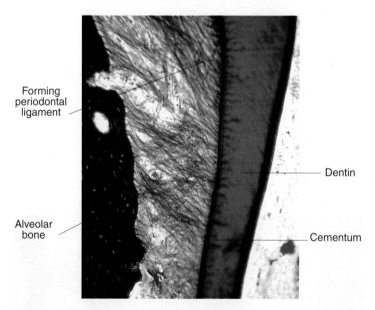

Forming
periodontal
ligament

Alveolar
bone

Dentin

Cementum

Fig. 6.**29** Differentiation of periodontal ligament fibers.

Development of the Alveolar Process

The alveolar bone develops as the tooth develops. Initially, this bone forms a thin eggshell of support, termed the tooth crypt, around each tooth germ (Fig. 6.**30**). Gradually, as the roots grow and lengthen, the alveolar bone keeps pace with the elongating and erupting tooth and maintains a relation with each tooth root (Figs. 6.**27** and 6.**31**).

Development of the alveolar process begins in the eighth week in utero. At that time, within the maxilla and the mandible the forming alveolar bone develops a horseshoe-shaped groove. The bony groove, or canal, is formed by growth of the facial and lingual plates of the body of the maxillae or mandible and contains the developing tooth germs together with the alveolar blood vessels and nerves (Fig. 6.**30**). At first, the developing tooth germs lie free in the groove. Gradually, bony septa develop between teeth, so that each tooth is eventually contained in a separate crypt (Fig. 6.**30**). The actual alveolar process develops during eruption of the teeth (Figs. 6.**28** and 6.**31**).

During uterine life, the dental alveolus, like the rest of the skeleton, is formed from an embryonic type of bone composed of tiny, bony spicules (Figs. 6.**30** and 6.**31**). This embryonic bone is of two types, woven bone and coarse bundle bone. Both types contain collagen bundles in their matrix. The main difference, however, is that in woven bone the bundles of collagen run in various directions in the matrix, while in coarse bundle bone, the collagen bundles are thicker and usually follow a parallel course in the matrix. The matrix of embryonic bone contains more glycosaminoglycans and glycoproteins than that of mature bone.The embryonic bone is, however, of temporary existence being gradually replaced by mature or lamellar bone of the compact or spongy type.

Mature bone is composed of layers (lamellae) arranged in an orderly manner. It is also characterized by its fine fiber arrangement, its fewer cells, and histologically by its uniform density and by the fact that its matrix stains evenly and lightly.

The bone between the roots of adjacent single-rooted or multirooted teeth is termed the interdental septum. The bone between the roots of a multirooted tooth is known as interradicular bone or septum (Fig. 6.**32**).

In its mature form, the alveolar bone is composed of two parts, the alveolar bone proper and the supporting

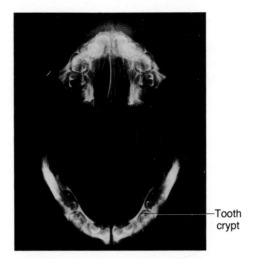

Tooth crypt

Fig. 6.**30** Formation of alveolar bone.

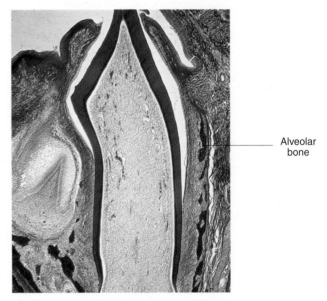

Alveolar bone

Fig. 6.**31** Bone development around erupting tooth.

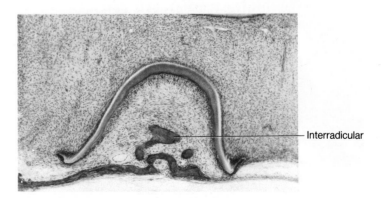

Interradicular

Fig. 6.**32** Development of interradicular bone.

Clinical Application

Alveolar bone resorption occurs more readily than permanent tooth root loss. Resorption of alveolar bone and primary tooth roots is necessary, however, before permanent tooth eruption can take place.

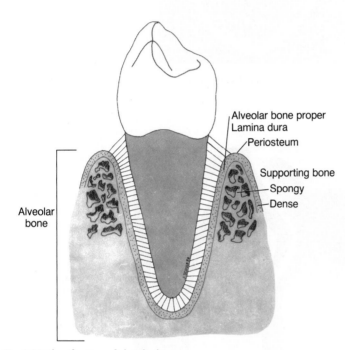

Fig. 6.**33** Classification of alveolar bone.

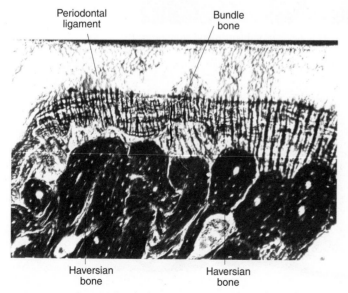

Fig. 6.**34** Histology of alveolar bone proper: Haversian and bundle.

bone (Fig. 6.**33**). The alveolar bone proper is a thin lamella of compact bone that lines the root socket, and in which the periodontal fibers are embedded. It is known radiographically as the lamina dura. The supporting bone consists of both spongy and dense (compact) bone and functions in support of the alveolar bone proper. The cortical plate, or covering of the mandible or maxilla, furnishes the compact portion of the supporting alveolar bone (Fig. 6.**33**).

The alveolar bone proper is a specialized type of dense bone composed of bundle bone and Haversian bone that appears noticeably radiopaque on X-ray and is therefore called the lamina dura. The bundle bone is so named because it is penetrated by bundles of periodontal ligament fibers (Fig. 6.**34**). The alveolar bone proper is formed by osteogenic cells in the outermost layer of the dental follicle. These differentiate into osteoblasts and lay down the bone matrix or osteoid in which some osteoblasts become embedded as osteocytes. The matrix then calcifies to form mature bone.

In all bony tissues a system of cell-to-cell communication exists between adjacent bone cells, for example osteogenic cells, osteoblasts, and osteocytes. This cell-to-cell communication takes place by three means.

1. Presence of junctional complex (gap) between the different cells.
2. Presence of cytoskeleton at opposing points of adjacent cells.
3. Presence of small nerve fibers in the periosteum.

These may work together to produce effective cell communication and coordination of cellular activity.

Summary

Root development begins after enamel formation nears completion and has reached the cementoenamel junction. An extension of the enamel organ has an important role in root development by forming the epithelial root sheath, which consists of an epithelial extension of the cervical loop (Fig. 6.**35**). The epithelial diaphragm is the bent first-formed part of the root sheath.

The inner cells of the sheath induce the adjacent mesenchymal cells to differentiate into odontoblasts, which form the root dentin. The cells of the root sheath also form a thin, structureless layer of cementum on the dentin and then begin to degenerate. As a result, three types of epithelial rests develop: proliferating, resting, and degenerating. These rests are present in the periodontal ligament along the root surface throughout life.

Development of the supporting tissues of the tooth and root development occur simultaneously. The cementum, periodontal ligament, and bone of the inside lining of the crypts or alveoli have a common origin, the cells of the dental follicle.

Root and cementum development may be divided into four phases (Fig. 6.**36**). Phase I is the formation of root sheath. In phase II, as the dentin is formed internal to the root sheath, a layer of intermediate cementum is deposited. The function of the root sheath is then complete and the sheath breaks up into rests. In phase III, mesenchymal cells appear and differentiate into cementoblasts that lay down the first layer of cementum. Periodontal ligament fibers, called perforating or Sharpey's fibers, become enmeshed in the cementum along the root surface. They will become the means of attachment of the principle fibers of the periodontal ligament. In phase IV, further layers of cementum are deposited. Finally, the epithelial rests move farther from the root, into the periodontal ligament.

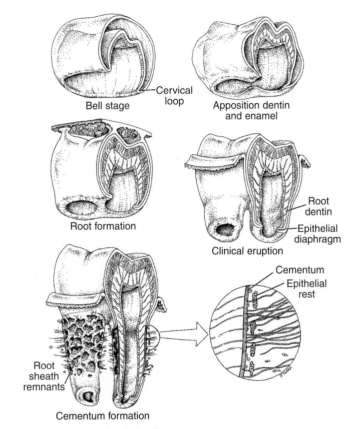

Fig. 6.**35** Summary of root development.

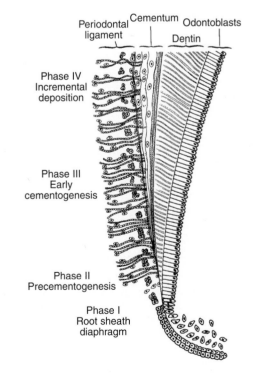

Fig. 6.**36** Summary of cementum formation.

Self-Evaluation Review

1. Describe the reduced enamel epithelium.
2. What cells are responsible for initiation of root development?
3. Define the root trunk.
4. Describe and define the furcation zone.
5. Describe two differences between the cervical loop and epithelial diaphragm.
6. What is the origin of the layer of intermediate cementum?
7. Define the dental follicle and name several of its functions.
8. Describe the arrangement of the principle fiber bundles.
9. Name a possible reason for the development of an accessory canal?
10. How does eruption compensate for root growth?

Suggested Readings

Davidson D, McCullooch CAG. Proliferative behaviour of periodontal ligament cell populations. J. Periodont. Res. 1986;21:444.

Gemenov VV. Histological characteristics of the rests of Malassez in the human periodontium. Stromatology. 1980;59:9.

Lindskog S. Formation of intermediate cementum I: early mineralization of aprismatic enamel and intermediate cementum in monkey. J. Craniofac. Genet. Dev. Biol. 1982;147–160.

Lindskog S. Formation of intermediate cementum II: a scanning electron microscope study of the epithelial root sheath of Hertwig in monkey. J. Craniofac. Genet. Dev. Biol. 1982;2:161–169.

Lindskog S. Formation of intermediate cementum III: 3H RTryptophan and 3H proline uptake into epithelial root sheath of Hertwig in vivo. J. Craniofac. Genet. Dev. 1982;2:171–177.

Melcher AH, Bowen WH, eds. The Biology of the Periodontium. New York, NY: New York Press inc.; 1969.

Sims MR. Ultrastructure of the mocrofibril components of mouse and human periodontal oxytalan fibers. Connect Tissue Res. 1984;13:59–67.

Stern IB. Current concepts of the dentogingival junction: the epithelial and connective tissue attachment to the tooth. J. Periodont. 1981;9:465–475.

Van der Linden FPGM, Duterloo HS. Development of the Human Dentition. New York, NY: Harper and Rowe; 1976.

Wise G, Marks Sandy C Jr., Cahill D, Dorski P. Ultrastructural features of the dental follicle and enamel organ prior to and during tooth eruption. Z. Davidovich (ed), Biological mechanisms of tooth eruption and root resorption. Birmingham: EBSCO Media; 1988:243–251.

Yamasaki A, Rose CG, Pinero G, Mahan CJ. Microfilaments in human cementoblasts and periodontal fibroblasts. J. Periodont. 1987;58:40–45.

7 Tooth Eruption and Shedding

Nagat M. ElNesr and James K. Avery

Introduction

Eruption is the movement of the developing teeth within and through the bone and the overlying mucosa of the jaws to appear in the oral cavity and reach the occlusal plane. Eruptive movements begin with the onset of root formation, well before the teeth are seen in the oral cavity. The emergence of the tooth through the gingiva is merely the first clinical sign of eruption. Following emergence, the teeth erupt at a maximum rate to reach the occlusal plane; they then continue to erupt at a slower rate to compensate for jaw growth and occlusal wear.

Movements leading to tooth eruption can be divided into three phases: the preeruptive phase, the prefunctional eruptive phase or eruptive phase, and the functional eruptive or posteruptive phase. All three can usually be observed at the same time in the various teeth in a dentition.

Objectives

The objective of this chapter is to familiarize you with tooth eruption by describing its three phases: preeruptive, prefunctional, and functional. You will obtain information on initial growth of the tooth relating to compensational changes in the crypt and on the development of the supporting fiber system. Later, during functional occlusion, minute changes taking place apically and elsewhere in the support system are described.

Movements Leading to Tooth Eruption

Preeruptive Phase

The preeruptive phase of tooth movement is preparatory to the eruptive phases. It consists of the movements to the developing and growing tooth germs within the alveolar process before root formation (Fig. 7.**1**). During this phase, the growing teeth move in various directions to maintain their position in the expanding jaws. This is accomplished by both bodily movement and eccentric growth. Bodily movement is a shift of the entire tooth germ, which causes bone resorption in the direction of tooth movement and bone apposition from behind (Figs.

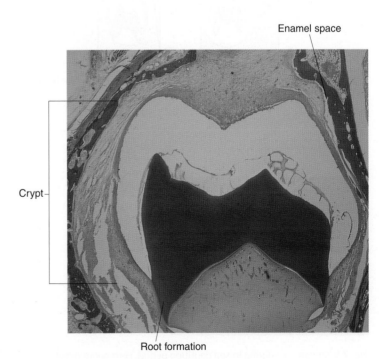

Fig. 7.**1** Preeruptive phase of tooth eruption.

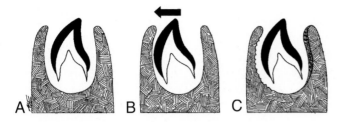

Fig. 7.**2 A–C** Bodily movement of crown during preeruptive phase.

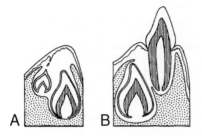

Fig. 7.**3** Relative position of primary and permanent teeth in **(A)** preeruptive and **(B)** eruptive phases.

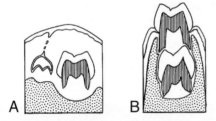

Fig. 7.**4** Relative position of primary molar and permanent premolar teeth in **(A)** preeruptive and **(B)** eruptive phases.

7.**2A–C**). These movements occur continuously as the jaws grow. Eccentric growth refers to relative growth in one part of the tooth, while the rest of the tooth remains constant. As a result, the center of the tooth changes. These movements relate to the adjustments that each crown must make in relation to its neighbor, and to the jaws as they increase in width, height, and length. The primary teeth in the alveolar process therefore move in a facial and occlusal direction or in the direction of the growth of the face. At the same time, there is some mesial as well as distal movement. The permanent teeth also move within the jaws to adjust their position in the growing alveolar process.

Early in the preeruptive phase, the successional permanent teeth develop lingual to, and near the incisal or occlusal level of, their primary predecessors (Figs. 7.**3A** and 7.**4A**). At the end of this phase, the developing anterior permanent teeth are positioned lingually and near the apical third of the primary anterior teeth (Fig.7.**3B**). The premolars are located under the roots of the primary molars (Fig. 7.**4B**). The change in position of the permanent tooth germs is mainly the result of the eruption of the primary teeth and the coincident increase in height of the supporting tissues, and not of the apical movement of the permanent tooth germs. The permanent molars, having no primary predecessors, develop without this kind of relation. The upper molars develop in the tuberosities of the maxilla, with their occlusal surfaces slanting distally (Fig.7.**5**). The lower molars develop in the base of the mandibular rami, and their occlusal surfaces slant mesially (Fig. 7.**5**). The permanent molars undergo considerable eccentric movement, adjusting their positions as the jaws and the alveolar processes grow. Note that all movements in this phase take place within the crypts of the developing and growing crowns before root formation. The preeruptive and prefunctional phases overlap to some extent, but proceed in the following order: preeruptive, prefunctional, functional.

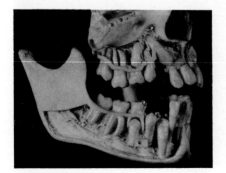

Fig. 7.**5** Human jaws during mixed dentition period. Permanent maxillary molar in tuberosity.

Prefunctional Eruptive Phase

The prefunctional eruptive phase begins with the initiation of root formation and ends when the teeth reach occlusal contact. Five major events take place during this phase.

1. The secretory phase of amelogenesis is completed just before the onset of root formation and prefunctional eruption. There is a relation between the cessation of mineralization and activation of the epithelial cells beyond the enamel-forming area.
2. The intraosseous stage occurs when the root formation begins as a result of the proliferation of both the epithelial root sheath and the mesenchymal tissue of the dental papilla and dental follicle (Fig. 7.**6**).
3. The supraosseous stage begins when the erupting tooth moves occlusally through the bone of the crypt and the connective tissue of the oral mucosa, so that the reduced enamel epithelium covering the crown comes into contact with the oral epithelium (Fig. 7.**7**). As this occurs, the reduced enamel epithelium of the crown proliferates and forms a firm attachment with the oral epithelium. A fused, double epithelial layer over the erupting crown is then formed (Fig. 7.**8**).
4. The tip of the crown enters the oral cavity by breaking through the center of the double-layered epithelial cells. This breakthrough is accomplished by the cusp tip

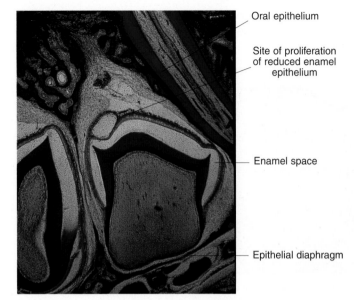

Fig. 7.**6** Prefunctional eruptive phase in formation of root.

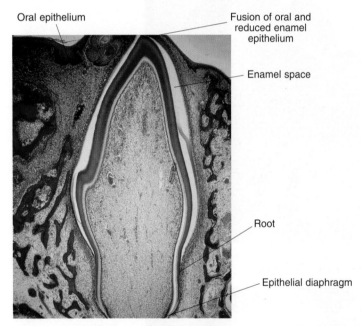

Fig. 7.**7** Crown tip approaching oral epithelium.

Fig. 7.**8** Contact and fusion of reduced enamel epithelium and oral mucosa.

Clinical Application

In infants, tooth eruption may be accompanied by a slight temperature increase, mild irritation of the gums, and general malaise. Any severe general symptoms, however, should not be associated with teething, although some systemic disturbance at the time of tooth eruption should be expected. An altered tissue space or compartment overlying the tooth becomes visible as an inverted, funnel-shaped area (Fig. 7.**11**). In the periphery of this zone, the follicle fibers direct themselves toward the mucosa and are defined as the gubernaculum dentis or gubernacular cord (Figs. 7.**10** and 7.**12**). Some authors believe that this structure guides the tooth in its eruptive movements.

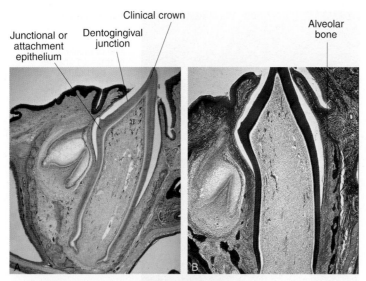

Fig. 7.**9** Clinical appearance of the crown.

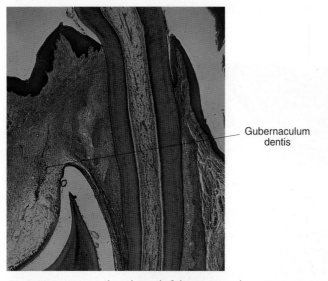

Fig. 7.**10** Primary tooth at the end of the eruptive phase. Permanent successor in preeruptive phase.

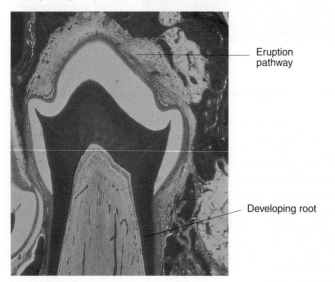

Fig. 7.**11** Development of eruptive pathway overlying the crown.

causing degeneration of the membrane, and is the beginning stage of clinical eruption (Fig.7.9). The crown erupts further, and the lateral borders of the oral mucosa become the dentogingival junction (Fig.7.**9B**). The reduced enamel epithelium, now surrounding the crown like a cuff, becomes known as the junctional or attachment epithelium. When the tip of the crown appears in the oral cavity, about one-half to two-thirds of the roots are formed (Fig. 7.**9A**).

5. The erupting tooth continues to move occlusally at a maximum rate, and there is gradual exposure of more of the clinical crown (Fig. 7.**10**). Occlusal movement is the result of active eruption. As the tooth moves occlusally, gradual exposure of the clinical crown is accomplished through separation of the attachment epithelium from the crown and the resulting apical shift of the gingiva. The clinical crown is the part of the tooth (coronal to the attachment epithelium) exposed in the oral cavity, and differs from the anatomic crown, the part of the tooth covered by enamel. The prefunctional eruptive or eruptive phase is also characterized by significant changes in the tissues overlying the teeth, around the teeth, and underlying the teeth.

Changes in tissues overlying teeth.

The initial change seen in the tissues overlying the teeth before eruption of the crown, is the alteration of the connective tissue of the dental follicle to form a pathway for the erupting tooth. Usually, this is more prominent in erupting permanent teeth. Histologically, the coronal part of the dental follicle becomes heavily populated by numerous monocytes in parallel with osteoclasts to participate in bone resorption and formation of the eruption pathway. The monocyte influx is enhanced by the increased secretion of colony-stimulating factor 1 receptor protein (CSF-1) and by the chemotactic action of the transforming growth factor beta-1 (TGF-beta-1). The future eruption pathway appears as a zone in which connective-tissue fibers have disappeared, cells have degenerated and decreased in number, blood vessels have become fewer, and terminal nerves have broken up and degenerated. These changes are probably the partial result of the loss of blood supply to this area, as well as the release of enzymes that aid in degradation of these tissues. Clinically, tooth eruption may be accompanied by discomfort or pain, irritability, and/or a slight temperature increase.

For successful tooth eruption, there must be some resorption of the overlying bony crypt (Fig. 7.**12**), which is in a constant state of remodeling as the tooth germ enlarges and the face grows anteriorly and laterally. The eruptive process can be considered part of this remodeling growth. Osteoclasts differentiate and resorb a portion of the bony crypt overlying the erupting tooth. The eruption pathway, which at first is small, increases in dimension, allowing movement of the tooth to the oral mucosa (Fig. 7.**12**). Although the eruption of most permanent teeth is similar to that of primary teeth, the overlying primary teeth are an additional complication. The eruptive pathway of permanent incisors and cuspids is lingual to the corresponding primary teeth. This area shows a pronounced enlargement to accommodate the advancing crown.

Small foramina in the mandible and maxilla are evidence of eruption pathways of the anterior permanent teeth. These openings, the gubernacular foramina, are found lingual to the anterior primary teeth and are the sites of the gubernacular cords (Fig. 7.**13**). The premolars are located between the roots of the primary molars. Root resorption in primary teeth proceeds in much the same manner as bone resorption (Fig. 7.**14**). When the roots are fully resorbed, the attachment of the primary crown is lessened and the crown is shed. This produces an eruption pathway for the premolars. Most roots resorb completely; the primary pulps degenerate as well. During the period of mixed dentition (around 6 to 12 years of age), when both primary and permanent teeth are in the mouth, the phenomena of root resorption and tooth formation proceed side by side (Fig. 7.**14**). These changes occur while teeth still maintain chewing efficiency.

When the tooth nears the oral mucosa, the reduced enamel epithelium comes into contact with the overlying mucosa (Fig. 7.**7**). Simultaneously, the oral epithelial cells and reduced enamel epithelial cells proliferate and fuse into one membrane (Fig. 7.**15**). Further movement of the tooth stretches and thins the membrane over the crown tip (Fig. 7.**15**). At this stage the mucosa becomes blanched because of a lack of blood supply to the area. Eruption is a gradual, as well as an intermittent, process. The tooth will erupt slightly, remain stationary for some time, and then erupt again. In this manner, the supporting tissues are able to make adjustments to the eruptive movements. Each eruptive movement results in more of the crown appearing in the oral cavity and further separation of the attachment epithelium from the enamel surface (Figs. 7.**9** and 7.**10**). Recent observations of human premolar eruption revealed eruptive activity occurring mostly at night, with a marked slowing or cessation during the day.

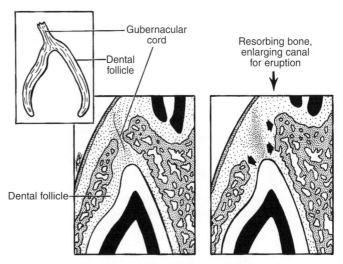

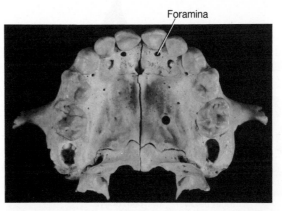

Fig. 7.**12** Developing eruption pathway and gubernaculum dentis.

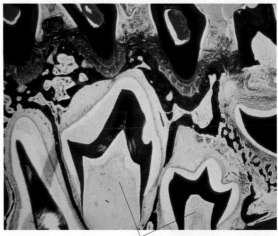

Fig. 7.**13** Eruption sites of permanent teeth (gubernacular foramina) lingual to the primary crowns. Note the tip of the lateral incisor in the foramen.

Fig. 7.**14** Microscopic appearance of the relation of primary and permanent teeth.

▬ Clinical Application ▬

Eruption of the teeth is more genetically determined than environmentally susceptible. Only cases of severe malnutrition, for example, cause delayed eruption.

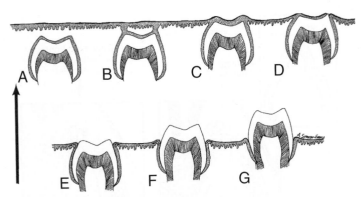

Fig. 7.**15** Summary diagram of fusion and rupture of reduced enamel epithelium and oral epithelium in tooth eruption.

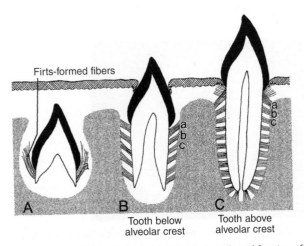

Firts-formed fibers

Tooth below
alveolar crest

Tooth above
alveolar crest

Fig. 7.**16** Development of periodontal fibers and modification of alveolar bone during tooth eruption. **A** Early fiber formation. **B** Bone changes. **C** Further fiber development, near occlusion, with fibers more dense.

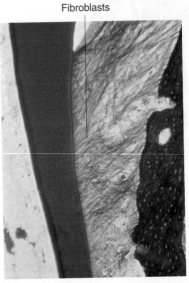

Fibroblasts

Fig. 7.**17** Histology of the periodontal ligament of the erupting tooth.

Changes in tissues around teeth.

The tissues around the teeth also undergo change during tooth eruption. Initially, the dental follicle is composed of delicate connective tissue. Gradually, as eruptive movements commence, collagen fibers become prominent, extending between the forming root and the alveolar bone surface. The first noticeable periodontal fiber bundles appear at the cervical area of the root and extend at an angle coronal to the alveolar process (Fig. 7.**16A**). At the same time, the alveolar bone of the crypt is remodeled to accommodate the forming root. As the large crown moves occlusally, the bone fills in to conform to the smaller root diameter (Figs. 7.**16B** and **C**). As eruption proceeds, other collagen fiber bundles become visible along the forming root (Figs. 7.**16B** and **C**). The area becomes more densely populated with fibroblasts (Fig. 7.**17**). A special type of fibroblast, the myofibroblast, is said to have contractile capabilities. It has been reported to be present in the periodontal ligament. If present, the myofibroblast could aid in the force needed in tooth eruption. All ligament cells and fibers are currently believed to be important in the eruptive process. During eruptive movements, collagen formation and fiber turnover are very rapid (possibly 24 hours). Very early in the eruptive process, perforating fibers attach to the cementum on the root surface and to the alveolar bone. Some fibers release as the tooth moves, then reattach to stabilize the tooth. In this manner, the tooth-stabilizing process is performed by the same groups of fibers throughout tooth eruption. The fibroblasts are the cells active in formation and degeneration of collagen fibers. Alveolar bone remodeling is continuous during eruption. As the tooth moves occlusally, the alveolar bone increases in height and changes shape to accommodate passage of the crown (Fig. 7.**18**). The tooth crown, as seen in Figure 7.**18**, has migrated occlusally, which results in new bone being deposited around the root to reduce the size of the crypt. Above and around the crown, osteoclastic and osteoblastic action occurs. These actions are coordinated during the entire eruption process, as well as throughout life.

Changes in tissue underlying teeth.

Changes also occur in the follicular tissue underlying the developing tooth. These changes take place in the soft tissue and the fundic bone (bone surrounding the apex of the root). As the tooth erupts, space is provided for the root to lengthen, primarily because of the crown moving occlusally and the increase in height of the alveolar bone. Changes in the fundic region are believed to be largely compensatory to the lengthening of the root. During the preeruptive and early eruptive phases, the follicular fibroblasts and fibers lie in a plane parallel to the base of the root (Fig. 7.**19**). The tooth moves more rapidly in the socket during prefunctional eruption than at any other period. Fine bony trabeculae appear in the fundic area. They compensate for tooth eruption and provide some support to the apical tissues (Fig.7.**19**). Some authors describe this as a bony ladder. The ladder becomes more dense as alternate layers of bone plates and connective tissue are laid down (Fig. 7.**20**). At the end of the prefunctional eruptive phase, when the tooth comes into occlusion, about one-third of the enamel remains covered by the gingiva (Fig. 7.**16B**), and the root is incomplete. At this time, the bony ladder is gradually resorbed, one plate at a time, to make space for the developing root tip. Root completion continues for a considerable time after the teeth have been in function; this process takes from 1 to 1.5 years in primary teeth and from 2 to 3 years in permanent teeth.

Functional Eruptive (Posteruptive) Phase

The final, functional, eruptive phase begins when the teeth reach occlusion, and continues for as long as each tooth remains in the oral cavity. During the early phase of this period, the alveolar processes increase in height and the roots continue to grow. The teeth continue to move occlusally, which accommodates jaw growth and allows for root elongation. The most marked changes occur as occlusion is established. Alveolar bone density increases, and the principle fibers of the periodontal ligament establish themselves into separate groups oriented about the gingiva, the alveolar crest, and the alveolar surface around the root.

Clinical Application

A missing tooth may result in tipping of adjacent teeth into the space created by this loss. Premature loss of a primary tooth resulting in this condition may prevent eruption of the permanent tooth or cause its impaction.

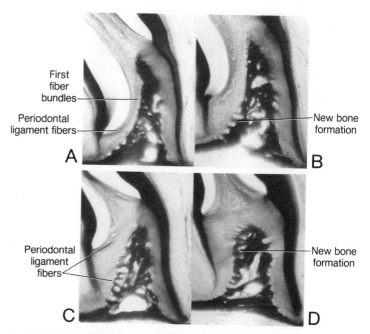

Fig. 7.**18** Principal fiber development in erupting teeth. Note the change in the relations of follicle fibers **(A–D)**, from tooth to bone.

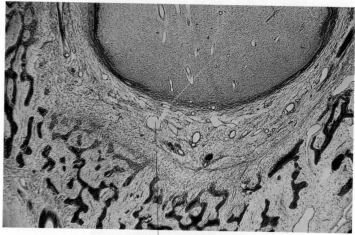

Fig. 7.**19** Changes in fundic bone during eruptive movement.

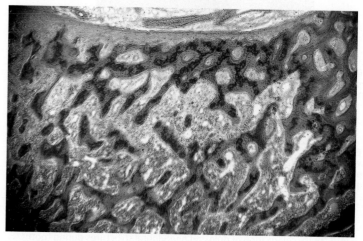

Fig. 7.**20** Formation of bone ladder in the fundic region.

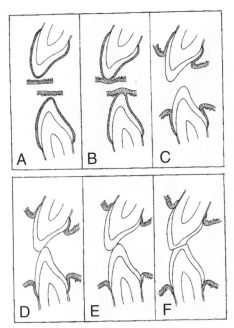

Fig. **7.21** Formation of the junctional epithelium. **A, B** Preeruptive. **C** Prefunctional eruptive phase. **D–F** Functional occlusion.

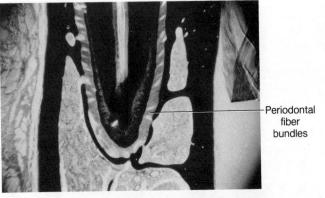

Fig. **7.22** Increased density of periodontal ligament fibers during eruption.

Periodontal fiber bundles

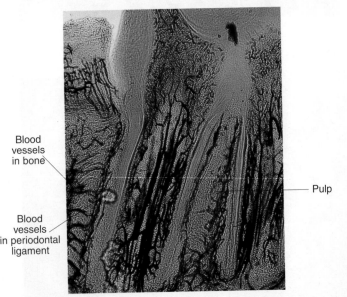

Fig. **7.23** Vascularization of pulp and periodontal structures during tooth eruption.

Blood vessels in bone

Blood vessels in periodontal ligament

Pulp

The diameter of the fiber bundles increase from delicate, fine groups of fibers to heavy, securely stabilized bundles (Fig. 7.**22**). Arteries are established circumferentially and longitudinally, with respect to the tooth, in the central zone of the periodontal ligament. Figure 7.**23** is a photomicrograph of a developing root. India ink outlines each of the blood vessels in the pulp, as well as in the periodontal ligament. Then the tissue is cleared to reveal the vessels. Observe the numerous vessels that enter the ligament from the alveolar bone. Nerves for sensing pain, heat, cold, proprioception, and pressure organize in the periodontal ligament and course alongside these blood vessels. From apex to gingiva, both myelinated and nonmyelinated nerves traverse the central region of the ligament along with the blood vessels (Fig. 7.**24**). When the root canal narrows, as a result of root tip maturation, apical fibers develop to help cushion the forces of occlusal impact (Fig. 7.**22**). Later in life, attrition may wear down the occlusal surfaces of the teeth (Fig. 7.**21**). The teeth erupt slightly to compensate for loss of tooth structure and to prevent occlusal overclosure (Fig. 7.**25**). If the occlusal wear is excessive, cementum is deposited on the apical third of the root (Fig. 7.**25**); it is deposited in the furcation region of molars to compensate for hypereruption of these teeth. Some bone apposition occurs at the alveolar crests. In addition to slight occlusal movement, the teeth tend to move anteriorly. This is termed mesial drift and results in bone resorption on the mesial wall of the socket and bone apposition on the distal wall.

Theories of Tooth Eruption

Many factors related to tooth eruption have been studied, and several appear to be important to the eruptive process. It was once thought that root growth and pulpal pressure were fundamental factors, until cases of eruption of rootless teeth were reported. The idea that the fundic bone area and bony ladder formation were caus-

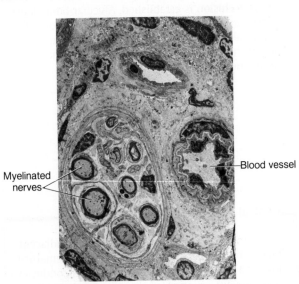

Myelinated nerves

Blood vessel

Fig. **7.24** Ultrastructure of interstitial space in periodontal ligament along with nerves and blood vessels.

es was discounted as measurements of the eruption pathway and the timing of its appearance revealed that these factors are more likely to be a result, rather than a cause of, eruption. Vascularity has long been considered to play a role in tooth eruption. For example, resection of the sympathetic nerves causes vasodilation and results in earlier eruption of teeth. Localized hyperemia, as a result of periodontitis, also causes increased vascularity of periodontal tissues and increased eruption of adjacent teeth. Other factors, such as hypopituitarism, decrease vascularity and also retard eruption.

Important to the discussion of causes of tooth eruption is the tooth at the cap and bell stage. It has been shown that follicular cells migrate from near the surface of the enamel organs and dental papillae to give rise to the cementum, periodontal ligament, and alveolar bone. Because these cells affect the resorption of bone in eccentric growth and bodily movement of the teeth, they probably play a role in tooth eruption. These cells may cause enzymatic degeneration of the tissues overlying the teeth and may contribute to the formation of tissues surrounding and underlying the teeth. Recent studies studies have shown the dental follicle to be of prime importance in tooth eruption. Removal of the dental follicle causes cessation of eruption. The main role of the dental follicle in tooth eruption is the formation of the eruption pathway ahead of the advancing tooth. The follicle also provides the osteoblasts that form the bone trabeculae apical to the tooth. Also, these events all take place at precise times during tooth eruption.

Biochemical analysis revealed that the dental follicle reaches its maximum weight at the time eruption begins. Collagen content increases by 25% and proteoglycans by 45% during eruption. Transforming growth factor beta 1(TGF-beta 1) is a member of a protein family with diverse biologic activities, which stimulates the fibroblast of the dental follicle to secrete an extracellular matrix needed for its development into a peridontal ligament. To date, the role of the epidermal growth factor (EGF) during eruption is not clear. It is, however, said that it stimulates the differentiation of periodontal ligament fibroblasts.

Decreased pressure overlying a tooth and increased pressure around and under it are major factors in tooth eruption. First, the eruption pathway begins development when root formation commences (Fig. 7.**26**). In fact, several investigators have shown that this pathway will develop even when the tooth is mechanically prevented from eruption. Second, remodeling of tissues surrounding the teeth occurs during both prefunctional and functional eruptive periods. As the periodontal ligament fibers increase in number and change position, the alveolar bone remodels and thus limits the soft-tissue space around the teeth. At the same time, the periodontal fibroblasts proliferate and the vascular supply increases (Fig. 7.**27**). All these changes bring about increased pressure around and under the erupting teeth.

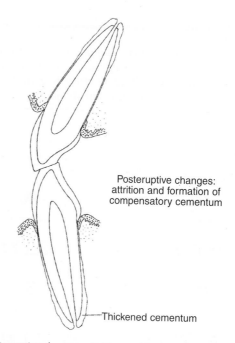

Posteruptive changes: attrition and formation of compensatory cementum

Thickened cementum

Fig. 7.**25** Posteruptive changes: attrition and compensative formation of cementum.

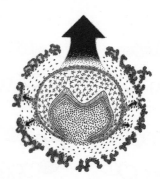

Fig. 7.**26** Cells lying near the outer enamel epithelium migrate into the follicle and aid in periodontal development and eruption of the tooth.

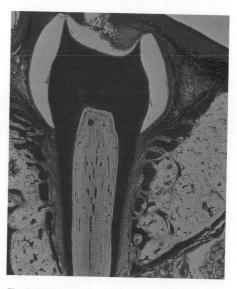

Fig. 7.**27** Increase in cell activity in periodontal ligament during eruption.

Clinical Application

The "six/four" rule for primary tooth emergence means that from birth four teeth will emerge for each 6 months of age. Thus, age 6 months = 4 teeth, 12 months = 8 teeth; 18 months = 12 teeth; 24 months = 16 teeth; and 30 months = 20 teeth.

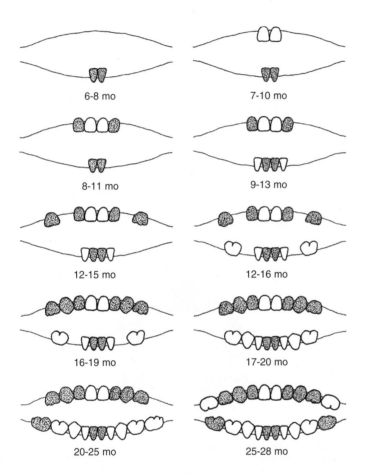

6-8 mo   7-10 mo

8-11 mo   9-13 mo

12-15 mo   12-16 mo

16-19 mo   17-20 mo

20-25 mo   25-28 mo

Fig. 7.**28** Eruption time and sequence of the primary dentition. Shaded teeth erupt earlier than the corresponding teeth in the opposing arch (see Table 7.**1**).

Chronology of Tooth Eruption

The eruption sequence of the primary dentition is presented in Figure 7.**28** and Table 7.**1**; the eruption sequence of the permanent dentition is shown in Figure 7.**29** and Table 7.**2**. In the primary dentition, eruption occurs earlier in boys than in girls. In the permanent dentition, however, eruption in girls usually precedes that in boys. There are no differences in the eruption sequence of the primary teeth.

In general, the mandibular teeth precede the maxillary teeth in the permanent dentition. Only the mandibular central incisors and, occasionally, the mandibular second molars precede the corresponding maxillary teeth in the primary dentition (Table 7.**1** and Fig. 7.**30**). Under normal conditions, teeth tend to be delayed rather than early in eruption. A difference of 1 or 2 months on either side of the noted range (Table 7.**1**) should not be considered abnormal. Homologous teeth in the same arch appear in close approximation of time. Infants who attain the incisor teeth early usually erupt the remaining teeth early. On the other hand, if the incisor teeth are delayed, the remaining teeth may not arrive late. A tooth generally takes from 1.5 to 2.5 months from the beginning of clinical eruption until it reaches the occlusal plane. Canines usually take the longest time to erupt.

Primary teeth eruption is generally characterized by interproximal or physiologic spacing. This occurs in about 70% of infants; the remaining 30% show no spaces between the teeth. There is more spacing between the maxillary than the mandibular teeth.

There is no physiologic spacing after the eruption of the primary teeth. An infant has either a spaced or closed dentition. The chances of there being no crowding with permanent teeth are higher in children with a spaced primary dentition than in those with a closed dentition.

Table. 7.**1** Chronology of development of the primary dentition

Primary teeth in order of eruption (sequence)	Beginning calcification (mo in utero)	Crown completed postnatally (mo)	Appearance in the oral cavity (eruption time) (mo)	Root completed time (y)	Root resorption begins (y)	Shedding (y)
Lower central incisor	3-4	2-3	6-8	1-2	4	7
Upper central incisor	3-4	2	7-10	1-2	4	7
Upper lateral incisor	4	2-3	8-11	2	5	8
Lower lateral incisor	4	3	9-13	1-2	5	8
Upper first molar	4	6	12-15	2-3	6	10
Lower first molar	4	6	12-16	2-3	6	9
Upper canine	4-5	9	16-19	3	8	11
Lower canine	4-5	9	17-20	3	7	9
Lower second molar	5	10	20-26	3	7	10
Upper second molar	5	11	25-28	3	7	10

The normal range of eruption times indicates a wide varation. A difference of 1 o 2 months on either side of the normal range would not necessarily mean that a child's eruption time schedule is abnormal. Only deviations considerably outside this range should be considered abnormal.

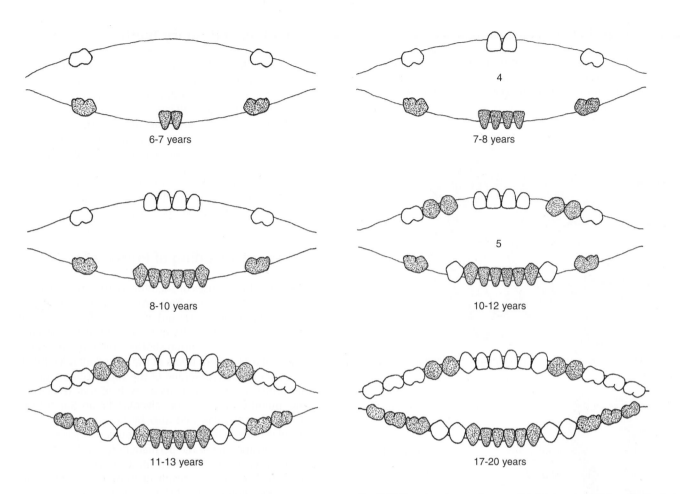

Fig. 7.**29** Eruption time and sequence of the permanent teeth. Shaded teeth erupt earlier than the corresponding teeth in the opposing arch (see Table 7.**2**).

Table. 7.**2** Chronology of development of the permanent dentition

Permanent teeth in order of eruption (sequence)	Beginning calcification	Crown completed (y)	Appearance in eruption time (y)	Root completed time (y)
Lower first molar	Birth	3-4	6-7	9-10
Upper first molar	Birth	4-5	6-7	9-10
Lower central incisor	3-4 mo	4	6-7	9
Upper central incisor	3-4 mo	4-5	7-8	10
Lower lateral incisor	3-4 mo	4-5	7-8	9-10
Upper lateral incisor	10-12 mo	4-5	8-10	10-11
Lower canine	4-5 mo	5-6	8-10	12-13
Upper first premolar	1-2 y	6-7	10-12	12-14
Lower first premolar	1-2 y	6-7	10-12	12-14
Upper second premolar	2-3 y	7-8	10-12	13-14
Lower second premolar	2-3 y	7	11-13	14-15
Upper canine	4-5 mo	6-7	11-13	14-15
Lower second molar	2-3 y	7-8	11-13	14-15
Upper second molar	2-3 y	7-8	11-13	15-16
Lower third molar	8-10 y	12-16	17-20	18-25
Upper third molar	7-9 y	12-16	17-20	18-25

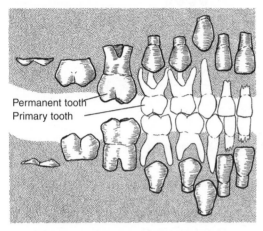

Fig. 7.**30** Relation of primary teeth to permanent teeth during mixed detention stages.

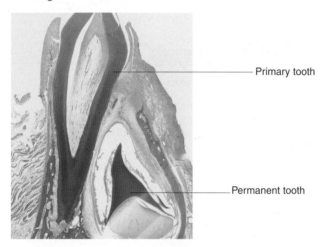

Primary tooth

Permanent tooth

Fig. 7.**31** Early stages in root resorption of primary tooth, caused by pressure of the growing permanent tooth germ.

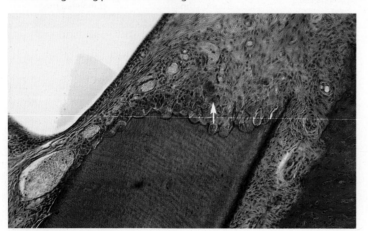

Fig. 7.**32** Histology of active resorption of the primary tooth root. The arrow points to resorption lacunae.

Shedding of Primary Teeth

Like most mammals, humans are dipyodont creatures—that is, they possess two sets of teeth: a primary set and a permanent set. The teeth of the primary set are small and fewer, to fit the small jaws of the infant. Because the teeth, once formed, cannot increase in size, it follows that the primary set must be shed or exfoliated to be replaced by the larger jaws of adults (Fig. 7.**30**).

Shedding is the exfoliation of the primary teeth caused by physiologic resorption of their roots. The permanent successors will then take their place.

Causes of Shedding of Primary Teeth

There are three causes of shedding of the primary teeth.
1. Loss of root: Pressure from growing and erupting permanent teeth (Fig. 7.**31**) induces the differentiation of osteoclasts, which results in resorption of the primary roots (Fig. 7.**32**). Resorption shortens the roots and causes loss of attachment fibers of the periodontal ligament.
2. Loss of bone: Weakening of the supporting tissues of the primary teeth occurs as a result of root resorption and modifications of the alveolar bone. Supporting structures are weakened also by facial growth of the alveolar bone, which occurs to provide sufficient space for the positioning of the permanent teeth (Fig. 7.**30**).
3. Increased force: Increased masticatory forces on the weakened teeth are a result of muscular growth. This amplifies compression of the periodontal ligament and promotes resorption of teeth and alveolar bone (Fig. 7.**33**).

Root and Bone Resorption

The process of resorption is initiated by osteoclasts or odontoclasts, which originate from the fusion of circulating blood monocytes after their escape from the blood vessels. Osteoclasts are generally large, multinucleated cells that appear in cup-shaped depressions of the resorbing front of any hard tissue (Fig. 7.**32**). The cup-shaped depressions are called Howship's lacunae (Fig. 7.**33**). Under the light microscope, the osteoclast appears as a large cell containing six to 12 nuclei. It has a vacuolated cytoplasm and a striated or brush border adjacent to the resorbing hard tissue. (Fig. 7.**34**). The electron microscope reveals a ruffled border consisting of deep invaginations of the cell membrane forming numerous intermingled villus–like processes. These differ in diameter not only from one another but also along the course of individual villi. The cytoplasm of the ruffled border is almost devoid of organelles. Between the ruffled border and the nuclei, the cytoplasm is extremely rich in mitochondria (Fig. 7.**34**). Still deeper and closer to the nuclei, many Golgi stacks are present surrounded by electron-dense granules and smooth and coated vesicles. The electron-dense granules are membrane-bound granules with a central electron-dense core surrounded by a pale halo. They are specific granules characteristic of osteoclasts and their precursors. They appear spherical or elongated and are found in monocytes as well. Acid phosphatase has been demonstrated in them. As for the nuclei, their ultrastructural appearance differs according to whether the osteoclast is young or old. In young osteoclasts, the nuclei are ovoid and euchromatic (pale) with smooth nuclear membrane. In older osteoclasts, the nuclei become heterochromatic (dark) showing wrinkled outlines, and may be pyknotic.

An osteoclast is the result of fusion of cells rather than the product of repeated nuclear division. Mononuclear osteoclasts may be fully functional, multinucleation is also possible for improved performance and regulation. Recently, studies confirmed the hemopoietic origin of osteoclasts from circulating monocytes. Some investigators have demonstrated that odontoclast precursors become fully differentiated and develop prominent ruffled borders only when they come into direct contact with mineralized dentin to be resorbed. They also observed that concomitant with the ruffled border formation, odontoclasts exhibit extensive synthesis and storage of acid phosphatase in many vacuoles and vesicles.

Current information indicates that hard-tissue resorption occurs in two phases. The extracellular phase involves the initial breakdown of a small area of hard tissue into partially dissolved fragments. In the intracellular phase, the osteoclast appears to ingest and complete the dissolution of the breakdown products. Resorption of hard tissue occurs near the ruffled border of the osteoclast. The cell appears to surround the resorption site with a modified or clear zone of cytoplasm (Figs. 7.**34B** and **D**), which suggests that the seal increases the effectiveness of its hydraulic enzymes. As the osteoclast

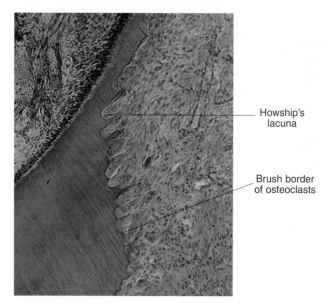

Fig. 7.**33** Osteoclasts on the surface of the tooth root.

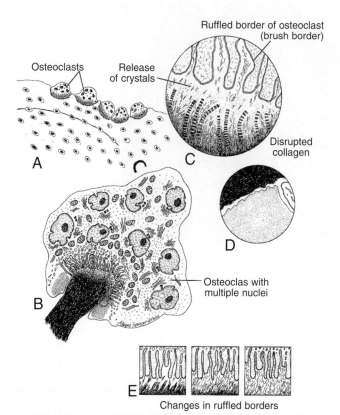

Fig. 7.**34** Osteoclast activity in Howship's lacunae. **A** Osteoclasts in lacunae. **B** Multinucleated osteoclast with brush border contacting spicule. **C** Ruffled border of osteoclast with mineral intracellularly and collagen extracellulary. **D** "Clear zone" of osteoclast. **E** Constant flux of ruffled borders during the resorption process.

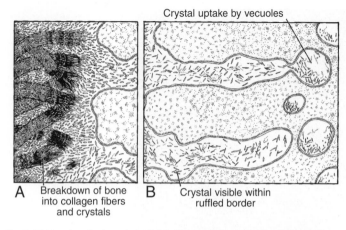

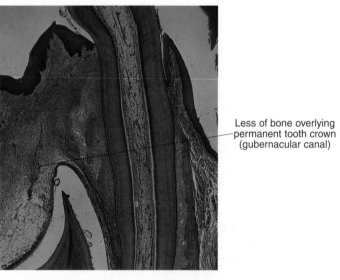

Fig. 7.**35** Uptake of mineral crystals in intracellular vacuoles. **A** Crystals appear within cytoplasmic extensions of the osteoclast. **B** Development of vacuoles in osteoclast cytoplasm.

Fig. 7.**36** Histology of permanent incisor crown to primary tooth.

attacks the hard-tissue matrix, the collagen meshwork is disrupted and crystals are released (Fig. 7.**34C**). The banding pattern characteristic of collagen fibrils at this stage can be seen with electron microscopy. Free crystals appear to be taken into cytoplasmic vacuoles of the osteoclast, and are gradually digested within it (Fig.7.**35**). The disrupted collagen fibrils are destroyed by fibroblastclasts, cells in the peridontal ligament capable of both degradation and synthesis of collagen.

During the process of resorption, the pressure of the erupting permanent tooth is first directed to the bone separating the crypt of the permanent tooth from the alveolus of the primary tooth (Fig. 7.**36**). After this area is resorbed, the eruptive force is directed at the root of the primary tooth, which results in resorption of the cementum and dentin.Osteoclasts resorb mineralized but not unmineralized tissues.

Osteoblastic cells play a key role in bone resorption by secreting neutral proteases, including collagenase to degrade the unmineralized organic matrix or osteoid that lines most bony surfaces. This process brings about direct contact of osteoclasts with bone mineral, which is a stimulus for resorptive activity. Whether cementoid tissue is first removed by a similar mechanism is not known.

Resorption, like eruption, is not a continuous process; periods of activity alternate with periods of rest. During periods of rest, repair may take place by apposition of bone and cementum in limited areas of the root, which results in partial reattachment of the tooth. This explains why children experience periods when primary teeth alternate between looseness and fixation. Resorption usually proceeds faster than repair and ultimately results in the tooth being shed.

Resorption Pattern of Anterior Teeth

Resorption of the primary anterior teeth begins at about 4 to 5 years for the incisors and 6 to 8 years for the canines, depending on whether they are mandibular or maxillary canines. At these times, the crowns of the permanent successors are completed and situated in their own crypts lingual to the apical third of the roots of the corresponding primary teeth (Fig. 7.**36**).

With the onset of eruptive movement of the permanent teeth, which proceeds in an incisal and labial direction, pressure is first directed at the bone separating the crypts of the permanent successors and the alveolus of the primary roots. With the loss of the separating bone, pressure is then directed at the primary roots (Fig. 7.**37A**). Therefore, resorption of the primary anterior teeth first occurs along the lingual surface of the apical third of the root. It then proceeds labially until the crown of the erupting permanent tooth comes to lie directly apical to the primary tooth root (Fig. 7.**37B**). Resorption then proceeds horizontally in an incisal direction, causing the primary root to exfoliate and the permanent one to erupt in its place (Fig. 7.**37C**).

Sometimes, particularly in the region of the mandibular incisors, the labial movement of the permanent teeth does not cause complete loss of the primary roots. This may result in the primary incisors remaining in the jaw, attached to the labial alveolar bone. Then, when the crowns of the permanent incisors emerge through the gingiva, they appear lingual to the primary ones that are still in place (Fig. 7.**38**). Prompt removal of the primary crown and remaining root assists the permanent ones in correcting their positions.

In the maxillary jaw, however, if the permanent canines appear in a misplaced position, they usually do so labial to the existing primary canines. Again, prompt removal is beneficial. It is rare to see a maxillary permanent canine erupting lingual to a primary one, as the permanent canine could then become embedded in the heavy bone of the palate.

Resorption Pattern of Posterior Teeth

The growing premolar crowns are initially located between the roots of the primary molar teeth (Fig. 7.**39A**). The first signs of resorption around these crowns occur in the supporting interradicular bone. This is followed by resorption of the adjacent surfaces of the primary tooth roots (Fig. 7.**39B**). Meanwhile, the bony alveolar processes increase in height to compensate for the lengthening roots of the permanent teeth (premolars). As this occurs the primary molars emerge occlusally, which positions the premolar crowns more apical to the primary molar roots. The premolars continue to erupt as the primary molar roots further resorb, and these teeth then exfoliate (Fig. 7.**39C**). The premolars then erupt in place of the primary molars.

Abnormal Behavior of Primary Teeth

Retained Primary Teeth

The most common causes for retained primary teeth are absence or impaction of the permanent successor. The teeth most often affected are the upper lateral incisors; next affected are the lower second molars; the teeth least often affected are the lower central incisors. Retained primary teeth often remain functional for many years among the permanent teeth before they are lost through resorption of their roots. Their loss is believed to be contributed to by heavy masticatory forces of adult life on the small roots and by the continued active eruption and progressive elongation of the clinical crown of such teeth at the expense of root length.

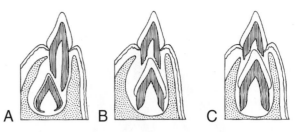

Fig. 7.**37** Relative position of a permanent anterior tooth to its primary predecessor during the process of shedding.

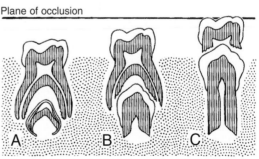

Permanent central incisors erupting lingually

Fig. 7.**38** Clinical view of eruption sites of permanent teeth lingual to primary crowns.

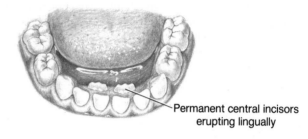

Plane of occlusion

Progressive resorption and exfolation of primary tooth as permanent tooth develops

Fig. 7.**39** Relative position of a premolar to a primary molar during the process of shedding.

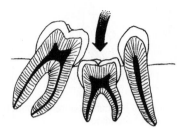

Fig. 7.**40** Diagram of submerged primary tooth.

Clinical Application

Ankylosis is a hard-tissue union between bone and tooth. It probably occurs as a result of disturbance in the interaction between normal resorption and hard-tissue repair during shedding. Primary molars are the teeth mostly affected, where ankylosis occurs mainly at the furcation area.

Submerged Primary Teeth

Sometimes, primary teeth become anklosed. Such teeth are prevented from active eruption and become submerged in the alveolar bone as a result of the continued eruption of adjacent teeth and the increase in height of the alveolar ridge (Fig. 7.**40**). Submerged primary teeth should be removed as soon as possible, particularly when their permanent successors are present. The major difference between retained and submerged primary teeth is that the latter are fused to the alveolar bone (ankylosed), whereas the former are not. Deeply submerged teeth suggest that the ankylosis occurred early during childhood.

Remnants of Primary Teeth

Remnants of primary teeth are parts of the roots of the primary teeth; these parts escape resorption during the process of shedding. Such root remnants remain embedded in the jaw, are most frequently seen in the interdental septa in the region of the lower second premolars, are usually asymptomatic, and, if observed on X-ray, should not be disturbed. Root remnants may exfoliate if they are near the surface of the jaws, or they may undergo resorption and become replaced by bone, thus disappearing completely.

Preprimary Teeth

In very rare cases, preprimary teeth appear in the oral cavity of newborn of neonatal infants. They are commonly found on the alveolar ridge of the mandible, in the incisor region, and usually number two or three. Because they possess no roots, they are not firmly attached. Frequently, they are shed during the first few weeks of life. They should be removed as soon as possible, however, to prevent discomfort to both the mother and the baby during suckling. Removal of the preprimary teeth does not affect the primary teeth. Sometimes, however, the teeth seen in the mouth of a newborn baby are premature primary teeth. Therefore, they are not replaced after they fall out, and their place remains patent until the corresponding permanent teeth erupt.

Summary

Eruption is the movement of the teeth through the bone of the jaws and the overlying mucosa, to appear and function in the oral cavity. These eruptive movements can be divided into three phases: preeruptive, prefunctional eruptive, and functional eruptive.

Active eruption is the result of occlusal movement of the tooth. After emergence of the tooth through the gingiva, active eruption is accompanied by gradual exposure of the clinical crown by separation of the attachment epithelium and the apical shift of the gingiva.

Clinical eruption begins with the appearance of the crown tip in the oral cavity and continues until the tooth comes into occlusion. During this period, the tooth moves faster than at any other time. Figure 7.**41** indicates many of the changes occurring at this time. The periodontal fibers are organizing to stabilize the erupting tooth, the root dentinogenesis follows as the bone in the fundic region organizes in response to the changes in root length.

Like most mammals, the human is a diphyodont creature—that is, possessing two sets of teeth: primary and permanent. The teeth of the primary set are small and fewer, to fit the small jaws of the infant. Because the teeth, once formed, cannot increase in size, the primary set of teeth must exfoliate and be replaced by the larger, more numerous teeth of the permanent set to accommodate the larger jaws of the adult.

Shedding of the primary teeth is the result of progressive resorption of their roots through the activity of the osteoclasts or odontoclasts. Hard-tissue resorption occurs in two phases: the extracellular, during which the matrix fragments and dissolution begins, and the intracellular, during which complete digestion of the products of resorption occurs. The process of resorption is not continuous; periods of activity alternate with periods of rest. Disturbance of the resorption process results in abnormal behavior of the primary teeth; some primary teeth may be retained because of the absence or impaction of their permanent successors, others may be ankylosed and submerged.

In rare cases, teeth may appear in the oral cavity of newborn or neonatal infants, and are called preprimary teeth.

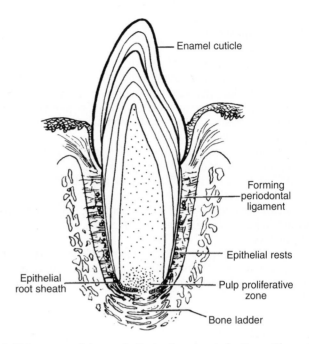

- Enamel cuticle
- Forming periodontal ligament
- Epithelial rests
- Epithelial root sheath
- Pulp proliferative zone
- Bone ladder

Fig. 7.**41** Summary of changes in the tooth and periodontium with eruption modification of alveolar bone and organization of ligament with root growth.

Self-Evaluation Review

1. What is the purpose of crown movements during the preeruptive phase of tooth eruption?

2. What are the characteristics of the intraosseus and supraosseus stages of the prefunctional phase of tooth eruption?

3. What is the relation of the secretory phase of amelogenesis to the beginning of root formation?

4. What is the cause of periods of looseness and fixation during the eruption and shedding of the primary teeth?

5. What are three causes believed to be important in shedding of the primary teeth?

6. Describe the two phases of bone resorption, indicating which cells are believed to be responsible for each phase. What are their functions?

7. Explain the "six/four" rule for emergence of the primary teeth.

8. What are some of the possible causes of tooth eruption?

9. Explain the rule of "fours" for development of the permanent teeth.

Acknowledgements

The author wishes to recognize the following contributions: Dr David C Johnsen of the University of Iowa for providing Figure 7.**16**; Dr Roger Noonan, Program Director of the Department of Pediatric Dentistry, Lyola University, for providing the clinical applications of the rule of "fours" and "six/fours"; Dr Sol Bernick (deceased) of the University of Southern California, for providing Figure 7.**23**.

Suggested Readings

Andreason JO. External resorption: Its implication in dental traumatology, paedodontics, orthodontics, and endodontics. Int Endo J.1986: 67–70.

Berkowitz, BKB, Moxam BJ, Newman HN. Periodontal ligament and physiologic tooth movement. In: BKB Berkowitz , BJ Moxaam, HN Newman, eds. The Periodontal Ligament in Health and Disease. New York, NY: Pergamon Press; 982:215–247.

Gorski JP, Marks SC Jr. Current concepts of the biology of tooth eruption. Crit. Rev. Oral Biol Med. 1992:3:185–206.

Marks SC Jr, Gorski JP, Cahill DR, Wise CG. Tooth eruption, a synthesis of experimental observations. In Davidovich Z, ed. The Biological Mechanism of Tooth Eruption and Resorption. Birmingham, Ala: EBSCO Media; 1988: 161–169.

Moxham BJ. The role of the periodontal vasculature in tooth eruption. In: Davidovich Z, ed. The Biological Mechanism of Tooth Eruption amd Root Resorption. Birmingham, Ala: EBSCO Media; 1988;107–233.

Profitt WR. The effect of intermittent forces on eruption. In: Davidovich Z, ed. The Biological Mechanisms of Tooth Eruption and Resorption. Birmingham, Ala: EBSCO Media; 1988:187–191.

Steedle JR, Proffit WR. The pattern and control of the eruptive tooth movements. Am J Orthodont. 1985;87:56–66.

Thesleff I. Does epidermal growth factor control tooth eruption? J. Dent. Child. 1987; 84:321–329.

Topham RT, Chiego DJ Jr., Smith AJ, Huton DA, Gattone VH II, Klein R. Effects of epidermal growth factor on tooth differentiation and eruption. In: Davidovich Z, ed. The Biological Mechanism of Tooth Eruption and Resorption. Birmingham, Ala: EBSCO Media; 1988:117–131.

Wise GE, Marks SC, Cahill DR. Ultrastructrural features of the dental follicle associated in the eruption pathway in the dog. J. Oral Pathol. 1985;14:15–26.

Zajick G. Fibroblast cell kinetics in the periodontal ligament in the mouse. Cell. Tissue Kinet. 1974;7:479–492.

8 Agents Affecting Tooth and Bone Development

James K. Avery

Introduction

Certain vitamin and hormone deficiencies, if present during tooth formation will adversely affect formative cells and the matrix that they produce. Reduced organic matrix content results in production of hypoplastic tissue. Excessive levels of tetracycline or fluoride may become incorporated into mineralizing teeth and interfere with the mineralization process. Should both situations occur, a hypoplastic matrix that is also hypomineralized would result. The extent of the defect is dependent on the nature of the substance, the degree of excess or deficiency, and the developmental time frame. Vitamins A, C, and D, parathyroid hormone, tetracycline, and fluoride are discussed in terms of their relation to matrix development, and dentin and enamel mineralization in developing teeth. Most experiments have been conducted on the continuously developing rodent incisors, which adequately records developmental defects. Tooth development may be affected by many substances. The examples cited are those most frequently studied in animal and human research.

Objectives

After reading this chapter you should be able to describe in detail the effects of vitamins A, C, and D, parathyroid hormone, sodium fluoride, and tetracycline on developing teeth.

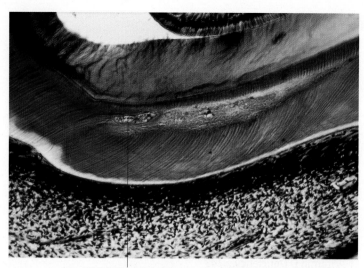

Vascular inclusions

Fig. 8.1 Histology of vitamin A deficiency reveals enamel matrix deficiency and related dentinal defects at the DEJ.

Vitamin A Deficiency

Although tissues of ectodermal origin—that is, the epidermis—are primarily affected in vitamin A deficiency, bones and teeth also record this deficiency. Hypovitaminosis A is evidenced by marked metaplasia of the enamel organ, which results in defective enamel and dentin formation (Fig. 8.1). Likewise, bone is laid down in abnormal locations, and its remodeling sequences seem to be affected. Both osteoclasts and osteoblasts have been shown to be affected by this disease process. Dentinal irregularities associated with vitamin A deficiency in developing teeth appear as areas characterized by either excessive osteodentin deposition (bonelike, with cell inclusions) or insufficient dentin depositions (Figs. 8.1 and 8.2). Alterations of the differentiated odontoblasts appear to be associated with these conditions. Some investigators, however, ascribe the primary effects of vitamin A deficiency to oral epithelial cells. This view originates from histologic changes seen initially in the oral mucosa and extending to the degeneration of the epithelial-derived ameloblasts, which results in a hypoplastic enamel matrix. If the vitamin A deficiency is severe, ameloblast cells will become completely atrophied, which results in an absence of enamel formation.

In less severe cases, the columnar ameloblasts apparently shorten, and adjacent enamel exhibits hypoplasia. An example can be seen in Figure 8.2. Several authors have described bone defects due to vitamin A deficiency. Most have noted that the defects are attributable to impaired endochondral ossification and faulty bone modeling. Figure 8.2 shows shortened ameloblasts and defective enamel and dentin formation. The normal appositional rhythm of dentin deposition may be altered. Vascular inclusions sometimes are seen in the dentin (Figs. 8.1 and 8.2). If the vitamin A deficiency is relieved during subsequent tooth development, normal dentin and enamel are produced, although defective tissue is not repaired (Fig. 8.2). Figure 8.3 illustrates enamel hypoplasia induced by vitamin A deficiency.

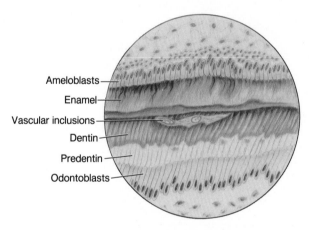

Ameloblasts
Enamel
Vascular inclusions
Dentin
Predentin
Odontoblasts

Fig. 8.2 Illustration of vitamin A deficiency indicates shortened ameloblasts, enamel matrix deficiency, and vascular inclusions in dentin at the DEJ.

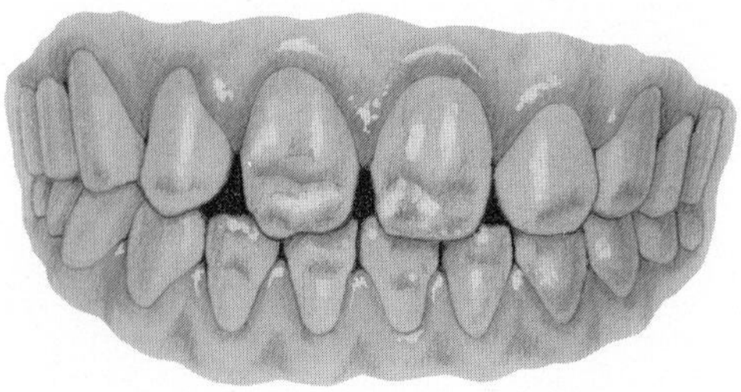

Fig. 8.3 Illustration of clinical view of defective enamel resulting from vitamin A deficiency.

Clinical Application

Clinically, vitamin C deficiency is manifested orally by gingival bleeding and loosening of the teeth. Weakness, anemia, bone loss, and susceptibility to hemorrhage may also be associated with this deficiency.

Vitamin C Deficiency

Ascorbic acid deficiency has been described in guinea pigs, monkeys, and humans. Because none of these species synthesize vitamin C, they must depend on a dietary supply to maintain health. Scurvy, the disease resulting from vitamin C deficiency causes bone, dentin, and cementum deposition to cease and formative cells to atrophy, if severe. Vitamin C is required for collagen formation. It is necessary for the hydroxylation of the amino acids proline and lysine; an absence or deficiency of vitamin C during dentinogenesis results in defective dentinal tissue development. Dentinal tubules become irregular and reduced in number, vascular inclusions become apparent, and those odontoblasts present are short, with some taking on a spindle-shaped fibroblast–like appearance. Compare the appearance of normal dentin, in Figure 8.**4**, with that of dentin formed while vitamin C was deficient, in Figure 8.**5**. Figure 8.**6** is an illustration of characteristics associated with vitamin C deficiency. Embryologically, vitamin C is essential for proper development of all mesenchymally derived structures, including bone, dentin, and cementum. Clinically, vitamin C deficiency is manifested by gingival bleeding and loosening of the teeth due to bone resorption. Weakness, anemia, and susceptibility to hemorrhage also may be evident. Administration of vitamin C results in rapid elimination of the symptoms associated with this deficiency.

Vitamin D Deficiency

Vitamin D is essential for deposition of calcium and phosphorus in hard tissues. Its presence increases the absorption of dietary calcium and maintains proper levels of calcium and phosphorus in the blood. Primary deficiency of vitamin D results from insufficient exposure to the sun and insufficient dietary intake. Secondary deficiencies result from abnormal intestinal resorption. Secondary deficiencies may be overcome by alteration of dietary intake of calcium and phosphorus. A severe vitamin D deficiency in children results in rickets, a condition characterized by insufficient deposition of calcium salts in bony tissue. Hypoplasia of the enamel also may be evident. Although vitamin D deficiency is less common among adults, it is manifested by decreased mineralization of the bone matrix. Insufficiently mineralized bones, especially the weight-bearing long bones, are prone to bending and distortion.

Normal dentin

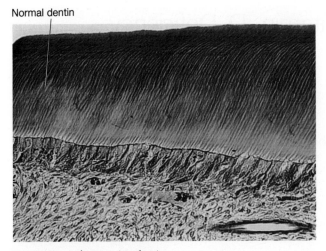

Fig. 8.**4** Normal-appearing dentin.

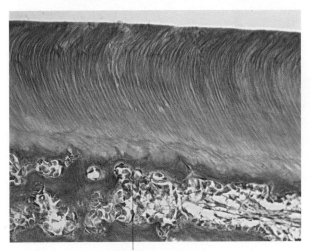

Vascular inclusions

Fig. 8.**5** Appearance of defective dentin formation resulting from vitamin C deficiency, with vascular inclusions and degenerated odontoblasts.

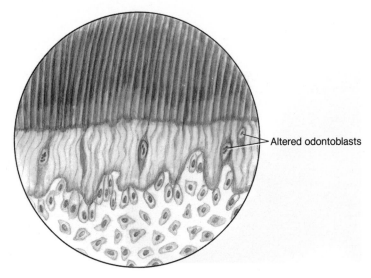

Altered odontoblasts

Fig. 8.**6** Illustration of vascular inclusions and altered odontoblasts resulting from vitamin C deficiency.

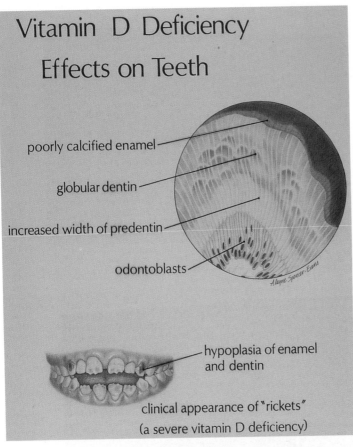

Vitamin D Deficiency
Effects on Teeth

poorly calcified enamel

globular dentin

increased width of predentin

odontoblasts

hypoplasia of enamel and dentin

clinical appearance of "rickets" (a severe vitamin D deficiency)

Fig. 8.**7** Illustration of histology and clinical view of vitamin D deficiency.

In Figures 8.**7** and 8.**8**, note the abnormally wide non-mineralized zone of predentin and the interglobular spaces in the dentin. Figure 8.**8** also shows areas of enamel affected by hypoplasia and hypomineralization. Results of a study of children with rickets indicated that as many as 25% exhibited enamel hypoplasia. It has been reported that hypomineralization of cementum is frequently found in these children. No other vitamin deficiencies have such notable effects on tooth formation as do vitamin A, C, and D deficiencies.

Parathyroid Hormone

The parathyroid glands regulate calcium balance in the body. An imbalance, either deficiency or excess, of parathyroid hormone (PTH) may affect bone and tooth formation. Excess PTH (hyperparathyroidism) causes mobilization of calcium from the skeleton into the blood stream. Calcium ions may then be excreted in urine, feces, and sweat. PTH may influence all of these mechanisms. Calcium excretion results in hypocalcemia or decreased levels of blood calcium. The bone, in turn, mobilizes more calcium. When calcium resorption is greater than deposition, osteoporosis results. Osteoporosis may then, for example, weaken the supporting alveolar bone of the teeth.

As shown in Figure 8.**9**, calcium mobilization in bone results in decreased bone density around the tooth, which is seen as a thinning of the lamina dura. Inactive parathyroids (hypoparathyroidism) results in low blood concentrations of ionized calcium, which causes an increase in gland activity. Bone density increases, which results in increased thickness of the lamina dura and an increased density of bone trabeculae (osteoperosis).

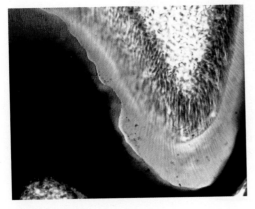

Fig. 8.**8** Histology of vitamin D deficiency. Globular dentin is indicated by irregular staining of the matrix and by wide predentin.

Clinical Application

Osteoporosis results when calcium loss because of resorption is greater than calcium deposition. This may be evident orally with loss of alveolar bone and loosening of the teeth.

Calcium is not released from mature teeth as it is from bone; so the structure of teeth is not affected by hyperparathyroidism and hypoparathyroidism, except during development.

Hyperparathyroidism will cause an initial hypocalcification of the forming dental tissue, followed by hypercalcification due to excessive blood calcium. Calcium excretion by the kidneys follows. The effect of hypoparathyroidism and hyperparathyroidism on teeth is illustrated in Figure 8.**9**. A section of defective dentin clearly shows the effects of both hypoparathyroidism and hyperparathyroidism (Fig. 8.**10**). The horizontally stained bands accentuate the hypocalcified and/or hypercalcified zones. A series of injections of parathyroid hormone into experimental animals were given to achieve this effect. Therefore, both hyperparathyroidism and hypoparathyroidism produce calcium imbalance, which results in hypocalcified bands in the forming dentin. A loss of mineral in the supporting bone occurs with hyperparathyroidism, and increased deposition of mineral takes place with hypoparathyroidism.

Tetracycline and Fluoride

Tetracycline and fluoride, if available during the mineralization phases, may be incorporated in dentin, enamel, cementum, and bone. They are very different compounds. Fluoride is a binary compound of fluorine, useful as an anticaries substance. Tetracycline, on the other hand, is used as an antibacterial agent. Both are deposited along with minerals in developing hard tissues. Tetracycline is derived from a yellow-gold fungus whose color is maintained in the purified antibiotic and trans-

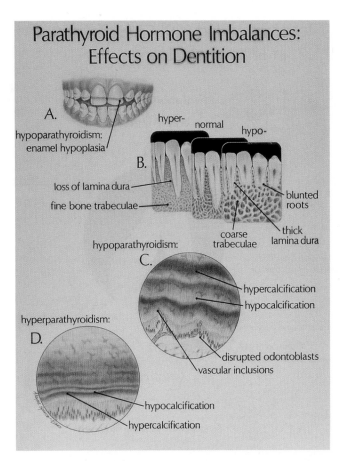

Fig. 8.**9 A** Illustration of the clinical effects of parathyroid hormone. **B** Diagrams of radiographs indicate altered supporting bone. **C** and **D** Histologic appearance of alternating bands of hypocalcified and hypercalcified dentin. These bonds may demonstrate the clinical appearance of hypocalcified tooth and bone.

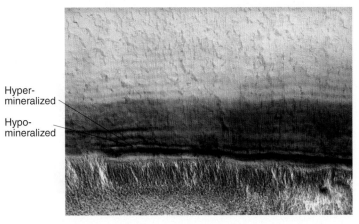

Fig. 8.**10** Alternating hypomineralized and hypermineralized dentin due to parathormone injections seen as bonds of decreased and increased mineralization of the matrix.

Clinical Application

Effects of tetracyclines include staining of teeth, hypoplasia, and loss of enamel. Most of the staining is in the dentin, which is seen through the translucent enamel.

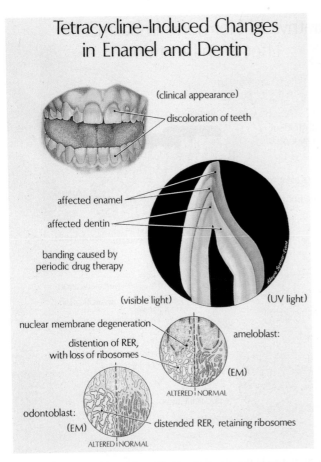

Fig. 8.11 Effects of tetracycline in human teeth result in staining and hypoplastic enamel. Staining is evident in first-formed dentin. Both ameloblast and odontoblast endoplasmic reticula are altered.

ferred to the hard tissues in which it is incorporated. On prolonged exposure to light, tetracycline-stained dental tissue will change color to a brown to gray (these shades of discoloration are eventually seen in the teeth) (Fig. 8.**11A**). Other effects of tetracyclines include hypoplasia or absence of enamel. Staining is most observable in the dentin, especially in the first-formed dentin at the dentinoenamel junction (DEJ). Notable staining of the crown is primarily from discolored dentin being seen through the translucent, and relatively unaffected, enamel (Fig.8.**11B**). Figure 8.**12** is an example of a patient to whom tetracycline was given during early infancy. Staining is not visible in the central incisors, as the crowns were formed after cessation of treatment with tetracycline. The diffuse staining seen on the lateral incisors and cuspids indicates that they were undergoing development at the time. Tetracycline staining is more noticeable under ultraviolet (UV) light (Fig. 8.**11B**). The amount of damage is directly related to the magnitude and duration of the dosage; any defects caused by the tetracycline may be compounded by the effects of the illness itself.

The precise mechanism of tetracycline incorporation into mineralizing tissue is not yet known, but it is believed that a chelate of calcium and tetracycline forms. At higher concentrations, cells may be altered, as is seen in Figure 8.**11C**. In both ameloblasts and odontoblasts, the cisternae of the endoplasmic reticulum become dilated, and protein synthesis is impaired. This, in turn, will result in hypoplasia of the enamel and dentin matrix.

Tetracycline and, to a limited extent, sodium fluoride cross the placental barrier and are available to the human fetus. If a pregnant female consumes fluoridated water during mineralization of the fetal teeth, the teeth will incorporate this compound. Such teeth exhibit higher resistance to dental caries. Compared with fluoride blood levels in the maternal circulation, fluoride blood levels in the fetus are relatively low. If on the other hand, tetracycline antibiotics are administered to the mother during the period of tooth mineralization, the deciduous teeth may later be stained. Tetracycline staining of teeth is permanent; staining of bone is not permanent because bone is remodeled continuously.

The period marked by mineralization of crowns extends from approximately 5 months in utero to 12 years of age, and include the mineralization of both primary and permanent dentitions.

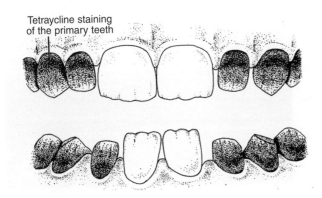

Fig. 8.**12** Illustration of tetracycline staining in teeth indicates that staining of these teeth developed when the injections were performed.

The teeth shown in Figure 8.13 exhibit brown staining of the incisal one-third of the central incisors. This staining is due to tetracycline therapy that occurred during the initial phases of mineralization of these teeth; otherwise, the teeth would have been stained more cervically. Cervical staining is more characteristic of tetracycline because this agent deposits primarily in the dentin. The lateral permanent incisors, on the other hand, began mineralization after drug therapy and were not affected.

Figure 8.14A is a photograph of mottled enamel caused by sodium fluoride. Mottled enamel describes the scattered sites of pigmentation and hypoplasia. Sodium fluoride when taken into the body in concentration of 5 ppm (which occurs in some naturally fluoridated areas in the United States) is anticariogenic, but often causes mottled enamel. The mottled areas may or may not be mineralized (Figs. 8.14C and D). The enamel rods follow an irregular course through these areas. Despite their unsightly appearance, these teeth are completely free of caries. Fluoride is most beneficial to the teeth in concentrations of approximately 0.5 to 1 ppm of water. Concentration of 0.5 ppm may not prevent caries. Higher concentrations, such as 5 ppm, cause mottling and hypoplasia of the enamel and hypomineralized dentin, with increased interglobular spaces.

As hydroxyapatite crystals form, they may incorporate fluoride either by an exchange with the hydroxyl groups or by simple adsorption. The hydroxyl group exchange is slower and less reversible than adsorption. In the latter process, the fluoride may be adsorbed to the surface of hydroxyapatite crystals. This adsorptive process involves weak electrostatic bonding. Adsorption is believed to be rapid, though reversible (Fig. 8.15).

It is believed that fluoride found in inner enamel is absorbed mainly during the secretory stage of amelogenesis and that fluoride found in the outer 30 to 50 μm of enamel occurs during the maturative stage. Because the latter stage lasts longer, there is time for more fluoride to be deposited in the outer enamel. The maturative stage lasts from 1 to 2 years in primary teeth and from 4 to 5 years in permanent teeth. This may be the reason for less fluoride being found in primary teeth than in permanent teeth.

When histologic examination is conducted on teeth from areas of high fluoride concentration, the enamel is found to be more altered than the dentin. Enamel rod formation is affected and zones of hypoplasia are commonly found. Figure 8.16, a photomicrograph, shows an area of hypoplasia and staining in the central fissure of a molar tooth; this area was caused by a high concentration of fluoride. Note that the inner enamel is stained less than the outer enamel. This is because the inner enamel is deposited prenatally, when less fluoride is available for incorporation.

Tetracycline was first discovered to be present in human teeth and bones when traces were detected in bones viewed under UV light. This observation provided a new method of marking bones and teeth for following

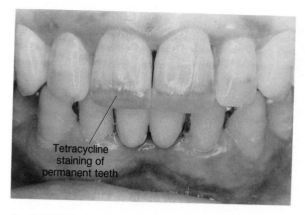

Fig. 8.13 Clinical appearance of tetracycline staining.

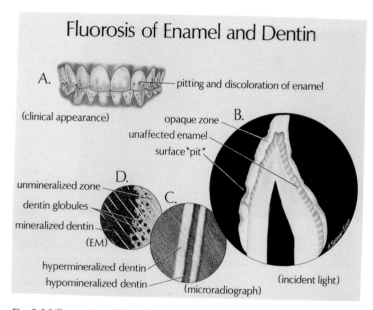

Fig. 8.14 Illustration of the effects of sodium fluoride on developing teeth. **A** Clinical picture reveals brown-stained hypoplastic pits. **B** Appearance of these pits in a ground section of the tooth seen in (**A**). **C** Altered incremental zones of the encircled zone in (**B**). **D** Hypocalcified dentin of the encircled zone in (**C**), at higher magnification of the electron microscope.

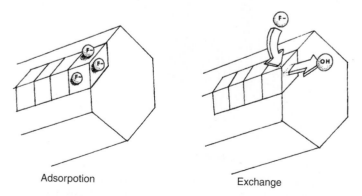

Fig. 8.15 Diagram of two mechanisms of uptake of fluoride in enamel.

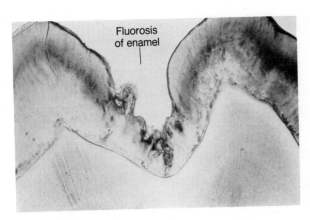

Fig. 8.**16** Histology of fluorosis of enamel indicates hypoplastic pits and altered brown-stained enamel.

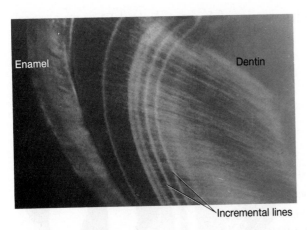

Fig. 8.**17** A series of lines of tetracycline staining in dentin mark the time of uptake. In enamel, there is less discrete staining. Photograph under UV light.

their development. An example of this procedure is shown in Figure 8.**17**, in which the slab of dentin was photographed under UV light. The photograph shows that tetracycline had been incorporated into new dentin that was mineralizing. This created the vertical arched lines marking separate injections of the tetracycline compound.

Tetracycline compound initially is deposited in the predentin as it mineralizes into dentin. Evidence of this marking is demonstrated in the increasing distance between new predentin formed and the area of fluorescent dentin. Because the therapeutic dosage level and visual tissue-labeling levels coincide, tetracycline has been widely used to visually record growth in experimental animals. The daily deposition rate of dentin can thus be recorded by measuring the width of dentin between each fluorescent line. In Figure 8.**17**, five discrete lines of tetracycline staining in dentin are seen. One is more widely spaced than the rest. In this instance, tetracycline injections were made on days one, six, seven, nine, and 11. Experimentally, if a second drug was administered on day one, the effect of this compound could be measured on dentinogenesis by comparing the banding patterns in the dentin with those of a control animal to which only tetracycline was administered. Some tetracycline is deposited in the dentinal tubules, which accounts for the near-horizontal fluorescent lines seen in Figure 8.**17**. Tetracycline can be used also to evaluated tooth movement by revealing bone and dentin formation (Fig.8.**18**). This diagram shows two lines in the dentin of a crown, which indicates the time between injections. In this case, the crown was in the early stages of formation, prior to eruption. Observe that there is no line in the root dentin, but that there are two vertical lines in the alveolar bone on the right of the roots and in the bifurcation zone. These lines were formed during a different time period, before the roots were formed. The tooth moved to the left, and the alveolar bone that formed behind the moving roots was clearly labeled by

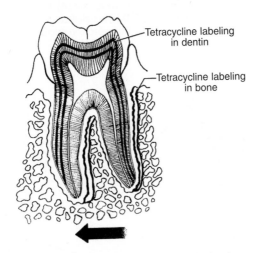

Fig. 8.**18** Diagram of tetracycline labeling during tooth development indicates lines in developing dentin and newly formed bone. Arrow indicates the direction of tooth movement.

Clinical Application

Brown staining or a defect in the enamel of the incisal third of crowns indicates the presence of a toxic substance in the body, at the time of initial mineralization of the teeth. Location of staining in the cervical area relates to introduction of a toxic substance at a time of final crown mineralization.

fluorescence.

In Figure 8.**19**, a UV photomicrograph of the tooth roots and the periodontium, there is heavy fluorescence in the roots and the alveolar bone. The tetracycline was absorbed by both sites of hard-tissue deposition, which indicates that both the roots and the supporting bone were undergoing development at the time tetracycline was injected. As can be demonstrated, tetracycline labeling is a valuable procedure for studying the development of teeth and bones.

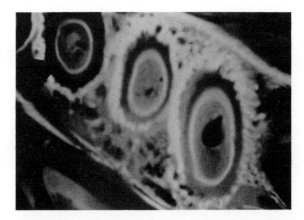

Fig. 8.**19** Histologic section shows tetracycline fluorescence in roots and alveolar bone (cross section). Photographed under UV light.

Summary

As noted on the left of Figure 8.**20**, the sectioned tooth exhibits normal-appearing ameloblasts, odontoblasts, enamel, dentin, and predentin. Compare this panel with the next, which illustrates the degenerative changes in the ameloblasts and affected enamel development associated with vitamin A deficiency. Observe the altered appearance of the adjacent first-formed dentin.

In the next panel, vitamin C deficiency is seen to primarily affect connective tissue-forming cells, such as the odontoblasts, fibroblasts, and osteoblasts. As a result, the tissues for which these cells are responsible will also be adversely affected. Vitamin D deficiency, which is indicated in the following panel, is seen affecting mineralization of teeth. Increased areas of globular dentin result with corresponding interglobular spaces. There is also an increased width of predentin.

On the far right of Figure 8.**20**, parathormone deficiency can be observed having similar effects. Hyperparathyroidism results in hypomineralized dentin, while hypoparathyroidism contributes to hypermineralized dentin.

If replacement therapy is provided, normal dentin deposition will resume in each of these thyroid deficiencies. Defective areas in the teeth are not restored, however, as is the case in bone that will be remodeled. All of the effects discussed are produced only during tooth development, not in fully developed teeth. Tetracycline and fluoride are absorbed during the mineralization phase of enamel and dentin formation; both can penetrate the maternal barrier in utero. Tetracycline can cause staining and hypoplasia of enamel, but with therapeutic doses staining is usually most evident in the first-formed dentin. This antibiotic registers a mark on dentin and bone, which is only visible under UV light. Therefore, it is used for measuring mineralized tissue growth. Excessive fluoride causes brown staining and hypoplasia in enamel (Figs. 8.**21A** and **B**), but the enamel is caries resistant. The hypoplasia may appear as pits or be in broad areas of the crown. One part per million affords maximum caries protection and minimal hard-tissue alteration.

Suggested Readings

Cohlan SQ. Tetracycline Staining of Teeth. Teratology.1977;16:27.

Fejerskof O, Thylstrup A, Larsen MJ. Clinical and structural features and possible pathogenetic mechanisms of dentinal fluorosis. Scand. J. Dent. Res. 1977;85:510.

Goodman AG. Pharmacologic Basis of Therapeutics. New York, NY: Macmillan; 1980.

Gregg JM, Avery JK. Studies of alveolar bone growth and tooth eruption using tetracycline induced fluorescence. J. Oral Therap. Pharmacol. 1964;1:268.

Horowitz HS, Thylstrup A, Driscoll WS, Glenn FB. Perspectives on the use of prenatal fluorides: a symposium. J. Dent. Child. 1981;48:101.

Humerinta K, Thesleff I, Saxon L. In vitro inhibititon of mouse odontoblast differentiation by vitamin A. Arch. Oral Biol. 1980;25:385.

Irving JT. A comparison of the influence of hormones, vitamins and other dietary factors on the formation of bone, dentin and enamel. Vitam. Horm. 1957;24:291.

Kallenbach E. Microscopy of tetracycline induced lesion in rat incisor enamel organ, Arch. Oral Biol. 1980:24:869.

Kawasaki K, Fernhead RW. On the relationship between tetra cycline and the incremental lines in dating. J. Anat. 1975;119:49.

Kruger BJ. Dose dependent ultrastructural changes induced by tetracycline developing dental tissues of the rat. J. Dent. Res. 1975;54:822.

Moffert JM, Cooley RO, Olsen NH, Heffernew JJ. Prediction of tetracycline induced tooth discoloration. J. Am. Dent. Assoc. 1974;88:547.

Pindborg JJ. Pathology of the Dental Hard Tissues. Philadelphia, Pa.: Saunders; 1970.

Shaw JH. A Textbook of Oral Biology. Philadelphia, Pa: WB Saunders; 1978.

Thylstrup A. Is there a biological rationale for prenatal fluoride administration? J.Dent. Child. 1981;48:103–108.

Thylstrup A. A distribution of dental flurosis in the primary dentition. Oral Epidemiol. 1978;6:329.

Thylstrup A, Fejerskof O. Appearance of dental flurosis in permanent teeth in relation to histologic changes. Community Dent. Oral Epidemiol. 1978;6:315.

Walton RE, Eisenman DR. Ultrastructural examination of dentin formation in rat incisors following multiple fluoride injections. Arch. Oral Biol. 1975;20:485.

Werstergaard J, Nylen NV. Dose and age dependent variations in effect of tetracycline on enamel formation in rat. Scand J. Dent. Res. 1975;82:209.

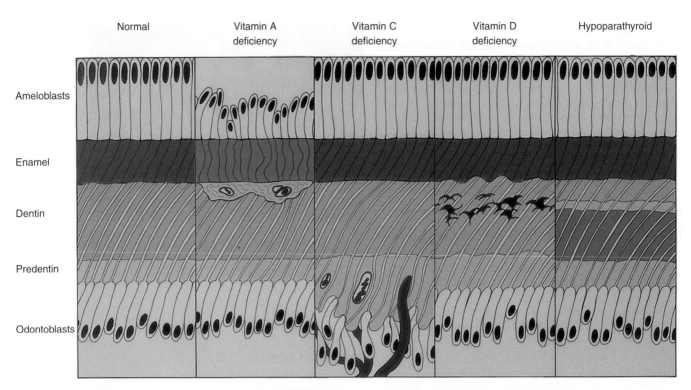

| Normal | Vitamin A deficiency | Vitamin C deficiency | Vitamin D deficiency | Hypoparathyroid |

Ameloblasts

Enamel

Dentin

Predentin

Odontoblasts

Fig. 8.**20** Summary of effects caused by vitamin A, C, and D deficiencies and hypoparathyroidism.

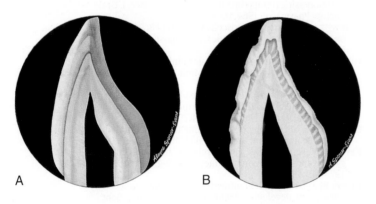

A   B

Fig. 8.**21** Summary of the effect of uptake of tetracycline **(A)** and fluoride **(B)**.

Clinical Application

Fluoridation of water supplies throughout the United States is dentistry's most successful preventative program. When mottled enamel was first noted there was an association with the lack of dental caries. Sodium fluoride was found to be the cause of this phenomenon when present in the water supply at a level of 5 ppm of water. Later, it was found that 0.5 ppm prevented caries and did not cause mottled enamel.

Self-Evaluation Review

1. Do tetracycline and fluoride cross the placental barrier?
2. When and in what form are tetracycline and/or fluoride deposited in hard tissues?
3. Do clinical doses of tetracycline and high levels of fluoride produce an effect on human teeth? If so, what are the clinical symptoms?
4. Enumerate advantages of hard-tissue labeling with tetracycline when one evaluates the effects of agents on tooth and bone development.
5. Compare differences between fluoride and tetracycline by contrasting the manner in which dentin and enamel are stained.
6. What tissues in the body are primariily affected by deficiencies of vitamins A, C, and D?
7. How is each of these deficiencies clinically characterized in the teeth?
8. Describe the effects of both deficiency and excess of parathormone on tooth formation.
9. Why are these effects limited to developing teeth and bones?
10. What are the periodontal symptoms of vitamin C deficiency?

SECTION III
Structure and Function of the Teeth

9 Histology of Enamel

Nicholas P. Piesco and James Simmelink

Introduction

Enamel is a highly mineralized tissue covering the tooth crown, unique because it is totally acellular and is produced as a result of both the secretory and resorptive activity of epithelial cells. Additionally, the enamel matrix consists of unique matrix proteins and lacks collagen, the main matrix constituent of mineralized tissues arising from mesoderm or ectomesenchyme. As a dental covering, enamel is highly adapted to withstand the forces of mastication and to resist wear. It is 96% mineral by weight and has a singular crystalline structure in comparison to other mineralized tissues. Enamel is unique since its hydroxyapatite crystals are extremely large, highly oriented, and packed into rod–like structures. The orientation of the enamel rods and the crystals within rod and interrod enamel makes it less brittle and provides it with a certain degree of flexibility, enabling it to withstand shearing forces. Enamel crystals are composed of hydroxyapatite, but also contain trace minerals (fluorapatite and carbonated apatite) and trace elements. These additional crystal components can make enamel crystals more or less susceptible to acid attack. The distribution of certain components within the crystal also explains the peculiar manner in which enamel crystals dissolve in acidic solutions. The orientation of crystals in rod and interrod enamel also contributes to etching patterns in carious lesions.

The structural features of enamel can be classified as those associated with the dentinoenamel junction (DEJ) and initial enamel formation, those associated with appositional growth, those associated with changes in enamel rod orientation, and those associated with the surface of the tooth. Enamel spindles, tufts, and lamellae arise at the DEJ. Of these, spindles are mesenchymally-derived structures representing extensions of dentinal tubules into the enamel matrix. Tufts and lamellae represent hypomineralized regions in the enamel, and are generally believed to be associated with structural weaknesses. Tufts are regular structures and extend from the DEJ through one-third to one-half of the thickness of enamel. Their regular appearance indicates that they may be an integral component linking enamel and dentin. Lamellae occur less frequently, extend from the DEJ to the enamel surface, represent areas of significant weakness, and are susceptible to fracture. Structures related to the appositional growth of enamel include cross striations and Retzius' striae. In ground sections of teeth, cross striations extend over the enamel rod with regular frequency giving the enamel rod the appearance of a ladder with the cross striations representing the rungs. The amount of enamel between cross striations is believed to be formed in 1 day. Retzius' striae are hypomineralized, occur less frequently, and display varying degrees of prominence. They represent incremental lines spaced 5 to 10 days apart; areas of enamel rod constriction and irregular crystal packing; and are formed as a result of differential deposition of rod and interrod enamel. The most pronounced stria is the neonatal line. Where the striae meet the surface of the tooth they are associated with grooves called perikymata or imbrication lines of Pickerill. Microscopic features associated with undulations of the enamel rod are gnarled enamel and Hunter-Schreger bands. Gnarled enamel is associated with the highly twisted enamel rods that occur in cusps and is believed to have increased resistance to shearing forces. Hunter-Schreger bands are alternating light and dark bands observed in ground sections, and represent patterns of reflected light from cross-sectioned and longitudinally sectioned enamel rods. Surface structures on enamel can be developmental or acquired. Developmental structures include the enamel cuticle, which is the product of cells of the enamel organ (primary cuticle) or the cells themselves (secondary cuticle). Acquired coatings include the salivary pellicle (accumulated salivary proteins), plaque (accumulation of bacteria in a soft dextran matrix), and calculus or tarter (mineralized plaque).

A thorough understanding of the development, structure, and physical properties of enamel as outlined in this chapter provides the conceptual basis for the dental treatment of carious lesions; for example, preventive measures (fluoride treatments, sealants, etc.), the design of cavity preparations, choice of restorative materials. Furthermore, understanding the factors that relate to the development of tooth color (aging, developmental defects, staining, etc.) is important for functional as well as aesthetic considerations.

Objectives

After reading this chapter, you should be able to describe the physical features of enamel, which make it an ideal covering for the tooth's surface, as well as the structure of the enamel rod and its relationship to other rods within the enamel in different areas on the tooth (from cusp tips to cervical areas). Furthermore, you should be able to describe other structural features of enamel that make it resistant or susceptible to caries and/or fracture.

Physical Characteristics of Enamel

The physical characteristics of enamel make it an excellent covering for the tooth crown and are appropriate for its primary functions, to enable mastication and protect the underlying dentin and pulp. It is the hardest and most mineralized tissue of the body. Indentation tests have shown that the average Knoop hardness number for enamel is approximately 343, making enamel five times harder than dentin, the second hardest tissue in the body. Enamel acquires these characteristics because, with maturity, it gains in mineral content what it loses in both organic material and water. Mature enamel is able to withstanding abrasion because of its extremely high mineral content (Table 9.**1**). As a hard, highly mineralized matrix, it could be assumed that enamel is extremely brittle and highly susceptible to fracture. Enamel's ability to withstand fracture is allayed, in part, because of the arrangement of its exceptionally large interlocking hydroxyapatite crystals into enamel rods and its firm support by the underlying, more pliant dentin. The scarcity of organic components in mature enamel makes it difficult to study their distribution and functional properties even in carefully prepared, demineralized histologic sections. It appears that the organic components of mature enamel play minor roles, if any, in conferring strength to enamel. Their primary function

Table. 9.**1** Comparison of enamel and dentin

Composition	Enamel	Dentin
By weight	96% inorganic 1% organic 3% water	70% inorganic 20% organic 10% water
By volume	89% inorganic 2% organic 9% water	47% inorganic 32% organic 21% water
Organic	Amelogenins (removed during development) Enamelins (tightly bound to the enamel crystals)	Collagen types I and II Phosphoproteins Carboxyglutamate-containing (GLA) proteins (osteocalcin and matrix gla) Acidic glycoproteins Plasma proteins Lipids Growth-related factors
Inorganic	Calcium phosphate (hydroxyapatite) large crystals Calcium carbonate Magnesium Potassium Sodium Fluoride	Calcium phosphate (hydroxyapatite) small crystals Trace amounts of fluoride and carbonate

Physical properties
  Color
  Hardness
  Compressive strength
  Elasticity
  Specific gravity
	Bluish-white tint
	Hardest tissue in the body
	Low tensile strength brittle
	
	High modulus of elasticity
	
	High specific gravity 2.8-3.1 g/ml refractive index 1.62
		Yellow color
		Harder than bone and cementum
		Greater tensile and compressive strength than enamel
		lower modulus of elasticity than enamel 5.21 g/ml

Structural characteristic	Enamel rod formed by Tomes' process. No processes are present in mature enamel	Dentinal tubule may contain an odontoblastic process and sometimes a nerve fiber
Permeability	Relatively impermeable	Permeable

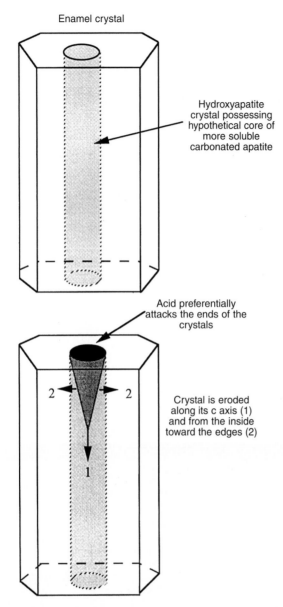

Enamel crystal

Hydroxyapatite crystal possessing hypothetical core of more soluble carbonated apatite

Acid preferentially attacks the ends of the crystals

Crystal is eroded along its c axis (1) and from the inside toward the edges (2)

Fig. 9.**1** Schematic view of an enamel crystal. The shaded area indicates the presence of a core consisting of soluble carbonated apatite.

Clinical Application

The color of enamel is due to its thickness, translucency, and the color of the underlying dentin. Enamel also becomes stained. Agents responsible for the most significant staining of enamel are beverages such as coffee, tea, and tobacco products (smoked and chewed). Before the era of home dental care products, in the 15th Century, acids (such as nitric acid, also called aqua fortis) were applied to whiten teeth by barber surgeons. This irreversibly damaged the teeth, causing significant loss of enamel. Dentifrices with high abrasive content also whiten teeth, but again remove significant amounts of enamel. Loss of cervical enamel (due to its thinness) and cementum on exposed root surfaces with the use of abrasives or improper brushing techniques exposes dentin and increases dental sensitivity.

appears to be to initiate and direct crystal growth during enamel development. Areas within enamel having a high organic content are generally associated with structural weaknesses. Furthermore, the low organic content of enamel makes it better adapted to withstand acid attack by cariogenic bacteria.

The color of a tooth is due to the thickness and opacity of the enamel. Bluish enamel is seen when the enamel layer is thick. Enamel with a bluish tinge can also be seen at the incisal edges of newly erupted teeth (where light passes through in absence of underlying dentin). The white color of deciduous teeth in comparison to permanent teeth is due to the opacity of their enamel covering. The yellowish tinge typical of secondary teeth is due to both the thinness and translucency of enamel, as well as the color and thickness of the underlying dentin.

Enamel is relatively impermeable in comparison to dentin. Pores, as such, do not exist in enamel. However, minute gaps exist between the crystals that may contain organic material and/or water. Surface enamel is more mineralized and harder than deeper enamel. It follows that the increase in mineral content occurs at the expense of the minute gaps between the crystals. Therefore, surface enamel is less permeable than inner enamel. Occlusal or incisal enamel has also been said to be harder and less permeable than cervical enamel.

Crystalline Component of Enamel

The mass of mature enamel consists of 96% inorganic material; this component is comprised almost entirely of hydroxyapatite crystals. The unit cells of hydroxyapatite crystals have the formula $Ca_{10}(PO_4)_6(OH)_2$. In addition to hydroxyapatite, enamel also contains carbonates and other trace metals. Because there is no turnover of enamel, trace elements to which the individual is exposed during the period of tooth development become incorporated and remain in the mineralized substance of the tooth. Some of these trace elements have cariostatic potential, the most notable being fluoride. Others minerals with suggested cariostatic potential are boron, barium, lithium, magnesium, molybdenum, strontium, and vanadium. Other trace elements and molecules make the tooth more susceptible to caries. These would include carbonate, cadmium chloride, iron, lead, manganese, tin, zinc, and magnesium. It is also important to note that during the formation of the enamel crystal, the first-formed mineral is a carbonated apatite. Furthermore, the core of the mature enamel crystal is thought to contain more carbonate than the peripheral regions. The presence of carbonated apatite in the crystal core makes the crystal more susceptible to dissolution from the central regions of its ends and along its core than from its sides (Fig. 9.**1**).

The hydroxyapatite crystals of enamel are the largest in the body and are easily resolved in the electron microscope. Their dimensions are approximately 30 nm in width and 90 nm in thickness. Determination of their exact length has been problematical. First, it is difficult to get a section perfectly parallel to the long axis of the crystal and secondly, the crystals fracture readily when sectioned. Some researchers believe that the crystals may extend several millimeters or throughout the entire thickness of the enamel. Direct measurements, using ground sections and the technique of ion etching to make the enamel thin enough to view with the electron microscope, have shown that crystals attain lengths of at least 100 μm. By contrast, the crystals of dentin and bone are only 3–6 nm thick and up to 60 nm long. This indicates that the hydroxyapatite crystals of enamel are approximately 10 times wider and thicker and over a thousand times greater in length than those of bone, dentin, and cementum. Their great length is achieved through the activity of ameloblasts and the interaction of the growing crystals with enamel matrix proteins (see Chapter 5). The orientation of the crystals in rod and interrod regions of mature enamel was established during the formation of the enamel matrix. Recalling that the crystals in the newly formed enamel matrix lie roughly perpendicular to the ameloblast membrane, the direction of crystals within these regions is easily explained. It is the inclination of the distal portion of Tomes' process, in relation to the proximal portion, that gives the variations of crystal directions in rod and interrod enamel (see Figs. 5.**19**–5.**21** and Fig. 9.**2**).

Organic Matrix of Enamel

Organic material is a minor component of the mature enamel tissue (less than 1%). The low abundance of organic material in mature enamel, compared to that of developing enamel, highlights the fact that the role of organic components are primarily to direct the growth of the enamel crystals. The remaining organic material apparently has an insignificant role in the structure of enamel per se. However, it has been speculated that since this material, along with water, is distributed between the hydroxyapatite crystals, its role may be to cement together the crystals or enamel rods. As can be seen in the transmission electron micrographs, the space between the crystals is small (Figs. 9.**3** and 9.**4**), but is greater in the arcade regions of the enamel rod (prism) sheaths, indicating that more organic matrix is present

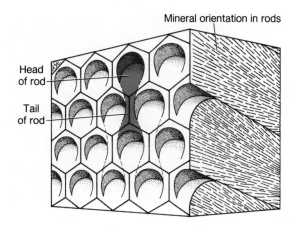

Fig. 9.**2** Diagram of the shapes of enamel rods and of mineral orientation in rods. Borders of ameloblasts are indicated by the hexagonal shapes. Arcuate pits demonstrate the relationship of Tomes' process with the enamel rod.

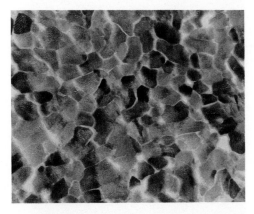

Fig. 9.**3** Transmission electron micrograph of enamel crystals seen as irregular hexagons in cross section (x 150 000). Note the small spaces between the crystals.

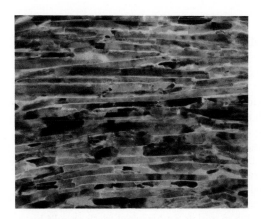

Fig. 9.**4** Enamel crystal sectioned longitudinally. Note the spaces between the crystals.

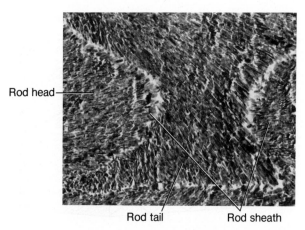

Fig. 9.**5** Transmission electron micrograph of the rod sheath prior to decalcification. Note the increased spacing between the crystals in the sheath area.

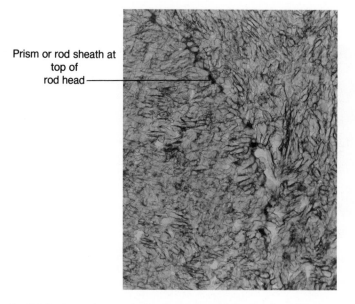

Fig. 9.**6** Electron micrograph of mature enamel following decalcification. Note the increased organic material in the sheath area.

Clinical Application

Bleaching agents approved by the American Dental Association (ADA) that reduce staining rely on the oxidizing power of peroxides. Scanning electron micrographs of bleached teeth show that bleaching increases the porosity of enamel, but these areas may remineralize rather quickly. It is possible to overbleach (or overwhiten) teeth and give them an unnaturally bright appearance. It is not possible to quickly reverse the overwhitening process. Additionally, oxygen trapped in enamel pores following bleaching may affect the set of some composite materials. For this reason, the use of composite restorative materials on bleached teeth should be postponed (2 weeks to 1 month).

in these areas (Figs. 9.**5** and 9.**6**). During enamel development degradation products of an enamel protein, sheathlin, preferentially accumulate in the arcades or prism boundaries. As a result, the area of the prism sheath has wider intercrystalline dimensions than those of corresponding prismatic or interprismatic areas and is the last area to mineralize. Therefore, the crystals in mature enamel are not as closely packed in the prism sheath as in the rod or interrod areas. Following decalcification, larger spaces are apparent in these areas (Fig. 9.**6**). The role of the organic matrix as "cementing material" may decrease the tendency of the crystals to fracture (within the rod or interrod regions) or separate (primarily along the rod sheaths) and strengthen the enamel.

The organic matrix is primarily composed of proteins and lipids. Components of the organic matrix of mature enamel consist mostly of products liberated by ameloblasts. However, exogenous components from the blood, saliva, and oral flora also become incorporated within the enamel. The most common exogenous component is serum albumin, which becomes incorporated into the enamel matrix during the maturation phase of enamel development. Lipids in the enamel matrix may represent membranous remnants pinched off from Tomes' process during the secretory stage of amelogenesis. In addition to lipids and proteins from oral bacteria, salivary secretions appear to become part of the organic matrix of enamel during or following eruption.

Structural Features of Enamel

The structural features of enamel can be classified as those associated with: the DEJ and initial enamel formation, appositional growth, changes in enamel rod orientation, and the surface of the tooth. The structural features of enamel and their clinical significance, if any, discussed below are summarized in Table 9.**2**.

Enamel Rod: Basic Structural Unit of Enamel

Calcified sections of teeth can be prepared with a diamond saw or carborundum disk, and ground and polished until they are thin enough to transmit light. Such undecalcified ground sections can be viewed by reflected or transmitted light. Sections can be made either along the longitudinal plane or as cross sections (parallel to the occlusal plane, Fig. 9.**7**). From these types of preparations, the structure of enamel was studied and described over 150 years ago by investigators like Purkynê, Fraenkel, Tomes, Retzius, and the Linderers. However, interpretations of how these structures arose and their clinical significance have only been elucidated more recently. This came about principally from improved histologic techniques (e.g., scanning and transmission electron microscopy), improved biochemical techniques (improved preservation and extraction techniques), and developments in molecular biology.

Table. 9.**2** Structural Features of Enamel

Structural feature	Developmental origin	Clinical relation
Enamel rod	Secretory product of one ameloblast from the distal or interdigitating portion of Tomes' process	Confers strength to the enamel Paths are important in cavity preparations
Enamel spindle	Extension of an odontoblast process and tubule across the basal lamina during the initial stage of matrix formation	No major clinical significance but may confer additional permeability to the deeper layers of enamel
Enamel tufts	Hypomineralized areas of enamel (rich in enamelin) near the DEJ formed during the initial stages of matrix secretion; resemble "tufts of grass"	No major clinical significance, but represent areas of enamel weakness
Enamel lamellae	Hypomineralized areas of enamel extending from the DEJ for considerable distances into the enamel	Represent a significant weakness in the structure of enamel and is susceptible to cracking
Cracks	May occur naturally, especially in hypomineralized areas between enamel rods; may be the result of lamellae; may be distinguished from lamellae in that they arise from the enamel surface and contain salivary proteins	Significant weakness in enamel; prone to breaking and caries
Hunter-Schreger bands	Viewed in ground sections with incident light and represent differences in the pattern of sectioning of enamel rods	Of no clinical significance
Gnarled enamel	Twisting of enamel rods in the cusps of teeth due to the small radius of rotation of ameloblasts during secretion	May confer some strength to the enamel
Enamel pits	Found between cusps; represent thin areas of enamel matrix due to the crowding of ameloblasts during development	Significant area of caries development; difficult to clean; areas are often treated with sealants
Incremental lines: 1. Neonatal line 2. Rezius' striae 3. Cross striations	All are formed due to the cyclical activity of ameloblasts ; represent hypomineralized areas or are due to small variations in rod orientation; during significant physiologic changes (birth and illnesses) these lines are accentuated or hypomineralized; cross striations have been explained as being due to sectioning of enamel rods across rows	Banding patterns formed during illnesses will show up on contralateral teeth which are developing at the same time Patterns of enamel hypoplasia on a single tooth or on one side indicate trauma or a localized rather than systemic infection
Perikymata	Represent the external boundary of Retzius' striae	No real clinical significance
External layer of prismless enamel	Formed during the latter stages of enamel secretion by the proximal part of Tomes' process after the distal portion is lost; this layer is thicker on primary teeth	This layer must be removed by acid etching to create "tags" prior to the application of orthodontic appliances or bonding agents
Enamel cuticle	Formed by the remnants of the reduced enamel epithelium and its secretory products; it is quickly lost	Of no major clinical significance
Enamel pellicle	Formed after the tooth is in the oral cavity; acquired from saliva and the oral flora	May contain factors which hinder the attachment of bacteria to tooth surfaces

The use of the scanning electron microscope and its improved resolution to view ground sections of enamel has substantiated the observations of these early dental histologists. Using the scanning electron microscope and following a brief etching period with dilute acids, enamel rods can be viewed in ground or fractured teeth. The orientation of the rods as seen following this procedure is depicted in Figures 9.**7**–9.**9**. The enamel rod represents the "mineralized trail" taken by the ameloblast and its distal (Tomes') process as it migrates outwardly during the process of amelogenesis. Since an initial thin layer of aprismatic enamel is formed at the DEJ, the enamel rods only extend approximately from the DEJ to the surface of the enamel (Fig. 9.**8**). Additionally, the path taken by the ameloblast during the elaboration of enamel is not straight. Enamel rods cross one another and follow an undulating course as they progress from the DEJ toward the surface of the enamel. Therefore, the length of the enamel rod is greater than the thickness of the enamel to which it is related. However, its length is directly proportional to the thickness of the enamel. In areas where the enamel is thin, such as near the cervix of the tooth and at the base of fissures, the rods are extremely short. The diameter of a rod corresponds to the diameter of the columnar ameloblast from which it was formed.

Examination of cross-sectioned enamel rods reveals an alternating series of arcades or rod sheaths in the

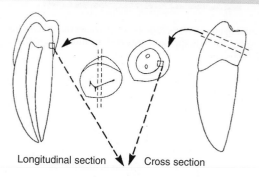

Longitudinal section   Cross section

Fig. 9.**7** Sketch showing sections of enamel depicted in Figures 9.9 and 9.10.

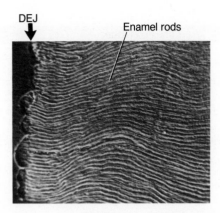

Fig. 9.**8** Scanning electron micrograph of enamel sectioned longitudinally following an acid etch. Note: the enamel rods are linear structures.

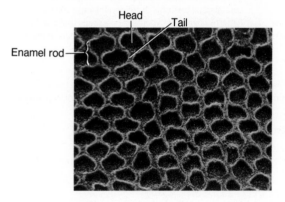

Fig. 9.**9** Scanning electron micrograph of cross-sectioned enamel after an acid etch. Note: the rods appear as pits and the interrod enamel forms the borders of the pits.

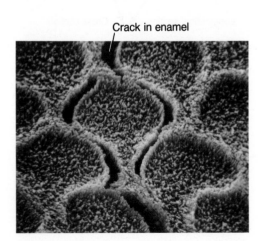

Fig. 9.**10** Scanning electron micrograph of enamel showing the staggered array of enamel rods. Note also the cracks that run between the enamel rods.

enamel (Figs. 9.**2** and 9.**9**–9.**11**; called pattern 3 enamel). When the arcades are connected to one another, enamel rods have the appearance of keyholes or paddles (Figs. 9.**2** and 9.**10**–9.**12**), with the convex surface of the arcades (or heads of the keyholes) oriented in a cuspald or incisal direction. Alternatively, the thinner neck and tail of the keyhole is oriented in an apical or cervical direction (Fig. 9.**13**). Although this view helps to explain the rod patterns observed in sectioned enamel, it does not account for the existence of interrod enamel. Investigators now favor the view that the head of the keyhole corresponds to the enamel rod (formed by the distal portion of Tomes' process during the secretory stage of amelogenesis) and the neck and tail of the keyhole correspond to the interrod enamel.

In order to understand enamel rod morphology, it is necessary to briefly re-examine the relationship of the ameloblast and Tomes' process to the developing enamel. The relationship is described and depicted in Chapter 5 (Figs. 5.**19**–5.**22**). However, in Fig. 9.**2** the hexagonal outlines represent the boundaries of ameloblasts in relation to the forming enamel in the secretory stage of amelogenesis. From this perspective it can be observed that it takes four ameloblasts to form the keyhole structure, one to form the head (the true enamel rod) and three to form the neck and tail (interrod enamel). Therefore, each ameloblast forms one enamel rod and some of the surrounding interrod enamel.

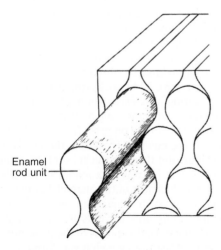

Fig. 9.**11** Diagram showing the relationship of enamel rod units (keyholes of rod and underlying interrod enamel) to one another. This relationship is typical pattern 3 enamel.

An aspect of rod structure that should be appreciated by the clinician is that enamel is more susceptible to fracturing or separation along rod boundaries (the arcades). The fracture lines are depicted in the scanning electron micrograph in Figure 9.10. The reason for the preferential cleavage is an abrupt change in the orientation of crystals at the arcade boundaries, and a more subtle shift in crystal orientation from the enamel rod and its cervically located interrod enamel (Figs. 9.**2** and 9.**14**). This observation has been used to advantage by clinicians when they refine cavity preparations. Through the use of fine chisels, clinicians can remove groups of rods that may be unsupported by dentin.

Although the typical pattern seen in cross sections of human enamel is the alternating series of arcades, as previously discussed (pattern 3), other patterns are frequently observed. These atypical patterns are due to changes in the shape of the Tomes' process from those typically described in textbooks. These variations usually occur when the Tomes' process is initially formed and, therefore, are observed near the DEJ. These rod outlines

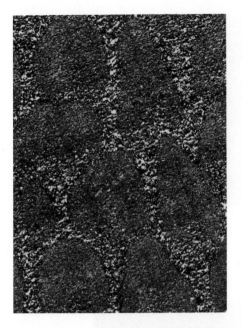

Fig. 9.**12** Transmission electron micrograph of enamel showing the typical type 3 pattern. Compare the crystal orientation in the rod and interrod enamel (cf. Figs. 9.**2** and 9.**14**).

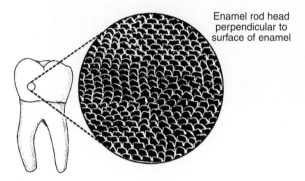

Enamel rod head perpendicular to surface of enamel

Fig. 9.**13** The appearance of enamel rods at the surface of the tooth.

Clinical Application

Enamel rods follow an undulating or spiral course running almost the full thickness of the enamel. They are more inclined in areas of the cusps and almost vertical near the cervix of the tooth. Their direction is an important consideration in the preparation of restorations. Enamel rods that are supported by hard restorative material rather than more pliant dentin are more likely to fracture. Fracturing of unsupported enamel rods in poorly designed restorative preparations causes loss of enamel around the margins of the filling material. This results in marginal leakage and makes the tooth more susceptible to carious attack. Additionally, it is also important to note that the inclination of rods differs in permanent and primary teeth and must be accounted for in the preparation of restorations.

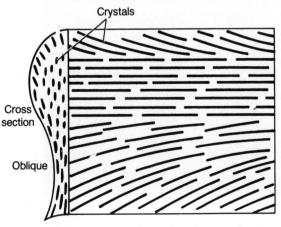

Crystals

Cross section

Oblique

Fig. 9.**14** Diagram of the orientation of crystals in the enamel rod.

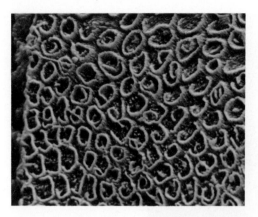

Fig. 9.**15** Irregular rod pattern. Some rods can be seen as circular structures (pattern 1).

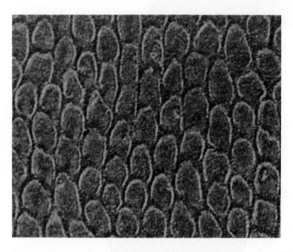

Fig. 9.**16** Vertical rod alignment (pattern 2) found near the DEJ.

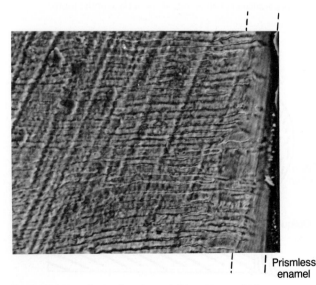

Prismless enamel

Fig. 9.**17** Layer of prismless enamel, 20 to 40 mm thick, seen near the DEJ.

take on many unusual forms near the DEJ, including circular (Fig. 9.**15**). Circular enamel rods (pattern 1) are more typical in some animal species. The enamel outside the circular rods is termed interrod or interprismatic enamel. As the ameloblasts move from the DEJ they become more oriented, and the rods they form may exhibit a stacked pattern in which the arcades appear in vertical rows (pattern 2; Fig. 9.**16**). This pattern changes into the typical alternating pattern 3 (Figs. 9.**2**, 9.**10**, and 9.**12**) as the ameloblasts retreat from the DEJ.

The enamel rods run nearly all the way to the surface of the tooth, stopping at the final layer of aprismatic enamel. This prismless layer is approximately 20 to 40 mm thick and is thicker in deciduous teeth than in primary teeth (Fig. 9.**17**). The layer is formed following loss of the distal portion of Tomes' process. All the crystals in this layer are oriented with their long crystallographic c-axis perpendicular to the enamel surface.

Dentinoenamel Junction

The DEJ represents the interface between two very different mineralized matrices, one originating from ectoderm and the other from ectomesenchyme. Its scalloped nature and resulting increased surface area enables these two dissimilar matrices to interlock. The proteins found at the DEJ (Fig. 9.**17**) are believed to provide nucleation centers for mineralization, and possibly serve as a cementing substance for dentin and enamel.

Enamel Spindle

Enamel spindles originate from the DEJ and are formed during the differentiation stage of amelogenesis. At this time, odontoblast processes cross the epithelial boundary formerly occupied by the basement membrane and their ends become insinuated between inner dental epithelial cells (preameloblasts). As the initial enamel layer is formed, the enamel spindles become represented as terminal extensions of the primary dentinal tubule into the enamel matrix. In the mature tooth enamel, spindles are bulbous structures found at the DEJ (Fig. 9.**18**). Enamel spindles do not exhibit any preferential alignment with enamel rods nor do they appear to be periodically spaced along the DEJ. They appear to be more numerous in enamel associated with the incisal edges or cusps of teeth than along the sides and cervix of the tooth. Spindles are better observed in longitudinal (coronal or sagittal) sections than in cross sections of the tooth.

Since spindles are not surface features, they are not sites for initiation of dental decay. However, once the incipient lesion approaches the DEJ, decay may proceed more rapidly in areas that have a higher porosity or organic content, such as enamel spindles.

Enamel Tufts

Enamel tufts also originate from the DEJ and are so called because of their similarity in appearance to tufts of grass. Tufts extend one-third to one-half of the thickness of the enamel matrix (Fig. 9.**19**). They are formed during the development of the Tomes' process and during the elaboration of the initial enamel of the enamel rod. As such, they represent protein-rich areas in the enamel matrix that failed to mature.

Unlike enamel spindles, enamel tufts are a frequent, regular, and periodic feature of the junctional area. They appear in rows, emanate from the scalloped crests of the DEJ, and are seen to persist following acid demineralization of enamel (Fig. 9.**20**). Tufts appear to lie in the interprismatic areas as undulating sheets associated with the sheaths of enamel rod groups. Due to their relatively high organic content, tufts have been viewed as "faults" that exist within the enamel matrix. While this may be true, it is equally possible that they may function to anchor dentin to enamel. Evidence for this view is speculative, but is based on observations that enamel tufts appear regularly along the DEJ. Since teeth are necessary for feeding and have evolved from integumental derivatives as highly adapted structures, it is unlikely that such "regular weaknesses or faults" would be selected during the process of evolution. It is plausible that these structures serve some useful purpose, such as anchoring enamel to dentin or distributing forces of mastication to prevent cracking or separation of enamel and dentin.

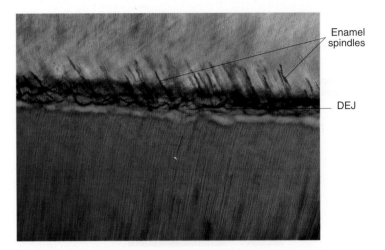

Fig. 9.**18** Enamel spindles are extensions of the primary dentinal tubule into the initial enamel matrix.

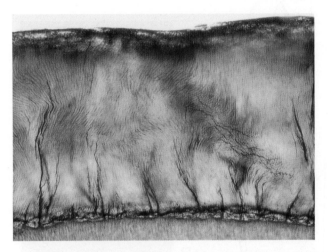

Fig. 9.**19** Enamel tufts are seen as "tufts of grass" extending from the DEJ.

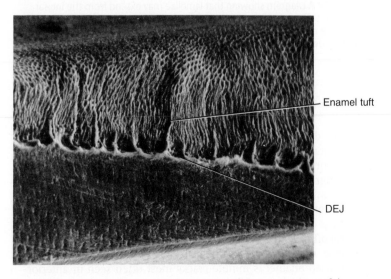

Fig. 9.**20** Enamel tufts as seen with the scanning electron microscope following a brief etch. Tuft proteins are acid resistant.

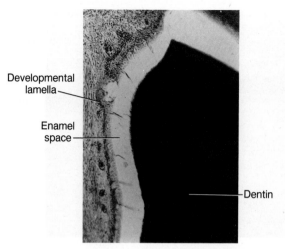

Fig. 9.**21** Lamellae can be seen as organic strands in the enamel space following demineralization.

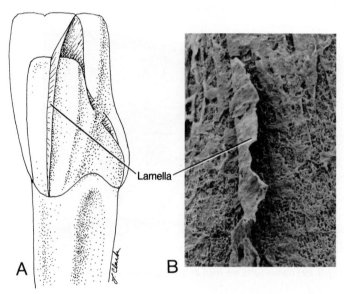

Fig. 9.**22 A** Diagram showing that lamellae may extend from the incisal edge to the cervix of the tooth. Although they appear as strands in sections, they are really sheet–like. **B** Scanning electron micrograph of a lamella following decalcification.

Clinical Application

The development of cracks or fractures can be a very serious dental complication requiring a crown and endodontic treatment. It is important to recognize fractures before they progress to a level below the gingiva or through the pulpal floor. Should this occur, the tooth would be unrestorable. Symptomatically, patients will experience pain upon biting on hard objects. Cracks or lamellae can often be seen in the dental office by transillumination with the use of fiber optics. It is also important to distinguish cracks from crazed enamel. Crazed enamel is minute cracks most often seen in anterior teeth, which are of little consequence.

Enamel Lamellae and Cracks

Enamel lamellae were first described and named by Bödecker almost 100 years ago. Lamellae consist of thin sheets of organic material that extend throughout the thickness of the enamel (Figs. 9.**21** and 9.**22A** and **B**) and run vertically from incisal or cuspal areas toward the cervix of the tooth. They can be readily demonstrated in acid decalcified whole mounts as lamellar sheets on the DEJ (Fig. 9.**22B**). It is believed that lamellae are formed as the result of local failure of the maturation process. Therefore, water and enamel matrix remnants remain in these areas. It has also been proposed that failure of the maturation process may be due to stresses that develop within the enamel matrix during the mineralization process. These stresses may trap or prevent the flow of water and enamel matrix and, therefore, inhibit their removal by ameloblasts.

Cracks have the same appearance as lamellae in ground sections and often appear as artifacts during the processing of teeth. Organic material found in cracks consists primarily of oral products that did not originate from the tissues of the developing tooth. Their composition would more closely resemble that of the salivary pellicle and, additionally, may include bacterial plaque or food debris.

Besides being areas prone to the initiation of cracks, there is some evidence that lamellae may also represent an area of permeability by which bacteria may gain access to the DEJ. This may explain some cases of the condition known as hidden caries. In this condition, the surface may differ greatly from the condition of the dentin deep below.

Structures Related to the Appositional Growth of Enamel

Cross Striations

Cross striations run at right angles to the axis of the enamel rods and, therefore, can only be observed in sections running parallel to the axis of the enamel rod. Cross striations were recognized in enamel long ago and were then proposed to be related to the 24-hour cyclical activity of ameloblasts. The observations of these early dental histologists have stood the test of time. Ultrastructural evidence suggests that regularly spaced undulations occur in the enamel prism. These cross striations are found to occur in human teeth as repeating structures 2 to 6 mm apart and are in agreement with the measured deposition rate of enamel. The regular periodicity of these structures gives enamel rods the appearance of a ladder, with the cross striations representing the rungs (Fig. 9.**23**). It has also been reported that in thick ground sections of teeth, superimposition of certain structures within the enamel, caused by undulations or varicosities of the enamel rod, might also give the appearance of cross striations.

Cross striations may also represent areas of cyclical variation in organic and/or mineral content or density of the enamel rod. Variations in carbonate and sodium content have been reported to occur along the length of the enamel rod at regular intervals. The spacing of these variations is in the order of the distance between cross striations. Cross striations may also represent areas within the enamel rod where there is altered packing of enamel crystals, that is where crystals abut one another with increased spacing and intervening organic material.

Retzius' Striae

Retzius' striae seen in ground cross sections are similar in appearance to the concentric growth rings found in cross sections of trees (Figs. 9.**24** and 9.**25**). Like the growth rings of trees and the cross striations mentioned above, the Retzius' striae also represent lines of incremental growth. However, similar to the rings of a tree, the striae are not really lines at all but only appear as such in sections. The rings of a tree can be visualized as a series of successively larger cylinders, one inside the other, because cells of the cambial layer proliferate and differentiate throughout the length of the stem. Because the growth of the tooth is limited and the deposition of enamel begins earlier in the cuspal and incisal regions, the Retzius striae can be thought of as the spaces between a series of successively larger cones stacked one inside the other. When cross-sectioned, striae appear as rings parallel to one another. In longitudinal sections, it is readily apparent that they are not parallel at all and some end at the enamel surface. The distance between successive striae is much greater and not as constant as that of cross striations. Therefore, they represent lines between layers of enamel deposited over a longer period of time, in the order of 5 to 10 days. Differences in mineral content occur in these areas, and are thought to be due to metabolic disturbances that occur during tooth formation.

The appearance of the Retzius striae is created during the secretory phase of amelogenesis and is most likely due to a periodic slowing of enamel matrix secretion. However, the release of enamel matrix is not uniformly slowed down at all points of the Tomes' process. Enamel matrix secretion slows down first at the distal portion of Tomes' process, and continues at a faster rate along the proximal or interameloblastic surfaces (Fig. 9.**25**). The effect of this altered release of enamel matrix is to increase the amount of interrod enamel in a localized

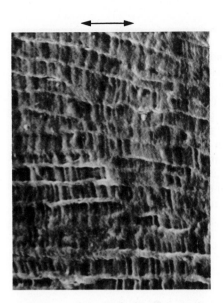

Fig. 9.**23** Scanning electron micrograph demonstrating cross striations or vertical incremental lines in enamel.

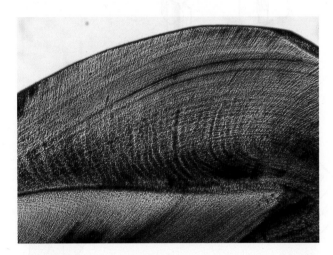

Fig. 9.**24** Light micrograph of a ground section of a tooth showing Retzius' striae.

Enamel surface

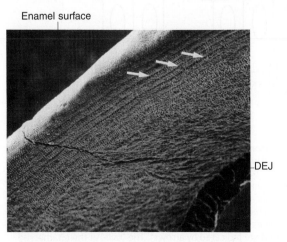

DEJ

Fig. 9.**25** Scanning electron micrograph of Retzius' striae. The pattern is accentuated due to the presence of fewer crystals and a change in crystal orientation in these areas (arrows).

Clinical Application

Caries spreads more rapidly in dentin than enamel. The reason for this spread is not strictly the mineral content, because in acid solutions enamel demineralizes more quickly than dentin. The low organic content of enamel does not provide a nutrient source for the growth of bacteria or production of acid. In dentin, exposed and degraded collagen can serve this purpose. Additionally, in enamel the Retzius' striae (or lines) are planar structures of increased organic content. These striae have been proposed as preferential areas for the spread of caries within the enamel. However, the change in crystal direction at these sites may actually impede the progress of caries.

area. The local increase in the thickness of interrod enamel in turn constricts the base of the distal portion of Tomes' process. When secretion speeds up, the distal portion of Tomes' process has to "squeeze through" the restricted area as it forms the enamel rod. Therefore, the enamel rod is constricted at the Retzius striae (Fig. 9.**26**). The altered shape of the enamel rod may interfere with the removal of organic elements (possibly sheathlin), and the changing orientation of the crystals may affect the packing of crystals in this area.

As seen with the scanning electron microscope, the packing of hydroxyapatite crystals is also more irregular within the Retzius striae than between them. Therefore, fewer enamel crystals are found within the Retzius striae (Fig. 9.**25**). The greater the physiologic disturbance, the more pronounced the line. The neonatal line is one such pronounced Retzius' stria. This is due to nutritional and hormonal changes that occur at birth. Fevers, vitamin deficiencies, metabolic diseases, etc. can also induce pronounced striae. No real clinical significance has been attributed to the Retzius' striae. However, it has been proposed that they may impede the progression of caries in enamel.

When the Retzius' striae reach the surface, they form a series of fine horizontal ridges on the enamel surface (Figs. 9.**27** and 9.**28**). Surface manifestations are known as perikymata or imbrication lines of Pickerill. Pickerill was the first to correlate their appearance with the Retzius' striae. They are formed at the boundary between one group of ameloblasts that stopped secreting and another that continued secreting more enamel matrix. Perikymata are particularly prominent on the facial side of newly erupted teeth. They are especially prominent in the middle to cervical portions of the crown. Because of the erosion that occurs with aging following eruption, they are less apparent in older teeth. When perikymata are properly illuminated, they give the enamel surface a finely corrugated appearance.

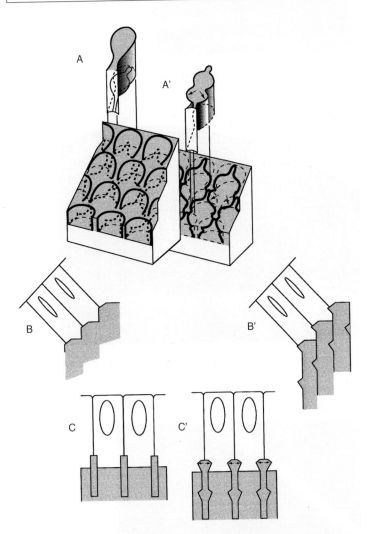

Fig. 9.**26** Proposed formation of Retzius' striae. **A** Shows the typical arcade structure of enamel with pits similar to those in Figure 9.2. The dotted lines indicate the pattern of formed enamel. Rod enamel is indicated in green and interrod enamel in pink. The image shows a sagittal and coronal section through ameloblasts and their Tomes' processes. Enamel rods and interrod enamel appear as alternating pink and green bands. **B, C** Enamel formation in Retzius' striae. Note the increased deposition of interrod enamel (widened pink areas are indicated by arrows). The "tails" of the enamel rod units thicken, constricting the base of the distal portions of the Tomes' processes as seen in sagittal and coronal sections (**B'** and **C'**). Modified after Risnes (Anat. Rec. 1990;226:135).

Additional Features of Enamel

Gnarled Enamel and Hunter-Schreger bands

Another group of structural features of enamel results from the changing courses or shifts in the orientations the enamel rods take as they pass through the enamel layer. In keeping with our analogy to wood, enamel, also shows a "grain pattern." Most enamel rods follow an undulating pathway from the DEJ to the tooth's surface. In the cusp tips of molars, groups of enamel rods twist about one another. This "grain pattern" is known as gnarled enamel (Fig. 9.**29**). These deposition patterns are thought to strengthen enamel, making it more resistant to fracture during the stress of mastication.

Hunter-Schreger bands are best seen in reflected light. They can easily be seen in a ground section with oblique illumination with the use of a hand lens, and appear as an alternating series of curved light and dark bands extending at an angle from the DEJ to the enamel surface. This interesting pattern is caused by the way in which sectioned enamel rods reflect light. The dark bands correspond to cross-sectional enamel rods and are known as diazones, while the lighter bands representing longitudinally sectioned rods are known as parazones (Figs. 9.**30** and 9.**31**). Shifts in rod orientation corresponding to Hunter-Schreger bands can be clearly demonstrated with the scanning electron microscope (Fig. 9.**32**).

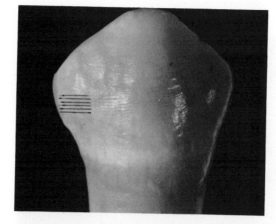

Fig. 9.**27** Perikymata or imbrication lines (of Pickerill) on the tooth surface are external manifestations of Retzius' striae.

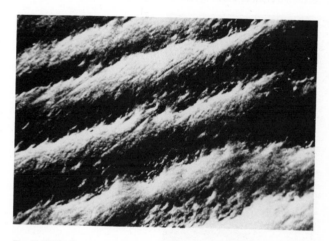

Fig. 9.**28** Perikymata as seen with the scanning electron microscope.

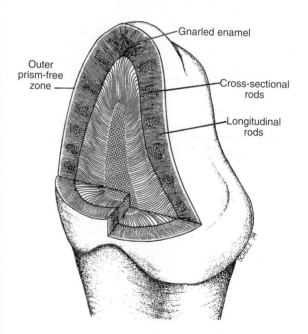

Fig. 9.**29 A** Diagram showing longitudinal and cross sections of enamel rods (Hunter-Schreger bands) as well as gnarled (twisted) enamel rods at the incisal or cuspal areas of the tooth.

Outer prism-free zone

Gnarled enamel

Cross-sectional rods

Longitudinal rods

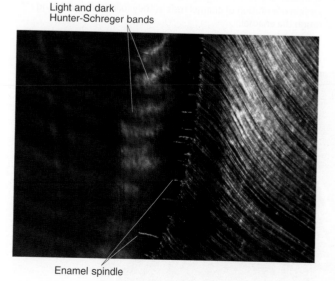

Light and dark Hunter-Schreger bands

Enamel spindle

Fig. 9.**29 B** The alternating light (parazones) and dark (diazones) bands in the enamel as viewed in reflected light are Hunter-Schreger bands.

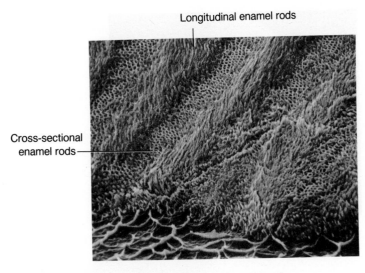

Fig. 9.**30** Sectioned enamel showing Hunter-Schreger bands.

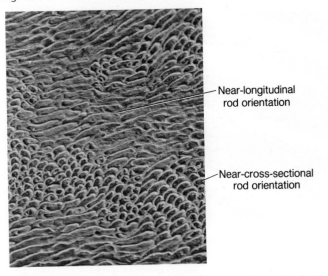

Fig. 9.**31** Scanning electron micrograph of Hunter-Schreger bands. Banding is due to varying orientation of enamel rods as they follow an undulating course through the enamel.

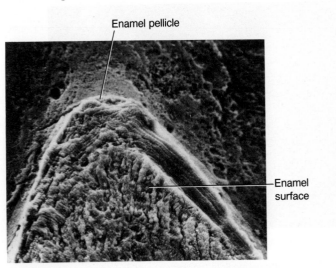

Fig. 9.**32** Scanning electron micrograph of an organic pellicle on the enamel surface.

Surface Coatings of Teeth

Surface coatings can be classified according to their origin. Developmental coatings are formed as a consequence of the normal development of teeth. The epithelial covering of reduced enamel epithelium, which is sometimes called the secondary dental cuticle, is lost soon after eruption due to abrasion. It is the same as Nasmyth's membrane which is an integumentary covering on the tooth surface derived from the enamel organ. The dental cuticle, sometimes called the primary acellular dental cuticle, is the epithelial attachment or the organic matrix responsible for binding the epithelium to the tooth. It is essentially the basal lamina material formed by the epithelium. Coronal cementum is found naturally on the occlusal surface of the teeth of many herbivores. If the reduced enamel epithelium should degenerate prior to eruption, cementum can be deposited on the surface of the crown by the cells of the dental follicle.

Acquired coatings are obtained in the environment of the oral cavity. They are briefly described in the order of their appearance. Following a cleaning the first coating to form is the salivary pellicle (Fig. 9.**32**). It is a thin film of organic material consisting of salivary proteins (mucoproteins and sialoproteins). Dental plaque is a soft adherent coating consisting of bacteria embedded in a matrix of bacterial and salivary products. Plaque is easily removed by brushing and flossing. If not removed, plaque can become calcified as calculus or tartar. It consists of 70–80% calcium phosphate salts. Since calculus becomes calcified, it is more difficult to remove than plaque.

Demineralization of Enamel

The demineralization pattern of enamel, whether it is through a pathological process or induced by exposure to etching materials applied by the clinician, is interesting and has some important clinical consequences. The "etching pattern" is due to two of the features of enamel. The first arises from the fact that as enamel crystal is nucleated, it is formed as a carbonated apatite. With crystal growth, the central regions of the crystal are richer in this carbonated apatite. This carbonated apatite is more susceptible to acid demineralization than hyroxyapatite or fluorapatite, and when exposed to acids the enamel crystals preferentially dissolve at their ends. More specifically, the mineral is removed first in the central regions of the ends and then progresses along the core of the crystal (Figs. 9.**33A** and **B** and 9.**34A** and **B**). The crystal appears to dissolve from the inside out. In sectioned carious enamel or acid demineralized enamel, cross-sectioned crystals in the early phases of demineralization have the appearance of doughnuts. In sections of obliquely sectioned crystals, they have the appearance of hairpins and are called hairpin defects (Fig. 9.**33B**). Secondly, the crystals in enamel are highly oriented in the rod and interrod regions. Crystals with their "sensitive ends" pointing toward the surface will be the first to be attacked. When enamel is etched in order to create a bond, the acid preferentially attacks crystals with exposed ends. Crystals running at an angle to the surface are more resistant and dissolve much later. Acid etching increases the surface area available for bonding by creating "enamel tags" due to the differential etching of rod and interrod enamel (Figs. 9.**35** and 9.**36**). Of course, the initial aprismatic layer of enamel would have to be removed first because all the crystals run in the same direction and are etched uniformly.

Plaque accumulates in areas that are not cleansed effectively (molar fissures, interproximal spaces, etc.), and bacteria that underlie dental plaque produce acids as products of their normal metabolism. The falling pH causes the enamel to dissolve and become porous. Initially, the porosity appears as a white lesion or spot. Demineralization progresses beneath an intact enamel surface. Collapsing of the surface structure or cavitation occurs with progressive demineralization. However, the removal of plaque (carbohydrate, food particles, and bacteria) and the buffering capacity of salivary secretions can prevent the demineralization process. Additionally, reversal of the process or remineralization can occur. Remineralization may take place as minerals from oral secretions return to the partially demineralized enamel. The frequency and length of the respective stages in this cycle (demineralization vs remineralization) and the complex interactions (bacterial metabolism, salivary composition, diet, hygiene, etc.) will determine whether or not a carious lesion develops. Fluoride also seems to play an important role in the remineralization process.

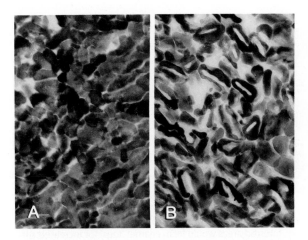

Fig. 9.**33** Cross-sectional enamel crystals. **A** Normal cross-sectional crystals. **B** Partial demineralization along the c-axis of the crystal. Note that some of the crystals exhibit the typical "hairpin" pattern when sectioned obliquely. See also Figure 9.**1**.

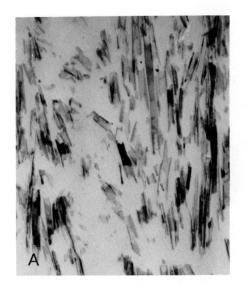

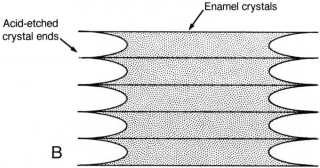

Fig. 9.**34 A** Longitudinal view of partially demineralized crystals. **B** Diagrammatic representation showing shortening of crystals due to erosion at their ends.

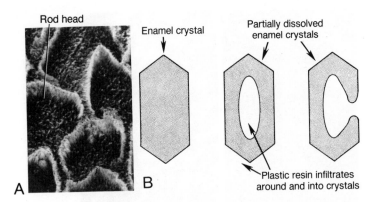

Fig. 9.**35 A** Acid etched enamel showing loss of rod structure and retention of interrod areas. Interrod areas would form enamel "tags" for increased surface area bonding. **B** Etching pattern is due to dissolution of enamel crystals at their ends and along their core.

Since fluoroapatite and hydroxyapatite are more resistant to demineralization than carbonated apatites, surfaces remineralized with fluoride are probably more resistant to decay. This is due to replacement of more easily dissolved carbonates with fluoro- and hydroxyapatite. Fluoride acts in two important ways: first, as an inhibitor of crystal dissolution during a carious attack, and second by enhancing the remineralization process that produces a surface veneer of resistant fluoroapatite material. Fluoride, at sufficient concentrations, can also inhibit the formation of plaque and acid.

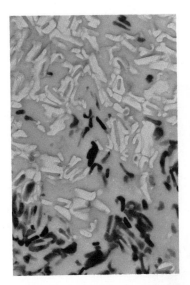

Fig. 9.**36** Transmission electron micrograph showing areas of crystal demineralization (white areas). The black areas represent intact crystals and the gray areas represent embedding material.

Summary

Enamel is a highly mineralized substance, thoroughly adapted to withstand the forces of mastication. Enamel crystals are the largest crystals found in the body and are over one thousand times larger that those of dentin, bone, or cementum. The primary structural unit of enamel is the enamel rod. Enamel rods are formed as a result of the secretory activity of ameloblasts. Ameloblasts play an important role in the maturation process regulating the removal of almost all of the matrix liberated during the secretory phase of amelogenesis. The orientation of crystals and the distribution of organic matrix materials remaining in the enamel matrix are responsible for the structural properties of enamel. The structural features of enamel can be categorized as those associated with the DEJ, the appositional growth of enamel, enamel rod orientation, or the surface of enamel. The structural features of the DEJ—increased surface area due to scalloping, presence of tufts and spindles—are believed to be important in joining enamel and dentin, initiating mineralization during development, or contributing to structural weakness of the enamel. Structures related to appositional growth include cross striations (daily growth lines) and Retzius' striae. These form as a result of cyclical activity of ameloblasts, and are enhanced during times of physiologic stress. Perikymata surface features are related to appositional growth.

Surface features of enamel include those which arise during development, the primary and secondary cuticle, and those that are acquired, the salivary pellicle, plaque, and tarter or calculus. The effect of acids on the enamel can be explained from knowledge of the formation of enamel crystals, their composition, and their orientation or distribution in the enamel. Demineralization — remineralization cycles play an important role in the formation of caries. Removal of food particles and plaque by cleaning, salivary buffering, and topical fluoride tend to favor the remineralization process and inhibit enamel destruction.

Clinical Application

Acid etching agents are used to improve bonding of composite materials to enamel and dentin. The mechanism of composite bonding differs in enamel and dentin. In enamel, the etching agents etch the enamel nonuniformly, creating enamel tags. The bond strengths of some cements, used to place orthodontic brackets on teeth, can be so strong that a significant amount of enamel is removed with the bracket. Etching is also used prior to the application of sealants. Sealants protect cavity-prone areas of the tooth, especially the enamel pits.

Self-Evaluation Review

1. Describe the physical properties of enamel that make it an excellent covering for the tooth.

2. Describe the orientation of crystals in rod and interrod enamel.

3. How are crystal composition and orientation related to patterns of demineralization?

4. Describe the courses and types of incremental lines that are found within the enamel. How are they formed and how do disease, diet, or other physiologic stressors affect their appearance?

5. Describe the orientation of enamel rods in different areas of the crown (occlusal surface, cusp tips, lateral surfaces, and near the cervix).

6. How do enamel rod patterns explain Hunter-Schreger banding?

7. What is the relationship between lamellae and cracks? How might they be distinguished from one another?

8. Where is prismless enamel found on the tooth?

9. What factors determine the color of the tooth? How can teeth be whitened?

10. What is the importance of the DEJ? What types of enamel features arise there?

11. How are enamel pits formed and how are they treated clinically?

Suggested Readings

Berkovitz BKB, Holland GR, Moxham BJ. Color atlas and textbook of oral anatomy, histology and embryology. St. Louis: Mosby Yearbook Inc.; 1992.

Boyde A. Structure and development of mammalian enamel. Ph.D. Thesis, Department of Anatomy, London Hospital Medical College, 1964.

Boyde A. A 3-D model of enamel development at the scale of one inch to the micron. Adv. Dent. Res. 1987;1:135–140.

Boyde A. Microstructure of enamel. In: Dental Enamel. CIBA Found Symp. 1997;205:18–31.

Boyde A, Fortelius M, Lester KS, Martin LB. Basis of the structure and development of mammalian enamel as seen by scanning electron microscopy. Scaning Microsc. 1988;2:1479–1490.

Dalcusi G, Kerebel B. High-resolution electron microscope study of human enamel crystallites: size, shape, and growth. J Ulrastruct Res.1978;65:163–172.

Fearnhead RW, Stack MV, eds. Tooth Enamel II: Its Composition, Properties, and Fundamental Structure. Bristol, UK: John Wright & Sons; 1971.

Fearnhead RW, Suga S, eds. Tooth Enamel IV. New York, NY: Elsevier Science Publishers; 1984.

Fearnhead RW, ed. Tooth Enamel V. Yokohama, Japan: Florence Publishers; 1989.

Fincham AG, Hu Y, Lau E, Pavlova Z, Slavkin HC, Snead MC. Isolation and partial characterization of a human amelogenin from a single fetal dentition using HPLC techniques. Calcif Tissue Int. 1990;47:105–111.

Fincham AG, Moradain-Oldak J, Simmer JP. The structural biology of the developing dental enamel matrix. J. Struct. Biol. 1999;126:270–299.

Goldberg M, Carreau JP, Arends J. Biochemical and scanning electron microscope study of lipids chloroform-methanol extracted from unerupted and erupted human tooth enamel. Arch. Oral Biol. 1987;32:765–772.

Harding AM, Zero DT, Featherstone JDB, McCormack SM, Shields CP, Proskin HM. Calcium fluoride formation on sound enamel using fluoride solutions with and without lactate. Caries Res. 1994;28:1–8.

Kodaka T, Natajima F, Higashi S. Structure of the so-called 'prismless' enamel in human deciduous teeth. Caries Res. 1989;23:290–296

Listgarten MA. Structure of surface coatings on teeth. A review. J Periodontol. 1976;47:139–147.

Newman HN, Poole DFG. Observations with scanning and transmission electron microscopy on the structure of human surface enamel. Arch. Oral Biol. 1974;19: 1135–1143.

Nygaard VK, Simmelink JW. Ultrastructural study of the resin infiltration zone in acid-treated human enamel. Arch. Oral Biol. 1978;23:1151–1156.

Nylen MU, Termine JD, eds. Tooth enamel III: its development, structure, and composition. J Dent Res. 1979;58:675–1031.

Massler M, Schour I. The appositional life span of the enamel and dentin-forming cells. I Human deciduous teeth and first permanent molars. J. Dent. Res. 1946;25:145–150.

Risnes S. Structural characteristics of staircase-type Retzius lines in human dental enamel analyzed by scanning electron microscopy. Anat. Rec. 1990;226:135–146.

Risnes S. Enamel apposition rate and the prism periodicity in human teeth. Scand. J. Dent. Res. 1986;94:394–404.

Risnes S. A scanning electron microscope study of the three-dimensional extent of Retzius lines in human dental enamel. Scand. J. Dent. Res. 1985;93:145–152.

Schroeder HE. Oral Structural Biology. New York, NY: Thieme; 1991:38–85.

Schour I, Poncher HG. Rate of apposition of enamel and dentin, measured by the effect of acute fluorosis. Am. J. Dis. Child. 1937;54:757–776.

Scott DB, Simmelink JW, Nygaard VK. Structural aspects of dental caries. J Dent. Res. 1974;53:165–178.

Simmelink JW. Mode of enamel matrix secretion. J Dent. Res. 1982;61:1483–1495.

Simmelink JW, Nygaard VK. Ultrastructure of striations in carious human enamel. Caries Res. 1982;16:179–188.

Simmelink JW, Nygaard YK, Scott DB. Theory for the sequence of human and rat enamel dissolution by acid and by EDTA: a correlated SEM and TEM study. Arch. Oral Biol. 1974;19:183–197.

Simmer JP, Fincham AG. Molecular mechanisms of dental enamel formation. Crit. Rev. Oral Biol. Med. 1995;6:84–108.

Stack MV, Fearnhead RW, eds. Tooth Enamel: Its Composition, Properties and Fundamental Structure. Bristol, UK: John Wright & Sons; 1965.

Ten Cate, AR. Oral Histology Development, Structure, and Function. 4th Ed. St. Louis: C.V. Mosby; 1998.

Termine JD, Belcourt AB, Christner PJ, Conn, KM, Nylen MU. Properties of dissociatively extracted fetal tooth matrix proteins. J Biol. Chem. 1980;255:9760–9768.

Tinanoff N, Glick PL, Weber DF. Ultrastructure of organic films on the enamel surface. Caries Res. 1976;10:19–32.

Walker, BN, Makinson OF, Peters MCRB. Enamel cracks. The role of enamel lamellae in caries initiation. Aust. Dent. J. 1998;43:110–116.

Weher DF. Sheath configurations in human cuspal enamel. J Morphol. 1975;141:479–490.

Whittaker DL, Richards D. Scanning electron microscopy of the neonatal line in human enamel. Arch. Oral Biol. 1978;23:45–50.

10 Histology of Dentin

Nicholas P. Piesco

Introduction

Dentin is primarily formed from the secretory products of the odontoblasts and their processes. It is the hard tissue that constitutes the body of each tooth, serving as both a protective covering for the pulp and as a support for the overlying enamel (Fig. 10.1). Unlike enamel, dentin is a vital tissue containing the cell processes of odontoblasts and neurons. Odontoblasts perform a structural role in the formation of the dentinal matrix, and neurons convey sensory information. The primary component of the dentinal matrix, collagen, imparts the resiliency necessary for the crown (enamel as well as dentin) to withstand the forces of mastication. The color of the crown of the tooth is partially due to the color and thickness of the underlying dentin as well as to the thinness and translucency of the enamel.

Although dentin resembles bone in composition, true dentin differs from bone in that contains no trapped cells or blood vessels and also, unlike bone dentin, is not continuously remodeled. Therefore, dentin has a limited capacity for repair. New physiologic or reparative dentin can only be added on its inner aspect so that as the tooth ages, the bulk of dentin increases as the pulp chamber decreases in volume. Also, unlike bone, coronal dentin is covered with enamel and radicular dentin is covered with cementum.

Objectives

After reading this chapter you should be able to: recognize and classify the various types of dentin; discuss the developmental origin of the various types of dentin; describe the organic and mineral components of the dentinal matrix; and explain the roles of the primary organic components of the dentinal matrix. Furthermore, you should be able to describe the effects of natural (environmental, physiologic, or pathologic) and clinician-induced (iatrogenic) factors that alter dentin composition and permeability.

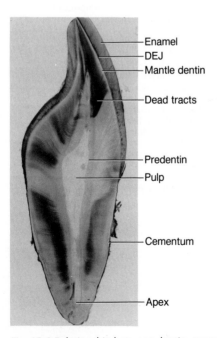

Enamel
DEJ
Mantle dentin

Dead tracts

Predentin
Pulp

Cementum

Apex

Fig. 10.1 Relationship between dentin, enamel, and the pulp. DEJ: dentino-enamel junction.

Dentinal Matrix Composition: Inorganic and Organic Constituents

Mature dentin is about 70% mineral, 20% organic matrix, and 10% water on a weight basis and about 50% mineral, 30% organic, and 20% water on a volume basis. Dentin does not have a uniform composition throughout the tooth. It can vary in organic composition as well as hardness and mineral content in different areas of the tooth. This may be related to anatomic location, degree of dental sclerosis, or both. Unlike enamel, the high organic content of dentin enables it to deform slightly under compression. Another factor contributing to the resiliency of the dentin may be the fluid within the dentinal tubules. The fluid-filled dentinal tubules may function as "hydraulic shock absorbers" dissipating the forces of mastication. Dentin therefore provides a "cushion" for the overlying brittle enamel.

Inorganic Matrix

Although trace amounts of calcium carbonate, fluoride, magnesium, zinc, and other minerals (e.g., metal phosphates and sulfates) are found in dentin, hydroxyapatite, $Ca_{10}(PO_4)_6(OH)_2$, is the principal inorganic component of the dentinal matrix. The hydroxyapatite crystals are in the form of flattened plates with the approximate dimensions of 60 to70 nm in length, 20 to 30 nm in width, and 3 to 4 nm in thickness. The calcium: phosphate ratio (by weight) varies in peritubular (1:2.14) and intertubular (1:2.10) dentin, but overall averages 1:2.13. Extensive sclerosis or deposition of peritubular dentin (sclerosis) that can occur with aging makes the dentin brittle and less resilient.

The high mineral content of dentin makes it harder than cementum or bone, although softer than enamel. In the laboratory, hardness can be measured by the Knoop hardness test in which a small diamond point is dropped from a known distance onto a polished dentinal surface. These indentation tests have shown that the average Knoop hardness test (Knoop hardness number) is approximately 68 for dentin and approximately 343 for enamel, making enamel five times harder than dentin (Table 10.**1**). Basically, there is little or no difference in the range of the Knoop hardness test between teeth of

Table. 10.**1** Classification of dentin by location, patterns of mineralization, and development

Location	Pattern of mineralization	Developmental pattern
Intertubular dentin: found around and between dentinal tubules.	**Globular dentin:** formed from calcospherites.	**Primary dentin:** formed prior to and during active eruption
Intratubular dentin: found and formed within dentinal tubules; also called peritubular dentin.	**Interglobular dentin:** hypomineralized dentin between mantle and circumpulpal dentil; normally only found in coronal dentin	**Secondary dentin:** formed when the tooth first comes into occlusion
Mantle dentin: formed initially in the crown; outer coronal dentin.	**Tomes granular layer:** hypomineralized layer in root dentin; similar to interglobular dentin in the crown.	**Tertiary dentin:** formed as a result of a pathologic response; may be *reactionary* or *reparative*.
Circumpulpal dentin: nearest to the pulp; formed in crown after mantle dentin has been deposited.	**Sclerotic dentin:** hypermineralized, occluding intratubular dentin.	

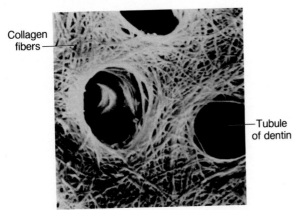

Collagen fibers

Tubule of dentin

Fig. 10.**2** Scanning electron micrograph of decalcified dentin showing collagen fibers and dentinal tubules.

Table. 10.**2** Comparison of the hardness of enamel and types of dentin

Matrix	Knoop hardness number
Enamel	343
Orthodentin	68
Sclerotic dentin	80
Carious dentin	25

different types or between root and coronal dentin of the same tooth. Variations may occur, however, under the various environmental influences discussed previously. Sclerotic dentin is harder, having a Knoop hardness test of approximately 80. Carious dentin or dead tracts are partially demineralized and have a reduced Knoop hardness test of approximately 25.

Organic matrix

The bulk of the organic matrix of dentin (85–90%) consists of collagen (Fig. 10.**2**). Most of the collagen is type I with minor amounts of type V and VI. Although type III collagen may be found in the pulp and in the initial predentinal matrix of developing teeth, it does not appear to be a secretory product of mature odontoblasts.

The noncollagenous macromolecules of dentin can be classified into several broad categories (Table 10.**2**): phosphoproteins, γ-carboxyglutamate-containing (Gla) proteins, miscellaneous acidic glycoproteins, growth–related factors, serum-derived proteins, lipids, and proteoglycans. Among the noncollagenous proteins, dentin phosphoprotein (DPP or phosphophoryn) is the major contributor, comprising 50% of all noncollagenous proteins. It has been found to associate with collagen at the mineralization front but is not found in the predentinal matrix. *In vitro* experiments have shown that collagen reconstituted with DPP readily mineralizes. It has been suggested that DPP resides in "hole" regions of collagen fibers (between tropocollagen molecules) and serves as a nucleator of mineralization. The presence of highly repetitive Asp-Ser-Ser (dss) motifs in DPP is primarily responsible for this function. In vivo most of the serine residues exhibiting these motifs, in the region of the protein, are phosphorylated. Due to its high electronegative charge and charge repulsion, of phosphate and carboxyl groups, this region of the molecule exists in an extended state and also serves as a "cationic sink" for binding of calcium ions.

Dentin sialoprotein (DSP) is a phosphorylated, highly glycosylated protein containing high amounts of sialic acid. Both DPP and DSP are tooth-specific products. However, synthesis of DPP has been detected transiently in preameloblasts and odontoblasts. Recent genetic evidence indicates that these two proteins (DPP and DSP) are transcribed as a bicistronic gene product and are parts of the same protein, dentin sialophosphoprotein (DSPP). However, they are not present in the dentinal matrix in the expected 1:1 ratio. The ratio is closer to 10:1 or 7:1 (DPP:DSP). Changes in the ratio may occur during post-translational modifications (phosphorylation and glycosylation reactions) or further intracellular or extracellular processing of the proteins. It is interesting to note that root or cementum–associated dentin only has one half of the phosphoprotein content of the coronal or enamel–associated dentin. The functional significance of this difference is not known.

The results of early radioautographic experiments using $^{32}PO_4$ to trace the synthesis of dentin phosphoproteins demonstrated that the phosphate label was preferentially deposited at the mineralization front, suggesting that the intracellular trafficking of phosphoproteins differs from that of proteins comprising the predentinal matrix (like collagen). The latter is released by the odontoblastic cell body or near the base of the odontoblastic process while phosphoproteins appear to be carried along the odontoblastic process, and deposited at the mineralization front.

Gla proteins are so named because they contain a unique amino acid, γ-carboxylated glutamic acid. The carboxylation reaction is vitamin-K dependent, and the addition of these carboxyl groups enables these proteins to bind calcium. Gla proteins are not specific to dentin. Bone Gla protein, or osteocalcin, and matrix Gla protein have both been found in dentin. Gla proteins of the osteocalcin type have been localized in odontoblastic processes and it has been suggested, because of their anionic character and calcium-binding abilities, that they play a significant role in mineralization. Matrix Gla protein has been found in dentin in levels similar to those of bone. Recent evidence seems to favor the view that they may serve as negative regulators of mineralization rather than nucleators.

Proteoglycans with dermatan, chondroitin, and keratin sulfate containing glycosaminoglycans have also been found in dentin. Decorin, a small proteoglycan often associated with collagen fibers and biglycan, a proteoglycan containing two glycosaminoglycan side chains, have both been found in dentin. Proteoglycans found in predentin are considerably larger than those found in dentin. The ability of some proteoglycans to associate with collagen suggests that they may play a role in fibrillogenesis (fiber morphology and size). Proteoglycans, such as chondroitin sulfate, can inhibit mineralization. Other proteoglycans bind calcium relatively nonspecifically and can induce hydroxyapatite formation in vitro.

Acidic glycoproteins are carbohydrate-rich and contain acidic groups such as acidic amino acids (e.g., aspartic and/or glutamic acids) and sialic acid (DSP and DSPP also belong to this group). The two most prominent proteins in this group are osteonectin and osteopontin. Osteonectin/SPARC (secreted protein acidic and rich in cystine) originally found in bone, has since been found in most other mineralized and nonmineralized tissues. It has been demonstrated in predentin and dentin. It binds strongly to calcium and surfaces of hydroxyapatite, inhibiting mineralization. It also binds nonspecifically to collagen. Osteopontin, a phosphorylated glycoprotein, contains an arginine-glycine-aspartic acid integrin receptor-binding sequence. Integrins are receptors found on the cell's surface that serve as receptors for extracellular matrix molecules. The 95 kDa is present in higher amounts in root (cementum–associated) dentin than in crown (enamel–associated) dentin.

Growth factors have the ability to stimulate the differentiation of undifferentiated cells. Members of the transforming growth factor β (TGF-β) have been observed in bone, cartilage, and dentin. In addition, insulin–like growth factors and fibroblast growth factors (FGFs) have also been found in dentin. A unique bone morphogenetic protein able to induce cartilage formation from fibroblasts has also been discovered in dentin. These growth factors most likely play important roles in the response to injury by inducing the formation of new odontoblasts during repair. It is of particular interest that small amounts of cartilage-specific proteins have been found to be secreted by reparative odontoblasts. This transient activity resembles the formation of a cartilaginous callus formed during the healing of a fractured bone in response to cartilage inducing factors present in the matrix. This indicates a basic similarity of these two tissue types.

Lipids exist as a minor component of the dentinal matrix. There are no unique lipids associated with the dentinal matrix. Phospholipids may participate in mineralization through formation of calcium-phospholipid complexes.

Another minor component of the organic matrix are the serum proteins. Serum albumins and α2HS-glycoprotein have been found in dentin. The functional significance of these proteins in dentin is not currently known.

Role of Matrix Vesicles in the Mineralization of Dentin

Matrix vesicles are membranous structures that arise by budding form cells, for example, from chondrocytes, osteoblasts, or odontoblasts. In these tissues matrix vesicles serve as nucleation sites for calcium phosphate. The internal portion of the bilayered lipid membrane is enriched in phosphotidylserine. Additionally, the vesicle contains nucleotides and a number of proteins including annexin V and alkaline phosphatase. In the presence of calcium, annexin V binds rapidly and with high affinity to phosphotidylserine, forming ion channels. Annexin V serves to mediate the flow of calcium into the vesicle. Phosphate ions recruited from phospholipids and nucleotides within the vesicle are liberated by the action of alkaline phosphatase. The association of phosphate ions with intravesicular calcium results in the formation of octacalcium phosphate crystals inside the vesicle near the membrane. Besides its role in the formation of ion channels, annexin V also serves as a collagen receptor. In this regard annexin V serves to bind matrix vesicles to the collagen and sequesters them in the predentinal matrix.

Clinical Application

Latent growth factors within the dentinal matrix assume important roles in tissue repair. When a tooth is injured due to infection or trauma the resulting release of proteolytic enzymes and the acidic environment cause dissolution of the extracellular matrix. Growth factors within the extracellular matrix and within platelets from the blood exist in latent forms. The conditions near the injured site, such as proteolysis and low pH, serve to activate some of these factors, especially TGF-ß. The active growth factors are able to induce growth and differentiation of cells.

Dentinal Structure and Classification

Orthodentin, true dentin, is a calcified tissue that lacks cells, contains tubules, and is organized by odontoblasts (Figs. 10.**1**–10.**3**). The most prominent features of dentin are the dentinal tubules. In the crown, the direction of the dentinal tubules extends in an S-shaped curve from the dentinoenamel junction (DEJ) to the mineralization front or dentin–predentin junction. The two bends, making up the S-shape, are called the primary curvatures. The first curve (nearest the DEJ) bends toward the occlusal or incisal surface of the tooth and the second toward the apex of the root (Figs. 10.**1**, 10.**4A**, and 10.**5**). These curves become less pronounced in the cervical region and the tubules are rather straight in the root (Figs. 10.**1** and 10.**4A**). Smaller secondary curvatures are visible microscopically (Fig. 10.**4B**). Primary curvatures represent the path taken during the inward migration of the odontoblasts. Secondary curvatures may be the

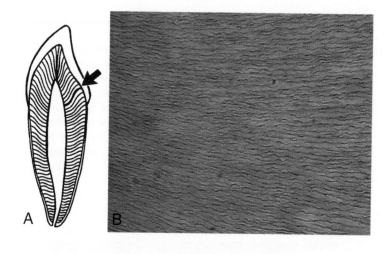

Fig. 10.**4 A** "S" curvature or primary curvatures of the dentinal tubules. **B** Secondary curvatures represented as undulations of the dentinal tubule.

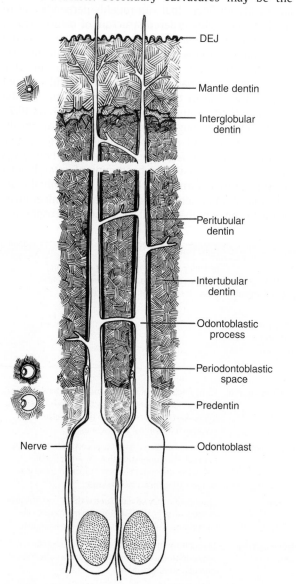

- DEJ
- Mantle dentin
- Interglobular dentin
- Peritubular dentin
- Intertubular dentin
- Odontoblastic process
- Periodontoblastic space
- Predentin
- Odontoblast
- Nerve

Fig. 10.**3** Relationship between the odontoblastic process and dentinal tubule.

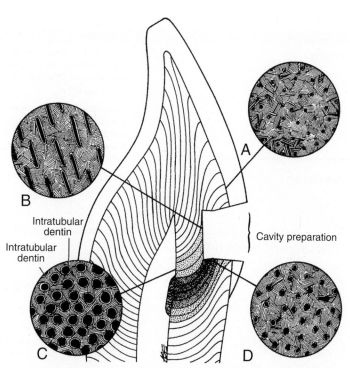

Intratubular dentin
Intratubular dentin
Cavity preparation

Fig. 10.**5** Location and size of dentinal tubules at the DEJ (**A**) and the pulp (**C**). Relationship between tubules in the cavity floor (**B** and **D**) and pathway of caries through dentin.

Clinical Application

The increase in the number and size of the dentinal tubules as the pulp chamber is approached is important for several reasons. First, when cutting into dentin, deeper cuts expose more tubules and damage more odontoblasts and their processes than shallower cuts. Secondly, the application of potentially harmful substances to the dentin can damage the pulp. Both the proximity and increased diameter of the tubules make diffusion of harmful materials such as bacteria or bacterial products as well as clinically applied liners, bases, or even pulpal obtundents more likely.

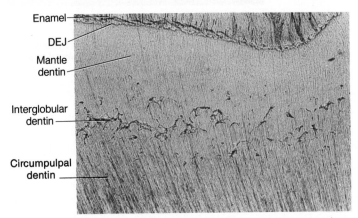

Fig. 10.**6** Interglobular spaces lie between the mantle dentin (above) and circumpulpal dentin (below) in the crown.

result of small spiraling undulations of the odontoblastic process during matrix formation and mineralization. Tubules, like the odontoblastic processes, are tapered and branched. The narrowest part and the most pronounced branching occur near the DEJ. As the odontoblasts produce more dentinal matrix, they migrate centrally and become more crowded. Therefore, dentinal tubules are more numerous and closer together nearer the pulp (40 000/mm²) than in the outer or mantle dentin (20 000/mm²).

Dentin can be classified into distinct types based on location, matrix composition, structure, and developmental pattern (Table 10.**3**). Dentin nomenclature is not necessarily exclusive and often is self-descriptive. The dentin nearest the DEJ of the crown is formed first and is called mantle dentin (Fig. 10.**6**). At the DEJ, mantle dentin and enamel interdigitate, giving the DEJ a scalloped appearance. Mantle dentin consists of relatively large collagen fibers that run roughly perpendicular to the DEJ. The highly ordered structure of mantle dentin makes it positively birefringent in polarized light. In the root, unlike the crown, the collagen fibers in the first formed dentin lie parallel or oblique to the DEJ. Therefore, no true mantle layer exists in radicular or root dentin. The bulk of the dentin underlying the mantle dentin is called circumpulpal dentin (Figs. 10.**6** and 10.**7**). Collagen fibers throughout this dentinal layer are smaller in diameter and more randomly oriented than in mantle dentin. The region separating these two layers has a characteristically high amount of interglobular dentin (Fig 10.**6**), formed as the result of the initial rapid mineralization of dentin. Initially, dentin is mineralized by the fusion of numerous calcospherites. Calcospherites

Table. 10.**3** Organic components in dentin and their possible functions

Component	Comments	Function
Collagen	Major organic component (91—92%). Type I predominates with minor amounts of type V; Type III found in the pulp and during early dentinal matrix formation.	May play a role in initiating mineralization. Provides the structural framework for dentin, giving it strength and resilience.
Phosphoproteins	Major noncollagenous proteins; deposited at the mineralization front; not found in predentin. Dentin sialoprotein and dentin phosphoprotein have recently been found to be cleavage products of a larger protein.	May play an important role in mineralization.
Proteoglycans	Dermatan, chondroitin, and keratin sulfates; decorin and biglycan are present.	Some inhibit mineralization and others bind calcium nonspecifically. Presence may thus control the mineralization process. Those that associate with collagen may control fibrillogenesis.
γ-carboxyglutamate-containing proteins, Matrix Gla and bone Gla (osteocalcin) proteins	Carboxylation reaction is vitamin K dependent.	Role in mineralized tissues is uncertain but they can bind calcium suggesting that they may initiate or control the mineralization process in some way by regulating local calcium levels.
Acidic glycoproteins	Osteopontin, 65 and 90 kDa glycoproteins.	Osteopontin may be associated with the odontoblastic process serving as a link between matrix and cell membrane. Roles of other proteins are unknown.
Growth factors	Transforming growth factor β, cartilage-inducing factors, insulin-like growth factors, and platelet-derived growth factors.	May control the proliferation and differentiation of new odontoblasts following injury or a pathologic process. Stimulate repair.
Lipids	No unique lipids are found in dentin.	Phospholipids may be involved in initiation of mineralization.

represent spherical foci of hydroxyapatite formed from calcium-phosphate nucleating sites. This mineralization pattern is often called globular mineralization. These spherical foci of mineralizing dentin are also termed globular dentin. These regions eventually fuse to form a mineralization front. The matrix between the fusing calcospherites is often hypomineralized (undermineralized). As a result, areas of hypomineralized dentin called interglobular dentin persist in the areas between fusing calcospherites. Increased amounts of interglobular dentin can be formed because of fluorosis or vitamin D deficiency. The junction between dentin and predentin during globular mineralization of dentin is irregular, showing numerous rounded profiles as opposed to the smooth profile of normal dentin. In the scanning electron microscope these profiles are see as round projections extending from the mineralization front after digestion of the predentin (Fig 10.**8**).

The dentin surrounding and nearest to each tubule in dentin is hypermineralized and lacks collagen as an organic component of its matrix. Historically, this dentin has been termed peritubular dentin because it seems to surround the tubule. Developmentally speaking, this dentin is really formed within the existing tubule and the term intratubular dentin is more appropriate (Figs. 10.**9**–10.**11**). Deposition of intratubular dentin begins shortly after formation of the mantle dentin is complete. The organic matrix is deeply basophilic, metachromatic with toluidine and methylene blue (pH 2.6 and 3.6), and stains deeply with alcian blue (pH 2.6), indicating a high content of acidic glycosaminoglycans. Intratubular dentinal matrix products are synthesized in the cell body of the odontoblast, transported via the cytoskeletal network through the odontoblastic process, and are liberated laterally into the dentinal tubule. Intratubular dentin is found throughout the dentinal matrix except in areas of interglobular dentin and in about the first 100μm of mineralized dentin (mantle dentin). In these areas the tubule lacks a hypermineralized layer. Upon demineralization intratubular dentin mostly disappears, leaving only traces of organic material (Fig. 10.**10B**). The remainder of the dentinal matrix, which lies between the tubules, is described as intertubular dentin. The zone between the intertubular dentin and intratubular dentin is hypomineralized and has been called the sheath of Neuman (Fig 10.**10B**). Although no true sheath seems to exist, the boundary between these two distinct matrices is distinct (differing in mineral and collagen content) and may mark the outer extent of the dentinal tubule, as it first existed during its development. Historically, the sheath of Neuman referred to the space between the odontoblastic process and the wall of the dentinal tubule by demineralization. Therefore, it was formerly equated with the intratubular dentinal space. With increased formation and mineralization of intratubular dentin, the tubule may eventually become occluded and the resulting dentin is termed sclerotic, transparent, or translu-

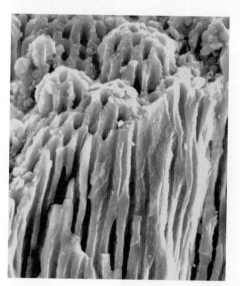

Fig. 10.**7** Circumpulpal dentin comprises most of the dentin of the tooth. Note the neonatal line.

Fig. 10.**8** Scanning electron micrograph of the pulpal surface of dentin depicting globular dentin.

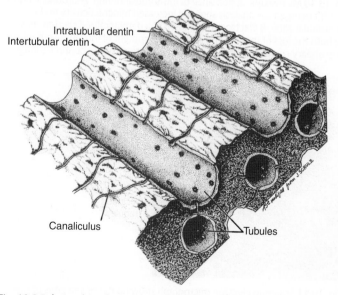

Fig. 10.**9** Relationship of intertubular and intratubular dentin and canaliculi between tubules.

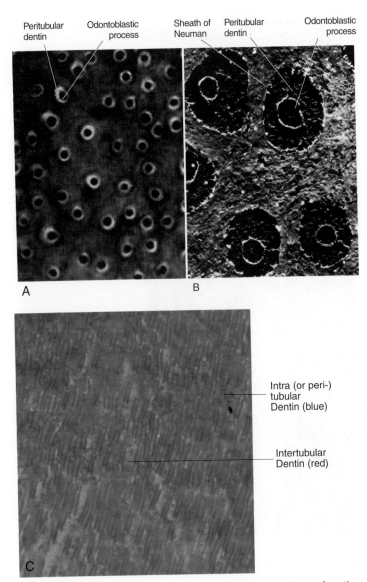

Peritubular dentin   Odontoblastic process   Sheath of Neuman   Peritubular dentin   Odontoblastic process

A   B

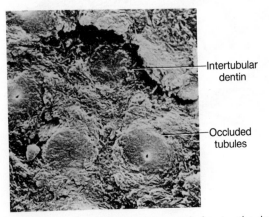

Intra (or peri-) tubular Dentin (blue)

Intertubular Dentin (red)

C

Fig. 10.**10** Microscopic appearance of intratubular dentin. **A** Ground section of soft Roentgen-ray analysis showing increased mineral density in the intratubular zone. **B** Electron micrograph of a demineralized section showing both the loss of mineral and low organic content of intratubular dentin. **C** Secondary curvatures represented as undulations of the dentinal tubule.

Intertubular dentin

Occluded tubules

Fig. 10.**11** Scanning electron micrograph showing the closed ends of sclerosed dentinal tubules.

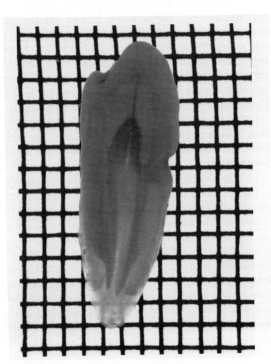

Fig. 10.**12** Sclerotic dentin in the apical area of root dentin from a ground section of a tooth. The absence of tubules (by filling with sclerotic dentin) causes this transparent appearance.

cent dentin (Figs. 10.**11** and 10.**12**). When immersed in water, the high mineral content of sclerotic dentin gives it a transparent or glassy appearance. This type of dentin is commonly found in the roots, especially near the apex (Fig. 10.**12**).

Dentin deposition begins with the formation of the pulp chamber and continues as long as the pulp remains vital. Dentin can be classified as developmental, when it is formed during development as a result of embryonic interactions, or physiologic, when it is formed as the result of responses to environmental stimuli. Primary dentin is developmental dentin that is formed before and during eruption. Secondary and tertiary dentin may be thought of as physiologic dentin. They are formed as the result of normal physiologic and pathologic stimuli, respectively. Formation of secondary dentin normally begins when root development is completed and after the teeth come into occlusion. However, secondary dentin deposition has been reported to occur in impacted (unerupted) third molars. The rate of secondary dentin deposition is generally slower than the rate of primary dentin deposition, and the rate depends upon diet and the occlusal forces to which the crown is subjected. Abrasive foods and greater chewing forces provide stronger stimuli for secondary dentin deposition. There is an abrupt change in the course of the dentinal tubules in the shift from deposition of primary to secondary dentin. The tubules are also more irregular in secondary dentin (Fig 10.**13**). It should be obvious that secondary deposition does not occur uniformly in all areas of the crown. Areas subjected to the most stimuli have higher rates of secondary dentin deposition. The pulp chamber, which roughly outlines the shape of the crown during development and the formation of primary dentin, assumes a different shape due to the asymmetric deposition of secondary dentin. The junction between primary and secondary dentin can also be distinguished by a slight change in the direction of the dentinal tubules (Fig. 10.**13**). With increased deposition, the pulp chamber becomes reduced in sized and there is further crowding of odontoblasts. Some odontoblasts may disappear (by apoptosis) and their tubules may become occluded (sclerotic). As mentioned previously, tubules are believed to become sclerotic by the progressive deposition of intratubular dentin. Electron micrographs have revealed mineralization occurring within the odontoblastic process during the formation of sclerotic dentin. This is not a normal process and is most likely due to cell injury or death. The calcium that enters the damaged process most likely precipitates due to the presence of phosphate groups (adenosine triphosphate, adenosine diphosphate, phosphoproteins, or any other phosphate-containing molecule) present in the cytoplasm.

Unlike secondary dentin, which is formed as a result of normal physiologic stimuli, tertiary or reparative dentin is formed as a result of a pathologic process such as caries. Deep caries stimulates odontoblasts to form dentin at a rapid rate (Fig. 10.**14**). Operative procedures, which are needed to restore decayed tooth surfaces, can also provide a stimulus or damage to the underlying odontoblasts. When the odontoblastic layer has been destroyed, cells in the underlying pulp migrate to this site and differentiate and rapidly deposit an irregular or disorganized dentinal matrix. Often cells become trapped in this matrix during its early stages of formation. When this occurs, the dentin appears to resemble bone and is called osteodentin. The boundary between secondary and tertiary dentin is abrupt (calciotraumatic line). Paths of the dentinal tubules usually are interrupted at this juncture due to the death of old odontoblasts

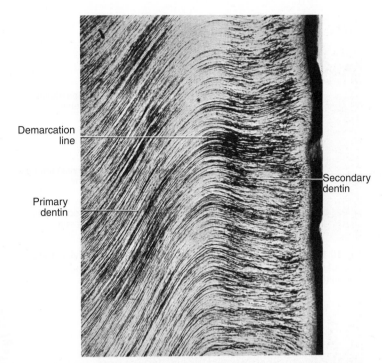

Fig. 10.**13** Ground section of dentin showing dentinal tubules bend sharply as they pass into secondary dentin. The dentinal tubules are somewhat irregular secondary dentin that is closer to the pulp.

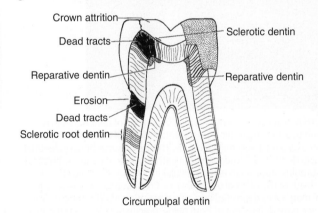

Fig. 10.**14** Diagram of root caries showing dead tracts and sclerotic and reparative dentin.

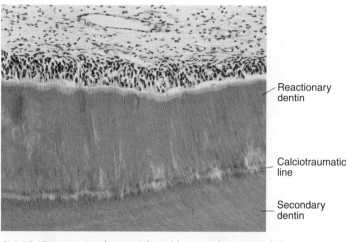

Fig. 10.**15** Reparative dentin. Odontoblasts can be seen underlying a thick layer of reactionary dentin. Between the reactionary and secondary dentin there is a pronounced calciotraumatic line.

and the development and differentiation of new odontoblasts. With the death of the initial odontoblasts, a new disorganized tubular matrix is formed by new odontoblasts. If the death of the odontoblasts is rapid, the dentinal tubules associated with the former odontoblasts have little chance of becoming sclerotic. In ground sections, these tubules are filled with air and look black in transmitted light and white in reflected light. These areas are called dead tracts (Figs. 10.**15** and 10.**16**). Tertiary dentin has numerous synonyms, such as irregular, irritation, reactionary, and reparative dentin. The distinctions between the types of tertiary dentin have been clarified. Reactionary dentin is tertiary dentin, formed by preexisting or primary odontoblasts in response to the pathologic stimulation. On the other hand, reparative dentin is formed by newly differentiated odontoblasts following the death of the original cells. Since the

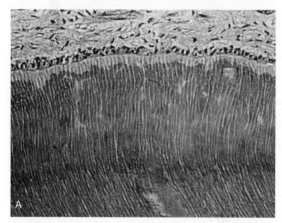

Fig. 10.**16 A** Reactionary dentin. Note a large zone of dentinal matrix deposited by surviving original postmitotic odontoblasts that had been stimulated by a relatively mild stimulus. This tubular reactionary dentinal matrix was deposited immediately beneath the area of dentin submitted to the stimulus. appears to exhibit cellular inclusions. A strong stimulus lead to death of the original odontoblasts. Consequently, the reparative dentinal matrix was deposited by a new generation of odontoblast–like cells which have differentiated from pulpal precursor cells as a reparative mechanism for tissue repair.

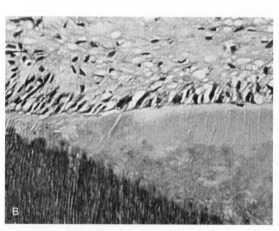

B Reparative dentin. Note the dystrophic and atubular dentinal matrix that appears to exhibit cellular inclusions (osteodentin). Consequently, the reparative dentinal matrix was deposited by a new generation of odontoblast–like cells which have differentiated from precursor cells as a mechanism for tissue repair.

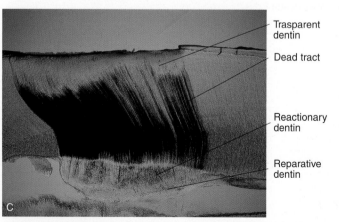

C Ground section showing cervical caries. Note the transparent dentin underlying the dead tract. Inset area showing reactionary dentin with sparse tubules overlying atubular reactionary dentin by polarized microscopy. Note the dark border between reactionary and reparative dentin.

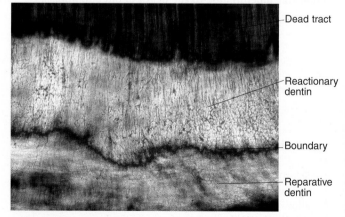

formation of reparative odontoblasts cannot be induced by an epithelial layer, the inductive stimulus is likely to come from growth factors found within the overlying dentinal matrix. Dentinal matrix has been shown to contain growth factors such as bone morphogenic proteins (BMPs, members of the TGF-β family), insulin–like growth factors (IGFs), and FGFs. These growth factors are capable of stimulating cell proliferation, differentiation, and matrix secretion.

In the roots of teeth, near the cementodentinal junction, is the Tomes' granular layer (Figs. 10.**17** and 10.**18**). The granular nature of this layer, as observed in ground sections, is the result of either small hypomineralized areas of dentin or small entrapped spaces that form around the dentinal tubules. These spaces may be the result of the disorientation of odontoblastic processes that are being formed as the tooth erupts. The results are tubules in which the terminal parts are twisted. The twisted ends appear as dark "granules" in ground sections.

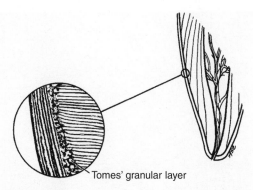

Fig. 10.**17** Diagram of the appearance and location of the Tomes' granular layer in the root dentin along the cementodentinal junction.

Contents of the Dentinal Tubule

The odontoblastic process is the primary occupant of the dentinal tubule. Fine cytofilaments are the most characteristic finding in the odontoblastic process. These may be the only cytoplasmic structures found in the small branches and terminal ends of the process. Microtubules are another common cytoskeletal feature of the odontoblastic process. Mitochondria and vesicles (coated vesicles, lysosomes, and secretion granules) are found closer to the cell body that is nearer the mineralization front at the predentin–dentin junction. The extent of the odontoblastic process within the tubule of the mature tooth has been controversial. Initially, transmission electron microscopy revealed the presence of an odontoblastic process within the tubule only in the inner third of the dentin. This is now believed to be due to considerable shrinkage that occurs during fixation, dehydration, and embedding. With improved methods of fixation, scientists have shown that the odontoblastic process extends further into the tubule and that some may reach the DEJ. Immune staining of dentin with anti-tubulin antibodies and anti-actin antibodies also indicated that the processes of many odontoblasts extend to the DEJ. Scanning electron micrographs of demineralized and collagenase-treated teeth has also provided evidence that a few processes may extend to the DEJ. However, in teeth that have been in occlusion for some time it is unlikely that many, if any, of the processes reach the DEJ.

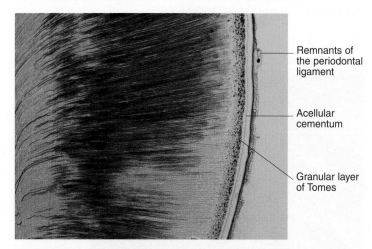

Remnants of the periodontal ligament

Acellular cementum

Granular layer of Tomes

Fig. 10.**18** Histologic appearance of the Tomes' granular layer (center) and cementum.

Clinical Application

The thickness of the dentinal layer increases with age due to the deposition of secondary and tertiary dentin. The color of the tooth is related to the translucency of the enamel and the thickness of the dentin. The increased thickness of the dentin contributes to the "yellowing" of the teeth with age. Increased thickness of dentin also serves to insulate the dental pulp, making vitality testing more difficult.

The deposition of localized secondary and tertiary dentin not only reduces the volume of the pulp chamber but also alters its shape. This makes endodontic procedures more difficult and increases the possibility of iatrogenic accidents, for example, perforations. Pulp stones form in coronal and radicular pulp due to trauma and age. This process further complicates the anatomy of the pulp chamber.

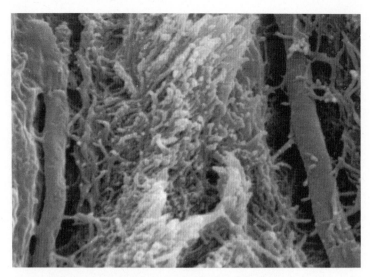

Fig. 10.**19** A scanning electron micrograph of an odontoblastic process with side branches that project into canaliculi.

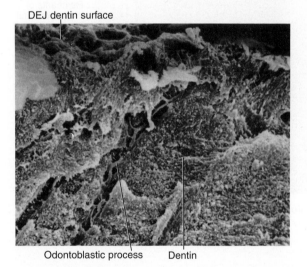

Fig. 10.**20** A scanning electron micrograph of an odontoblastic process at the DEJ. Enamel is above.

Clinical Application

The degree of dental sclerosis can influence the choice of dental surface treatment techniques for adhesive materials. Resin from composite materials flows into open (nonsclerotic) tubules more readily and forms resin tags. Formation of resin tags results in better adhesion. In sclerosed dentin there is less potential for these tags to form. On the contrary, intertubular dentin may be etched more readily than intratubular dentin, and sclerotic "tubules" may actually project from the surface of the intertubular dentin. Therefore, retention of some composite materials may be adversely affected when applied to sclerotic dentin. Dentin exposed to the oral cavity has increased resistance to acid attack, possibly due to incorporation of fluoride and the mineralizing effect of saliva (eburnation).

Branches of the main process extend laterally in smaller tubules (lateral branches). The smallest branches lie in canaliculi (Figs. 10.**3**, 10.**8**, 10.**19**, and 10.**20**). It has recently been shown by several investigators that the odontoblastic process has numerous side branches that exist in the lateral branches of the dentinal tubules throughout dentin. This is best shown in the odontoblastic process after the dentin has been cleared (Fig. 10.**21**).

Besides the odontoblastic process, the other cellular processes found in the dentinal tubules are nerve fibers. Nerve endings are a variable feature of the dentinal tubule (Fig 10.**22**). When present, these fibers often partially encircle the odontoblastic process. Nerve fibers do not extend as far as the odontoblastic process and form no discernible junctions, gap junctions or synapses with it. Unmyelinated nerve fibers have been shown to be occasionally present in the outer dentin at the DEJ of young teeth. There appears to be a relationship between the nerve endings and the odontoblastic process in the dentinal tubule in which the nerve terminal indents the process. In this way, a greater surface area is created between the nerve terminal and the odontoblastic process. In addition, these terminals usually exhibit a cleft or space between the ending and the cell process, about 200 to 250 Å wide. This space is comparable to a synaptic cleft in thickness, as found elsewhere in the body. However other features of a synapse, specializations of the presynaptic and postsynaptic membranes and the presence of synaptic vesicles, are either lacking or are poorly developed. It is not known whether this cellular relationship functions as a rudimentary synapse.

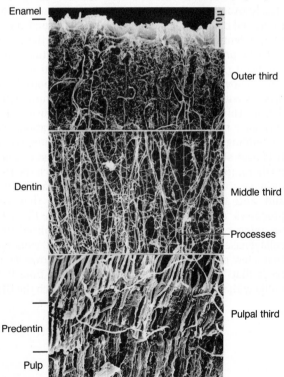

Fig. 10.**21** A scanning electron micrograph of an odontoblastic process decalcification and removal of the organic components of dentin. Top, near DEJ; center, at mid-dentin; bottom, along the pulp border.

Some nerve endings in the dentinal tubules have singular enlargements while others have alternating dilations and constrictions with the odontoblastic processes. Both types exhibit a similar vesiculated appearance, contain a few mitochondria, and have a characteristic cleft surrounding them (Figs. 10.**22** and 10.**23**).

The other feature of the dentinal tubule is the presence of an organic coating or inner lining consisting mostly of glycosaminoglycans. This coating has the appearance of a membrane in decalcified stained sections and by light microscopy, and can easily be confused with the outer cell membrane of the odontoblastic process. This layer represents hypomineralized intratubular dentin, and has been termed the internal hypomineralized layer. The term "limiting membrane" or "lamina limitans" has been applied to this layer.

Incremental Nature of Dentinal Deposition

The daily deposition of dentin can be measured through the use of labeling agents. A labeling agent is a substance that is visibly incorporated into the dentinal matrix. This agent is given initially, and after a specified period of time (1 week to 10 days) the process is repeated. The tooth is removed some days later, sectioned, and microscopically examined. The distance between the labeled bands divided by the time represents the amount of matrix formed per unit time, usually days. Labels that are commonly used bind to hydroxyapatite, such as fluorescent markers like tetracyclines or calcium stains like procion and alizarin red. Radioactive precursors that are incorporated into the dentinal matrix have also been given to measure matrix synthesis. Microradiographs, through their demonstration of alternating densities in the mineralization pattern of dentin, also indicate the

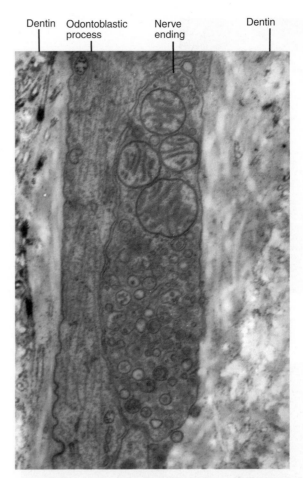

Fig. 10.**22** Nerve fiber found within a dentinal tubule. Note the presence of mitochondria in the nerve fiber and their absence in the odontoblastic process.

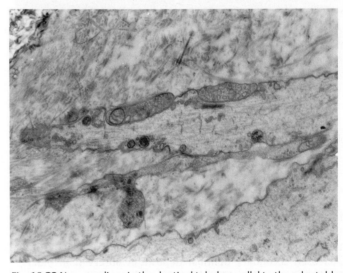

Fig. 10.**23** Nerve endings in the dentinal tubule parallel to the odontoblastic process. Below is a nerve ending extending lateral to the tubule in a canaliculus.

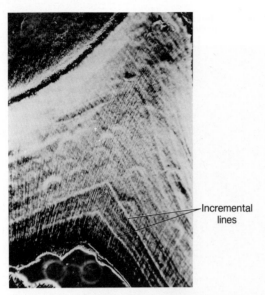

Fig. 10.**24** Microradiograph of incremental lines in dentin that depict the rhythmic recurrent deposition of mineral.

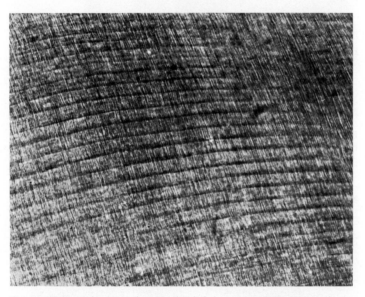

Fig. 10.**25** Ground section showing the daily incremental deposition of dentin (Imbrication lines of von Ebner).

Clinical Application

Increased secondary dentinal deposition results in changes of the pulp chamber shapes as well as changes in size and location of the apical foramina. During endodontic therapy the increased secondary dentinal deposition observed in older teeth makes it more difficult to access the pulp chamber and locate the coronal orifices of the root canals due to constriction. However, increased secondary dentinal deposition decreases the amount of instrumentation needed during root-canal therapy. Additionally, increased secondary dentin at the apical foramen leads to development of more definite apical stops and achievement of a better apical seal.

incremental nature of dentinal deposition (Fig. 10.**24**). Based on these measurements, dentin is believed to be deposited at a rate of about 4 to 8 µm per day. Dentinogenesis is thought to occur in a rhythmic manner, possibly due to the circadian rhythmic activity of neurons that control the flow of nutrients to odontoblasts. The imbrication lines of von Ebner represent daily changes in odontoblast activity (Fig. 10.**25**). More pronounced incremental lines, contour lines of Owen, represent normal physiologic alterations in the pattern of mineralization, which occur at less frequent intervals (Fig. 10.**26**). Exaggerated contour lines may be the result of a sudden change or pathologic process. The neonatal line represents an exaggerated contour line of Owen and typifies the changes in physiology (nutritional, hormonal, etc.) that occur at birth (Fig. 10.**7**). These neonatal lines are seen in the primary teeth and the first permanent molars. The dentin distal to this line (nearer the DEJ) was formed prior to birth, and the dentin proximal to it (nearer to the pulp) was formed after birth.

There are no reversal lines because dentin does not remodel in the same manner as bone. For odontoclastic activity to occur, the odontoblastic layer would have to be disrupted. Bone resorption is mediated by osteoblasts. Factors that cause bone resorption, such as parathyroid hormone and interleukin-1b, do so indirectly by binding to receptors on osteoblasts, causing them to retract from bone surfaces. Odontoblasts have branched processes that extend for great distances into the dentin and are tightly joined to one another by terminal bars and other junctions (see Chapter 11). Therefore, it is not easy for them to separate from the predentral surface to allow for dentinal remodeling. Furthermore, these cells may be incapable of responding to these hormones due to a lack of receptors. However, there is evidence of minimal remodeling by odontoblasts. Endocytic activity has been demonstrated along the odontoblastic process in dentinal tubules as well as at the mineralization front. Ultrastructural evidence of intracellular collagen degradation also suggests that odontoblasts may participate in predentral matrix turnover to a minimal degree. The extent of remodeling is insignificant compared to that seen in bone.

Dentinal Fluid, Permeability, and Sensitivity

Dentin is composed of tubules and, unlike enamel, is relatively permeable. Fluids can readily flow across or through the dentinal tubule complex from the pulp to the DEJ or, when the enamel is damaged, from the DEJ to the pulp. Fluid arising from the cut surface of the dentinal tubules has a similar composition as plasma and, in fact, is formed as a transudate of plasma. Fluid from the blood flows through the fenestrations and intercellular clefts of pulpal capillaries (see Chapter 11). Once this fluid leaves the capillaries it penetrates through the odontoblastic predentral layer, where it may be combined with the secretory products of odontoblasts. The

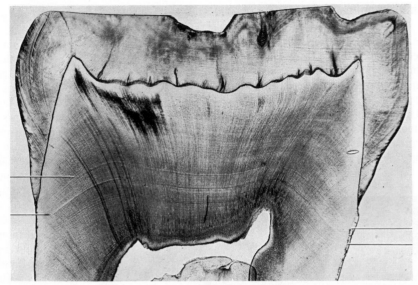

Lines of Owen

Lines of Owen

Fig. 10.**26** Ground section showing accentuated incremental lines, contour lines of Owen.

fluid then enters the periodontoblastic space within the dentinal tubule (Figs. 10.**3**, 10.**19**, and 10.**22**). The fluid is always under a slight positive pressure.

Bacterial products (endotoxins) can enter the pulp through the dentinal tubules and create an inflammatory response. As a result of inflammation, there is an increase in the permeability of blood vessels in the pulp. The increased pulpal pressure and production of dentinal fluid tends to cleanse the tubules and hinder bacteria from entering the pulp. Reduction in the size of dentinal tubules, due to sclerosis or restorative materials, reduces dentin permeability. The application of potassium oxalate and calcium hydroxide containing restorative materials at the base of cavity preparations reduces the permeability of cut dentinal tubules. Liners and varnishes also seal the dentinal tubules. The formation of dentinal fluid under cavity preparations can adversely affect the bonding of restorative agents to the dentin.

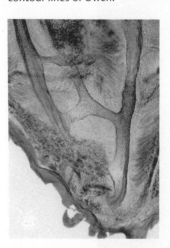

Fig. 10.**27** Section showing accessory root canals in dentin at the root apex. Note that the canals have interconnecting channels.

Furthermore, toxins and bacterial products can gain entry to the pulp or periodontal ligament through lateral or accessory canals found in the dentin of the root (Fig. 10.**27**). The pulpal periodontal relationship through these canals shows that pulpal infections can affect the periodontal ligament and vice versa.

Dentin is a sensitive tissue. This is particularly true in root dentin that may be exposed with gingival recession. Cementum covering this dentin may be absent or removed by vigorous tooth brushing. Exposed dentin is especially sensitive. However, the application of coating materials or increased deposition of intratubular dentin reduces both the permeability and sensitivity of this dentin. The theories explaining dentinal sensitivity will be discussed in Chapter 11.

Clinical Application

The smear layer, debris from instrumented dentin, also effectively reduces the permeability of dentinal tubules. Some debris enters the tubules forming smear plugs (Fig 10.28). The entry of smear into the dentinal tubules is dependent on both the size of the smear particles and the diameter of the dentinal tubules. Smear layers decrease dentinal permeability; they cannot be removed by irrigation but can be removed by acid treatment. The removal of smear by acids can damage the pulp.

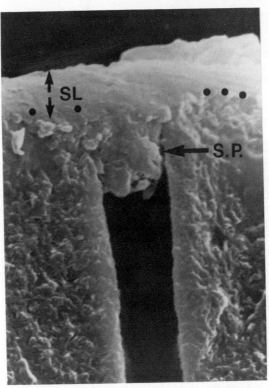

Fig. 10.28 A scanning electron micrograph showing a smear plug occluding a dentinal tubule. (S.P. smear plug; SL smear layer)

Summary

Dentin is a vital mineralized tubular tissue organized by odontoblasts. The dentinal tubules provide space for the odontoblastic process, tissue fluid, and sometimes nerve endings. The odontoblastic process plays an important role in maintaining the qualitative and quantitative differences in the dentinal and predentinal matrices, by controlling the release of phosphoproteins at the mineralization front and the formation of peritubular dentin. Dentin is incrementally deposited throughout life as circumpulpal dentin, unless environmental factors stimulate a localized production of reparative dentin. This incremental deposition coupled with a lack of internal remodeling effectively reduces the size and architecture of the pulp chamber with aging. Dentin types can be classified according to their developmental pattern and location. These common types are called primary, secondary, mantle, circumpulpal, reparative, interglobular, and the Tomes' granular layer in root dentin, as well as intertubular and intratubular (peritubular) zones. Dentinal composition may be altered by environmental and iatrogenic influences such as caries, sclerosis, dead tracts, and/or irregular reparative dentin.

Self-Evaluation Review

1. Describe the course of the dentinal tubule in the crown of the tooth. Include in your description primary and secondary curvatures. How do the diameter and branching pattern of the tubule change from the DEJ to the pulp?
2. What are incremental lines of von Ebner, contour lines of Owen? What are neonatal lines? What is developmental dentin? What are the differences between mantle and circumpulpal dentin? Do they represent developmental dentin?
3. Compare the location and composition of intertubular and intratubular dentin. What is the sheath of Neuman? What is interglobular dentin? How is it formed? Where is it characteristically located in the crown and root?
4. What is sclerotic dentin? How is it formed? What function does it serve?
5. What are the structural differences between primary, secondary, and tertiary dentin? What are osteodentin, reaction, irritation, and reparative dentin? How does the deposition of these types of dentin affect the anatomy of the pulp chamber?
6. What is responsible for the appearance of the Tomes' granular layer? Where is it found?
7. What are the contents of the dentinal tubule? What role does the odontoblastic process play in the deposition of the peritubular dentinal matrix and phosphophoryns?

8. How can dentinal deposition be measured? Why is it easier to measure dentinal deposition over long periods than bone?

9. What is the mineral and organic content of dentin as compared to bone, cementum, and enamel? How does dentin compare in hardness to these tissues? Is the organic component of the predential matrix the same as that of the dentinal matrix? Are there any qualitative differences?

10. Describe the functions of some of the organic components of dentin. What characteristics (functional groups) enable them to provide these functions?

11. What factors are responsible for limiting or increasing dentinal permeability? How is dentinal fluid formed? What influences its rate of formation?

Acknowledgements

We thank the following for permitting use of individual figures: Dr. Alan Boyde, University of London, for Figure 10.**2**; Dr. Martin Brannstrom and Wolfe Medical Pub. Inc. for Figure 10.**10**; Dr. AEW Miles, University of London, and Mosby Year Book, St. Louis, for Figure 10.**11** (in Orban's Oral Histology and Embryology, p.128); Dr. Gerrit Bevelander (University of Texas, Houston) and Mosby Year Book, St. Louis, for Figure 10.**12** (in Orban's Oral Histology and Embryology, p. 109); Dr. Keith Kelly for Figure 10.**19**; Dr. Takahide Gungi for Figure 10.**20**; Dr. I Schour and M Massler for Figure 10.**24** (J. Am. Dent. Assoc. 23:1946); Dr. David Pashley for Figure 10.**27** (Proc. Finn. Dent. Soc. 88(suppl. 1):225–242).

Suggested Readings

Aubin JE. New immunological approaches to studying the odontoblast process. J. Dent. Res. 1984;64(Special Issue):515–522.

Avery JK. Response of the pulp and dentin to contact with filling materials. J. Dent. Res. 1975;54:188–197.

Bergenholz G, Cox CF, Loesche WJ, Syed SA. Bacterial leakage around dental restorations and its effect on the dental pulp. J. Oral Pathol. 1982;11:439–450.

Boskey A. The role of extracellular matrix components in dentin mineralization. Crit. Rev. Oral Biol. Med. 1991;2:369–388.

Brannstrom M. Dentin and pulp in restorative dentistry. Wolfe Med. Pub. Ltd.; 1982.

Brannstrom M, Garberoglio R. Occlusion of dentinal tubules under superficial attrited dentin. Swed. Dent. J. 1980;4: 87–91.

Cox CF, Heys DR, Gibbons PK, Avery JK, Heys RJ. The effect of various restorative materials on the microhardness of reparative dentin. J. Dent. Res. 1980;59:109–115.

Frank RM, Steuer P. Transmission electron microscopy of the human odontoblast process in peripheral root dentin. Arch. Oral Biol. 1988;33:91–98.

Goldberg M, Boskey AL. Lipids and biomineralizations. Prog. Histochem. Cytochem. 1996;31:1–187.

Gorski JP. Is all bone the same? Distinctive distributions and properties of non-collagenous matrix proteins in lamellar vs. woven bone imply the existence of different underlying osteogenic mechanisms. Crit. Rev. Oral Biol. Med. 1998;9:201–223.

Gorter de Vries I, Quartier E, Van Steirteghem A, Boute P, Coomans D, Wisse E. Characterization and immunocytochemical localization of dentine phosphoprotein in rat and bovine teeth. Arch. Oral Biol. 1986;31:57–66.

Hawkinson RW, Eisenmann DR. Sclerosis in enamel-free rat dentin. Arch. Oral Biol. 1983;28:409–414.

Holland GR. The odontoblast process: Form and function. J. Dent. Res. 1984;64(SI):499–514.

Holland GR. Role of the odontoblast process. In: Inoki R, Kudo T, Olgart L (eds.). Dynamic Aspects of Dental Pulp: Molecular Biology, Pharmacology, and Pathophysiology. London: Chapman and Hall; 1990:73–96.

Kelley K, Bergenholtz G, Cox CF. The extent of the odontoblast process in Rhesus monkeys (Macaca mulatta) as observed by scanning electron microscopy. Arch. Oral Biol. 1981;26:893–897.

Linde A. Calcium metabolism in dentinogenesis. In: The Role of Calcium in Biological Systems. Boca Raton, FL: CRC Press; 1982.

Linde A. Dentin and Dentinogenesis. Vols. 1 and 2. Boca Raton, FL: CRC Press; 1984.

Linde A. Structure and calcification of dentin. In: Bonucci E (ed.). Calcification in Biological Systems. Boca Raton, FL: CRC Press; 1992;269–311.

MacDougall M. Refined mapping of the human dentin sialophosphoprotein (dspp) gene within the critical dentinogenesis imperfecta type iI and dentin dysplasia type II loci. Eur. J. Oral Sci. 1998;106(Suppl. 1):227–233.

MacDougall M, Simmons D, Luan X, Nydegger J, Feng J, Gu TT. Dentin phosphoprotein and dentin sialoprotein are cleav age products expressed from a single transcript coded by a gene on human chromosome 4: dentin phosphoprotein sequence determination. J. Biol. Chem. 1997;272:835–842.

MacDougall M, Zeichner-David M, Slavkin HC. Production and characterization of antibodies against murine dentine phosphoprotein. Biochem. J. 1985;232:493–500.

Mjor IA. Microradiography of human coronal dentin. Arch. Oral Biol. 1966;11:225–234.

Moss ML. Studies on dentin I. Mantle dentin. Acta Anat. 1974;87:481–507.

Pashley DH. Dentin permeability and dentin sensitivity. Proc. Fin. Dent. Soc. 1992;88(suppl. 1):31–38.

Pashley DH. Smear layer: Overview of structure and function. Proc. Fin. Dent. Soc. 1992;88(suppl. 1):225–242.

Pashley DH, Nelson R, Pashley EL. In vivo fluid movement across dentin in the dog. Arch. Oral Biol. 1981;26:707–710.

Rauschenberger CS: Dentin permeability: The clinical ramifications. Dental Clinics in North America. 1992;36:527–542.

Ritchie HH, Ritchie DG, Wang L-H. Six decades of dentinogenesis research historical prospective views on phosphophoryn and dentin sialoprotein. Eur. J. Oral Sci. 1998;106 (Suppl. 1):211–220.

Schour I, Massler M. The neonatal line in enamel and dentin of human deciduous teeth and first permanent molar. J. Am. Dent. Assoc.1936;23:1946.

Schour I, Poncher HG. The rate of apposition of human enamel and dentin as measured by the effects of acute fluorosis. Am. J. Dis. Child.1937;54:757.

Schroeder HE. Development and structure of the tissues of the tooth. In Oral Structural Biology. New York, NY: Thieme Medical Publishers, Inc.; 1991;4–184.

Stanley H, Pereira JC, Spiegel E, et al. Sclerosis, dead tracts and reparative dentin. J. Oral Pathol. 1983;12:257–289.

Szabo J, Trombitas K, Szabo I. The odontoblast process and its branches. Arch. Oral Biol. 1984;29:331–333.

Seltzer S, Bender IB. The Dental Pulp: Biologic Considerations in Dental Procedures. Philadelphia: JB Lippincott Co.; 1984.

Veis A. Acidic proteins as regulators of biomineralization in vertebrates. In: Davidovitch Z (ed.) Biological Mechanisms of Tooth Movement and Craniofacial Adaptation. Colombus: The Ohio State University; 1992:115–120.

Weinstock M, LeBlond CP. Radioautographic visualization of the deposition of a phosphoprotein at the mineralization front in the dentin of the rat incisor. J. Cell Biol. 1973;56:839–845.

Wigglesworth DJ, Longmore GA, Kuc IM, Murdoch C. Early dentinogenesis in mice :von Korff fibers and their possible significance. Acta Anat. 1986;127:151–160.

11 Histology of the Pulp

D. J. Chiego, Jr.

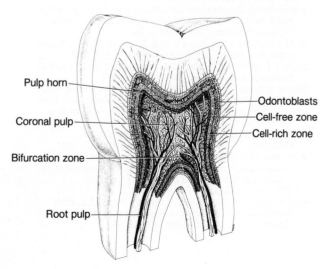

Fig. 11.**1** Diagram of the histology of pulp.

Introduction

The dental pulp consists of loose connective tissue derived from neural crest cells or ectomesenchymal cells and is confined within the pulp chamber and root canals of the tooth. The pulp contains cells that provide the mature pulp with odontogenic, nutritive, sensory, and defensive functions and allow for preservation of vitality during normal homeostatic maintenance and during wound repair after injury. The mature dental pulp can be divided into two compartments: the odontogenic zone and the pulp proper (Fig. 11.**1**). The odontogenic zone includes the odontoblasts, which are the cells responsible for the production and maintenance of predentin and dentin, the cell-free zone, the cell-rich zone, and the parietal plexus of nerves. The pulp proper includes the majority of the remaining area of the pulp and consists primarily of fibroblasts and ECM, blood vessels, and nerves. Before it is surrounded by dentin, the pulp is called the dental papilla. In the mature tooth, the pulp can be divided into the coronal and radicular chambers (root canals). As the pulp ages, the volume decreases with a corresponding increase in dentinal thickness.

The blood vessels and nerves of the pulp enter the root canals through the apical foramen. The nerve bundles are composed of myelinated and unmyelinated fibers surrounded by a connective-tissue sheath. The nerve fibers have been morphologically and physiologically described as sensory and postganglionic sympathetic nerves. As the large bundles of nerves reach the coronal pulp, branching occurs and a peripheral parietal plexus (subodontoblastic plexus) is formed. Unmyelinated nerves then traverse the cell-rich, cell-free, odontoblastic layer and enter the dentinal tubules along with the odontoblastic processes. The density of innervated tubules depends on the specific location within the pulp, with the pulp horns the most densely innervated and the root pulp the least densely innervated.

Objectives

After reading this chapter you should be able to discuss the cells, ECM, and vascular and neural elements of the mature dental pulp. You will also be able to describe the response of the dental pulp to factors such as aging, trauma, and clinical treatment. After further study, you should be able to discuss the origin and function of the nerves in the dental pulp and describe the various theories of pain transmission through the enamel and dentin.

Pulpal Architecture

The dental pulp can be divided into several compartments based on its location within the pulp chambers. The average volume of the dental pulp is 0.02 mL, the molar pulps having four times the volume of incisor pulps (Fig. 11.**2**). The coronal pulp extends occlusally into the pulp horns of each crown. Apically, the coronal pulp extends into the radicular or root pulp. The floor of the coronal pulp in multirooted teeth is the furcation zone. Accessory or lateral canals are connective-tissue connections between the pulp and the periodontal ligament and are found predominately at the apical third of permanent teeth and in the furcation zone of primary teeth. They are formed by a defective root sheath, which breaks down prematurely and then reforms, preventing the induction of odontoblasts on the dental papilla side of the epithelial root sheath and cementoblasts on the follicular side resulting in a tubular defect. Fibroblasts, blood vessels, and nerves can sometimes be found within the accessory canals. At the apical foramen, the pulpal tissue becomes continuous with the tissue of the periodontal ligament. As the erupting tooth enters functional occlusion, the cell-free and cell-rich zones become defined (Fig. 11.**3**). The cell-rich zone may be absent in older teeth. The cell-free zone separates the cell-rich and odontoblastic layers. The cell-rich zone is thought to contain progenitor odontoblasts that can be induced to differentiate into mature odontoblasts in response to wounding. The most peripheral aspect of the coronal pulp is lined by the columnar-shaped odontoblasts, whereas the odontoblasts in the radicular pulp and furcation zones are cuboidal or exhibit a flattened morphology (Fig. 11.**4**). The pulp proper, or central pulp, contains the large blood vessels of the pulp and nerve

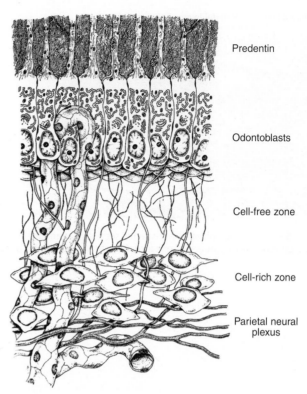

Predentin

Odontoblasts

Cell-free zone

Cell-rich zone

Parietal neural plexus

Fig. 11.**3** Diagram of odontogenic zone with odontoblasts, cell-free and cell-rich zones, and parietal layer of nerves.

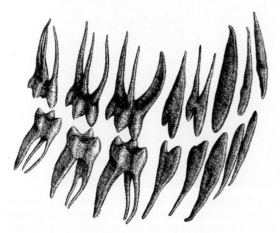

Fig. 11.**2** Pulp organs of permanent human teeth. Upper row, maxillary arch; left central incisor through third molar. Lower row, mandibular arch; left central incisor through third molar.

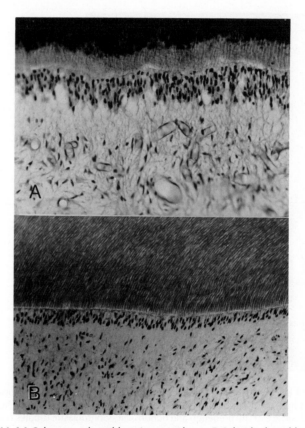

Fig. 11.**4 A** Columnar odontoblasts in coronal area. **B** Cuboid odontoblasts in radicular pulp.

Odontoblasts   Parietal layer of nerves

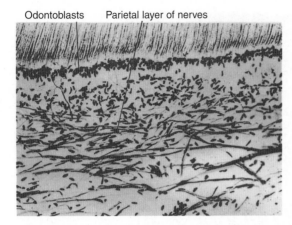

Fig. 11.**5** Photomicrograph of a silver-stained section of a human tooth demonstrating the odontogenic zone including the parietal plexus of nerves.

trunks. The veins in the pulp range from 100 to 150μm in diameter and arterioles from 50 to 150 μm in diameter. Myelinated and unmyelinated nerves are normally found in close association with the blood vessels (Fig. 11.**5**).

Cells of the Pulp

The most predominant cell type in the dental pulp is the fibroblast, but the pulp also contains odontoblasts, blood cells, perivascular cells, pericytes, Schwann cells, endothelial cells, and undifferentiated mesenchymal cells. Cells involved in the inflammatory and immune responses, such as lymphocytes, macrophages, mast cells, type II antigen processing cells (dendritic cells) and plasma cells can also be found in the pulp during periods of inflammation.

Odontoblasts

Odontoblasts are terminally differentiated, polarized, pulpal cells derived from the cranial (mesencephalic) neural crest, which are found in a peripheral layer of the pulp closely associated with the predentin (Fig. 11.**6**). The major function of odontoblasts is the synthesis and secretion of the fibers and extracellular matrix (ECM) of the predentin and biomineralization of the dentin (Fig. 11.**7**). The odontoblast also maintains the ECM of predentin and dentin throughout the life of the tooth. Dentin, unlike bone, does not remodel under normal, nonpathologic, circumstances. The cell body of the odontoblast contains all of the organelles that are para-

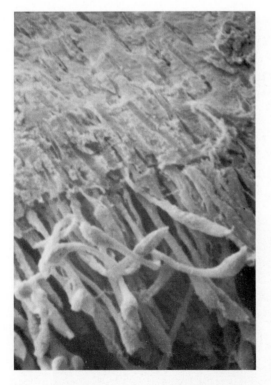

Fig. 11.**6** This high-magnification scanning electron micrograph demonstrates intact human odontoblasts and odontoblastic processes attached to the fractured surface of the predentin and dentin. Cut odontoblastic tubules containing odontoblastic processes can be seen above the cells.

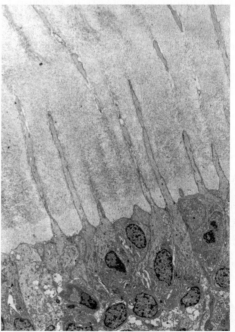

Fig. 11.**7** This low-magnification transmission electron micrograph shows the odontoblastic layer. The majority of the odontoblasts demonstrate a normal distribution of organelles and processes extending into the predentin and dentin. Tight junctional complexes can be seen at the neck of the odontoblast at the level of the cell and predentinal matrix.

mount to the cells' role in protein synthesis (Fig. 11.8). The nucleus of the odontoblast is basally located, with the rough endoplasmic reticulum (RER) and Golgi apparatus located supranuclear. Numerous mitochondria and lysosomes are found throughout the cytoplasm, as are various other cellular inclusions such as cytoskeletal elements, cilia, and secretory vesicles. The major protein produced by the odontoblast is type I collagen; which is secreted into the extracellular space at the predentin interface. Type I trimer and type V collagens have also been reported to be a minor component of the ECM. Non-collagenous components of the ECM of predentin and dentin, including proteoglycans, glycosaminoglycans, phosphoproteins, glycoproteins, and γ-carboxyglutamate-containing proteins, are also synthesized and secreted by odontoblasts. Other soluble molecules, such as members of the TGF-β superfamily—including the bone morphogenic proteins (BMP 2,4,7), epidermal growth factor and fibroblast growth factor—have been found in the odontoblast and sequestered in the ECM of predentin and dentin. This suggests that these molecules could play an important role during wound healing. Other molecules reported to be found in the odontoblast include substances that are important for organization and mineralization of the ECM, including dentin phosphoprotein (DPP) and dentin sialoprotein (DSP), dentin matrix proteins (DMP's), decorin, and biglycan. Since many of these molecules have specific functions, they are secreted at different levels where they can be the most efficient. Molecules such as biglycan and type I collagen are secreted at the odontoblast–predentin interface where biglycan has been reported to play a role in the organization of the collagen fibrils in the ECM (Fig. 11.9). Decorin and DPP are secreted at the mineralization front where decorin organizes and aids in the registration of the collagen fibrils allowing DPP to then bind Ca⁺⁺ to initiate mineralization of the predentin to dentin (Fig. 11.10). Other substances reported to be in the ECM of predentin and dentin, and which therefore have been synthesized by the odontoblast, include a variety of glycosaminoglycans (e.g., hyaluronic acid),

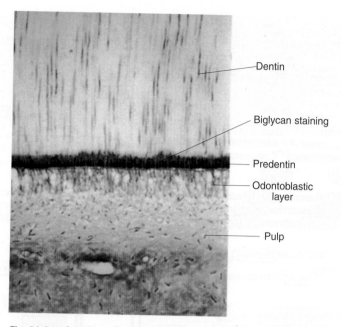

Fig. 11.9 In this photomicrograph, the proteoglycan biglycan is seen localized within the predentin. Biglycan is thought to be associated with organization of the extracellular matrix and is secreted at the odontoblast–predentin interface.

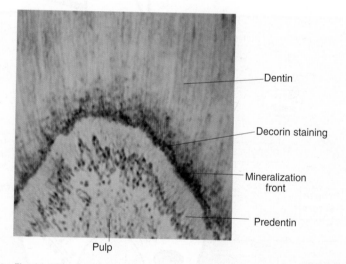

Fig. 11.10 In this photomicrograph the proteoglycan decorin is localized at the mineralization front between the predentin and the mineralized dentin. Decorin is thought to organize the collagen of the predentinal extracellular matrix and also maintain spacing between the type I collagen prior to displacement by dentin phosphoprotein. Decorin is secreted at the level of the mineralization front and therefore must be transported intracellularly through the cell body of the odontoblast and up the odontoblastic process to the mineralization front.

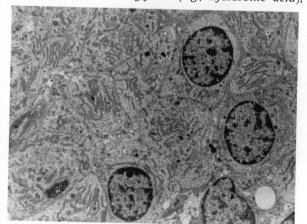

Fig. 11.8 This low-magnification electron micrograph demonstrates a cross-sectional view of the odontoblastic layer. The odontoblasts contain organelles typical of protein sythetic activity, including abundant RER, ribosomes, and mitochondria.

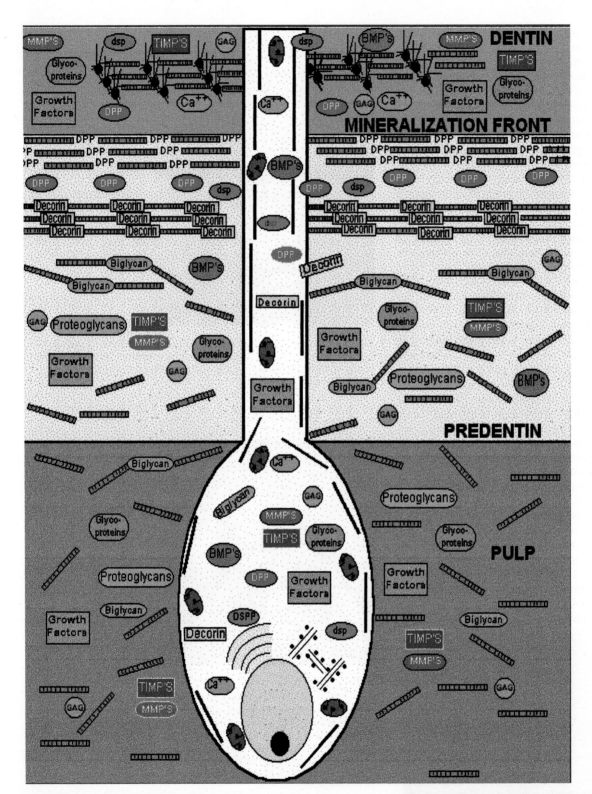

Fig. 11.**11** Summary of many of the ECM substances and their distribution, as discussed above. GAG: glycosaminoglycan. MMP: matrix metalloproteinase. TIMP: tissue inhibitor of metalloproteinase. DPP: dentin phosphoprotein. DSP: dentin sialoprotein.

matrix metalloproteinases (e.g., collagenase), tissue inhibitors of metalloproteinases, and glycoproteins (e.g., osteopontin and osteocalcin). A summary diagram of many of these ECM substances can be seen in Figure 11.**11**.

The odontoblast also has a process extending from the cell body to the dentinoenamel junction (DEJ) contained within a dentinal tubule. The odontoblast exhibits multiple processes at the time of terminal differentiation. By the time the mantle dentin layer has been completed, the cells normally exhibit only one main process. There are multiple lateral odontoblastic processes contained within the dentin that are maintained through the life of the odontoblast. The odontoblastic process may also contain mitochondria, secretory vesicles, microtubules, and intermediate filaments.

Odontoblasts are intimately associated with adjacent odontoblasts, cells of the cell-rich zone, and cells in the pulp proper through a series of junctional complexes including desmosomes, and tight, intermediate, and gap junctions (Fig. 11.**12**). The tight and intermediate junctional complexes are important for maintaining the integrity of the odontoblastic layer and preventing the ingress of foreign material, for example toxins and bacterial products, from the oral cavity (Fig. 11.**13**). The tight junctions provide mechanical attachment between adjacent odontoblasts. Intermediate junctions have been shown to extend around the perimeter of the odontoblasts as narrow bands.

The gap junctions are areas of reduced electrical resistance that also allow selective exchange of substances between odontoblasts. Gap junctions are characterized as circumscribed structures with 2-nm tubular channels surrounded by rings of proteins of adjacent plasma membranes that traverse the gap between cells and link the interior of adjacent odontoblasts. Each half of the gap junctional complex consists of a symmetrically equivalent hexamer of approximately 27 kD, and is termed a connexin. Various mechanisms have been proposed to explain how gap junctions are regulated, including changes in pH, calcium concentrations, and voltage changes. Opening of the gap junction allows small molecules and ions (<1 kD M.W.), such as c-AMP and Ca^2, to diffuse between the cells and initiate a cascade of events leading to an increase or decrease in cell activity. Gap junctions between odontoblasts, odontoblasts and cells of the cell-rich zone and cells of the pulp proper have been demonstrated at the light and electron microscopic levels using special staining techniques and immunohistochemistry, and by freeze fracture. It has been suggested that gap junctions play an important role in the regulation of cell growth and differentiation as well as coordinating cellular activity between odontoblasts—for example, dentinogenesis. As the tooth ages, the odontoblasts change shape from cuboidal to ovoid and become quiescent. Some odontoblasts are lost and not replaced. The functioning odontoblasts continue to produce predentin throughout the life of the tooth, although irregularly and at a reduced rate. Odontoblasts retain the ability to upregulate protein synthetic activity in response to trauma after aging; however, the response is initiated slower. The odontoblastic cell layer becomes discontinuous, and the cells vary in the amount of ECM being produced and subsequently mineralized in the older tooth.

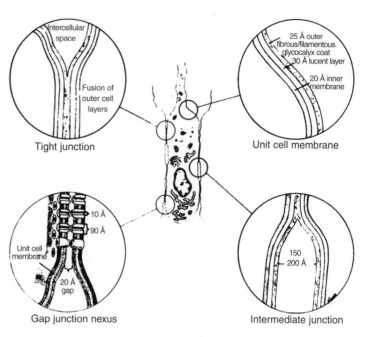

Fig. 11.**12** Diagram of odontoblasts, cell membranes, and types of junctional complexes.

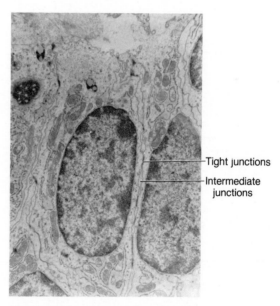

Fig. 11.**13** Ultrastructure of junctional complexes of odontoblasts in the region of the nuclei.

Clinical Application

Pulp stones are a normal resident of the mature dental pulp. In most cases pulp stones are asymptomatic unless they impinge on the pulpal blood supply or neurovascular bundle. However, if a patient presents with clinical symptoms that require endodontic therapy, a pulp stone that obstructs the root canals could complicate treatment.

Fibroblasts and Undifferentiated Mesenchymal Cells

Fibroblasts are the most numerous cells found in the dental pulp. They are stellate-shaped cells with long cytoplasmic extensions that contact adjacent fibroblasts or odontoblasts through gap-junctional processes. Fibroblasts can synthesize and secrete several types of collagen, including type III collagen, and other ECM components of the pulp, including proteoglycans and glycosaminoglycans. The fibroblast is also responsible for degrading the ECM, and can simultaneously synthesize and degrade the pulpal ECM. Collagen is the most abundant connective-tissue protein and occurs in several specific isotypes. Each is recognized as a specific genetic product differing in amino-acid composition. In the pulp, type III is the most abundant type of collagen with other types, such as IV and V, as minor constituents. As the dental pulp ages, there is a reduction in the numbers of fibroblasts and a concomitant increase in the number and size of the collagen fibrils, fibers, and bundles (fibrosis).

Fibroblasts or undifferentiated mesenchymal cells also play an important role in wound-healing mechanisms in the pulp. The resident cells of the cell-rich zone are thought to differentiate into odontoblasts after the right stimulus—for example, growth factors (e.g., TGF-β), bone morphogenic proteins (e.g., BMP-2, 4, or 7), cytokines (Il-1,6), or inflammatory mediators (prostaglandin E_1, $F_{2\alpha}$) released during wounding from the exposed predentin or dentin, or inflammatory cells that have migrated to the wound site.

There are many other cells found in a vital dental pulp and some are associated with a diseased pulp.

Perivascular cells are found in the dental pulp closely associated with the vasculature. These cells have been reported to be important in wound-healing mechanisms associated with pulpal repair mechanisms. Perivascular cells have also been shown to proliferate in response to an iatrogenic exposure of the dental pulp, and are thought to possibly provide replacement cells for the odontoblastic layer in wounds where the cell-rich layer has been destroyed.

Pericytes are another type of cell that are intimately associated with blood vessels in the pulp. They have cytoplasmic processes in contact with the basement membrane of the blood vessels. Pericytes are one type of resident cells of the dental pulp that have been suggested as progenitor cells for replacement odontoblasts.

Endothelial cells line the lumen of the pulpal blood vessels and contribute to the basal lamina by producing type IV collagen, an afibrillar collagen. They have been shown to proliferate after a pulp exposure in an attempt to neovascularize the wounded area during the process of wound healing.

Class II antigen processing cells have been demonstrated by immunohistochemical methods in both the normal and inflamed pulp (Fig. 11.**14**). These cells are commonly called dendritic cells because of multiple, long cytoplasmic processes that bind antigens and process them for presentation to macrophages and lymphocytes. Dendritic cells have been found within the walls of periapical granulomas after pulpal necrosis.

Other vascular-derived cells found in the pulp during an inflammatory condition include mast cells, B- and T-lymphocytes, polymorphonuclear neutrophils, and macrophages (Figs. 11.**15** and 11.**16**). These blood cells are of paramount importance in fighting infection in the pulp because of the substances they contain: histamine, serotonin, cytokines, growth factors, and other cellular mediators.

Schwann cells envelope nerve processes with a myelin sheath. The myelin is a lipid-rich substance synthesized and secreted by the Schwann cell and contained within the cytoplasm. Many Schwann cells are required to cover an individual axon, and therefore only a small portion of each axon is covered by one Schwann cell. The joint where two axons meet is called a Ranvier's node. Myelinated nerves contain many wrappings of myelin, whereas unmyelinated nerves are covered by a single wrapping of the Schwann cell's cytoplasm in an inflamed dental pulp.

Pulp stones (denticles) can be found in the dental pulp as a normal consequence of aging (Fig. 11.**17**). True pulp stones contain dentinal tubules within a mineralized

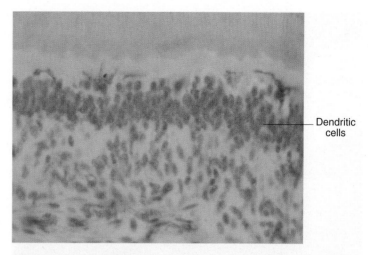

Fig. 11. **14** Immunohistologic localization of dentritic cells in the deep pulp under a pulp exposure and at the odontoblast–dentin interface where a series of dendritic cells was also localized.

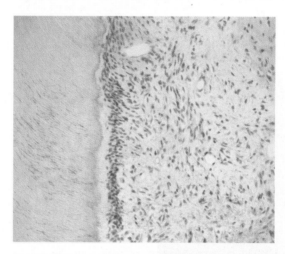

Fig. 11. **15** Immunohistochemically-stained T-lymphocyte in an inflamed dental pulp (Brown cytoplasm).

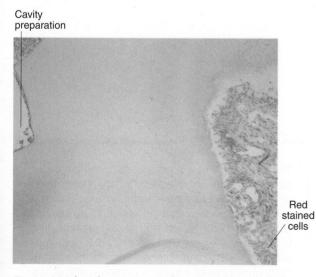

Fig. 11. **16** B-lymphocytes in an inflamed monkey pulp underlying a cavity preparation.

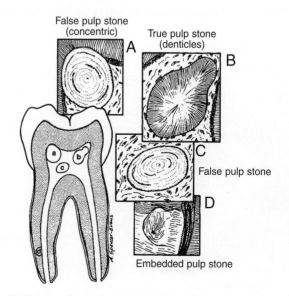

Fig. 11. **17** Diagram of pulp stones (denticles). **A** False attached denticle. **B** True denticle with tubules. **C** False, free denticle. **D** Embedded denticle.

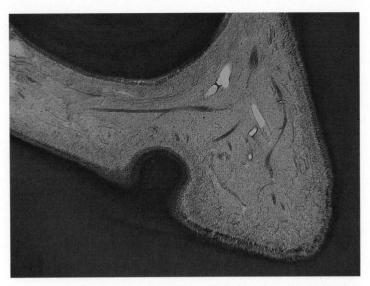

Fig. 11. **18** Photomicrograph of a false, attached pulp stone in coronal pulp.

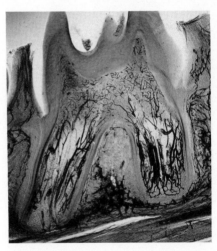

Fig. 11. **19** The vascular organization in the pulp (India-ink injection of vessels).

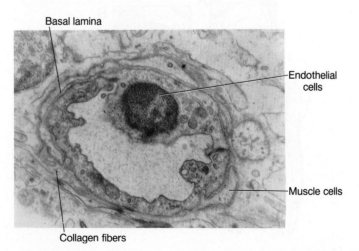

Fig. 11. **20** Transmission electron micrograph of a small arteriole in pulp, with endothelial cells and a cytoplasmic extension of a smooth muscle cell.

matrix and are surrounded by odontoblast–like cells. False pulp stones are composed of a mineralized matrix arranged in a series of concentric lamellae (Fig. 11.**18**). Flattened or spindle-shaped cells are occasionally seen on the surface of the tissue. Pulp stones can be found embedded within the dentinal matrix, attached to the predentin and dentin, or lying free within the stroma of the pulp proper. Pulp stones are usually asymptomatic unless they impinge upon a nerve or blood vessel. Pulp stones can cause problems during endodontic procedures when they lie over or within the radicular pulp. Occasionally, diffuse calcifications can be found in the coronal or radicular portion of the dental pulp, and are usually associated with the vasculature in a linear arrangement. These dystrophic calcifications are thought to be initiated by microtrauma to pulp in the areas where they are found.

Vasculature of Pulp

Blood vessels enter the pulp through the apical foramen in a connective-tissue compartment known as the central core (Fig. 11.**19**). The venules are between 100 to 150 µm and the arterioles are approximately 50 to 100 µm in diameter. Branches of smaller vessels are given off as the blood vessels proceed toward the coronal pulp and pulp horns (Fig. 11.**20**). The terminal capillaries and venules anastomose deep to the odontoblastic layer, where they provide nutrients and oxygen needed for cellular metab-

Clinical Application

The placement of a hard-set, calcium-hydroxide-containing material over deep cavity preparations or after a pulp exposure is standard clinical dental practice. How the hard-set, calcium-hydroxide-containing materials function to aid pulpal healing is not known. Recent work suggests that pulp-capping materials combining growth factors with an inert carrier can be equally, if not more, efficacious in promoting pulpal healing.

olism (Fig. 11.**21**) and remove the byproducts of cellular metabolism. The capillary loops are dense in the coronal and pulp horn aspect of the pulp and less dense in the radicular pulp. Continuous and fenestrated capillaries are present in the odontoblastic layer. The fenestrated capillaries have small pores that contain only a thin membrane covering composed of endothelial cell cytoplasm and a basement membrane (Fig. 11.**22**). These pores allow for rapid outward transport of substances and cells into the extracellular space, as well as removal of metabolic waste during times of pulpal insult. Arteriovenous and venous-venous shunts are also present in the pulp for rapid transfer of blood (Fig. 11.**23**). Both the arteriovenous shunt and the fenestrated capillaries have been suggested to function in reducing interstitial pressure in the pulp during inflammation. After a dental operative procedure, the capillaries underlying a cavity preparation will become leaky, allowing plasma and vascular cells into the extracellular spaces. Lymphatic vessels have also been reported to be located in the dental pulp. The lymphatic vessels are thin-walled, tubular structures that usually do not contain cellular elements. During the aging process, the blood vessels of the pulp exhibit changes similar to those seen in the rest of the body. Accumulations of cholesterol can be seen in the walls of the vessels. These cholesterol deposits can cause a localized inflammatory response, which in turn causes the intimal surface of the pulpal vessel to become adherent, allowing erythrocytes to adhere to the walls of the vessels. The reduced diameter of the vessels decreases the blood flow to those areas of the pulp, resulting in hypoxia. Eventually, a thrombus formed by the accumulation of erythrocytes can dislodge and cause an embolus, which will cause a localized pulp necrosis when it occludes a terminal capillary within the odontoblastic region or pulp proper.

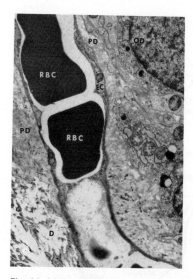

Fig. 11. **21** Transmission electron micrograph of a capillary coursing among odontoblasts. D: dentin. EC: endothelial cell. OD: odontoblast. PD: predentin. RBC: red blood cell.

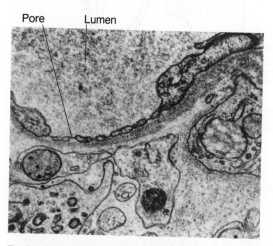

Fig. 11. **22** Transmission electron micrograph of a fenestrated capillary in the odontogenic zone.

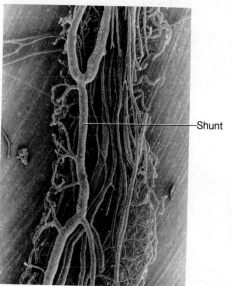

Fig. 11. **23** Scanning electron micrograph of a vein-to-vein shunt in the coronal pulp.

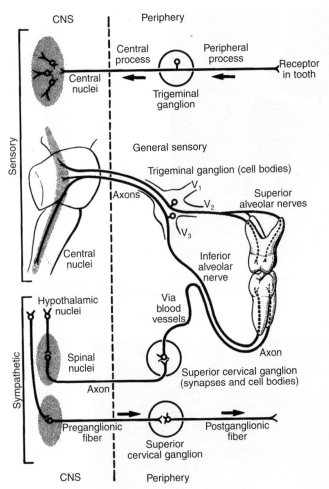

Fig. 11.**24** Summary of the sensory and autonomic nerve supply to the dental pulp.

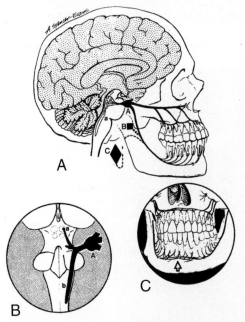

Fig. 11.**25** Peripheral and central innervation to teeth. **A** Pathways of the trigeminal nerve. Trigeminal ganglion (A); otic ganglion (B); superior cervical sympathetic ganglion (C); brainstem trigeminal nuclear complex. **B** Trigeminal ganglion (A) with mesencephalic nucleus (a) and brainstem trigeminal nuclear complex (b). **C** Transmedian collateral innervation.

Nerves In the Pulp

The sensory and postganglionic sympathetic nerves that innervate the dental pulp (Fig. 11.**24**) originate in the trigeminal and superior cervical ganglia and enter the teeth through the apical foramen. From the neural receptor in the pulp, the central process of a trigeminal sensory neuron traverses the trigeminal ganglion located in the floor of the middle cranial fossa (Figs. 11.**25**–11.**28**). The central process then synapses on a second-order neuron located in the subnucleus caudalis of the brainstem trigeminal complex. The majority of second-order neurons then decussate and ascend to synapse on neuronal cell bodies located in the ventroposteriomedial nucleus of the thalamus. The third-order neurons ascend to the area of the postcentral gyrus concerned with the orofacial region. The majority of sensory stimuli to the teeth are perceived by the patient as pain, although recent reports suggest that other sensory modalities may also be discerned, such as pressure and temperature. The mandibular teeth are innervated by the inferior alveolar nerve originating from the third division of the trigeminal ganglion. The maxillary teeth are innervated by the anterior, middle, and posterior superior alveolar nerves. The postganglionic sympathetic nerves form a plexus on the external carotid arteries and subsequently follow the terminal branches of this artery into the pulps of the mandibular and maxillary teeth.

Electrophysiology of Pulpal Nerves

Biophysical characterization of trigeminal neurons innervating the dental pulp, using dissociated trigeminal cell bodies previously labeled with a neuronal tracer, suggest that there are three types of neurons relative to the type of action potential generated after a current injection using the technique of whole cell patch clamping. Three types of action potentials have been found

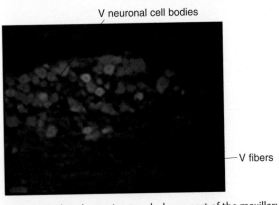

Fig. 11.**26** This photomicrograph shows part of the maxillary portion of the trigeminal ganglion. Each division of the trigeminal nerve (ophthalmic, maxillary, and mandibular) has neuronal cell bodies located somatotopically within the ganglion. Immunohistochemical-stained ganglion cells containing CGRP are the bright-yellow fluorescent cells interspersed within the ganglion.

after a series of hyperpolarizing and depolarizing current injections. Sharp action potentials, action potentials with an inflection on the descending limb and multiple firing neurons, in association with different ganglion cell diameters, suggest that the neurons innervating the dental pulp consist of a diverse population of neurons. Although the literature suggests that the neurons innervating the dental pulp carry only the modality of nociception, the diversity of these cells suggests that other functions could also be subserved. This is further supported by the large variety of neurotransmitters, neuromodulators, and neuropeptides that have also been reported to be associated with pulpal neurons (Figs. 11.**29**–11.**31**).

Branches of the inferior and superior alveolar nerves and sympathetic nerves enter the apices of the teeth as myelinated A-β and A-δ fibers or unmyelinated c-fibers. The majority of the myelinated fibers are associated with nociception, and the unmyelinated c fibers with post-ganglionic sympathetic nerves and nociception. Two or three branches enter the premolars and molars, and single trunks usually enter the incisors and canines. Some

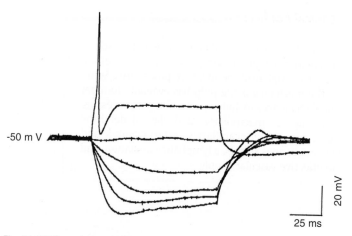

Fig. 11.**29** Sharp neuron: This neuron is typical of an Aβ or Aδ neuron. The action potential spike shows a fast rise and decline with no pronounced inflection on the falling phase.

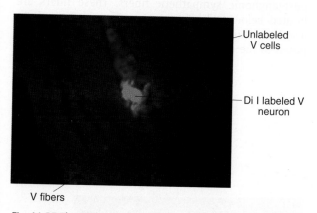

Fig. 11.**27** This photomicrograph is a DiI-labeled trigeminal ganglion cell that had the neurotracer DiI placed in an exposed first maxillary molar pulp 5 days earlier.

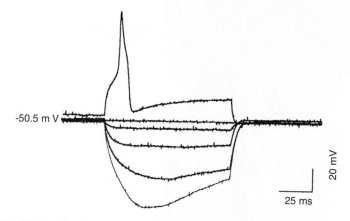

Fig. 11.**30** Humped neuron: This neuron is typical of a nociceptive, afferent Aδ or c-fiber. It demonstrates an inflection on the downward portion of the action potential spike.

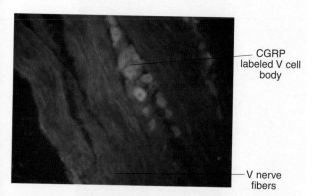

Fig. 11.**28** This photomicrograph demonstrates immunohistochemical staining for the neuropeptide CGRP. This cell corresponds to the cell in the previous figure that is also labeled with DiI and is therefore innervating the first maxillary molar dental pulp.

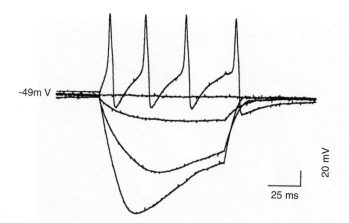

Fig.11.**31** Multiple humped neuron: This neuron fired multiple action potentials when a 20-mV depolarizing current was injected. The action potentials have broad spikes.

Clinical Application

The dental pulp has an inherent capacity to respond to environmental or iatrogenic trauma resulting from bacterial insult or operative procedures. Some of the mechanisms the pulp has available to meet these challenges include various antigen processing cells such as macrophages and class II dendritic cells, fenestrated capillaries, arteriovenous and venous-venous shunts, a lymphatic circulation, and an effective vascular supply.

terminal branches from the nerve trunks are given off within the radicular pulp, but most of the branches terminate in the coronal pulp in the pulp horns, and within the dentinal tubules. As the nerve trunks reach the sub-odontoblastic region they form a plexus in the coronal pulp deep to the cell-rich zone. The myelinated nerves then lose the myelin sheath and, together with the sympathetic nerves, enter the cell-rich layer, traverse the cell-free and odontoblastic layers, and enter the dentinal tubules of the predentin and dentin. Nerve terminals are found in all parts of the dental pulp, but the most dense area of innervation is in the pulp horns (Fig 11.**32**). The pulp horns are the most clinically susceptible areas for environmental trauma, which may explain the density of innervation. Approximately every 10th dentinal tubule contains a nerve terminal in the pulp horn region of the coronal pulp (Fig. 11.**33**). The nerves extend nearly 200 Ìm into the dentinal tubules through the predentin and dentin (Fig. 11.**34**).

The majority of the nerves located within the odontogenic zone of the mature dental pulp are unmyelinated A-δ or c fibers and are thought to be nociceptive fibers or postganglionic sympathetic fibers. These fibers are located below and between the odontoblasts and are also located in the dentinal tubules of predentin juxtaposed to the odontoblastic process. Most of the termi-

Dentin

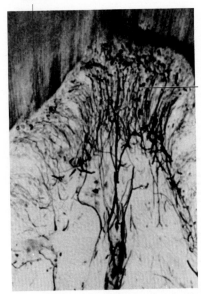

Nerves among odontoblasts

Fig. 11. **32** Nerves in the odontogenic zone of the pulp.

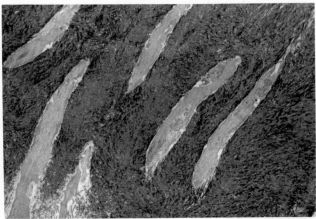

Fig. 11. **33** Transmission electron micrograph demonstrating a series of dentinal tubules in a pulp horn containing nerves and odontoblastic processes.

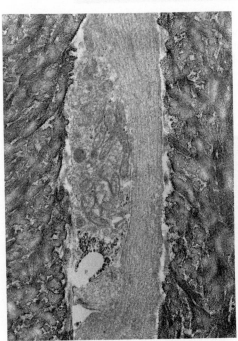

Fig. 11. **34** High-magnification transmission electron micrograph showing a nerve terminal and odontoblastic process in a dentinal tubule.

nals associated with the odontoblast and the odonto-blastic process contain a variety of electron-dense and/or electron-lucent vesicles (Fig. 11.**35**). Although the majority of nerve terminals located in the coronal or root pulp associated with the vasculature contain dense core vesicles that stain positively for catecholamines, other substances could also be colocalized within the same terminal, for example, substance P and vasoactive intestinal peptide (VIP). These nerve terminals are thought to be postganglionic sympathetic terminals for the regulation of pulpal blood flow (Fig. 11.**36**). There are terminals located in the odontogenic zone that contain a homogeneous population of dense core vesicles and are associated with capillaries. (Figs. 11.**37A** and **B**). However, their vascular stimulation function is unclear since capillary diameter is regulated by local humoral factors such as bradykinin, prostaglandins, and interleukins elaborated by cells involved in the inflammatory response. Several authors have reported that these dense core-containing terminals located in the odontoblastic region play a role in modulating the response of the sensory nociceptors by regulating the vascular supply to these terminals. Other investigators suggest that these nerve terminals play a role in modifying the response of the odontoblast to insult, in recruitment of progenitor cells after pulp exposure or deep cavity preparation, or in the regulation

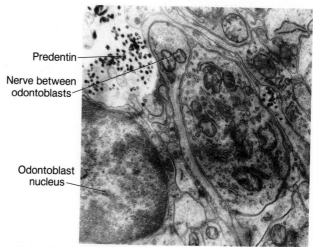

Fig. 11. **35** Ultrastructure of unmyelinated nerve extending between odontoblasts into predentin.

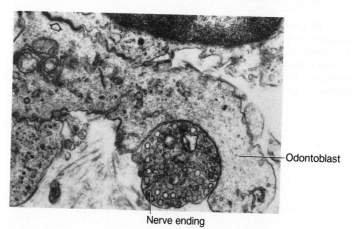

Fig. 11. **36** Ultrastructure of a nerve ending indenting an odoblastic process. Arrow: gap junction between adjacent odontoblasts.

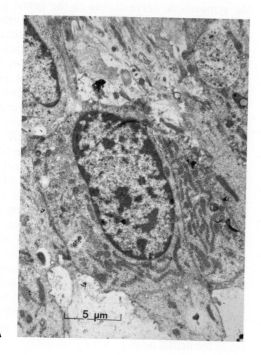

A

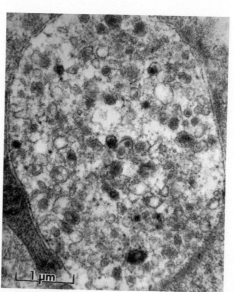

B

Fig. 11. **37** Ultrastructural transmission electron micrograph of odontoblasts **(A)** with a large nerve terminal **(B)** containing various sizes and types of membrane-bound vesicles.

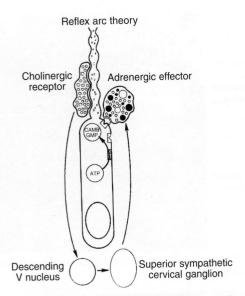

Fig. 11.**38** Schematic of reflex arc theory. Cell movement or deformation of the nerve terminal may stimulate the sensory terminal (cholinergic) to conduct an impulse to the main sensory nucleus in the central nervous system. A descending pathway may stimulate sympathetic stimuli to the effectory (adrenergic) on or near the odontoblast, which effects response of dentinogenesis and reparative dentin formation.

of odontoblastic metabolism (Fig. 11.**38**).

Many anatomic variations of nerves and nerve terminals have been reported to exist in the dental pulp as described morphologically, neurohistochemically, and immunohistochemically. These variations have raised questions as to the functional significance of these findings. Neurotransmitters such as calcitonin gene-related peptide (CGRP), enkephalin, neuropeptide Y, vasoactive intestinal peptide, substance P, somatostatin, serotonin, acetylcholine, and norepinepherine have been reported to be associated with nerves innervating the dental pulp. Presumably, these putative neurotransmitters are contained in the vesicles of the nerve terminals adjacent to the odontoblasts. However, there are no ultrastructural studies characterizing the contents of the vesicles within nerve terminals juxtaposed to the odontoblasts of the dental pulp or in the dentinal tubules located within the predentin or dentin. In addition, there are no studies demonstrating that the odontoblastic plasma membrane contains receptors for any of these putative neurotransmitters. Do these different conformations of nerve terminals and different neurotransmitters function only during the transmission or modulation of nociceptive mechanoreception, or do they have other roles, such as modifying the responsiveness of the odontoblasts to iatrogenic or environmental insult? The answer to these questions are unknown at present, but recent evidence suggests that CGRP-containing nerves in the periosteum and marrow of bones can increase osteoblastic activity. CGRP-containing nerves have also been found in the dental pulp in close proximity to odontoblasts, which were in the process of forming reparative dentin.

Reports of adrenergic sympathetic nerves located in the dental pulp of various species of animals suggest that the sympathetic nerve supply to the dental pulp has multiple functions. One function that is well established is the response of the vasculature of the dental pulp to sympathetic stimulation. Many investigators have shown that the adrenergic sympathetic nerves function to control in intravascular and interstitial pressures within the pulpal tissues. Electrical stimulation of the superior sympathetic trunk and/or ganglion results in a decrease in pulpal blood flow, but does not result in a change in diameter of the blood vessels located in the dental pulp. The use of sympathomimetics decreases the flow rate. Several investigators have reported changes in the pulpal blood flow rate after injection of specific cholinergic agonists, suggesting that there is a population of autonomic nerves in the dental pulp that use acetylcholine as the postganglionic neurotransmitter. These studies corroborate light-microscopic studies in which acetylcholine esterase has been localized in the odontogenic zone and adjacent subodontoblastic plexus where the nerve supply is most dense. These results present a perplexing problem that needs to be further elucidated, considering there are very few morphologic reports in the literature of a parasympathetic nerve supply to the dental pulp.

Theories of Pain Transmission through Dentin

At present there are three major theories that have been suggested to explain how pain is transmitted through the dentin (Fig. 11.**39**). Confusion arises as a result of several factors, including the lack of synaptic specializations between nerves and odontoblasts, the multiplicity of neurotransmitters found in the dental pulp, and the technical difficulties in recording electrophysiologically from an intact pulp. Currently, the hydrodynamic theory predominates, although each theory has positive and negative points.

Hydrodynamic Theory

The movement of the fluid contained in the dentinal tubules, in response to iatrogenic or environmental trauma, is the basis of the hydrodynamic theory. When the fluid in the dentinal tubules, a derivative of the blood plasma, is perturbed, the nerve terminals within the dentinal tubules and the odontoblast layer are deformed and initiate an action potential. Numerous studies have demonstrated that rapid movement of the dentinal fluid will cause pain whether the stimulus is osmotic, chemical, temperature-related, or mechanical.

Transduction Theory

The transduction theory is based on several experimental criteria suggesting that the odontoblast can transduce a mechanical stimulus and transfer that signal to a closely opposed nerve terminal. This theory is supported by reports showing odontoblasts to be derived from neural crest cells, to be closely associated with nerve terminals, and to contain gap junctions that electronically couple adjacent odontoblasts. Arguments against the odontoblast transduction theory are that there have been no reports of synaptic specializations between odontoblasts and nerve terminals, and therefore no means of chemical transmission, and that odontoblasts are not excitable cells, and therefore are unable to produce an electrical response.

Direct Innervation Theory

The direct innervation hypothesis is the oldest theory of dentinal innervation and is based on the belief that dentinal nerve terminals extend to the DEJ. When the dentin is penetrated the nerve terminal is deformed directly by mechanical perturbation and initiates an action potential. Presently, the evidence suggests that nerve terminals extend between 200 and 300 µm into the predentin–dentin, which is too close to the pulp to support this theory.

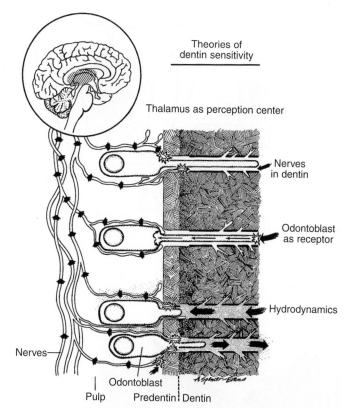

Fig. 11.**39** Summary of information on function according to three theories of dentinal innervation.

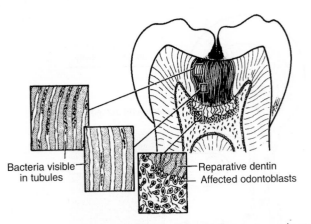

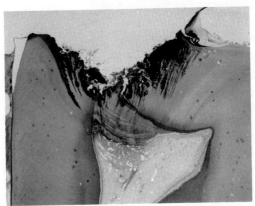

Fig. 11. **40** Diagram of dental caries in tubules and inflammatory pulp exposure.

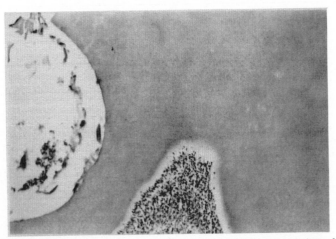

Fig. 11. **41** Histology of caries in dentin with underlying reparative dentin and inflammatory pulp response.

Fig. 11. **42** Autoradiographic demonstration of the pattern of labeling of I^{125}-fibrinogen 10 minutes after a class V cavity preparation was completed.

Pulp Response to Environmental and Iatrogenic Trauma

Caries

Dentin affected by a carious insult will initiate an inflammatory response from the dental pulp as a result of invasion of the pulpal tissue by bacterial toxins (Fig. 11.**40**). Initial disruption of the odontoblasts due to edema breaks down the junctional complexes between odontoblasts and allows access of the pulpal tissue by the bacteria and other oral contaminants (Fig. 11.**41**). The capillaries begin to leak plasma, and vascular cells will become extravasated (Fig. 11.**42**). The acute inflammatory cells release various chemotaxic factors, cytokines, and growth factors. The inflammatory response consists of a rapid accumulation of neutrophils, histiocytes, and monocytes. Prolonged inflammation results in a chronic inflammatory response that includes B- and T-lymphocytes and plasma cells. With the presence of chronic inflammation, focal necrotic lesions develop that may lead to total pulpal necrosis, possibly due to anaerobic bacterial invasion and the subsequent release of degradative enzymes by these virulent bacteria.

Healing after Cavity Preparation

Experimental evidence suggests that wound healing in the rat dental pulp begins after mechanical or thermal trauma caused by the cavity preparation, injures the odontoblast, opens the dentinal tubules, and displaces the nerves and nerve terminals adjacent to the odontoblasts and odontoblastic processes within the dentinal tubules. The distortion of the nerve terminals causes them to rapidly release neuropeptides contained within their vesicles, such as substance P and VIP. Disruption of the odontoblastic layer and injury to the cells as a result of the cavity preparation initiate chemotactic signals recruiting inflammatory cells to the area. The inflammatory cells respond by releasing various cellular mediators—histamine, serotonin, and prostaglandins—into the surrounding tissue, thus potentiating the inflammatory response. The junctional complexes between adjacent odontoblasts are disrupted, allowing an influx of ionic calcium from the extracellular dentinal fluid into the injured odontoblast, and possibly from intracellular sequestration because of injury, causing disruption of gap-junctional complexes. The intercellular spaces become filled with fluid and proteins derived from the plasma leaking from the permeable capillaries, effectively preventing intercellular communication. Concomitantly, the clotting cascade is initiated, decreasing the permeability of the dentin and preventing further ingress of irritants into the dental pulp. Within 1 day, in shallow cavity preparations, the odontoblasts reorganize and re-establish their plasma membranes that were damaged during the operative procedure. These odontoblasts begin to secrete collagen and other ECM components in an attempt to repair the damage effectively. However, at 3 days their metabolic functions are not synchronous because the tight-junctional and gap-junctional complexes have not been re-established between adjacent cells. At 5 days after the initial trauma, the gap junctions and tight-junctional complexes re-establish, and reparative dentinogenesis has reached the point where the amount of ECM produced by the odontoblasts begins to decrease. By 14 days, the inflammatory response is resolved, the odontoblastic cell layer is re-established, and reparative dentinogenesis and new collagen formation are diminished to the level of the controls.

Notes on How Inflammation Modifies Pulpal Responses

Inflammation in the dental pulp is accompanied by the release of a wide variety of chemical mediators, of which highly oxidative molecules—known as reactive oxygen species (ROS)—play a major role. As the name infers, ROS are unstable and more readily react with other compounds than their ground state derivatives.

Species that have mild thermodynamic properties can be used to the organism's benefit as messenger molecules. For example, the reactive oxygen species, nitric oxide ($NO^{\bullet}$) and superoxide ($O_2^{\bullet-}$) play key roles in inflammation. Nitric oxide has recently been discovered to be the endothelium-derived relaxing factor (EDRF) important for regulating vasodilatation. Superoxide aids neutrophil migration by activation of a superoxide-dependent chemoattractant.

ROS are produced in greater quantities by activated inflammatory cells as an aid in phagocytosis. This process is used by our defense cells as a mechanism to neutralize invading organisms. The respiratory burst found in stimulated macrophages is the best known example of this phenomena. However, it is also thought that overproduction of ROS may be harmful to normal host tissue as well. ROS have been shown to cause disruption at multiple cellular sites. Recently the role of nitric oxide and superoxide have been investigated in inflammation induced in dental pulp via cavity preparation. These studies have shown that both nitric oxide and superoxide levels increase with inflammation. These increases occurred not only in inflammatory cells but also in resident pulp tissue as well as surrounding endothelial/vascular structures.

To control ROS concentrations, an elaborate system of antioxidant enzymes are in place, of which superoxide dismutase (SOD) is a major component. SOD catalyses the dismutation (the simultaneous oxidation and reduction of two like molecules) of superoxide radicals to form H_2O_2 and O_2. In mammalian cells there are two major forms of the SOD enzyme, which differ by their intracellular locations and type of metal used at the enzyme's active site. Copper and zinc-containing SOD

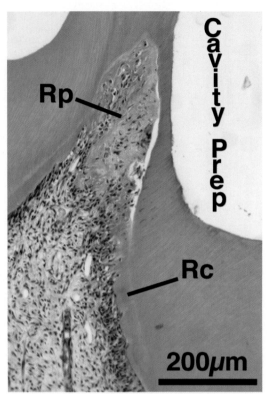

Fig. 11.43 Cavity preparation in the hrCuZnSOD-treated group results in minimal inflammation of the mesial pulp horns. In the deeper portions of the cavity preparation, the original odontoblasts have been destroyed. Replacement odontoblasts have produced an atubular reparative dentin (Rp). In the shallower portions of the preparation, the original odontoblasts survived and produced a regular, tubular, reactionary dentin (Rc).

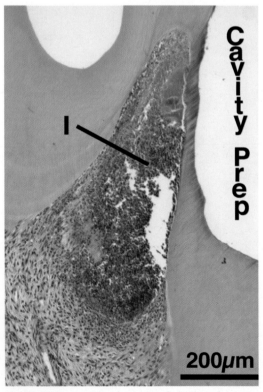

Fig. 11.44 Deep cavity preparation from the saline control group left unrestored for 5 days results in leukocytic infiltration (I) that obliterates the normal cellular architecture in the pulp.

(CuZnSOD) is found primarily in the cytosol of the cell, and manganese-containing SOD (MnSOD) is located mainly in the mitochondrial matrix and the nucleus. Recently, CuZnSOD activity has been demonstrated in animal and human dental pulp. In addition, CuZnSOD activity increases with inflammation in extirpated human pulp tissue. Both CuZnSOD and MnSOD immunostaining increases dramatically with inflammation in pulp tissue surrounding a leukocytic infiltration.

Indirect evidence that increased ROS concentrations are deleterious to the pulp comes from a recent study in which the effects of superoxide radical scavenging was investigated on pulpal inflammation 5 days after a standardized cavity preparation. Inflammation and repair were compared histomorphometrically between animals treated with exogenous administration of a human recombinant CuZnSOD antioxidant enzyme versus saline-vehicle controls. There was a significant reduction in area of inflammation involvement in those animals treated with hrCuZnSOD as compared to controls (Figs. 11.**43** and 11.**44**). Pulp repair was measured by the amount of reparative dentin (the dentin produced by replacement odontoblasts after the original odontoblasts have been destroyed) and reactionary dentin (increased secondary dentin deposition produced by the original odontoblasts in response to an irritant) produced by the inflamed pulps. None of the inflamed pulps from the saline control animals demonstrated reparative dentin formation and only a small percentage produced reactionary dentin. Reparative and reactionary dentin, however, were observed in the majority of the SOD-treated animals. Exogenous administration of hrCuZnSOD promoted an environment within the pulp in which replacement odontoblasts could develop and deposit reparative dentin with a minimal inflammatory response compared to the saline-treated controls. The dentin–like matrix produced in the SOD-treated animals contained multiple cell body inclusions and, therefore, may be extremely permeable to oral irritants. Whether SOD treatment of these cavity-prepared rats would ultimately prevent pulp necrosis at longer time intervals is currently under investigation.

Clinical Application

The high density of nerves in the dental pulp has been reported to function in the transmission of nociceptive stimuli (pain) and in regulating the response of the odontoblast and pulp to trauma. Various investigators have shown that mitotic activity and reparative dentinogenesis can be altered when the sensory or postganglionic sympathetic nerves are resected. The nervous system has also been reported to modulate immunologic responses in various tissues. The regulation of vascular tone by the postganglionic sympathetic nerves is also important in maintaining interstitial fluid pressure in the pulp as well as in modulating the response of the nociceptive nerve terminals within the dental pulp. Recent evidence demonstrates that axon reflexes also play a key role during inflammation.

Immediate Pulp Exposure and Direct Pulp Capping

Numerous studies have demonstrated that the dental pulp has an inherent capacity to respond to wounding in the absence of other inflammatory insults (Fig. 11.**45**). Experimental evidence has shown that using clinically acceptable criteria, an uninflammed and exposed dental pulp will form a dentin bridge by 2 weeks in a human and by 9 days in the monkey.

When an experimental pulp exposure is completed in a previously healthy tooth, portions of the odontoblastic layer and underlying cell-free and cell-rich layers and pulp proper are destroyed. Nerves and blood vessels are cut and extravasation of erythrocytes and plasma causes tissue edema and increased interstitial pressure in the surrounding pulp tissue. At 2 days after pulp capping with a calcium-hydroxide-containing medicament and restoration to the surface, the exposure site contains a clot composed of fibrin, platelets, and red blood cells (Fig. 11.**46**). Some polymorphonuclear leukocytes migrate from the blood vessels into the reorganizing pulp proper surrounding the exposure site. Fibroblasts begin to migrate into the periphery of the subjacent injured pulp (Fig. 11.**47**). The clot begins to reorganize. The previously terminally injured odontoblasts have completely degenerated whereas the adjacent uninjured pulp appears normal.

By 5 days after pulp exposure, the clot has been phagocytosed and stellate-shaped fibroblasts can be seen migrating into the injured area along the axial walls of the cut dentin and in the area below the exposure site

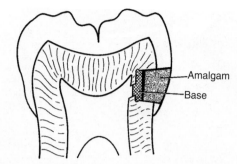

Fig. 11.**45** Diagram of cavity preparation and exposure of pulp.

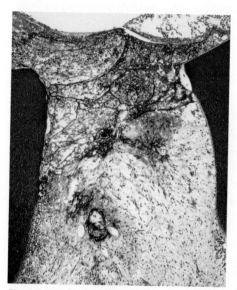

Fig. 11.**46** Pulp exposure with blood clot after 2 days.

Clinical Application

Today, individuals retain their teeth for long periods of time. Periodontal disease is currently prevalent. The gingiva and epithelial attachment migrate down the root surface of the teeth, exposing the cementum and root dentin, resulting in an increased incidence of root caries. Root odontoblasts have recently been reported to respond to root caries in the aging pulp in a manner similar to coronal odontoblasts, except that it takes longer to initiate reparative dentinogenesis and to complete the reparative process.

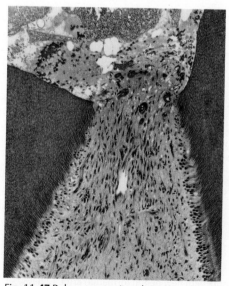

Fig. 11.**47** Pulp exposure in a rhesus monkey after 4 days. Observe the granulation tissue near the exposure site.

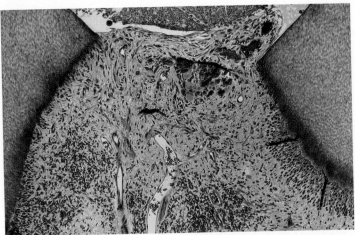

Fig. 11.**48** Pulp exposure, granulation tissue, and pulp growth into exposure site in a rhesus monkey after 5 days.

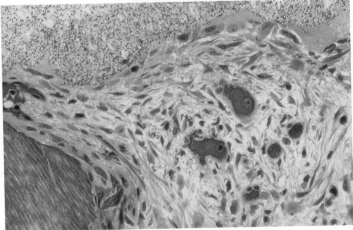

Fig. 11.**49** Pulp exposure after 9 days. Note the organization of cells along the exposure site.

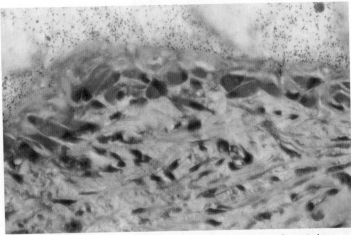

Fig. 11.**50** Site of pulp exposure with new dentin formation after 12 days.

(Fig. 11.**48**). Neoangiogenesis and a predominance of fibroblasts describe the granulation tissue occupying the wound site. Pulp tissue can be seen adjacent to the overlying medicament. Late in this stage of pulpal healing, the fibroblasts become oriented parallel to the medicament interface.

At 7 to 9 days, the fibroblasts begin to enlarge and polarize with their nucleus oriented basally (Fig. 11.**49**). These odontoblast–like cells then reorganize perpendicular to the pulp capping material. By 12 days, the cells have deposited and mineralized the secreted ECM, reparative dentin (Fig. 11.**50**). As reparative dentin formation continues, the tissue begins to resemble normal circumpulpal dentin and contains odontoblastic processes. This process continues until healing has been completed.

The clinical success of direct pulp capping depends on several factors including prevention of bacteria and bacterial products from entering the pulp during the operative procedures. Successful treatment includes the formation of a permanent dentinal bridge by replacement odontoblasts that act, along with the restorative material, to prevent leakage of oral contaminants from affecting the pulp. The formation of a dentinal bridge is similar to reparative dentin formation under a cavity preparation or in the pulp horns resulting from occlusal attrition or trauma.

Summary

The dental pulp consists of a loose connective tissue enclosed by rigid predentin and dentin lining the coronal and radicular pulp. The most peripheral aspect of the dental pulp contains four layers of cells including the odontoblastic layer, the cell-free zone, the cell-rich zone, and the parietal plexus of nerves. Deep within these four layers is the pulp proper, composed of fibroblasts and an ECM. The pulp is densely innervated with sensory and postganglionic sympathetic nerves. Some nerves are associated with maintenance of vascular tone, whereas other nerves are associated with the conduction of nociceptive stimuli. The most dense innervation is in the pulp horns. Of the three theories of dentinal sensitivity, the hydrodynamic theory is the most viable. Arterioles, venules, and lymphatics vessels are also present. The pulp has an inherent capacity to respond to environmental as well as iatrogenic trauma resulting from restorative procedures by the upregulation of odontoblastic activity and the production, secretion, and subsequent mineralization of reparative dentin (Fig. 11.**51**).

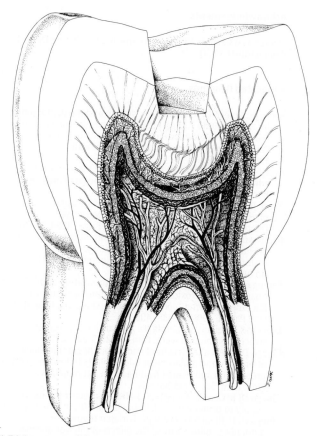

Fig. 11.**51** Summary of diagram of cavity preparation with underlying reparative dentin. Pulp organization with odontoblasts, cell-free and cell-rich zones, and parietal layer of nerves. Large myelinated nerve trunks appear in the central pulp and nonmyelinated nerves appear on vessel walls.

Self-Evaluation Review

1. What embryonic cell layer gives rise to odontoblasts?
2. Describe and discuss the junctional complexes between odontoblasts.
3. Discuss the pulpal fibroblast and its function during maintenance and repair of the dental pulp.
4. What vascular structures are important in reducing interstitial pressure during pulpal injury?
5. Which pulpal nerves function in the maintenance of vascular tone? How are pulpal capillaries controlled?
6. Which theory of pain transmission through dentin is the most popular? Give reasons to support your answer.
7. Discuss inflammation in the dental pulp, including the types of cells and sequence of events leading to pulpal healing.
8. Describe the aging process in the dental pulp.
9. Name three neurotransmitters found in the dental pulp and their functions.
10. Compare and contrast the ECM of predentin and dentin.

Acknowledgements

Figures 11.**43** and 11.**44** were generously provided by Dr. Kirk Baumgardner, Ph. D.

Suggested Readings

Avery JK, Chiego DJ Jr. Cholinergic system and the dental pulp. In: Inoki R, Kudo T, Olgart LM, eds. Dynamic Aspects of the Dental Pulp-Molecular Biology, Pharmacology and Pathophysiology. New York: Chapman & Hall; 1990:297–332.

Avery JK, Cox CF, Chiego DJ Jr. Presence and location of adrenergic nerve endings in the dental pulps of mice. Anat. Rec. 1980;198:59–71.

Avery JK, Cox CF, Chiego DJ Jr. The ultrastructure and physiology of dentin. In: Linde A, ed. Dentin and Dentinogenesis. Cleveland, Ohio: CRC Press; 1984:19–46.

Baumgardner KR, Sulfaro MA. The Anti-inflammatory Effects of Human Recombinant Copper-Zinc Superoxide Dismutase on Pulp Inflammation. J Endodont. 2001; (in press).

Baumgardner KR, Law AS, Gebhart GF. Localization and Changes in Superoxide Dismutase Immunoreactivity in Rat Pulp Following Tooth Preparation. Oral Surg. Oral Med. Oral Pathol. 1999;88:488–495.

Byers MR, Neuhaus SJ, Gehrig JD. Dental sensory receptor structure in human teeth. Pain. 1982;13:221–235.

Chiego DJ Jr. An ultrastructural and autoradiographic analysis of primary and replacement odontoblasts following cavity preparation and wound healing in the rat molar. Proc. Finn. Dent. Soc. 1993;88:243.

Chiego DJ Jr, Cox CF, Avery JK. H3-HRP analysis of the nerve supply to primate teeth. J. Dent. Res. 1980;59:736–744.

Chiego DJ Jr, Klein RM, Avery JK. Tritiated thymidine autoradiographic study of the effects of inferior alveolar nerve resection on the proliferative compartments of the mouse incisors formative tissues. Arch. Oral Biol. 1981;26:83–89.

Chiego DJ Jr, Klein RM, Avery JK. Neuroregulation of protein synthesis in odontoblasts of the first molar of the rat after wounding. Cell Tiss. Res. 1987;248:119–123.

Chiego DJ Jr, Fisher MA, Klein RM, Avery JK. Effects of denervation on 3H-fucose incorporation by odontoblasts in the mouse incisor. Cell Tiss. Res. 1983;230:197–203.

Chiego DJ Jr, Klein RM, Avery JK, Gruhl IM. Denervation induced changes in cell proliferation in the rat molar after wounding. Anat. Rec. 1986;214:348–352.

Contos JG, Corcoran JF, LaTurno SA, Chiego DJ Jr, Regezi JA. Langerhans cells in apical periodontal cysts. J. Endodont. 1987;13:52–55.

Fitzgerald M, Chiego DJ Jr, Heys DR. Autoradiographic analysis of odontoblast replacement following pulp exposure in primate teeth. Arch. Oral Biol. 1990;35:707–715.

Heys DR, Fitzgerald M, Heys RJ, Chiego DJ Jr. Healing of primate dental pulps capped with Teflon. Oral Surg. Oral Med. Oral Pathol. 990;69:227–237.

Holland GR. Lanthanum hydroxide labeling of gap junctions in the odontoblast layer. Anat. Rec. 1976;186:211–216.

Inoki R, Kudo T, Olgart LM, eds. Dynamic Aspects of Dental Pulp: Molecular Biology, Pharmacology and Pathophysiology. New York, NY: Chapman & Hall; 1990.

Law AS, Baumgardner KR, Meller ST, Gebhart GF. Localization and Changes in NADPH-Diaphorase Reactivity and Nitric Oxide Synthase Immunoreactivity in Rat Pulp Following Tooth Preparation. J. Dent. Res. 1999;78:1585–1595.

Linde A, ed. Dentin and Dentinogenesis. Vols. I and 2. Boca Raton, Fla: CRC Press; 1984.

Kim S. Regulation of pulpal blood flow. J. Dent. Res. 1985;65:602–606.

Klein RM, Chiego DJ Jr, Avery JK. Effects of chemical sympathectomy on cell proliferation in the progenitive compartment of the neonatal mouse incisor. Arch. Oral Biol. 1981;26:319–325.

Pashley DH. Dentin-predentin complex and its permeability: physiological overview. J. Dent. Res. 1985;64:613–620.

Palmer RM, Ferrige AG, Moncada S. Nitric oxide release accounts for the biological activity of endothelium-derived relaxing factor. Nature (London) 1987;327:523–526.

Rutherford RB, Wahle J, Tucker M, Rueger D, Charette M. Induction of reparative dentine formation in monkeys by recombinant human osteogenic protein-1. Arch. Oral Biol. 1993;38:571–576.

Turner DF, Marfurt CF, Sattelberg C. Demonstration of physiological barrier between pulpal odontoblasts and its perturbation following routine restorative procedures: a horse radish peroxidase tracking study in the rat. J. Dent. Res. 1989;68:1262–1268.

Ushiyama J. Gap junctions between odontoblasts revealed by transjunctional flux of fluorescent tracers. Cell Tissue Res. 1989; 258:611–616.

12 Comparison of Primary and Permanent Teeth

David C. Johnsen

Introduction

A comparison of the morphology and histology of primary and permanent teeth is important, as they differ in a number of ways. Clinical problems in the developing jaw of the growing child, as compared with the jaw in the adult, are related to characteristics of developing primary and permanent teeth and their supporting structures. As described in Chapter 7, there are differences in the number of teeth; there are 20 in the primary dentition and 32 in the permanent dentition. As also discussed previously, the anterior 20 permanent teeth replace the primary dentition and are thus defined as successional. These teeth are closely related in the timing of their exfoliation and in the development of the successional dentition. The remaining 12 permanent teeth develop posterior to the 20 primary teeth as the jaws continue to grow in length (Fig. 12.**1**). Both primary and permanent teeth proceed through the same stages of development. This chapter describes differences in tooth size, shape of crowns, roots, and pulp chambers, the microscopic structure of enamel and dentin, as well as interdental spacing, tooth inclination, and arch shape.

Objectives

After reading this chapter you should be able to discuss the similarities and differences between primary and permanent teeth and to describe how these characteristics relate to clinical treatment.

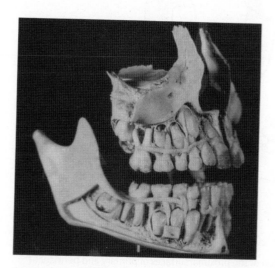

Fig. 12.**1** Mixed dentition period as seen in the cadaver specimen of a child about 9 years of age.

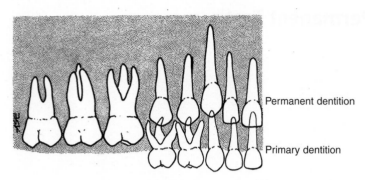

Fig. 12.**2** Size and positional relation of primary and permanent teeth.

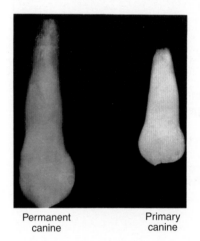

Fig. 12.**3** Comparison of size and shape of permanent and primary canines.

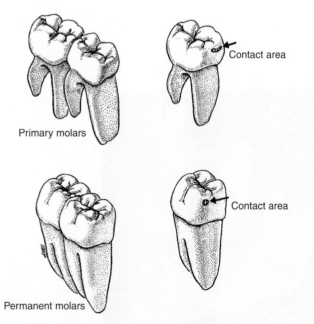

Fig. 12.**4** Comparison of the proximal surfaces of primary and permanent crowns. Primary molars have a flat surface with a contact line; permanent molars have a contact point.

Tooth Number and Size

Perhaps the most obvious difference between primary and permanent dentitions is the number of teeth. There are 20 teeth in the primary dentition, and the permanent teeth replacing them are called successional. There are 32 teeth in the permanent dentition, and the 12 permanent molars that have no predecessors are called accessional. As these permanent molars are added, arch length and total masticatory surface increase (Fig. 12.**2**).

Primary and permanent teeth differ in size and form. Several of these differences influence decisions about dental treatment. Crowns of primary teeth are smaller than crowns of their successors, with only a few key exceptions. Crowns of permanent incisors and canines are larger than their primary counterparts in all dimensions (Fig. 12.**3**), and although crowns of permanent molars are larger than crowns of primary molars, the latter have a larger mesiodistal diameter than crowns of the succeeding premolars. The difference between the cumulative mesiodistal diameters of the primary molars and canines and those of the premolars and permanent canines is called the leeway space. Roots of the primary teeth are shorter than those of permanent teeth.

Tooth shape

Primary teeth resemble permanent teeth in several ways. Both primary incisors and their respective permanent successors are single rooted and have incised edges. Both primary canines and their respective permanent successors have single roots and a single cusp. Primary molars, however, bear no resemblance to the premolars that will succeed them; instead, the second primary molar crown resembles the adjacent first permanent molar crown. The first primary molars bear little resemblance to any other tooth.

Crowns of primary teeth are shorter incisocervically than mesiodistally and have a short, thick-set appearance. Primary teeth have greater contour than permanent teeth, especially at the cervical portion of the crown. Contact areas differ for approximating molars. The approximating surfaces of the permanent molars are more rounded than those of the primary molars, which results in a contact point (Fig. 12.**4**). Primary molars have flattened approximal surfaces, which results in a contact line. This difference has clinical significance in caries patterns on approximal surfaces and in cavity design for caries removal. Interproximal carious lesions will be cervical to the contact areas and of similar shape. A second difference in molar crown shape involves cusp height. Permanent molars and premolars have steeper cusps than their primary counterparts, and interdigitation is more flexible with primary molars than with permanent ones.

Roots of primary molars are more divergent than roots of permanent molars. The flat, curved roots of the primary molars permit development of the underlying premolars. Radiographs (Fig. 12.**5**) demonstrate the positions of the premolars underlying the primary molars. The widely divergent primary molar roots allow the premolar crowns to develop under them without displacing the primary teeth. As the premolar erupts, the roots of the primary molar will be resorbed along the interradicular surfaces. Resorption is indicated in a radiograph by increased radiolucency.

Root shape dictates pulp shape and is closely correlated with two important clinical considerations (Fig. 12.**6**). First, curved roots with thin walls make mechanical access to root canals more difficult in primary molars than in permanent molars. Second, the fat, ribbon–like root canal of the primary tooth is in sharp contrast to the oval, tube–like root canal of the permanent tooth. Significant developmental differences occur in the root canals of the primary molars; the root canal fills in unevenly with secondary dentin, which leaves calcified bridges. Extensions of pulpal tissues are then sheltered from instrumentation attempts. Filling-in of the pulp canals usually occurs at about the time that the first permanent molars erupt. In mandibular second primary molars there are two distal canals, one buccal and one lingual, which are connected by a maze of pulpal tissue (Fig.12.**6**).

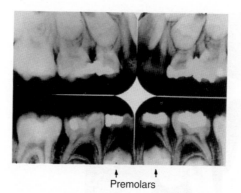

Fig. 12.**5** Radiograph of the position of premolars underlying divergent primary molar roots.

Tooth Development

Primary and permanent teeth have a similar process of development, but the time needed for development of the primary teeth is considerably shorter than that needed for development of the permanent teeth (Fig.12.**7**). In addition to formative events, primary teeth undergo root resorption and pulp degeneration. Primary tooth crowns begin mineralization in utero, with the crown completed shortly after birth. Permanent tooth crowns begin formation at or after birth, depending on the tooth. One clinical result is that prenatal systemic

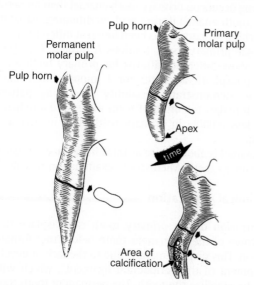

Fig. 12.**6** Comparison of primary and permanent pulp horns and root canals.

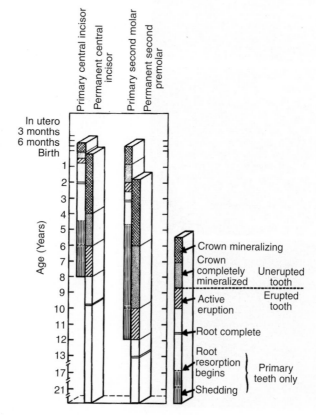

Fig. 12.**7** Comparison of the life of primary and permanent teeth in chronologic pattern.

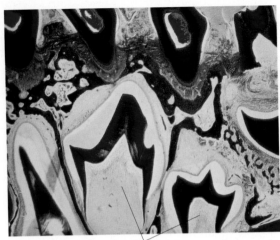

Permanent teeth

Fig. 12.**8** Eruption of permanent teeth and exfoliation of primary teeth during mixed dentition period.

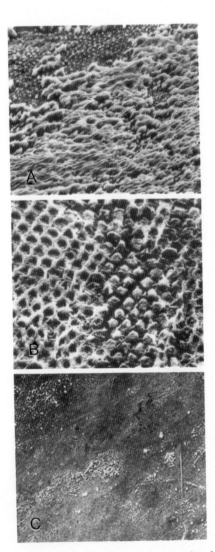

Fig. 12.**9** Scanning electron micrographs of the variation of etching pattern in the surface enamel of same primary teeth. **A** and **C** x400, **B** x1000.

disturbances can affect mineralization of the primary tooth crowns whereas postnatal disturbances can affect mineralization of the permanent tooth crowns.

Primary teeth function in the mouth approximately 8.5 years, and this time-span can be divided into three periods: crown and root growth, root maturation, and root resorption and shedding. The growth period lasts about a year, root maturation about 3.75 years, and root resorption and exfoliation about 3.5 years. On the other hand, some of the 32 permanent teeth may be in the mouth from the 5th year on, whereas others may be in the mouth from the 20th to the 25th year. The permanent teeth could thus function seven to eight times longer than the primary teeth; this time of function includes 12 years of development, which is three times longer in permanent teeth than in primary teeth.

Many separate events occur within the space of a few millimeters during dentition development. For a single primary tooth and its successor, two simultaneous events could be the eruption (with root formation) of the primary tooth and the crown mineralization of the permanent tooth. Another example could be root resorption of the primary tooth, which is concurrent with root formation of the permanent tooth. In a 6-year-old child, one or more formative processes can be occurring in 28 of 32 permanent teeth, while some degree of root resorption can be occurring in each of 20 primary teeth. Timing and coordination of myriad events permit continual function of and accommodation to the growing jaws (Fig. 12.**8**).

Tooth Structure

Primary and permanent teeth have a similar enamel prism structure, except at the tooth surface. Primary teeth are more likely to have a prismless surface zone than are permanent teeth. A difference in the surface reaction to conditioning agents is suspected because less etching occurs on primary tooth enamel than on permanent tooth enamel during acid conditioning. Variability in etching properties has been found at different sites on a single primary tooth. Sections A through C of Figure 12.**9** show different patterns for primary teeth after a 50% phosphoric-acid etch for 1 minute. These micrographs demonstrate variability in etching patterns, which makes retention of resin material unpredictable and less reliable in primary teeth than in permanent teeth.

Enamel is about twice as thick in permanent teeth as in primary teeth. Microscopic examination reveals fur-

Clinical Application

Intrusion of the primary tooth can displace the crown of the permanent tooth before root formation. This displacement is due to the lack of development of the periodontal ligament , which will later stabilize the tooth. The permanent tooth root then forms at an angle to the crown (dilaceration).

ther differences in the enamel of the primary and permanent teeth. Figure 12.**10** demonstrates the most prominent incremental line of Retzius in primary teeth, the neonatal line. This distinct incremental line is the result of metabolic trauma to the developing tooth at or near the time of birth. A view of an incremental (neonatal) line at higher magnification is seen in Figure 12.**11**. Enamel formed postnatally is more highly pigmented than enamel formed prenatally. Despite this pigmentation, the enamel of primary teeth is whiter than that of permanent teeth. This is believed to be because much of primary tooth enamel is formed prenatally and is not subject to some environmental factors.

Primary and permanent teeth have a similar basic dentinal structure. Dentin is thinner in the crown and the roots of primary teeth than in the crown and roots of permanent teeth. A comparison of the hardness of dentin reveals primary dentin to be slightly softer than permanent dentin (Fig. 12.**12**). Peripheral and circumpulpal areas are similar in hardness in both dentitions, but the central area of root and crown dentin is considerably harder in permanent teeth than in primary teeth. Hardness is believed to be due to the degree of mineralization. On this basis, permanent dentin is more highly mineralized. In both primary and permanent teeth, the hardness gradient is critical in attempting to differentiate pathologically soft dentin due to caries from physiologically soft dentin adjacent to the pulp (Fig. 12.**13**). Dentin immediately adjacent to the pulp is normally softer than dentin in the intermediate and outer portions. With a small carious lesion, differentiation of carious and sound dentin is not difficult. With a larger lesion close to to the pulp, however, differentiation of pathologically soft dentin from physiologically soft dentin is impossible on the basis of touch or mechanical manipulation alone. This phenomenon has significant implications in establishing protocol for management of deep caries.

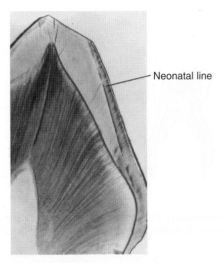

Fig. 12.**10** Neonatal line illustrates the comparison of prenatally and postnatally formed enamel. Prenatal enamel is less pigmented and more free of defects than postnatal enamel.

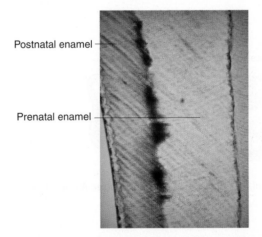

Fig. 12.**11** Prenatal enamel can be seen on the right in this higher magnification micrograph taken from Figure 12.10.

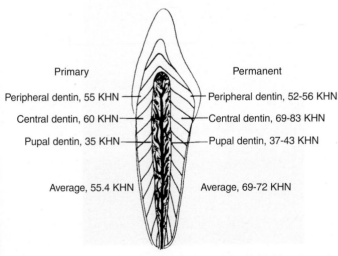

Fig. 12.**12** Comparison of the hardness of primary and permanent dentin.

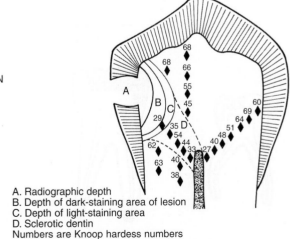

A. Radiographic depth
B. Depth of dark-staining area of lesion
C. Depth of light-staining area
D. Sclerotic dentin
Numbers are Knoop hardness numbers

Fig. 12.**13** Hardness of dentin adjacent to carious dentin.

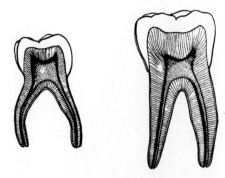

Fig. 12.**14** Comparison of relative pulp sizes in primary and permanent molars. There is relatively more pulp in the primary molar than in the permanent molar.

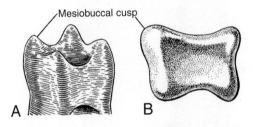

Fig. 12.**15** Pulp horns of the primary mandibular first molar. **A** Lingual view. **B** Occlusal view.

Pulp Size and Shape

There are a number of differences between the pulp of primary teeth and that of permanent teeth. The most significant difference is that in relation to the protective enamel and dentin, there is relatively more pulp in primary than permanent teeth. Because there is relatively more coronal pulp in primary than permanent teeth (Fig.12.**14**), cavity preparation is an important consideration. Primary-tooth pulp size and shape vary considerably. The coronal pulp chambers of the primary teeth have three to five pulp horns that are more sharply pointed than the outer cusp contour would indicate. The largest pulp horn in primary molars is the mesiobuccal; the second largest is the mesiolingual (Fig. 12.**15A**).

Because the primary molars are small and have large pulps, the bulk and the depth of restorations are limited. The mandibular first primary molar is different in that the pulp chamber is rhomboidal with four pulp horns (Fig.12.**15B**). Again, the mesiobuccal is the largest pulp horn and exhibits a ridge connecting it to the mesiolingual. The mesial area is thus susceptible to exposure. A comparison of class II restorations in a primary and a permanent first molar is shown in Figure 12.**16**. The primary molar restoration is several times smaller, especially in depth, than the permanent one.

Primary and permanent pulps are similar in basic histologic architecture (Fig. 12.**17**), and the vasculature, connective tissue, and odontoblastic and subodontoblastic zones are similar in appearance. There is some variation in the number of nerves in the two dentitions, although the permanent pulps generally have more nerves than the primary pulps. The plexus of Raschkow or the parietal-nerve plexus is not evident in early root-formation stages in primary teeth.

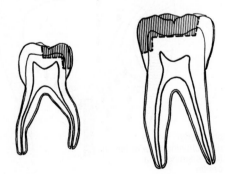

Fig. 12.**16** Comparison of the size of class II restorations in primary (left) and permanent (right) teeth.

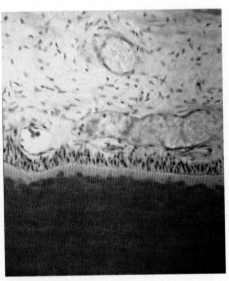

Fig. 12.**17** The odontogenic zone of the primary tooth is similar to that of the permanent tooth.

Accessory Root Canals

Primary and permanent teeth differ in the location of accessory canals. In primary molars, a few accessory canals are found in the area of the bifurcation dentin at the floor of the coronal pulp chamber. The canals can be seen along the inferior surface of the coronal pulp chamber. Accessory canals are much less frequent in this location in permanent teeth. According to one investigator, 20% of primary molars have accessory canals in this location (Fig. 12.**18**). Other authors found a higher percentage. Some canals enter the cementum and dentin and return to the periodontum without entering the pulp.

The usual location of accessory canals in root dentin of permanent teeth is near the apex of the root. In Figure 12.**19**, a view of a permanent molar root apex, two accessory canals can be seen connecting the two vertical root canals. Some have also been reported in the furcation region.

Arch Shape and Tooth Position

Four principal factors influence tooth alignment and adjustments in the arches of primary and permanent dentitions: interdental spacing, tooth inclination, sites of arch growth, and tooth size. The primary dentition has more spacing than the permanent dentition. Primary incisors normally have interdental spacing, whereas permanent incisors do not (Fig.12.**20**). The primary molars frequently have interdental spaces that close during later primary dentition. This movement has been called the early mesial shift.

Primary incisors and canines have a more upright orientation than do succeeding permanent teeth, and per-

Fig. 12.**18** Accessory root canals may appear in the bifurcation zone of a primary molar.

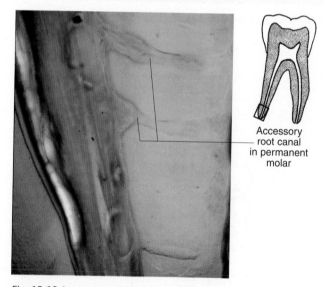

Accessory root canal in permanent molar

Fig. 12.**19** Accessory root canals usually appear near the root apex in a permanent tooth.

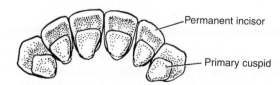

Permanent incisor

Primary cuspid

Fig. 12.**20** Comparison of interdental spacing of primary and permanent teeth.

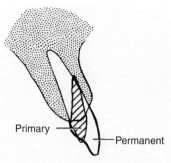

Fig. 12.**21** Comparison of inclination of anterior primary and permanent teeth.

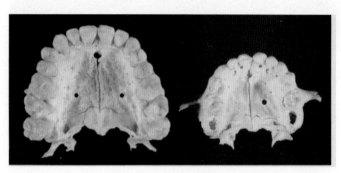

Fig. 12.**22** Comparison of dental arches of primary and permanent teeth.

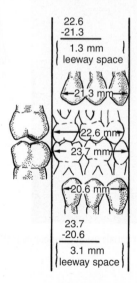

Fig. 12.**23** The leeway space is the difference in mesial-distal dimension of primary molars and succeeding premolars. Note that it is 1.3 mm in the maxillary arch and 3.1 mm in the mandibular arch.

manent tooth crowns have a more labial inclination (Fig. 12.**21**) than do primary tooth crowns. A common arch measurement is intercanine width, which is measured from the cusp tips. With use of these landmarks, the intercanine width is greater in the permanent dentition than in the primary dentition. The increase is somewhat misleading because different teeth are measured. Cingulum (basal-ridge) positions are approximately the same tor the two dentitions (Fig. 12.**21**).

Arch shape is similar in the anterior portion of the two dentitions, but the permanent dentition extends further distally. This is due to growth of the arches, mainly in the posterior aspects, with little growth occurring in the maxillary anterior areas and practically no growth occurring in the mandibular anterior areas (Fig. 12.**22**).

Differences in the characteristics if individual teeth are important in themselves and as a part of the entire dentition. Tooth-size differences are critical in the assessment of potential space for permanent teeth to erupt into good alignment. The succession of smaller primary incisors with larger permanent incisors has been called incisor liability. The size ratio of primary to permanent incisors means that spacing is favorable in the primary dentition if permanent incisors and canines are to have enough space to erupt into an acceptable alignment. In the posterior segments, the size ratio is reversed for primary and permanent teeth. This leeway space provides the opportunity for the premolars to erupt unobstructed by other teeth. The leeway space averages 1.3 mm in each maxillary quadrant and 3.1 mm in each mandibular quadrant (Fig. 12.**23**). The spaces then close by mesial movement of the permanent molars. This is called the late mesial shift. The lower arch shifts more mesially than does the upper arch. The two main results are a change in the molar relation, with the lower molars more forward, and a decrease in the arch circumference.

Clinical Application

The appearance of larger permanent incisors succeeding the primary incisors is termed incisor liability. Compensation in spacing is gained by the smaller premolars that succeed the primary molars; this is termed leeway space.

Root Resorption and Pulp Degeneration

Another major difference between primary and permanent teeth is that the roots of primary teeth normally resorb (Fig. 12.**24**). The process occurs simultaneously with the eruption of the permanent teeth. In the absence of a permanent tooth, primary-tooth resorption still occurs, but it occurs much more slowly. The primary tooth roots have a higher susceptibility to resorption than permanent teeth. The primary teeth have pressure from the permanent teeth exerted on their roots, but this is not the total cause of this susceptibility to resorption. As stated previously, even when a permanent tooth is missing, the primary roots will gradually resorb. The process of resorption is accompanied by gradual changes in the pulp. Figures 12.**25** and 12.**26** show the pulp during root resorption. The first sign is a reduction in the number of cells in the pulp; nerve trunks degenerate into patches of myelin, and some fibrosis occurs. Blood vessels remain until the tooth is exfoliated.

Cellular and fibrillar changes occur during the three phases in the root life of primary teeth: formation, completion, and resorption. During root formation, the young primary tooth pulp is highly cellular. As the roots are completed, fewer cells and more fibers are evident. The proliferation of fibers continues during the root resorption phase, and fiber bundles may be seen (Fig. 12.**27**).

The blood vessels that enter the pulp chamber through the forming roots are initially associated with the odontoblastic layer. They will later form a subodontoblastic network. As the roots are resorbed, these blood vessels exhibit some degenerative changes, although most are maintained until the tooth is lost.

Nerve fibers gradually organize in the pulp chamber of the primary tooth. As the tooth reaches occlusion, the nerve fibres form a plexus underlying the odontoblastic layer; this plexus is termed the parietal layer of nerve fibers. These nerve fibers are lost during resorption of the primary-tooth roots, which makes teeth insensitive to pulpal pain at the time of exfoliation.

The periodontal support of primary and permanent teeth is similar in basic architecture. Healthy gingiva of permanent teeth has been observed to be redder than the gingiva around primary teeth.

Clinical Application

Primary and permanent teeth differ in their response to trauma. Although both have similar kinds of outcomes when a blow is struck, such as tooth fracture, the permanent tooth has an additional sequela. When the primary tooth is dislodged, the permanent tooth may be damaged sufficiently to cause enamel hypoplasia or white spots.

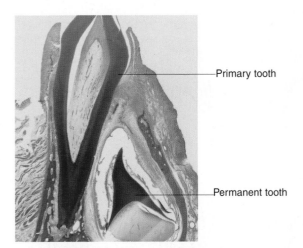

Fig. 12.**24** Relation between the exfoliating primary tooth and erupting permanent crown.

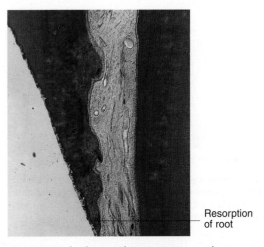

Fig. 12.**25** Pulp changes during primary-tooth root resorption. There is a reduction in cells, nerves, blood vessels, and various intercellular components.

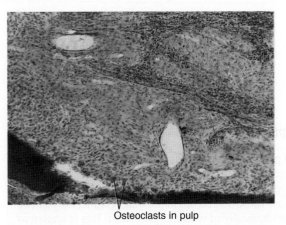

Osteoclasts in pulp

Fig. 12.**26** Histologic appearance of root resorption by osteoclasts.

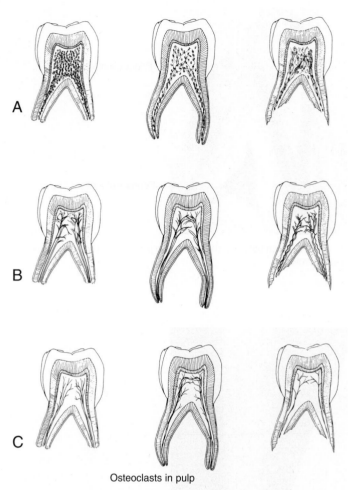

Osteoclasts in pulp

Fig. 12.**27** Pulp changes in the life cycle of the primary tooth. **A** Decrease in the number of cells. **B** Development of vascular nerves. **C** Development and loss of nerves. On the left is the root formation stage, in the center the root completion stage, and on the right the root resorption stage.

Sequela to Injuries

The differences between permanent and primary teeth extend to the area of dental trauma. Primary and permanent teeth differ in their response to trauma in one clinically significant aspect. Although both primary and permanent teeth can have similar kinds of outcomes when struck (fracture of the tooth, fracture of the crown, dislodgement of the tooth, etc.), the permanent tooth has the additional sequela of the indirect effect of a blow to the primary tooth. Early in enamel formation, there can be interruption of the enamel formation in the form of a mark on the tooth at the point where the root tip of the primary tooth strikes the facial surface of the developing permanent tooth crown. The clinical appearance can be a "white spot" or a frank enamel hypoplasia. Intrusion of the primary tooth can also displace the developing crown of the permanent tooth before root formation. The reason for the relative ease of displacement of the crown before root formation is that there is no ligament to stabilize the position of the permanent tooth crown. Once root formation begins, the periodontal ligament has a stabilizing effect on the orientation of the tooth. Once the permanent tooth crown is rotated in its sac, the permanent tooth root continues to develop in its original orientation. The result is disfigured angulation (or dilaceration) between the crown and root of the permanent tooth. Recognition of such disfigurements resulting from trauma can lead to clearer planning for treatment of the affected tooth.

Susceptibility to Enamel Defects

Enamels of primary and permanent teeth differ in their susceptibility to tooth defects. The greater susceptibility of the enamel from permanent teeth to hypomineralization is associated with the different environment for the tooth after birth. Permanent teeth are more susceptible to hypomineralization or "white spot" defects. Although the teeth are not at increased risk for dental caries or abrasion, there can be aesthetic concerns. Inference has been made to the apparent increased prevalence of white-spot lesions of incisors to the increased use of fluorides from multiple sources. It is interesting that the defects for the permanent teeth are located in the outer portions of the tooth enamel. Removal of the outer portions of the tooth enamel, either mechanically or with inorganic acid, can result in removal of the "white-spot" lesion. The technique has been described as microabrasion. Primary teeth, on the other hand, form for the most part before birth and in relative isolation from the mother. Primary teeth are therefore less likely to have defects unless there is a significant systemic insult affecting the unborn child.

Clinical Application

Enamels of primary and permanent teeth differ in their susceptibility to tooth defects. The permanent teeth are more susceptible to hypomineralization or "white spots" than primary teeth. Because these defects are in the outer enamel they can be removed mechanically or with inorganic acid. This is known as microabrasion.

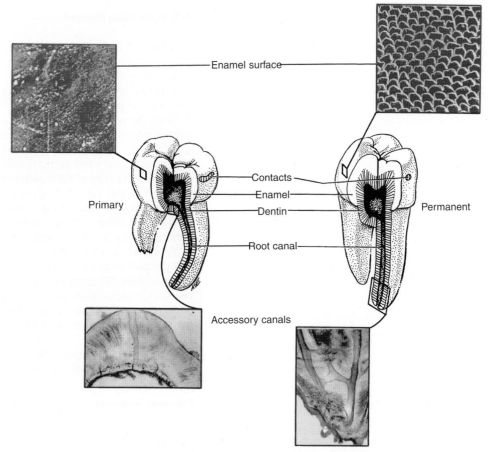

Fig. 12.**28** Summary comparison of primary and permanent teeth. Enamel thickness, enamel surface characteristics, contact points, dentin hardness, pulp size, root canal and root curvature, and location of accessory canals.

Summary

For the practitioner, primary and permanent teeth have several significant gross differences. Primary teeth are fewer and smaller in all dimensions than their successors, with one exception. Primary molars have a greater mesiodistal dimension than succeeding premolars. Primary-tooth crowns have a short and thick-set appearance and exhibit contour, especially near the cervical region. Primary molars form line contacts, whereas permanent molars form point contacts. Although primary and permanent teeth have similar processes of tissue formation, primary teeth take less time to form than permanent teeth. Enamel and dentin are thinner in primary teeth than in permanent teeth. Primary tooth enamel is more opaque than permanent tooth enamel and has a neonatal line. Surface enamel is more likely to be prismless in primary than permanent teeth; however, much variability occurs in primary teeth, from tooth to tooth and for different sites on the same tooth. Tooth pulps of primary molars are relatively large in the coronal portion and become ribbon–like to accommodate to the flat roots (Fig. 12.**28**).

Primary and permanent dentitions have several differences that influence tooth alignment in the arch. Interdental spacing is greater in the primary than in the permanent dentition. Primary anterior teeth are more upright than the more labially inclined permanent anterior teeth. Arch shape in primary and permanent teeth is similar in the anterior portion, but the permanent dentition extends further posteriorly.

Self-Evaluation Review

1. What are the differences in the shape of the primary and permanent molar roots and what is the clinical significance?
2. What is the difference in the formation time of the primary and permanent teeth?
3. State the differences in enamel and dentin thickness of primary and permanent teeth?
4. What are the differences in the surfaces of the enamel in primary and permanent teeth? What is the clinical significance of these differences?
5. Describe the potential effect on the permanent teeth by trauma to the primary tooth.
6. State the differences in hardness of the dentin at various depths of primary and permanent teeth?
7. Where are accessory canals located in the primary and permanent tooth roots?
8. Discuss the differences in size and shape of the pulp chamber in the primary and permanent molar teeth.
9. State four principal factors that influence tooth malalignment in the arches of the primary and permanent dentitions.
10. Define "incisor liability" and "leeway space," and state the clinical significance of each.

Acknowledgements

Figure 12.**6** was provided courtesy of Joe Camp, DDS; Figures12.**7** and12.**21** were provided courtesy of David Scott, DDS; Figure 12.**11** was provided courtesy of Rod Owen, DDS.

Suggested Readings

Avery JK. A possible mechanism of pain conduction in teeth. Acta Histochem. 1963;10:59–64.

Croll TP. Enamel microabrasion for removal of superficial demineralization and decalcification defects. J. Am. Dent. Assoc. 1990;120:411–415.

Enlow DH. Handbook of Facial Growth. Philadelphia, Pa: WB Saunders; 1975.

Gutmann Jr. Prevalence, location and patency of accessory canals in the furcation region of permanent molars. J. Periodontology. 1978;49:21–26.

Johnsen DC, Johns S. Quantitation of nerve fibers in the primary and permanent canine and incisor teeth in man. Arch. Oral Biol. 1978;23:825.

Kraus BS, Jordan RE. The Human Dentition Before Birth. Philadelphia, Pa: WB Saunders; 1965.

Pink JR, Pediatric Dentistry. Philadelphia, Pa: WB Saunders; 1999.

Rapp R, AveryJK, Strachan DS. Distribution of nerves in human primary teeth. Anat. Rec. 1967;159:89–103.

Wheeler RC. A Textbook of Dental Anatomy and Physiology. 4th ed. Philadelphia, Pa.: WB Saunders; 1965.

Yoshida H, Yakushijim, Sugihara A, Tanaka K, Taguchi M, Machida Y. Accessory canals at floor of the pulp chamber of primary molars. Shikwa and Bukuho Vol 75 Soc. 1975;75:580–585.

SECTION IV
Structure and Function of Supporting Tissues of the Teeth

13 Histology of the Periodontium: Alveolar Bone, Cementum, and Periodontal Ligament

James K. Avery

Introduction

The periodontium includes the three supporting structures of the teeth: the bony alveolar process, the root-covered cementum, and the intervening periodontal ligament. The gingiva may also be considered part of the periodontium and is described in Chapter 15. The *alveolar process* is the bony extension of the mandible and maxilla that provides the necessary support for the teeth and serves as a fibrous attachment for the periodontal ligament fibers. By resorption and deposition it also compensates for tooth movement. The *periodontal ligament* is also supportive, suspending the tooth in the socket and providing a cushion against various occlusal forces. Its nerve supply provides a delicate sense of touch and pressure to the tooth, and its blood vessels carry oxygen and nutrition to the ligament as well as to the periodontium and alveolar bone. *Cementum* covers the roots of the teeth and serves as an attachment for the periodontal ligament fibers. It provides compensation for occlusal wear by apical deposition and, at the same time, protection for the sensitive dentin (Fig. 13.**1**).

Objectives

After reading this chapter you should be able to describe the histologic structures and function of the periodontal tissues, the root-covered cementum, the alveolar bone, and the intervening periodontal ligament.

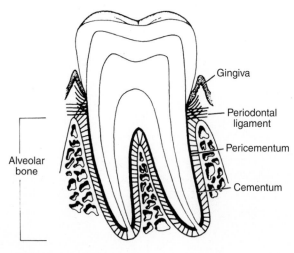

Fig. 13.**1** Diagram of periodontium.

Alveolar Process

The alveolar processes are those portions of the maxilla and mandible that support the roots of the teeth. They are composed of the *alveolar bone proper* and the *supporting bone*. The alveolar bone proper is the bone that lines the socket. In radiographic terms, it is referred to as the *lamina dura*. This process is the bony site of attachment of the periodontal ligament fibers. The supporting bone includes the remainder of the alveolar process, specifically the compact cortical plates on the outer surfaces of the alveolar processes and the spongy bone between the cortical plates and the alveolar bone proper (Fig. 13.**2**).

As discussed in Chapter 7, the alveolar process develops as a result of tooth root elongation and tooth eruption. Alveolar bone matures as the teeth gain functional occlusion; later, if the teeth are lost, the alveolar process disappears. Thus, the teeth are important in the development and maintenance of the alveolar bone. The alveolar bone proper is attached to the supporting cancellous and compact alveolar bone. Bone marrow containing blood vessels, nerves, and adipose tissue fills the space between the cortical plates and the alveolar bone proper (Fig. 13.**3**). The coronal border of the alveolar process is termed the alveolar crest (Fig 13.**2**). It is located about 1 to 1.5 mm below the cementoenamel junction, and is rounded in the anterior region and nearly flat in the molar area. If the teeth are in buccal or lingual position, the alveolar process will be very thin or partially missing. The area of an apical root penetrating the bone is known as a *fenestration*, and its occurrence at the coronal root zone is termed *dehiscence* (Fig. 13.**4**).

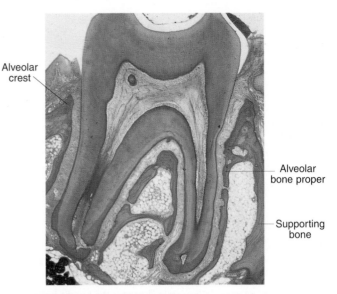

Fig. 13.**2** Histology of periodontium.

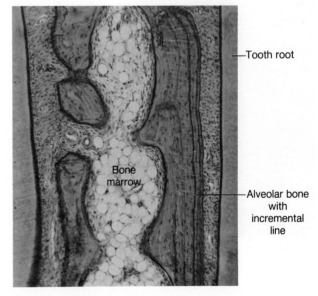

Fig. 13.**3** Histology of alveolar bone proper, with connective-tissue communication between the ligament and supporting bone shown.

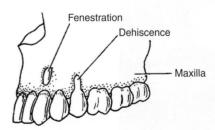

Fig. 13.**4** Diagram showing loss of alveolar bone adjacent to tooth. Bone loss near root apices is termed "fenestration," and bone loss in the region of the coronal root is termed "dehiscence."

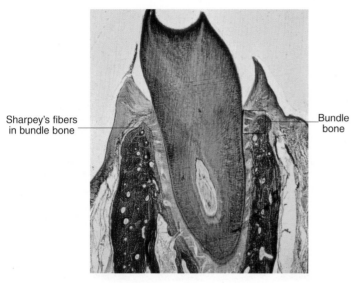

Fig. 13.**5** Alveolar bone proper. Silver stain illustrates the bundle bone. Outlined area is shown in Figure 13.6.

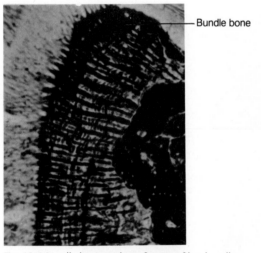

Fig. 13.**6** Bundle bone with perforating fiber bundles.

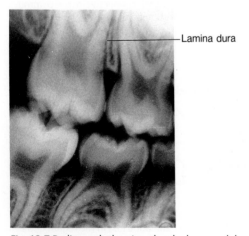

Fig. 13.**7** Radiograph showing alveolar bone and density of lamina dura.

Alveolar Bone Proper

On a histologic basis, there are two types of bone: cancellous (spongy) and compact. Alveolar bone proper is a modification of compact bone, as it contains perforating fibers (Sharpey's) (Fig. 13.**5**). These collagen fibers pierce the alveolar bone proper at right angles or oblique to the surface of the long axis of the tooth. This is the means of attachment for the periodontal ligament to the tooth. The fiber bundles originating from bone are much larger than the fiber bundles inserting in cementum. Perforating fibers occur elsewhere in the skeleton, wherever ligaments and tendons insert. Purely elastic perforating fibers are also found, but not in alveolar bone proper. Because the bone of the alveolar process is regularly penetrated by collagen bundles, it has been appropriately named *bundle bone* or alveolar bone proper (Figs. 13.**5** and 13.**6**) When this bone is viewed radiographically, it is referred to as the *lamina dura* (Fig. 13.**7**). The lamina dura appears more dense than the adjacent supporting bone, but this radiographic density may be due to the mineral orientation around the fiber bundles and the apparent lack of nutrient canals. Actually, there may be no difference in mineral content between the lamina dura and the supporting bone. The lamina dura is evaluated clinically for periapical or periodontal pathology.

Tension created by occlusal forces is believed to be important in the maintenance of this bone. In physiologic movement of teeth, this bone is readily resorbed in zones of compression and readily formed in zones of tension. Not all alveolar bone proper appears as bundle bone. At times, there are no apparent perforating fibers in the socket-lining bone (Fig. 13.**8**). Supporting bone constantly undergoes modification in adapting to minor tooth movements, and therefore fibers may be lost or replaced from time to time in some areas of root.

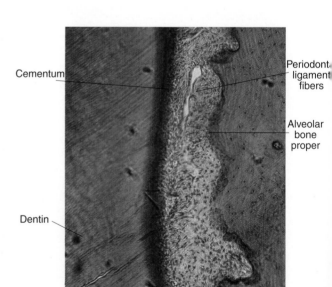

Fig. 13.**8** Organizing periodontal ligament.

Aging of Alveolar Bone

A comparison of young and old alveolar bone reveals a shift with age from alveolar processes with smoothly lined sockets, and active bone formation with numerous viable cells, to alveolar sockets that appear jagged and uneven. Marrow appears to have a fatty infiltration, and osteoporosis indicates loss of some bony elements (Fig. 13.**15**).

Edentulous Jaws

The changes in the jaws resulting from tissue loading, compression, tissue conditioning, and denture retention coupled with the aging processes have not been clearly elucidated. It is apparent, however, that with age the alveolar process in edentulous jaws decreases in size (Fig. 13.**16**); loss of maxillary bone is accompanied by an increase in the size of the maxillary sinus. The internal trabecular arrangement is more open, which indicates bone loss. From a common radiographic viewpoint, the location of various structures such as glands, fatty zones, muscle masses, and blood vessels varies little in the edentulous jaws.

Cementum

Cementum is the calcified tissue covering the roots of teeth (Fig. 13.**17**). It appears to be similar to bone and generally is of ectomesenchymal origin, although recent evidence indicates that the initial layer on the root surface is of epithelial cell origin. Cementum contains less mineral than bone or dentin, as is seen in Table 13.**1**. Its histologic appearance is similar to bone in that it contains cells within lacunae and exhibits incremental dep-

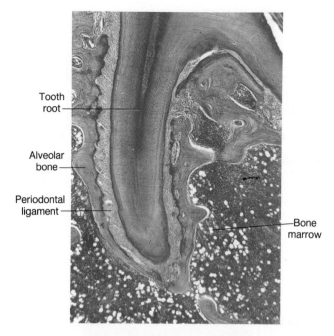

Fig. 13.**15** Aging alveolar bone illustrating scalloping of the alveolar bone proper.

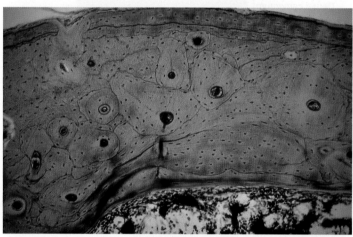

Fig. 13.**16** Edentulous jaw with loss of alveolar process. Remaining compact basal bone is seen.

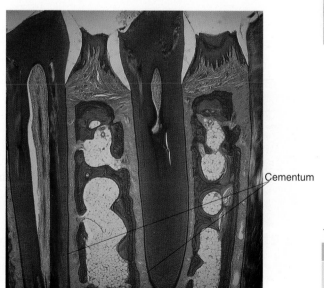

Fig. 13.**17** Relation of root to periodontium. Observe cementum on the apex (right).

Table. 13.**1** Comparison of composition of hard tissues

	Cementum (%)	Bone (%)	Dentin (%)
Organic	50-55	30-35	30
Mineral	45-50	60-65	65.5

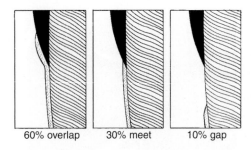

Fig. 13.**18** Relation of cementum to enamel at the cementoenamel junction.

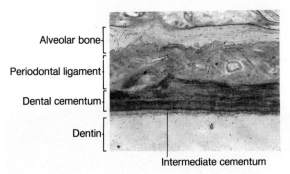

Fig. 13.**19** Histology of cementum on the root surface.

osition lines. Unlike bone, cementum contains no Haversion canals and has neither blood vessels nor nerves in the matrix. Cementum is thinnest (20 to 50 µm) at the cementoenemel junction and gradually increases in thickness (150 to 200 µm) toward the root tip, where it surrounds the apical foramen. Generally, cementum is limited to the root surface, although in 60% of teeth it overlaps enamel for a short distance. In 30% of teeth, cementum meets enamel at a sharp point; and in 10% there is a short gap between the two (Fig. 13.**18**).

Intermediate Cementum

Recent investigations have confirmed an intermediate layer of cementum on the surface of the roots, situated between the granular layer of Tomes and the "dental cementum." This thin layer appears nearly identical to aprismatic enamel, that product of ameloblasts which is 10 µm thick and covers the mantle dentin in the crowns of the teeth. It is best described as an amorphous layer of noncollagenous material containing no odontoblast processes or cementocytes. Because of the close similarity of this layer to the epithelial cell-originated aprismatic enamel, it has been suggested that intermediate cementum (Fig. 13.**19**) is formed by cells of the epithelial root sheath. If this process is accurate, deposition of this layer on the surface of the newly formed root dentin occurs shortly before these cells detach from the root surface and migrate into the periodontal ligament. The layer then mineralizes to an extent greater than that of either the adjacent dentin or the dental cementum. Intermediate cementum probably functions to seal the surface of the sensitive root dentin.

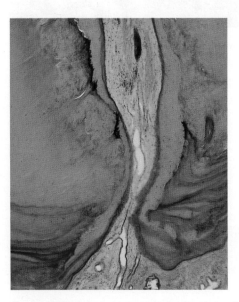

Fig. 13.**20** Thick cementum on root apices in an elderly person.

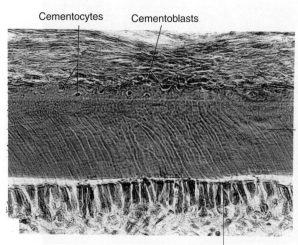

Fig. 13.**21** Early cementum deposited on root dentin.

Cellular and Acellular Cementum

The initial layer of cementum deposited on the intermediate cementum is acellular. It is a thin layer, and subsequent increments usually alternate, with some containing cells and others not (Figs. 13.**21** and 13.**22**). As a general rule, the thicker the cementum, the more lacunae are present. This rule is proven by the thick cementum at the root apex being highly cellular (Fig. 13.**20**). (Development of cementum is described in Chapter 6.) Cementum is incrementally deposited, with a new layer of cementoid being deposited as the preceding layer is calcified. Along the surface of the cementoid, numerous cementoblasts are observed (Fig. 13.**21**). The cementocytes found in the interior of the matrix appear polygonal (Fig. 13.**24**). As the cementoid calcifies, cementoblasts are incorporated into the cementum; these cells become cementocytes and are found in the lacunae. Near the surface they develop long processes that lie in canaliculi radiating from the cell body (Fig. 13.**23**). Their processes contact neighboring cell processes and may exhibit intercellular couplings by means of gap junctional complexes.

In contrast, cementocytes in the deeper layers of cementum display few organelles and are in stages of degeneration (Fig. 13.**24**). The deepest layers of cementum may contain empty lacunae. Both cellular and acellular cementum are laid down incrementally, with these lines being more highly mineralized than those in adjacent cementum. Incremental lines are best seen in decalcified sections (Fig. 13.**25**).

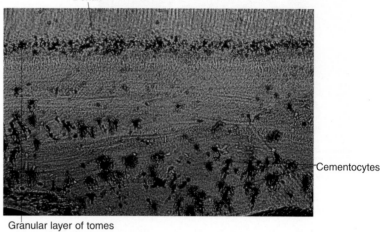

Fig. 13.**22** Histology of the granular layer of Tomes and lacunae in cementum.

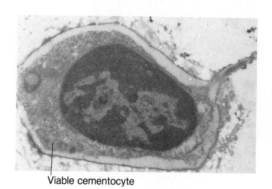

Fig. 13.**23** Ultrastructure of cemetocyte near cementum surface.

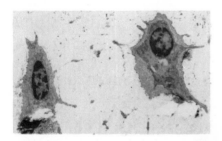

Fig. 13.**24** Ultrastructure of cemtocytes deep in cementum.

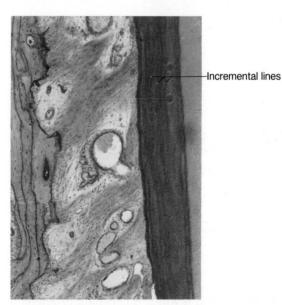

Fig. 13.**25** Principal fibers arising from cementum surface (right) and bone (left). Hematoxylin and eosin staining does not permit observation of penetrating fibers.

Clinical Application

Cementum is painless to scale and will repair itself by further deposition. Unlike bone, it is devoid of nerves, but like bone, it is a living tissue containing cells. Cementum serves to seal the ends of the dental tubules to prevent ingress of periodontally originated infections to the pulp.

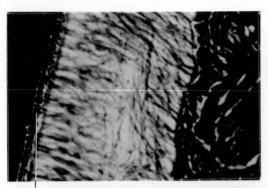

Periodontal ligament fibers penetrating cementum

Fig. 13.**26** Principal fibers arising from cementum and bone stained with silver to illustrate penetrating fibers.

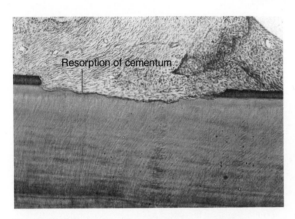

Resorption of cementum

Fig. 13.**27** Cemental loss by resorption.

Cementum Surface Characteristics

Cementum attaches the periodontal ligament fibers to the tooth. Its surface thus has the appearance of numerous fiber bundles. (Figs. 13.**25** and 13.**26**). Basally, fiber bundles appear over the entire surface of the root, although some zones of cementum appear less active than others in fiber attachment. Some fiber bundles penetrate deeply, through a number of increments of cementum, whereas others are embedded more superficially. In general, the thinner the cementum, the more superficially the fibers penetrate the matrix. Perforating fiber bundles are smaller in cementum than in bone.

One characteristic of cementum is its resistance to resorption. This is clinically significant, as it allows orthodontic tooth movement with resultant remodeling of alveolar bone. Some investigators claim to have isolated an autoinvasive factor in cementum that may contribute to this resistance.

The surface of cementum may reveal resorptive zones (Fig. 13.**27**). In some of these areas, cementum repair occurs and is an important feature of cementum. At the front, where resorption has ceased and repair by cementum has occurred, a *reversal line* is seen (Fig. 13.**28**). This line is so named because this is where the resorptive process has reversed. Periodontal fiber bundles attach to the newly formed cementum. One example of such an occurrence is an exfoliating tooth where, during root resorption, partial repair takes place. Because root loss is the eventual goal of physiologic resorption, repair may provide some support to the tooth until the advancing exfoliation is complete (Fig. 13.**29**).

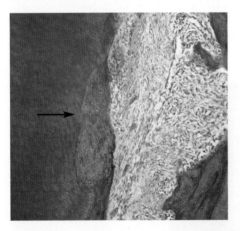

Fig. 13.**28** Reversal line in cementum (arrow): A healed root surface at an early stage.

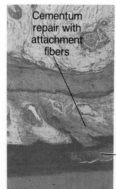

Cementum repair with attachment fibers

Resorption site

Fig. 13.**29** Cemental repair and fiber attachment. A healed root surface at a later stage.

_____ **Clinical Application** _____

Aging changes in the periodontium should be monitored. Changes in color, form, and density are signs of change. Gingival recession is seen along with changes in contour and stippling of the gingiva; this is why it is important to determine the normal appearance of the surface and its underlying structures.

Aging of Cementum

With aging, the surface of cementum becomes more irregular (Fig. 13.**30**). Generally, greater amounts of cementum may appear in the apical zone. An older root surface is less highly populated with fiber bundles than a younger root surface. Seen microscopically, only the surface layer of cementocytes appears viable. All other lacunae appear empty.

Cementicles

Cementicles are calcified bodies appearing on or in the cementum and in the periodontal ligament. They usually are ovoid or round with a similar appearance to the denticles, and they are classified as *free*, *attached*, or *embedded* (Figs. 13.**31** and 13.**32**). Cementicles are a response to either local trauma or hyperactivity and appear in increasing numbers in the aging person.

Periodontal Ligament

The periodontal ligament is the connective tissue located between the cementum and the alveolar bone proper (Fig.13.**33**). Its functions are formative, supportive, protective, sensory, and nutritive. This ligament serves as a periosteum to the alveolar bone proper and as a pericementum to the cementum. The periodontium is also an extension of the gingival connective tissues. The periodontal ligament is fairly consistent in thickness, although it ranges from 0.15 to 0.38 mm. This thickness characteristically decreases slightly with age, measuring 0.21 mm in the young adult (11 to 16 years of age), 0.18 mm in the mature adult (32 to 52 years of age) and 0.15 mm in the older adult (51 to 67 years of age). The thinnest part of the ligament is located in the midroot zone. The periodontal ligament is composed of collagen

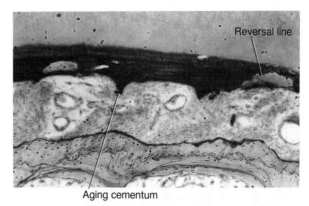

Fig. 13.**30** Aging cementum showing projection of spikes into ligament. Note the reversal lines (upper right).

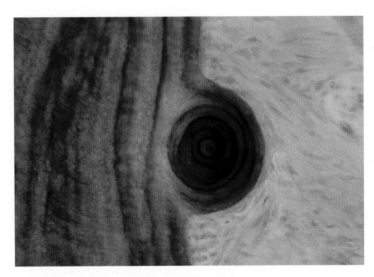

Fig. 13.**31** Attached cementicles on surface of cementum.

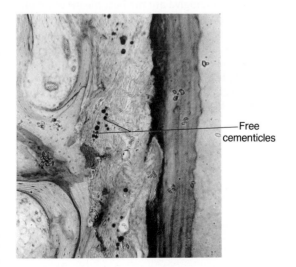

Fig. 13.**32** Appearance of free cementicles in the periodontal ligament.

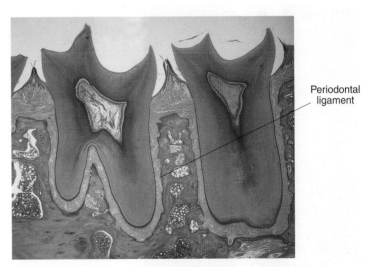

Fig. 13.**33** Histology of periodontium. Note the constant thickness of the periodontal ligament.

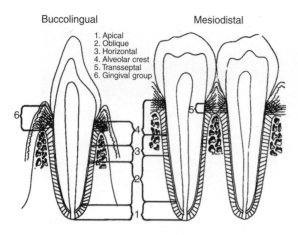

Buccolingual   Mesiodistal

1. Apical
2. Oblique
3. Horizontal
4. Alveolar crest
5. Transseptal
6. Gingival group

Fig. 13.**34** Principal fibers of the periodontal ligament.

fiber bundles connecting cementum and alveolar bone proper—hence the name ligament. This ligament is highly cellular and contains a rich nerve and blood supply. The terms "periodontal ligament" and "periodontal membrane" are used interchangeably, although the former term more aptly describes this tissue.

Principal Fibers

The fiber bundles that exit the cementum and alveolar bone proper to form the periodontal ligament are termed *principal fibers*. Groups of these fibers are named according to their location with respect to the tooth (Fig. 13.**34**). The *apical* fiber group is located at the *apical* area of the root and the *oblique* fibers immediately above. The *horizontal* fibers appear in midroot, and the *alveolar crest* fibers are situated in the cervical region. The gingival group contains *circumferential, transseptal, free,* and *attached gingival fibers,* which are described below. Table 13.**2** lists the function and the site of attachment for each of the principal fiber groups.

Table. 13.**2** Principal fibers

	Location of attachment	Function
Dentoalveolar fiber group		
Apical	Apex of root to fundic proper	Resist vertical force
Oblique	Apical one third of root to adjacent alveolar bone proper	Resist vertical and intrusive force
Horizontal	Midroot to adjacent alveolar bone proper	Resist horizontal and tipping force
Alveolar crest	Cervical root to alveolar crest of alveolar bone proper	Resist vertical and intrusive force
Interradicular	Between roots to alveolar bone proper	Resist vertical and lateral movement
Gingival fiber group		
Transseptal	Cervical tooth to tooth; mesial or distal to it	Resist tooth separation; mesial distal
Attached gingival	Cervical tooth to attached gingiva	Resist gingival displacement
Free gingival	Cervical tooth to free gingiva	Resist gingival displacement
Circumferential	Continuous around neck of tooth	Resist gingival displacement

Gingival Group

Histologic identification of these fiber groups is not difficult. Although the groups appear similar, their origin and location in the gingiva are the best means of identification. In the gingiva, the transseptal fibers extend to adjacent teeth on their mesial and distal surfaces (Fig. 13.**35**). The free and attached gingival fibers arise from the cervical cementum and end freely in the lamina propria of the gingiva. The circumferential fibers circle the necks of the teeth and appear as dots in a longitudinal section (Fig. 13.**35**).

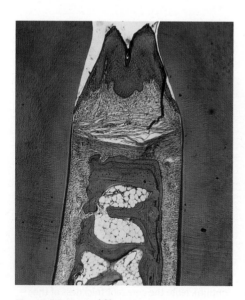

Fig. 13.**35** Gingival fiber group.

Dentoalveolar Group

The dentoalveolar group consists of *alveolar crest* fibers extending from the crest to the gingiva (Fig. 13.**35**), with *horizontal* fibers extending in a horizontal direction to the midroot alveolar bone proper (Fig. 13.**36**). *Oblique* fibers traverse above the apex and extend upward from the tooth to the bone (Fig. 13.**37**); apical fibers extend perpendicularly from the surface of the root to the fundic bone (Fig. 13.**37**); and *interradicular* fibers extend perpendicularly from the root surface to the interradicular alveolar bone proper in multi-rooted teeth (Fig. 13.**38**). In Figures 13.**35** to 13.**38**, the fiber bundles were prepared with silver stain to enhance viewing.

Vascular and Neural Supply

The principal fibers shown in Figures 13.**35** to 13.**38** were enhanced for viewing because of the spaces between fiber bundles termed *interstitial spaces*, which contain blood vessels, lymph channels, and myelinated and non-myelinated nerves. With these structures, the periodontal ligament maintains the vitality of the periodontium. The blood vessels and nerves encircle the tooth and connect with others that extend vertically from the tooth apex to the gingiva. The organization of these vessels can be seen in a cleared specimen after India-ink injection (Fig. 13.**39**). On the left side in Figure 13.**39** are vessels entering the ligament from the alveolar bone. Through the center a vascular plexus runs longitudinally in the ligament. On the right, this plexus is a clear zone, which is dentin. Further right are the blood vessels in the pulp.

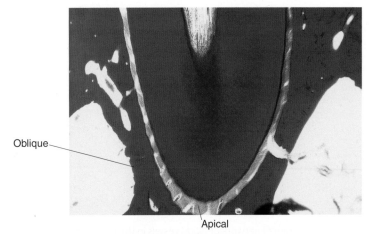

Fig. 13.**37** Oblique and apical fiber group in ligament.

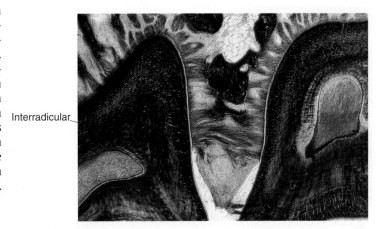

Fig. 13.**38** Interradicular fiber group of the periodontal ligament.

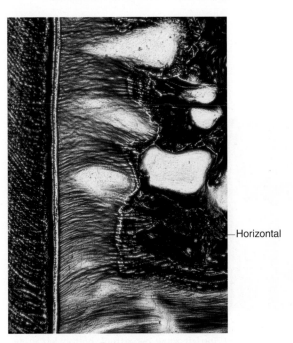

Fig. 13.**36** Horizontal fiber group in ligament.

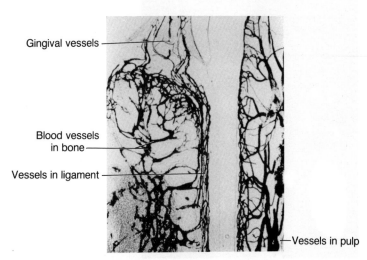

Fig. 13.**39** Cleared tooth and bone; blood vessels injected with India ink. Observe loops progressing from the bone into the periodontium and in the tooth pulp (right).

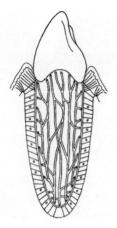

Fig. 13.**40** Diagram of network of blood vessels in the periodontium. Dots indicate the position between fiber bundles.

Figure 13.**40** shows how the circular and longitudinal vessels of the ligament provide a network functioning in nutrition and "dampening" the change in the shape of the ligament that occurs when the teeth are occluded. In Figure 13.**41**, the interconnecting channels in the ligament are seen in a section longitudinal to the root surface. When a cross section of a tooth is viewed, the regularity of the longitudinal vessels can be seen (Fig. 13.**42**). A longitudinal section through the periodontium illustrates the communicating branches of the longitudinal plexus (Fig. 13.**43**).

Nerve trunks also travel in the interstitial spaces. The larger trunks traverse the ligament in the central zone, as is seen in a longitudinal view of the ligament in Figure 13.**44**. Higher magnification of this section reveals sever-

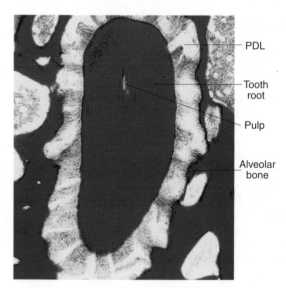

Fig. 13.**42** Histology of cross section of the root, with interstitial spaces between fiber bundles shown. PDL: peridontal ligament.

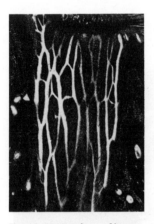

Fig. 13.**41** Histology of ligament in longitudinal section illustrating vascular and neural pathways.

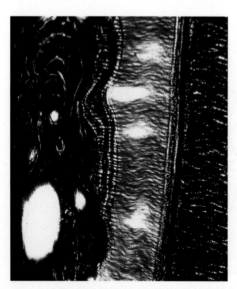

Fig. 13.**43** Histology of longitudinal section of the periodontal ligament, with spaces shown.

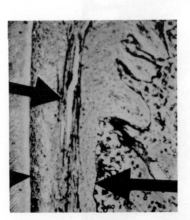

Fig. 13.**44** Longitudinal section of the nerve trunk in the periodontal ligament. Top left arrow, nerve trunk; bottom left arrow, surface of root; bottom right arrow, surface of alveolar bone.

al arteries and veins, as well as a nerve entering an interstitial space (Fig. 13.**45**). A clearer picture is seen under the electron microscope (Fig. 13.**46**). A few nerve endings, which appear to be pacinian pressure receptors, may also be viewed (Fig. 13.**47**). In this figure the organized nerve ending is enclosed in a delicate connective-tissue capsule.

Organization of Periodontal Ligament

The principal fibers make up the bulk of the ligament and perform the important function of support. When the ultrastructure of the periodontal ligament is examined, it is found to be a dense, supportive network of collagen fibers. Some investigators believe a secondary network of fine fibers aids in supporting the primary principal fiber system. The supporting fiber system has been termed the *indifferent fiber plexus*. Transmission electron microscopic observations illustrate the presence of fine fibers supporting the principal fiber of the ligament (Fig. 13.**48**). The dense population of principal collagen fibers shows the presence of large numbers of fibroblasts. Throughout the ligament are additional fine fibers, termed *oxytalan fibers*, that appear elastic–like. They appear to be located around vessel walls and generally run parallel to the long axis of the tooth (Fig. 13.**49**).

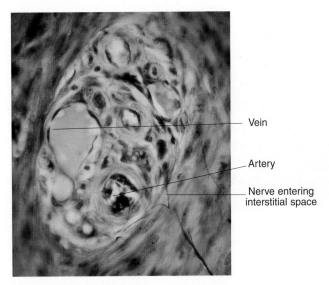

Fig. 13.**45** Interstitial space with vein, artery, and nerve.

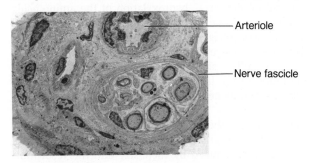

Fig. 13.**46** Ultrastructure of the interstitial space with nerve bundle (lower right) and arterioles (above).

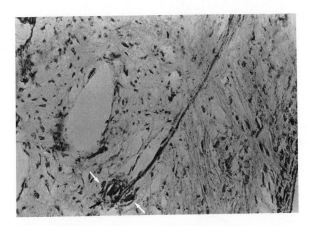

Fig. 13.**47** Nerve and nerve ending (arrows) in the periodontal ligament (silver stain).

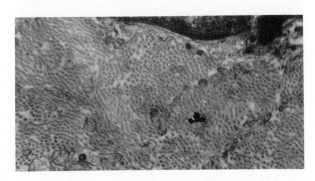

Fig. 13.**48** Electron micrograph of collagen fibers in the ligament.

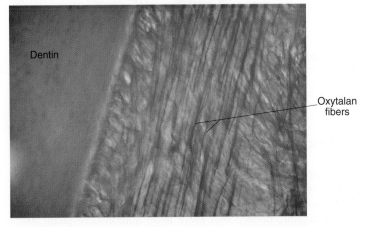

Fig. 13.**49** Histology of oxytalan fibers running longitudinally in the ligament.

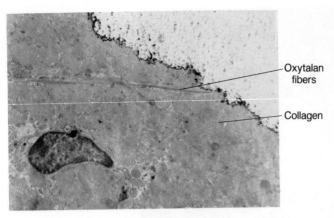

Fig. 13.**50** Ultrastructure of the periodontal ligament, with relation of collagen and oxytalan fibers shown.

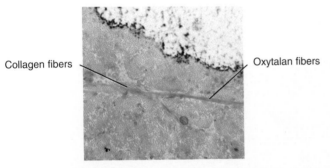

Fig. 13.**51** Ultrastructure of the periodontal ligament, with relation of collagen and oxytalan fibers shown.

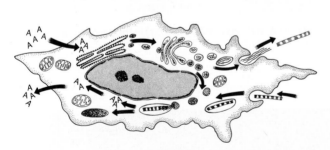

Fig. 13.**52** Diagram of fibroblast/fibroclast and, possibly, functional pathways.

Oxytalan fibers can only be highlighted with special stains (aldehyde fuchsin with preoxidation); around each, there appears to be both a fibrillar and an amorphous zone. These fibers are in parallel arrangement and are about 150 Å in diameter. Although their function is unknown, oxytalan fibers may be part of the support system of the principal fibers. Figures 13.**50** and 13.**51** are electron micrographs of associated oxytalan and collagen fibers.

Ligament Cells

There are numerous cells in the ligament, as in most other tissues of the body. The most important is the fibroblast, because of the high density of collagen composing this tissue. Recent evidence that the ligament collagen "turns over" rapidly has attached further importance to these cells. These cells are believed to function in resorption or destruction of the ligament collagen as well as in its formation. Moreover, there is evidence that a single cell, the fibroblast/fibroclast, can perform both functions (Fig.13.**52**). One end of the cell is active in phagocytizing collagen and contains a lysosomal system; the other end of the same cell is active in assembling the procollagen chains. These will then form the superhelix of the collagen molecule (Fig. 13.**52**). With the aid of vitamin C, hydroxylation of the amino acids proline and lysine occurs. The fibroblasts thus maintain a balance of collagen fibers in the ligament by balancing the rate of collagen formation and destruction.

Other cells in addition to blood vascular elements can be found in the ligament. Osteoblasts may exist along the alveolar bone proper, and cementoblasts may be seen. All may be called osteoclasts (Fig.13.**53**) because they carry out the same function. These large multinucleated cells originate from circulating monocytes and are easily recognized by their size and the resorption lacunae. Cementoclasts, although similar in appearance to osteoclasts, are rare, being seen only during exfoliaton of primary teeth, traumatic occlusion, or, possibly, tooth movement.

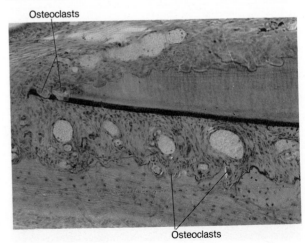

Fig. 13.**53** Periodontal ligament during period of resorption and repair.

Clinical Application

A characteristic of cementum is its resistance to resorption. This is clinically significant as it allows orthodontic tooth movement with resultant remodeling of alveolar bone. Some investigators believe that there is an autoinvasive factor in cementum that contributes to this resistance.

Epithelial Rests

Epithelial rests are a normal constituent of the periodontal ligament throughout life and are discussed in Chapter 6. The epithelial cells that originated from the root sheath may appear as lacy strands, networks, or isolated nests of active or inactive cells. Epithelial cells are described as either proliferating, resting, or degenerating. An example of one of these rests is seen in Figure 13.**54**.

Periodontal Disease

It is currently thought that periodontal disease is a result of periodontic bacteria coupled with specific host inflammatory response. The polymorphic nature of the immune system components may partially explain individual differences in susceptibility to periodontitis and disease progression. Genetic studies have identified alleles that may predispose persons to infectious disease or an unusual disease severity. These results have been found in recent immunogenetic studies of periodontal disease. Effective humeral and cellular responses are considered essential for defense against periodontitis causing bacteria.

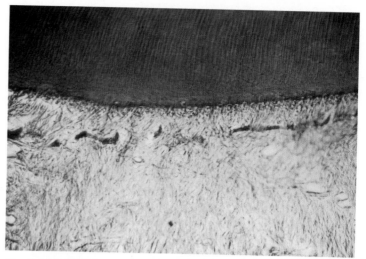

Fig. 13.**54** Epithelial rests in the ligament near the root surface.

Summary

Alveolar process. The alveolar process is the bone in the maxilla and mandible that supports the roots of the teeth. It is composed of the *alveolar bone proper*, which lines the sockets and attaches the ligament fibers to the bone. The remainder of the alveolar process is made up of supporting bone, the compact cortical plate, and the cancellous bone, with the compact cortical plate and the cancellous bone situated between the cortical plate and the alveolar bone proper. The alveolar bone is constantly being modified, but its period of maximal change is during facial growth and tooth growth. The alveolar process is guided in growth by both extrinsic factors generated by the teeth and extrinsic factors generated by growth of the face. Finally, the alveolar process ages, as do other bone in the body, although in some cases tooth loss means bone loss.

Cementum. The calcified tissue covering the roots of the teeth is composed of epithelial root sheath-originated cementum, termed "intermediate cementum." Cementum can also be formed by cementoblasts. The latter is less highly calcified than is bone to dentin. Cementum is thinnest at the cervical region, and thickest at the apical region. Cementoblasts incorporated into the cementum are termed "cementocytes." They appear as lacunae and are similar to bone cells. There are no Haversian systems in cementum, as in bone, because blood and nerves do not enter it. Cementum is resistant to resorption and, if resorbed, is likely to repair and form a reversal line. Cementum has free, attached, and embedded cementicles.

Periodontal ligament. The periodontal ligament is the pliant tissue located between the root surface and the alveolar bone proper. It has a fairly constant thickness. It is composed of five groups of dentoalveolar fibers: apical, oblique, horizontal, alveolar crest, and interradicular. Free and attached gingival, circular, and transseptal fiber bundles comprise the dentogingival group. Each fiber group has a specific function. The periodontal ligament "turns over" collagen rapidly and also has an active population of fibroblasts that both form and destroy collagen. The periodontal ligament is highly vascularized by vessels in the interstitial spaces. Nerves transmit through these spaces, and several types of terminals respond to touch, pain, and the pressures of mastication. Fine fibers aid in the support of the ligament, and some of these are termed *oxytalan* fibers. They transverse the ligament in the long axis of the teeth.

Self-Evaluation Review

1. The cortical plates of the maxilla and mandible are classified as what type of bone?

2. What is the function of this bone?

3. Describe the bone that lines the tooth sockets. What is its name?

4. Name five types of cells found in the periodontal ligament, in addition to blood cells.

5. Name five functions of the periodontal ligament, in order of importance.

6. What forces would the transseptal, free gingival, and the circular fiber groups resist?

7. What types of organized nerve endings have been found in the periodontal ligament? What is their function?

8. Describe the function of the attachment fibers in the periodontal ligament.

9. What is the name and function of the periodontal fibers found between the tooth roots?

10. What is the function of the oxytalan fibers in the periodontium?

11. Compare the appearance of a "healing" and "healed" root surface.

Suggested Readings

Alveolar Bone

Ash P, Loutit JF, Townsend KMS. Osteoclasts derived from hematopoetic stem cells. Nature. 1980;293:669.

Bonucci E. New knowledge on the origin, function, and fate of osteoclasts. Clin. Orthop. 1982;158:252.

Marks, BI. The microanatomy of the human edentulous maxillae. Aust. Dent. J.1978;23:69.

Marks SC Jr. The origin of osteoclasts; evidence of clinical applications and investigative challenges of an extraskeletal source. J. Oral Pathol. 1983;12:226.

Quelch KJ, Medlik RA, Bingham PJ, Mecuri SM. Chemical composition of human bone. Arch. Oral Biol. 1983;28:665.

Severson JA, Moffett BC, Kokich V, Selipsky H. A histologic study of age changes in the human periodontal joint (ligament). J. Periodontol. 1978;49:189.

Ten Cate AR, Mills C. The development of the periodontium: the origin of alveolar bone. Anat. Rec. 1972;173:369.

Cementum

Boyd A, Jones SJ. Scanning electron microscopy of cementum and Sharpey's fiber bone. Z. Zellforsch. 1968;92:536.

Bravman D, Eberhardt D, Stohl S. Antigens found in cementum exposed to periodontal disease. J. Periodontol. 1979;50:656.

Furseth R. The fine structure of the cellular cementum of young human teeth. Arch. Oral Biol. 1969;14:1147.

Furseth R, Johansen E. The mineral phase of sound and carious human dental cementum studied by electon microscopy. Acta. Odontol. Scand. 1970;28:305.

Held AJ. Cementogenesis and the normal and pathologic structure of cementum. Oral Surg. Oral Med. Oral Pathol. 1951;4:53.

Jande SS, Belanger LF. Fine structural study of rat molar cementum. Anat. Rec. 1970;167:439.

Jones SJ, Boyde A. A study of human root cementum surfaces as prepared for and examined in the scanning electron microscope. Z. Zellforsch. 1972;130:318.

Lisodeskog S, Hammerstrom L. Evidence in human teeth of anti-invasive factor in cementum or perio ligament. Scand. J. Dent. Res. 1980;88:1.

Listgarten MA, Karmin A. The development of a cementum layer over the enamel surface of enamel molars—a light and electron microscopic study. Arch. Oral Biol. 1969;14:961.

Schroeder HE. The gingival tissue. In: Scientific Foundations in Dentistry. Cohen B, Kramer RH, eds. London: Heinemann; 1976;Chap 37.

Schroeder HE. Development and structure of the dental attachment apparatus. Oral Struc. Biol. New York: Thieme Medical Publishers; 1991;187:290.

Selvig KA. An ultrastructural study of cementum formation. Acta. Odontool. Scand. 1964;22:1055.

Periodontal Ligament

Berkowitz BKB, Moxham BJ, Newman HN. The periodontal ligament and physiological tooth movements. In: The Periodontal Ligament in Health and Disease. Berkowitz BKB, Moxham BJ, Newman HN, eds. Tarrytown, NY: Pergamon Press; 1982;215–247.

Bernick S, Levy BM, Dreize S, Grant DA. The intraosseus orientation of the alveolar component of marmoset alveo dental fibers. J. Dent. Res. 1977;56:1409.

Bhaskar SN, ed. Orban's Oral Histology and Embryology. 11th ed. St. Louis, Mo: CV Mosby; 1991.

Cho Mi, Garnat PR. Mannose utilization by fibroblast of the periodontal ligament. J. Periodont. Res. 1987;21:64–72.

Edmunds RS, Simmons TA, Cox CF, Avery JK, Light and ultrastructural relationship between oxytalan fibers in the periodontal ligament of the guinea pig. J. Oral Pathol. 1979;8:109.

Fulmer HM, Lillie RD, The oxytalan fiber: a previously undescribed connective tissue fiber: J. Histochem. Cytochem. 1958;6:426.

Garant PR. Collagen resorption by fibroblasts, a theory of fibroblastic maintenance of periodontal ligament. J. Periodontol. 1976;47:380.

Griffin CJ, Harris R. Unmyelinated nerve endings in the periodontal membrane of human teeth. Arch. Oral Biol. 1968;13:1207.

Kobayashi Tetsuo, Ludo Vander Pol W, HaraKohji, van de Winkle GJ. IgFe receptor polymorphisms: genetic risk factors for periodontal disease in Oral Biology at the Turn of the Century. Zurich: Karger; 1998.

Levy BM, Bernick S. Studies on the biology of the periodontium of marmosets II. Development and organization of the periodontal ligament of deciduous teeth in marmosets. J. Dent. Res. 1978;47:27.

Marchi AH, Bowen WH. Secretory granules in cells producing fibrillar collagen . In: The Biological Mechanisms of Tooth Eruption and Root Resorption. Z Davidovich, ed. Birmingham, Ala: EBSCO Media; 1988;53–59.

Melcher AH, Bowen WH. The Biology of the Periodontium. New York, NY: Academic Press; 1969.

Nakamura,TK, Hanal H, Nakamura MT. Ultrastructure of encapsulated nerve terminals in human periodontal ligaments. Jpn. J. Oral Biol. 1982;24:126.

Ramfjord SP, Ash MM. Periodontology and Periodontics. Philadelphia, Pa: WB Saunders; 1979.

Simmons TA, Avery JK. Electron dense staining affinities of mouse oxytalan and elastic fibers. J. Oral Pathol. 1980;9:183.

Slavkin HC. Towards a cellular and mollecular under standing of periodontics. J. Periodontol. 1976;47:249.

TenCate AR, Deporter DA. The role of the fibroblast on collagen turnover in the functioning periodontal ligament of the mouse. Arch. Oral Biol. 1974;19:339.

14 Histology of the Oral Mucosa and Tonsils

Donald S. Strachan and James K. Avery

Introduction

The oral mucosa consists of two layers: an epithelium (stratified squamous epithelium) and an underlying layer of connective tissue, which is the lamina propria. Mucosa forms the lining of the oral cavity and shows regional modifications corresponding to functional needs. The keratinized palate and gingiva have a masticatory function. The dorsal (superior) surface of the tongue is specialized with regard to taste and masticatory functions. Numerous taste buds are located in the epithelium of the tongue, which is also keratinized. The remainder of the oral mucosa functions as a lining. The epithelium of the oral cavity is continually being replaced by basal cells that divide, migrate to the surface, and eventually wear off during normal functions of speech and mastication. Beneath select areas of the oral mucosa is a loose connective tissue, the submucosa.

The tonsils are found posterior to the oral and nasal cavities and form a ring of tonsillar tissue in this area. There are three tonsils: palatine, pharyngeal, and lingual. All contain lymphatic tissue and function in the production of lymphocytes, which are important in processing antigens for the production of immunocompetent T-cell and B-cell lymphocytes for the immune system.

Objectives

After reading this chapter you should be able to discuss the following material by: 1) Describing the structure and function of the various types of oral mucosa with a detailed description of the keratinocytes and nonkeratinocytes; 2) Explaining how epithelial cells can be replaced (turnover) and understanding the basic process of keratinization; 3) Identifying and describing the various papillae of the tongue as well as describing the morphology of the three types of tonsils and discussing their functions.

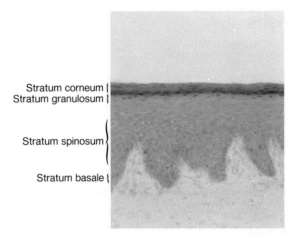

Fig. 14.**1** Light micrograph of keratinized oral mucosa. The lamina propria is below the stratum basale.

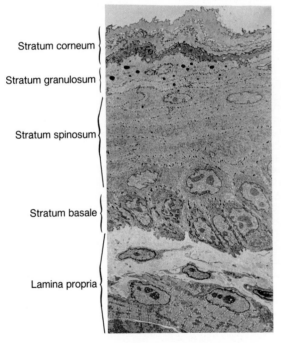

Fig. 14.**2** Electron micrograph of keratinized oral mucosa.

Development and Structure of Oral Epithelium

The epithelium of the oral cavity is derived from the embryonic ectoderm and is stratified squamous throughout. As is true of stratified squamous epithelium elsewhere, the cells vary from cuboidal or low columnar at the connective-tissue interface to flat squamous at the surface. Most of the mucosal surface of the oral cavity is lined by a nonkeratinized, stratified squamous epithelium, except for the gingiva, hard palate, and dorsal surface of the tongue where the epithelium is keratinized. From the underlying connective tissue of the lamina propria to the surface, the four layers in the nonkeratinized epithelium are: the stratum basale (basal layer), stratum spinosum (spinous layer), stratum intermedium (intermediate layer), and stratum superficiale (superficial layer). In keratinized epithelium there are also four layers or strata. The first two layers—the stratum basale and stratum spinosum—are the same as in nonkeratinized epithelium, and the next two layers are the stratum granulosum (granular layer) and stratum corneum (keratinized layer) (Fig. 14.**1**). Four layers of the epithelium can be clearly seen at the ultrastructural level in Figure 14.**2**.

Stratum Basale

The cells of the stratum basale are cuboidal or low columnar and form a single layer resting on the basal lamina at the interface of the epithelium and lamina propria (Figs. 14.**2** and 14.**3**). The epithelia of the oral mucosa are in a constant state of renewal, and the basal cells show the most mitotic activity.

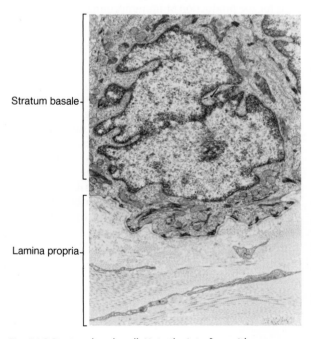

Fig. 14.**3** Stratum basale cell. Note the interface with connective tissue of the lamina propria.

Stratum Spinosum

The stratum spinosum usually is several cells thick, and mitotic figures can occasionally be seen in the layer adjacent to the basal cell layer. The stratum basale and the first layer(s) of the stratum spinosum are sometimes referred to as the stratum germinativum. This zone gives rise to new epithelial cells. The cells of the stratum spinosum are shaped like a polyhedron, with short cytoplasmic processes. At the point where the processes of neighboring cells meet, mechanical adhesions (desmosomes) can be seen coupling the cells (Fig. 14.**4**). Under the light microscope, the normal appearance of these stratum spinosum cells usually is accentuated by shrinkage artifacts produced during routine fixation, staining, and mounting. This has caused some observers to refer to this layer as the prickle cell layer (Fig. 14.**2**). These cells have an abundance of intracytoplasmic fibrils (tonofibrils) that project toward and attach to the desmosomes (Fig. 14.**4**). In the upper layers of the stratum spinosum, the cells contain a unique cytoplasmic inclusion in the form of dense spherical granules (Fig. 14.**5**). Because of the intimate association of these granules with the cell membrane, they are often referred to as membrane-coating granules. These granules fuse with the cytoplasmic membrane of the cell and exteriorize their contents into the intercellular spaces. Morphologic differences have been shown between the membrane-coating granules in keratinized and nonkeratinized epithelium. The precise nature and function of these granules is not yet known.

Stratum Granulosum

The cells of the stratum granulosum are flat and stacked in a layer three to five cells thick. This layer is prominent in keratinized epithelium but deficient or nonexistent in nonkeratinized epithelium. The cells of this layer have many dense, relatively large (0.5 to 1 µm) keratohyaline granules in their cytoplasm. Many microfilaments are closely associated with these granules (Fig. 14.**5**). Viewed under the light microscope the granules are basophilic (blue with a hematoxylin stain), and viewed under the electron microscope they are dense (appearing black). They are closely associated with ribosomes. There are many microfilaments throughout the cells of this layer. The keratohyaline granules help to form the matrix for the numerous keratin fibers found in the superficial layers. Recently, many studies have shown great heterogeneity in the types of cytokeratins synthesized in the oral epithelium of various locations. Variations in the cytokeratin patterns have been shown in pathologically changed oral mucosa. Some 27 cytokeratins have been identified.

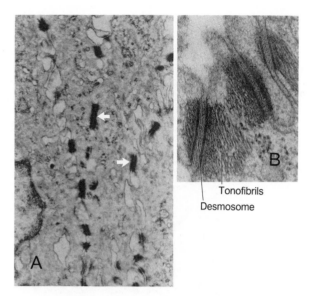

Fig. 14.**4 A** Cell-to-cell junctions between epithelial cells. These are termed desmosomes (arrows). **B** Desmosomes under high magnification. These are adhesion discs between plasma membranes. Desmosomes are anchored by tonofilaments located in the cell.

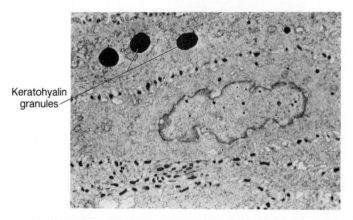

Fig. 14.**5** Ultrastructure of stratum granulosum cells with keratohyaline granules.

Clinical Application

For the clinician, astute observation and interpretation of the status of the oral mucosa and tongue have long been known to give a sensitive diagnosis of systemic disease and nutritional deficiencies. The oral mucosa can change according to various factors, including smoking, age, and disease.

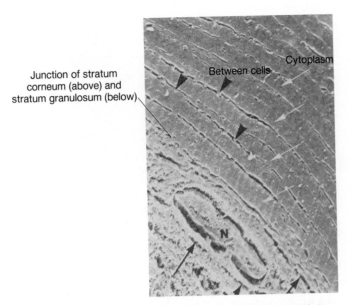

Junction of stratum corneum (above) and stratum granulosum (below)

Between cells

Cytoplasm

N

Fig. 14.**6** Ultrastructure of cells of stratum corneum (black arrows). Spaces between cells (black arrowheads) and cell cytoplasm (white arrows) in cells of the stratum corneum. N: nucleus.

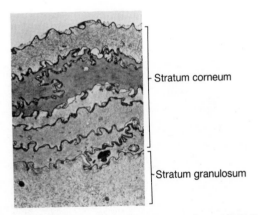

Stratum corneum

Stratum granulosum

Fig. 14.**7** Ultrastructure of the stratum corneum with interdigitation between cells.

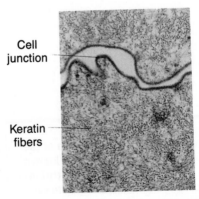

Cell junction

Keratin fibers

Fig. 14.**8** Ultrastructure of the stratum corneum. Note the cell junctions and keratin fibers.

Stratum Corneum

The junction between the nucleated cells in the stratum granulosum and the stratum corneum (superficial layer of keratinized cells) is abrupt, as can be seen in Figure 14.**6**. The cells of the stratum corneum are very flat, devoid of nuclei, and full of keratin filaments surrounded by a matrix. Figure 14.**7** shows the abrupt change between the stratum corneum (only four cell layers thick in this figure) and stratum granulosum. Note the interdigitation between cells in this electron micrograph. Greater magnification of two adjacent cells in the stratum corneum (Fig. 14.**8**) shows the abundance of keratin fibers throughout these cells.

The cells of the stratum corneum are squamous (flat), and superficially have various shapes. These surface cells are continually being sloughed and are replaced by the continual migration of cells from the underlying layers. Figure 14.**9** shows the surface of the stratified squamous epithelium of the hard palate; the boundaries between cells are prominent and the surface of the cells appears pitted.

Turnover of Oral Epithelium

Consistent with the day-to-day function of the oral epithelium and the histologic description presented previously, there is a high turnover rate of the cells of the oral epithelium. The concept of cells undergoing mitosis in the basal cell layer and eventually migrating to the free surface is sometimes difficult to appreciate on a static diagram or histologic slide. The dynamic nature of this epithelium is best appreciated when the cells are labeled experimentally with radioactive thymidine, which "tags" DNA at synthesis. With sampling of tissue at various times, the labeling substance appears first in the basal cell layer and later in the stratum corneum (Fig.

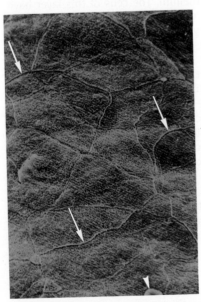

Fig. 14.**9** Scanning electron micrograph of surface view of epithelial cells. Note the cell junctions (arrows).

14.**10**). The technique used to view the labeled DNA is termed radioautography. Different areas of the oral epithelium change at varying rates. Sulcular epithelium takes 10 days to renew, whereas the general oral mucosa takes approximately 12 to 13 days. The basal cells move away from the basal layer perpendicularly and toward the surface of the epithelium.

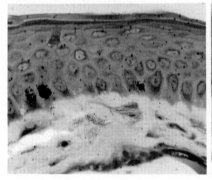 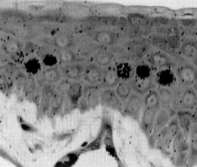 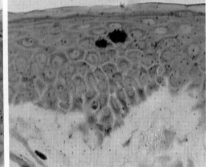

Fig. 14.**10** Turnover of epithelial cells revealed by |3H| thymidine labeling.

Functional Characteristics

The surface of stratified squamous epithelium has various characteristics, depending on the location and functional requirements of the oral mucosa. As the cells migrate from the basal cell layer to the surface layer, differentiation produces a surface layer that is either keratinized, parakeratinized, or nonkeratinized.

Nonkeratinized

In nonkeratinized epithelium, the surface cells retain their nuclei and the cytoplasm does not contain keratin filaments. The stratum corneum and granulosum is absent; this epithelium is composed of four layers (stratum basale, stratum spinosum, stratum intermedium, and stratum superficiale). This type of epithelium is associated with the "lining mucosa" in the oral cavity (Fig. 14.**11**).

Keratinized

As described previously, the keratinized surface results when the cells have lost their nuclei and the cytoplasm has been displaced by large numbers of the keratin filaments. This surface can only be present where there is a well-defined stratum granulosum. The surface of the gingiva and palate is usually of the keratinized type, as it is associated with "masticatory function" (Fig.14.**11**).

Parakeratinized

In parakeratinized epithelium, the surface cells have dark-staining pyknotic nuclei and the cytoplasm contains little if any keratin filaments. The stratum corneum and stratum granulosum are not found in pararkeratinized epithelium. Like nonkeratinized epithelium, the keratinized epithelium is composed of four layers. Usually, this epithelium is associated with the gingiva (Fig. 14.**11**).

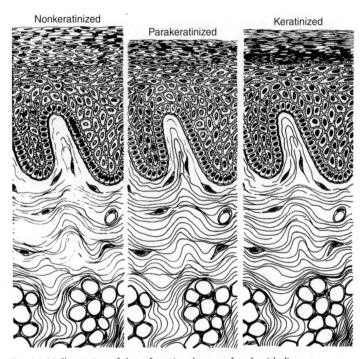

Fig. 14.**11** Illustration of three functional types of oral epithelium.

Clinical Application

Over 7% of the total number of cancers diagnosed in the United States are located in the oral and oropharyngeal areas. Many diseases affect the rate of division of the basal cells and the turnover rate of the epithelium. The process of keratinization can be altered in cancerous and precancerous lesions such as leukoplakia.

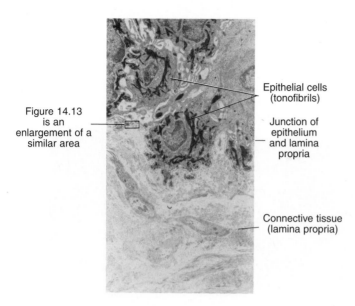

Figure 14.13 is an enlargement of a similar area

Epithelial cells (tonofibrils)

Junction of epithelium and lamina propria

Connective tissue (lamina propria)

Fig. 14.**12** Junction of oral epithelium and connective tissue.

Junction of Epithelium and Connective Tissue

The interface between the lamina propria and the epithelium is an interesting area (Fig. 14.**12**). Connective tissue, with its inductive properties, exerts control over the overlying epithelium. When viewed by light microscopy, the interface tissue termed the basement membrane can be observed. Electron microscopic magnification reveals the basement membrane to be composed of three parts: the lamina lucida, which is less dense and is toward the epithelial side; the lamina densa (basal lamina), the middle of the three parts; and the lamina reticularis, which is less dense than the lamina densa and is located next to the lamina propria. Type IV collagen and laminin, a glycoprotein, are major components of the lamina densa. The lamina reticularis contains fine reticular fibers. Basal cells of the epithelium are not attached to the connective tissue proper, but rather form mechanical adhesions with the basal lamina. These attachments are hemidesmosomes (Fig. 14.**13**). Hemidesmosomes are composed of an attachment plaque that possesses intracellular modifications of tonofilaments. These penetrate the plasma membrane of the cell, terminating in the basal lamina (Figs. 14.**13** and 14.**14**). Fine collagen fibers attach to this lamina on the connective-tissue side (Fig. 14.**14**). These fibers are anchoring fibers, composed of type VII collagen. This complex of fibers is found at intervals along the basal cell plasma membrane of the epithelial–connective-tissue interface.

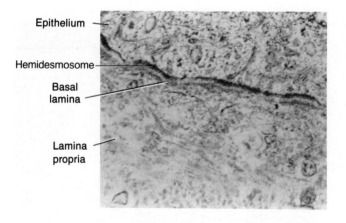

Epithelium

Hemidesmosome

Basal lamina

Lamina propria

Fig. 14.**13** Junction of oral epithelium (above) and connective tissue (below) separated by basal lamina and hemidesmosomes.

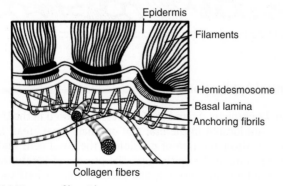

Epidermis

Filaments

Hemidesmosome

Basal lamina

Anchoring fibrils

Collagen fibers

Fig. 14.**14** Diagram of hemidesmosomes.

Clinical Application

Thinning of the epithelium occurs in relation to prosthetic devices covering the surface of the mucosa. Changes in salivary flow—due to age, radiation, or disease—disrupt the normal maturation and differentiation of the epithelial cell layers.

Lamina Propria

The lamina propria is the connective-tissue layer immediately below the epithelium (Fig. 14.**13**), which can be divided into the papillary layer and reticular layer. In the papillary layer, fingerlike projections of connective tissue extend into the deep surface of the epithelium (Fig. 14.**15**). The length of the papillae varies with location and functional requirements. An increase in the number and length of the papillae is seen in areas where mechanical adhesion between the epithelium and lamina propria is required (masticatory mucosa). In areas of lining mucosa, the reticular or subpapillary layer predominates (Fig. 14.**15**). The blood supply consists of a deep plexus of large vessels in the submucosa, which gives rise to a secondary plexus in the papillary layer of the lamina propria. Capillary loops extend into the connective-tissue papillae. The epithelium is avascular; therefore, its metabolic needs must come via the vessels of the lamina propria. The amino acids, peptides, carbohydrates, lipids, inorganic compounds, and salts required for the nutrition of the epithelium diffuse from the capillary beds through the connective tissue and basement membrane to enter the epithelium. In addition to the fibroblasts, cells of blood vessels and lymphatics (endothelial, pericytes, and smooth muscle cells), and of nerves (Schwann cells), many other cells are found in the lamina propria. Some of these cells are normal residents and others are present because of inflammation or trauma. Mast cells, macrophages, fat cells, plasma cells, eosinophils, undifferentiated cells, and other cells can be found in this tissue. Lymphocytes are a common cell found in the lamina propria of the gingiva. Lymphocytes are also often found in the epithelium itself, presumedly in transit to the surface.

Submucosa

In most areas of the mouth the submucosa is absent or limited and serves primarily as an attachment for the lamina propria to the underlying bone or skeletal muscle. Like the lamina propria, the submucosa is a connective-tissue compartment composed of cells and intercellular elements. The submucosa is found in the cheeks, lips, and parts of the palate, and is a less dense component than the lamina propria. It contains numerous large blood vessels, nerves, and lymphatics, and its functions are nutrition and defense. The submucosa is also the site containing adipose tissue and minor salivary glands in the oral cavity (Figs. 14.**16** and 14.**17**). In the bony areas with no submucosa, fibers of the lamina propria attach tightly to bone. The mucosa and lamina propria in these areas is generally referred to as mucoperiosteum.

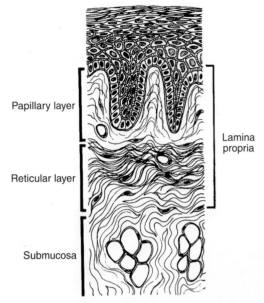

Fig. 14.**15** The lamina propria consists of the papillary layer and reticular layer, below which is the submucosa.

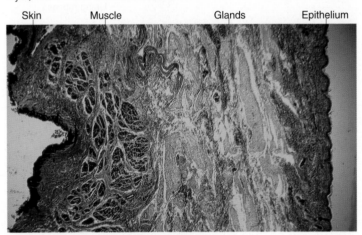

Fig. 14.**16** Full thickness of cheek. Skin is on the left; oral mucosa is on the right.

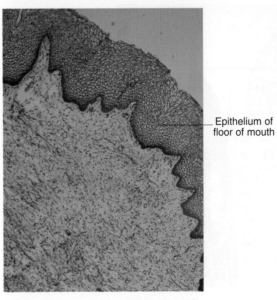

Fig. 14.**17** Lining mucosa of floor of mouth.

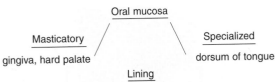

Fig. 14.**18** Classification of oral mucosa.

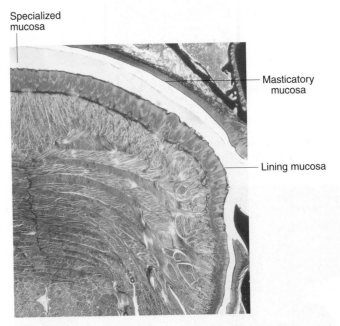

Fig. 14.**19** Cross section of tongue. Note the lining mucosa below and beside the tongue, the specialized mucosa over it, and the masticatory mucosa in the palate.

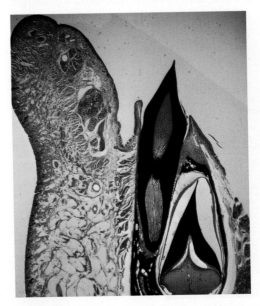

Fig. 14.**20** Lip with skin on outer surface and lining mucosa on inner surface.

Functional Types of Oral Mucosa

The three functional types of oral mucosa are the lining, masticatory, and specialized mucosa. These terms provide functional descriptions of the oral mucosa in specific locations (Fig. 14.**18**). Each type of oral mucosa can be recognized on visual inspection of the oral cavity. In Figure 14.**19**, a cross section through the molar area of the oral cavity, each of the three types of oral mucosa can be observed.

Lining Mucosa

The lining mucosa covers all soft tissue of the oral cavity except the gingiva, hard palate, and dorsal surface of the tongue. The epithelium is nonkeratinized, stratified squamous epithelium, and the lamina propria contains the typical collagenous, elastic, and reticular fibers found in other supporting connective tissues. These collagenous fibers are not as thick and tightly organized as those found in other types of oral mucosa. Lining mucosa is smooth and shiny. Oral epithelium is less pigmented than the epithelium of the skin and varies in color from light pink to darker pink or red. The hues are influenced by the underlying capillary network in relation to the free surface and by the amount of melanin pigment in the epithelial cells. The submucosa associated with most of the lining mucosa is loosely organized and allows for free mobility of the mucosa in relation to the underlying tissue.

Lip. Figure 14.**20** is a microscopic section of the lip in which the following structures can be identified: skin with hair follicles, sweat glands, mucous membrane, skeletal muscle, salivary glands, submucosa, and lamina propria. Near the inner surface of the lips and cheeks are many small salivary glands. Their ducts may be seen clinically by everting the lip and drying the surface. Small droplets of saliva will eventually become visible.

┌─ **Clinical Application** ─

Infections are few after oral surgical procedures and scarring is rare. The healing capacity of the oral mucosa is greater than that of the skin. Orthognathic surgery to move segments of the mandible and maxilla can be performed using an intraoral approach to take advantage of these characteristics.

Vermilion Border. The junction between the skin and mucous membrane is known as the vermilion border, which is apparent where the epithelium changes from the keratinized, stratified squamous epithelium of the oral cavity. The epithelium is thin, especially where the connective-tissue papillae are close to the surface (Fig.14.**21**). The red blood cells in the capillaries show through the thin epithelium, contributing to the vermilion color. Note the ink-injected specimen (Fig. 14.**22**). The thin epithelium in this region contains a protein, eleidin, which is more transparent than the protein keratin. The appearance of the vermilion border is therefore due to several factors: vascularized connective-tissue papillae situated close to the surface; the thin epithelium; and the transparent nature of eleidin in the epithelium, revealing the vermilion color of the red blood cells.

Frequently, ectopic (out of place) sebaceous glands are seen in the vermilion border at the corners of the mouth or, more laterally, in the cheeks opposite the molar teeth. These are termed Fordyce's spots. The presence of sebaceous glands at these sites is considered normal and should not be construed as a pathologic entity (Fig.14.**23**).

Soft Palate. The oral surface of the soft palate is covered by lining mucosa, which is more pink than the hard palate. This results from the highly vascularized lamina propria. A layer of elastic fibers separates the lamina propria from the underlining submucosa, the latter containing both muscles and mucous glands. Above the muscles are mixed glands underlying the respiratory epithelium of the nasal cavity (Fig. 14.**24**).

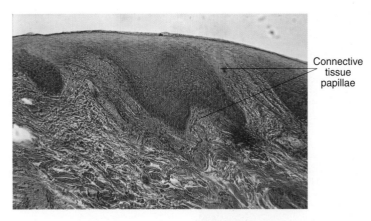

Fig. 14.**21** Vermilion border with its covering of clear eleidin.

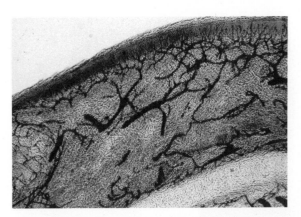

Fig. 14.**22** Blood vessels (injected) in connective-tissue papillae of vermilion border of lip. This illustrates the close relation of the vasculature to the surface of the vermilion border.

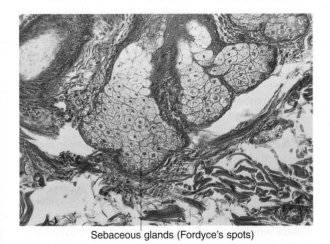

Sebaceous glands (Fordyce's spots)

Fig. 14.**23** Fordyce's spot (sebaceous gland) found at borders of mouth.

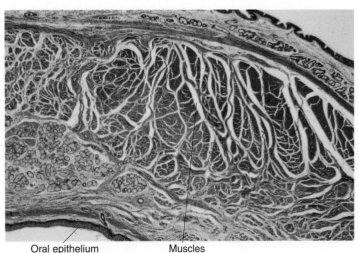

Oral epithelium   Muscles

Fig. 14.**24** Sagittal section of soft palate (anterior on the left). Note the muscle and glands in the submucosa. The respiratory epithelium of the nasal cavity is above.

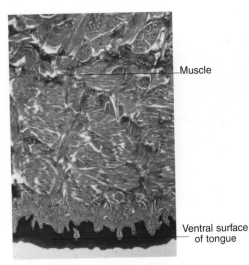

Fig. 14.**25** Muscle in submucosa of ventral surface of tongue.

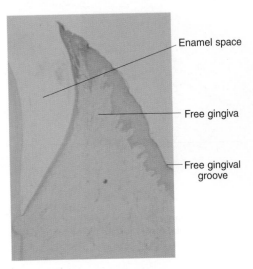

Fig. 14.**26** Boundary of gingiva. The enamel was lost during the decalcification process resulting in the enamel space.

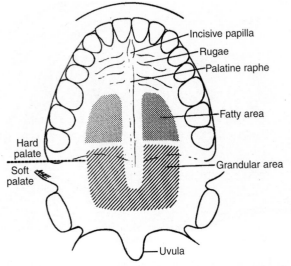

Fig. 14.**27** Diagram of regions of palate. Observe the location of the glandular and fatty zones.

Ventral surface of the tongue. This lining mucosa contains both a lamina propria and submucosa. The mucous membrane is smooth and thin with short but numerous connective-tissue papillae. The submucosa is not clearly distinguishable as it merges with the connective tissue that lies between the muscle bundles of the ventral tongue (Fig. 14.**25**).

Cheek. The lining mucosa of the check is stratified squamous and nonkeratinized epithelium. The underlying submucosa contains fat cells and small, mixed salivary glands intermingled with connective-tissue fibers that bind the mucous membrane to the underlying musculature. The presence of these mixed glands lodged between the muscle bundles in the submucosa is a characteristic of the cheek (Fig. 14.**16**).

Floor of the Mouth. The mucous membrane of the floor of the mouth is thin and loosely attached to the underlying structures. The connective-tissue papillae are short, and there is adipose tissue in the underlying submucosa as well as the sublingual mucous glands (Fig.14.**17**).

Masticatory Mucosa

Masticatory mucosa covers the gingiva and hard palate. In an edentulous mouth, masticatory mucosa covers the chewing surfaces of the dental arches. The epithelium is keratinized or parakeratinized. The connective tissue of the lamina propria contains collagenous fibers that bind the epithelium tightly to the underlying bone and are thicker and more organized than those fibers in the lining mucosa.

Gingiva. The gingiva is more often parakeratinized than keratinized and has no submucosal layer. The attached gingiva is normally stippled. Keratinized epithelium of the gingiva is represented by a thin, dark-stained border that changes at the junction with the nonkeratinized surface of the alveolar mucosa (Fig. 14.**26**). This continues as the lining of the vestibule. In this case, the enamel was lost because of decalcification. The gingiva is discussed in more detail in Chapter 15.

Hard Palate. The oral surface of the hard palate is covered with masticatory mucosa. The epithelium is bound to the underlying bone in anterior regions of the palate by connective tissue. In the anterior lateral regions of the hard palate the submucosa contains fatty tissue. The lateral regions of the posterior parts contain the palatine glands, which extend posteriorly into the soft palate (Fig. 14.**27**). These glands are pure mucous glands containing only mucous acini. The glands associated with the lingual tonsil are the only other pure mucous glands associated with the oral cavity and oropharynx. Although the surface of this mucosa appears to be uniform, it may be subdivided into several zones according to the nature of its submucosa. The midline of the hard palate is termed the median raphe. No submucosa is found in this area, and there is only dense fibrous attachment to the underlying bone (Fig. 14.**28**). This combination of epithelium and lamina propria is given the name mucoperiosteum. In the lateral regions of the palatine mucosa, both fatty and glandular tissue make up the submucosa.

Rugae appear in the anterior region of the hard palate, anterior to the *fatty* zones on either side of the midline. Rugae appear as a series of ridges running across the anterior palate (Fig. 14.**27**). They do not cross the midline but are easily seen and palpated, and can be felt with the tongue. In the midline, the papillae located about 1 cm posterior to the anterior incisors are the incisive papillae.

Three prominent palatine rugae appear in this sagittal section in Figure 14.**29**. Histologically, the palatine rugae are folds of epithelium that contain a dense connective-tissue lamina propria. The connective-tissue fibers pass directly from the papillary layer of the lamina propria into the underlying bone. These are termed traction bands and make the rugae immovable structures.

Figure 14.**29** is a histologic cross section of the palate at low magnification. Note that in the *median raphe* bone underlies the mucosa, so that no submucosa is found. Therefore, the dense lamina propria is directly attached to the underlying bone. This combination of epithelium and lamina propria is termed mucoperiosteum. In the lateral regions of the palatine mucosa, the submucosa comprises both fatty and glandular tissue.

Figure 14.**30** is a view of the lateral region of the palate near the maxillary molar tooth. There is no submucosal layer adjacent to the teeth overlying the alveolar bone, and the fibers of the lamina propria of the palate and gingiva are continuous. Observe the keratinized epithelium of the palate continuous with the gingiva.

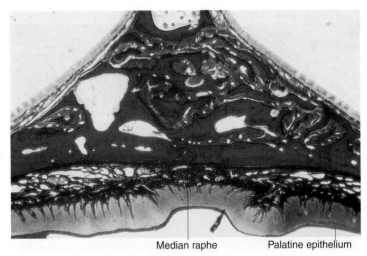

Fig. 14.**28** Median raphe. There is no submucosa along the median raphe.

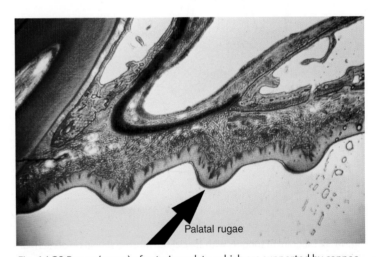

Fig. 14.**29** Rugae (arrow) of anterior palate, which are supported by connective-tissue fibers.

Clinical Application

The integrity of the interface between the oral epithelium and the post that extends from osseointegrated implants will determine the longevity of the implant. Much of the science and therapy of periodontics is focused on the integrity of the interface between the gingiva and the tooth.

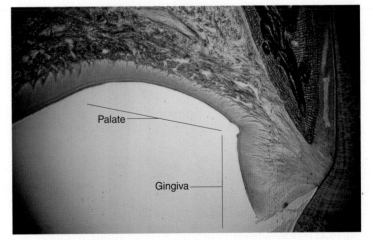

Fig. 14.**30** Lateral hard palate. There is no submucosa adjacent to the teeth.

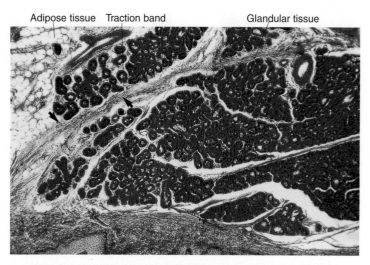

Fig. 14.**31** Hard palate, with junction of fatty zone on left and glandular zones on right. Arrows: traction band.

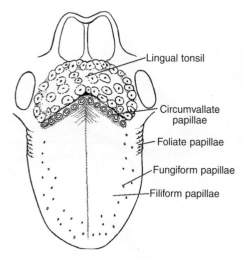

Fig. 14.**32** Diagram of tongue, with specialized mucosa shown on dorsum of tongue.

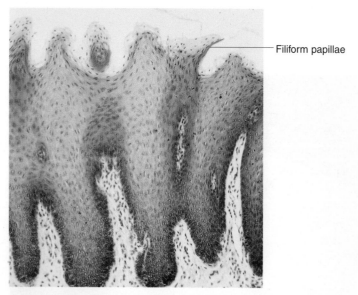

Fig. 14.**33** Light transmission micrograph of filiform papillae, which are pointed keratinized projections on the surface of the tongue.

Figure 14.**31** is a histologic section in the sagittal plane of the junction of the anterior fatty and posterior glandular zones of the hard palate. The anterior adipose tissue is on the left. Observe the lobules of dark-stained mucous cells on the right. Note the collagen bundles extending through the submucosa to the periosteum above; these are termed traction bands. They firmly attach the oral mucosa to the underlying bone. The arrows in Figure 14.**31** point to a traction band. The adipose tissue and glands are within the submucosa; the dark-staining lamina propia and epithelium are seen at the bottom of the picture.

Specialized Mucosa of the Tongue

Specialized mucosa covers the dorsum (superior surface) of the body or papillary portion of the tongue (Fig. 14.**32**). Epithelium on the anterior portion of the tongue is modified, keratinized, stratified epithelium covered with papillae. The great majority of papillae are the pointed filiform papillae, keratinized extensions of the epithelial cells. Occasional fungiform papillae are seen among the numerous *filiform papillae*, normally covered with a nonkeratiniazed epithelium. The connective tissue under the epithelium binds this mucosa to the underlying skeletal muscle of the tongue. At the posterior limit of the body of the tongue is a row of rounded papillae, the circumvallate papillae, and along the sides of the tongue are rows of foliate papillae (Fig. 14.**32**). Beneath the specialized epithelial layer of the tongue body is a layer of connective tissue, the lamina propria. Connective-tissue fibers of the lamina propria extend from the mucosa to deep within and between the muscle bundles of the tongue.

Filiform papillae. Filiform papillae, the most numerous papillae of the tongue, are pointed keratinized projections formed by overlapping sheets of the surface epithelial cells. Figure 14.**33** is a light transmission micrograph, and Figure 14.**34** is a scanning electron micrograph of these papillae. The papillae project toward the oropharynx. They are not associated with taste buds, are easily seen without magnification, and contribute to the rough surface of the tongue.

Fungiform papillae. Fungiform papillae can also be seen with the naked eye. There are fewer fungiform than filiform papillae, and the fungiform papillae are scattered over the surface of the tongue. They are rounded elevations above the surface of the tongue, about 2 mm in diameter and with a smooth surface. They contain taste buds on their superior surfaces. Their surface is not keratinized. Figure 14.**35** shows a light transmission micograph and Figure 14.**36** a scanning electron micrograph of a fungiform papilla situated on the surface of the tongue.

Circumvallate papillae. The circumvallate papillae are located at the junction of the anterior two-thirds and posterior one-third of the tongue (see Fig. 14.**32**). There are eight to twelve in number and are located at the junction of the base and body of the tongue. They are larger than the fungiform papillae and do not project above the surface of the tongue (Fig. 14.**37**). Taste buds line the lateral walls of the papillae. Ducts of the underlying serous glands open into the trenches surrounding the papillae, and their function is to flush out these areas to allow renewal of taste.

Foliate papillae. The foliate papillae are located in furrows along the posterior sides of the tongue (Fig. 14.**32**). Although they are not as prominent in the human tongue as in lower animals, the four to eleven vertical furrows containing the foliate papillae may be lined with taste buds.

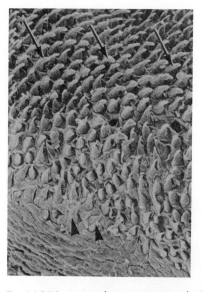

Fig. 14.**34** Scanning electron micrograph of filiform papillae (arrows and arrowheads).

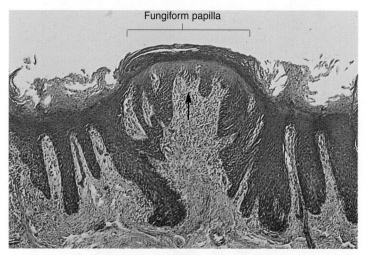

Fig. 14.**35** Light transmission micrograph of fungiform papilla. Taste buds are located in the oral surface of the papilla (arrow).

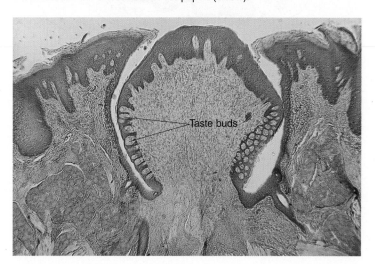

Fig. 14.**37** Circumvallate papillae with numerous taste buds in trench on wall of papilla.

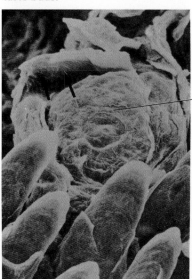

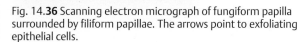

Fig. 14.**36** Scanning electron micrograph of fungiform papilla surrounded by filiform papillae. The arrows point to exfoliating epithelial cells.

Intraepithelial Nonkeratinocytes

The epithelium of the oral mucosa contains several types of nonkeratinocytes. In contrast to keratinocytes, nonkeratinocytes, when viewed in the light microscope, have a clear halo around their nuclei and are therefore termed clear cells. These cells comprise four different types: Langerhans' cells, Merkel cells, melanocytes (pigment-producing cells), and lymphocytes (Figs. 14.**38**–14.**41**). These cells possess none of the characteristic features of epithelial cells, except for the Merkel cells, which are joined to neighboring keratinocytes by desmosomes.

Lagerhans' Cells

Lagerhans' cells were first described over a century ago. They are related to similar cells found in the spleen, lymph nodes, and thymus, and also to the cells of the epidermis. These cells have long, thin extensions of the cytoplasmic membrane, called dendrites. Langerhans' cells are found in the stratum spinosum and, occasionally, in the stratum basale (Fig. 14.**38**). They can be distinguished from keratinocytes by the absence of desmosomes and tonofilaments, and from melanocytes by the absence of premelanosomes (Figs. 14.**38A–C**). The cells contain a unique organelle, the rod-shaped or racquet-shaped Birbeck granule, which allows for positive identification at the ultrastructural level (Fig. 14.**38A**). Langerhans' cells are antigen-presenting cells. They engulf antigens from the external environment, and the intracellualr lysosomes split the antigens into peptide components. These fragments are then transferred to T-lymphocytes, which are important cells in the immune system.

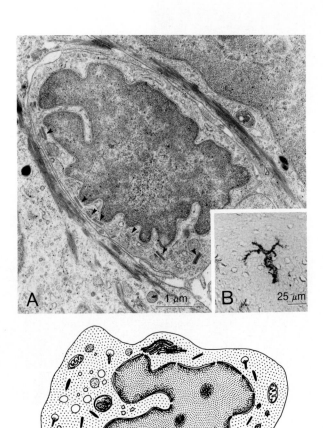

Fig. 14.**38 A** Ultrastructure of Langerhans' cell. Note the convoluted nucleus and lack of desmosomes. **B** Light micrograph of Langerhans' cell. Observe the dendritic nature of the cell. **C** Diagram of Langerhans' cell. Note the rod-like Langerhans' granules.

Merkel's Cells

Merkel's cells are situated in the basal layer of the gingival epithelium (Fig. 14.**39**), and possess occasional desmosomes and tonofilaments, which suggest that they may be of epithelial origin. They are usually associated with an axon terminal, and contain round, electron-dense granules polarized in the cytoplasm between the nucleus and associated axon (Fig. 14.**40**). The Merkel's cell and associated axon terminal form a complex that serves as a *touch receptor*. Merkel's cells are usually found in groups or clusters.

Melanocytes

Melanocytes are melanin-producing cells located in the basal layer of the gingival epithelium. These cells arise from the neural crest, and unlike their neighboring keratinocytes, lack tonofibrils, desmosomes, and hemidesmosomes (Fig. 14.**41**). Although these cells are highly dendritic in nature, this feature is rarely apparent in thin histologic sections. The most characteristic feature of the melanocyte is the melanosome granule found within the cytoplasm (Fig. 14.**41**). Melanosomes are also found in the cytoplasm of keratinocytes. It is thought that the melanocytes inject melanosomes into keratinocytes. A more heavily pigmented gingiva is due to the production of melanin and its subsequent uptake by the epithelial cells. There is great variability in the location and distribution of melanin in the oral cavity.

Lymphocytes

Lymphocytes are found in all epithelia associated with the oral cavity, nasal cavity, and digestive tract. They are more numerous in gingival epithelium and are described in Chapter 15.

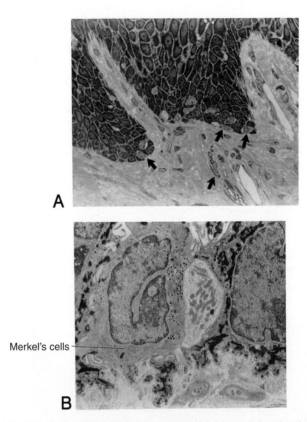

Fig. 14.**39 A** Merkel's cells located in the region of the stratum basale. They are lighter staining than epithelial cells (upper arrows). The axon is noted by the lower arrow. **B** Ultrastructure of Merkel's cell reveals dense vesicles in the cytoplasm of the cell adjacent to a nonmyelinated nerve terminal.

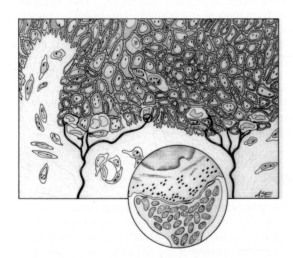

Fig. 14.**40** Diagram of a Merkel's cell showing the location and appearance of these cells in the oral epithelium. Note their relation to the nerves. The inset shows nerve terminal with vesicles in Merkel's cell adjacent to nerve.

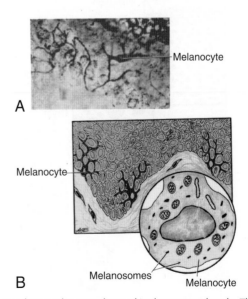

Fig. 14.**41 A** Dendritic melanocyte located in the stratum basale. The cell stains positive to dopa oxidase. **B** Diagram of several melanocytes in the basal region of the oral epithelium. Inset reveals the melanosome granules observed in this cell.

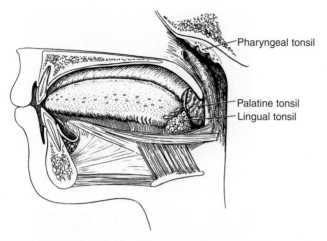

Fig. 14.**42** Diagram of location of three tonsillar groups: pharyngeal, palatine, and lingual.

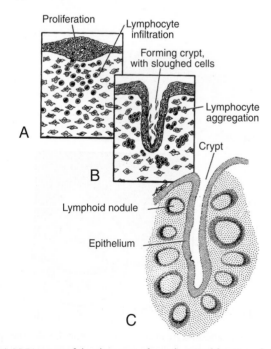

Fig. 14.**43** Clinical view of palatine tonsils (arrows). These tonsils are infected and appear swollen.

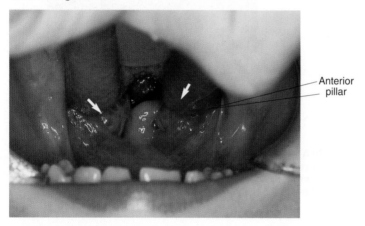

Fig. 14.**44** Diagram of development of tonsils. **A** Proliferation of epithelium. **B** Development of crypts. **C** Organization of lymphoid nodules.

Tonsils

Posteriorly the nasal cavity joins with the pharynx as the nasopharynx, and the oral cavity joins the pharynx as the oropharynx. At these junctions, tonsilar tissue is found as a wide circular band (Waldeyer's ring). The pharyngeal tonsil is in the superior aspects of the nasopharynx. In the oropharynx, the palatine tonsils are located laterally, and completing the ring inferiorly is the lingual tonsil (Fig. 14.**42**). The tonsils are part of the lymphatic system, which includes the lymph nodes, thymus, spleen, and diffuse lymphatic tissue. Tonsils, having a free surface covered by epithelium, are continuous with clefts or grooves. The tonsils contain many lymphocytes (which appear generally in nodules), some plasma cells, macrophages, and reticular cells. Lymphatic nodules with germinal centers are common both to the lingual and palatine tonsils. Tonsils and lymph nodes have efferent lymphatic vessels draining them. Unlike lymph nodes, the tonsils do not have afferent lymphatic vessels. Tonsils have a connective-tissue capsule of variable density and have associated glands underlying them. Figure 14.**43** shows a clinical view of the palatine tonsils.

Development

The tonsilar ring corresponds to the anterior limit of the embryonic foregut; hence the epithelium that gives rise to tonsils of endodermal origin. Tonsils develop by diffuse proliferation of the basal cells of the endodermal epithelium, with simultaneous subepithelial condensation of mesenchyme (Fig. 14.**44A**). The epithelail areas later evolve into nodular projections that extend into both the lamina propria and the oral cavity. These nodules become the foci of lymphocytic infiltration (Fig. 14.**44B**). The nodules grow into lymphoid tissue by mitotic division of existing lymphocytes accompanied by differentiation of mesenchymal cells. Additional lymphoid tissue aggregates around the crypt, completing the formation of the nodules (Fig. 14.**44C**). Connective tissue forms a capsule along the base of the glands and sends supporting projections into the folds of lymphatic tissue.

Growth of the tonsils is very rapid from birth to 3 years and then again from 7 to 12 years. Thereafter, the tonsils atrophy. The pharyngeal tonsils can occupy up to one half of the available space of the nasopharynx during childhood growth.

Types

Pharyngeal tonsil. The pharyngeal tonsil is located in the midline, in the posterior wall of the superior portion of the nasopharynx (Fig. 14.**42**). It may extend laterally around the opening of the auditory tube in the region of the torus tubarius (a raised projection above and to the sides of this opening). Tonsilar tissue in this location is referred to as the tubal tonsil. The pharyngeal tonsil when enlarged is referred to as the adenoids. This tonsil is covered by pseudostratified columnar epithelium (respiratory epithelium) with occasional patches of stratified squamous epithelium. The epithelial cells lining this surface are ciliated and contain numerous goblet cells (Fig. 14.**46**). There are no crypts associated with this tonsil; there are, however, folds in the mucosa. The pharyngeal tonsils are not highly characterized by lymphoid nodules and germinal centers, but occasionally these structures do occur. In general, the lymphoid tissue is diffusely arranged, as seen in Figure 14.**46**. In the lamina propria underlying the tonsil are mixed glands that drain on the surface of the respiratory epithelium (Fig.14.**45**). Deep to the lamina propria, the periosteum is attached to the sphenoid bone adjacent to the sinuses.

Palatine tonsils. The Palatine tonsils are largest in children, protruding into the oropharynx as large masses between the palatoglossus muscle (anterior pillar) and the palatopharygeus muscle (posterior pillar) (Fig.14.**43**). Most people refer to the palatine tonsils as "the tonsils." When patients have their "tonsils" out, these are the tonsils that are excised. Another name for the palatine tonsil is the faucial tonsil. The stratified squamous epithelium overlying these tonsils is similar to that of the adjacent oropharynx and oral cavity. The area immediately beneath the epithelium contains numerous lymphatic nodules with germinal centers (Fig.14.**47**). Septae of connective tissue support the masses of lymphatic tissue. Numerous branching crypts are present in the tonsilar tissue, and seromucous glands are found in the adjacent lamina propria. These crypts may contain plugs of dead lymphocytes and desquamated epithelium. The seromucous gland ducts do not open into the crypts; however; they open into the surface of the epithelium. The lack of flushing action in the crypts may account for an accumulation of foreign debris, causing inflammation of the tissues.

The epithelium in many areas of the crypts is discontinuous, and between the epithelial cells are cords and networks of lymphocytes and other nonepithelial cells. This type of epithelium is referred to as reticulated epithelium. There are intraepithelial passages from the lumen to the follicular tissue in the lamina propria. Not only are there disruptions in the surface epithelium, there are discontinuities in the basement membrane. The cells close to the surface of the epithelium are M cells (membrane cells); they initiate the action of processing antigens that come from the outside environment by way of the oral and nasal cavities. Dendritic cells similar to Langerhans' cells and other macrophages are present. Antigens are phagocytized by the cells, and the lysosomes of the cells break down the antigens into smaller peptides. These smaller fragments are then transferred to T cells to start the complex coding of antibodies for the body's immune system. The cells that process the antigens are called *antigen-presenter cells.* These cells in the tonsils are part of a large family of antigen-presenter cells found throughout the body.

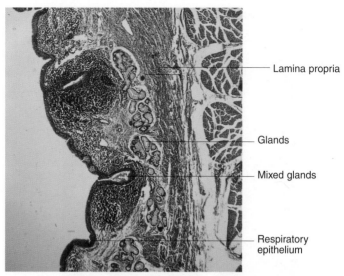

Fig. 14.**45** Histologic appearance of pharangeal tonsils with folds in the epithelium and with adjacent diffuse lymphatic tissue and seromucous glands underlying them.

Lamina propria

Glands

Mixed glands

Respiratory epithelium

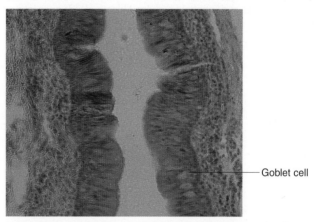

Fig. 14.**46** Histology of respiratory epithelium overlying the pharyngeal tonsils. At times, this epithelium may appear to be squamous.

Goblet cell

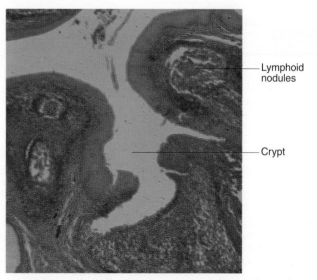

Fig. 14.**47** Histology of palatine tonsil tissue. Observe the overlying squamous epithelium, deep branching crypts, and organized lymphoid nodules.

Lymphoid nodules

Crypt

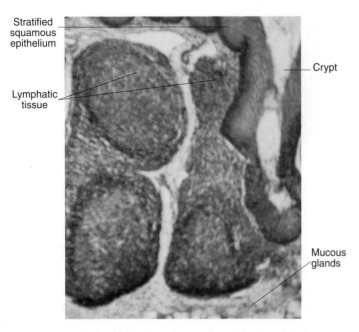

Stratified squamous epithelium

Lymphatic tissue

Crypt

Mucous glands

Fig. 14.**48** Histology of lingual tonsil. Note the overlying stratified squamous epithelium, short crypts, and lymphoid nodules. Mucous glands open into the crypts.

Lingual tonsils. The lingual tonsil is located on the posterior third of the tongue, extending from the circumvallate papillae posteriorly to the base of the epiglottis (Fig. 14.**42**). The surface epithelium of this tonsil is nonkeratinized stratified squamous epithelium similar to oral epithelium elsewhere. There are several dozen or more nonbranching crypts associated with this tonsil (Fig. 14.**48**). A connective-tissue capsule, some adipose tissue, and mucous glands are found under this tonsil. Most of its ducts enter the crypts and aid in the removal of trapped foreign material. Accumulation of debris or infection is rare in these tonsils, because they are washed by saliva as well as the mucous secretion that empties into the crypts. Underlying these mucous glands are the skeletal muscles of the tongue.

In Figure 14.**48**, which shows a section of lingual tonsil, the opening and base of a crypt lined by a nonkeratinized stratified squamous epithelium can be seen. Note the pure mucous acini of the glands and the well-organized lymphatic nodules. The apical cytoplasm is clear because the mucous is removed during tissue preparation.

Function

One function of tonsils is the formation of lymphocytes. Because of their location at the entrance of the alimentary and respiratory tracts, they are continuously exposed to a multitude of natural and foreign substances during breathing and eating. The lymphocytes protect the body against invasion of micro-organims. Allergens passing through the epithelium can be sensed by immunogenic cells of the lymphatic tissue, which start the complex process of coding for antibody production.

Table 14.**1** provides comparative information regarding morphologic features of the three tonsils.

Table. 14.**1** Comparison of tonsils

	Location	Lymphatic tissue organization	Epithelial covering	Crypts or folds	Capsules and septa	Associated glands and ducts	Lymphatic drainage
Palatine	Posterior lateral oral cavity between anterior and posterior faucial pillars	Arranged in rows of nodules with germinal centers	Nonkeratinous stratified squamous epithelium	Numerous and deep branching crypts	Fibrous connective-tissue capsule under tonsil, thin connective-tissue septa between segments	Mixed glands underlie tonsil, ducts open on free surface of epithelium, not in crypts	Drain to deep cervical nodes
Lingual	Dorsum of base of tongue	Row of nodules with terminal centers	Nonkeratinous stratified squamous epithelium	Wide-mouthed deep crypts with few branches	Thin capsule underlying gland, with few trabeculae separating lobules	Mucous glands open in crypts as well as on free surface of epithelium	Drain to deep superior cervical nodes
Pharyngeal	Medial posterior nasopharynx behind ostium of auditory tube	Aggregations of lymphoid tissue, few nodules and, occasionally, germinal center	Pseudostratified ciliated columnar epithelium with patches of stratified squamous epithelium	Folds of epithelium and lymphoid tissue, without crypts	Thin indistinct connective-tissue capsule, occasionally with septa	Seromucous glands open on free surface or in folds	Drain to retropharyngeal nodes

Summary

Oral mucosa consists of the epithelium and lamina propria lining all the surfaces of the oral cavity. There is continual turnover of the epithelial cells, with mitotic figures found in the basal layers. Migration of the cells to the surface occurs to replace the surface cells lost in the normal functions of mastication, speech, and swallowing. Both keratinized and nonkeratinized epithelia are found in the oral cavity and have a basal layer of cells (stratum basale) next to the lamina propria. These epithelia are characterized by prominent, numerous desmosones between the cells. In keratinized epithelium, there is a stratum granulosum with prominent spherical keratohyaline granules in these cells. The superficial layer of keratinized epithelium is the stratum corneum. These cells are full of keratin, and the nuclei have disappeared. In nonkeratinized epithelium the stratum granulosum is absent. In the superficial layers the nuclei are still present and the cells do not have the concentration of keratin found in keratinized epithelium.

The oral mucosa can be divided into three functional types: masticatory, specialized, and lining mucosa. The *masticatory mucosa* is a keratinized epithelium found on the gingiva and covering the hard palate. The *specialized mucosa* covers the dorsal surface of the tongue. The *lining mucosa* covers the remainder of the oral cavity and is a nonkeratinized epithelium.

The *lamina propria* varies extensively in the different areas of the mouth and may be tightly bound to underlying bone or freely movable as in the lips, vestibule, and cheeks. The presence of a submucosa varies, being absent in the gingival areas and large areas of the hard palate (anterior and midline).

The tonsils form a ring of lymphatic tissue at the posterior border of the oral and nasal cavities. The pharyngeal tonsils, also referred to as the adenoids, are located in the nasopharynx. The epithelium of these tonsils is composed of *respiratory epithelium* because it is ciliated at the luminal ends of the cells. Seromucous glands and diffuse lymphatic tissue are found in the lamina propria. The mucosa is folded and there are no crypts.

The palatine tonsils are located bilaterally between the anterior and posterior pillars at the posterior border of the oral cavity. These tonsils have deep branching crypts, and the surface epithelium is nonkeratinized stratified squamous epithelium. Many lymphatic nodules are located in these tonsils.

The lingual tonsil is situated on the posterior surface of the tongue in the oropharynx above the epiglottis. Several dozen single (nonbranching) crypts are found in it, and the epithelium is nonkeratinized stratified squamous epithelium. Lymphatic nodules along with many pure mucous glands are found in the lamina propria.

Self-Evaluation Review

1. Name the location and function of the masticatory, lining, and specialized mucosa.

2. In what areas of the oral mucosa are the glands located deep in the submucosa among the muscle fibers?

3. What is the name of the junction between the free and attached gingival mucosa?

4. Discuss the origin (development) of the oral mucosa.

5. Name the three factors responsible for the appearance of the vermilion border.

6. Where are the Fordyce spots located and what type of gland are they?

7. Name the four types of nonkeratinocytes and their functions.

8. Name and locate the three groups of tonsillar tissue.

9. What is the function of tonsillar tissue?

10. What is the name given to the tonsillar ring and what is its significance?

11. Which tonsillar mass is partially covered by respiratory epithelium and can also be ciliated?

12. Which tonsillar tissue is associated with deep, branching crypts and contains numerous germinal centers?

Acknowledgements

Figures 14.**2**–14.**8** are provided courtesy of Dr D MacCallum, Figures 14.**6**, 14.**9**, 14.**34**, and 14.**36** are provided courtesy of Dr. M Pirabazari. Figure 14.10 is provided courtesy of Dr. SS Han. Figures 14.**12**, 14.**13**, and 14.**39** are provided courtesy of Dr D Turner. Figure 14.**38B** is provided courtesy of Dr. Ian Mackenzie.

Suggested Readings

Barrett AW, Beymen AD. A histochemical study on the distribution of melanin in human oral epithelium. Arch. Oral. Biol. 1991;36:771–774.

Breusted A. Age induced changes in the oral mucosa and their characteristic consequences. Int. Dent. J. 1983;33: 272–280.

Dreisen S. The mouth as an indicator of internal nutritional problems. Pediatrician.1989;16:139–146.

Harris D, Robinson JR. Drug delivery via the mucous membranes of the oral cavity. J. Pharm. Sci. 1992;81:1–10.

Hoefsmit ECMM, Arkema JMS, Betjes MGH, et al. Heterogeneity of dendritic cells and nomenclature. In: Kamperdijk EWA, Wieuhuis P, Hoefsmit ECM, eds. Dendritic cells in Fundamental and clinical Immunology. New York, NY: Plenum Press; 1993.

Karchev T. Specialization of tonsils as analyzers of the human immune system. Acta Otolaryngol (Stockholm). 1988;Suppl. 454:53–59.

MacKenzie IC, Binnie WH. Recent advances in oral mucosal research. J. Oral Pathol. 983;12:389–415.

Perry ME, Jones MM, Mustafa Y. Structure of the crypt epithelium in human palatine tonsils. Acta Otolaryngol. (Stockholm). 1988;Suppl. 454:53–59.

Regauer S, Seiler GR, Barrandon Y, Easley LW, Compton CC. Epithelial origin of vitaneous anchoring fibrils. J. Cell Biol. 1990;1111:2109–2115.

Riebel J, Sorensen CH. Association between keratin-staining patterns and the structural and functional aspects of palatine tonsil epithelium. APMIS 1991;99:905–915.

Schroeder HE. Differentiation of Human Stratified Epithelia. Basel: Karger; 1981.

Schroeder HE. Oral Structural Biology. New York, NY: Thieme; 1991.

Schultz J, Ermich T, Kasper M, Raabe G, Schamann D. Cytokeratin pattern of clinically inatct and pathologically changed oral mucosa. In: J. Oral Maxillofac. Surg. 1992;21:35–39.

Slipka J. Palatine tonsils—their evolution and ontogeny. Acta Otolaryngol. (Stockholm). 1988;Suppl,454:18–22.

Squier CA. Oral Mucosa. In: Ten Cate AR, ed. Oral Histology and Development, Structure and Function. St Louis, Mo: Mosby; 1998:345–385.

Squier CA. The permeability of oral mucosa. Crit. Rev. Oral Biol. Med. 1991;3:13–32.

Yamoto Y, Okato S, Takahashi H, Takeda K, Magati S. Distribution and morphology of macrophages in palatine tonsils. Acta Otolaryngol. (Stockholm). 1988:Suppl. 454:83–95.

15 Histology of the Gingiva and Epithelial Attachment

James K. Avery

Introduction

The gingiva is that portion of the oral mucosa located around the necks of teeth, extending apically over the alveolar bone, and ending at the mucogingival junction. Like the palatine mucosa, it is keratinized and functions during mastication. The gingiva traditionally is divided into three zones (Fig. 15.1): the free or marginal zone, which circles the tooth and defines the gingival sulcus as the space between the tooth and the free gingiva; the attached zone, which is joined to the tooth by a unique junctional epithelium and is firmly attached to the underlying alveolar bone: and the interdental zone, which occupies the space between two adjacent teeth apical to the contact area. The free gingiva often is separated from the adjacent attached gingiva by a minute intervening groove termed the *free gingival groove*, which runs parallel and slightly apical to the free gingival margin (Fig. 15.1).

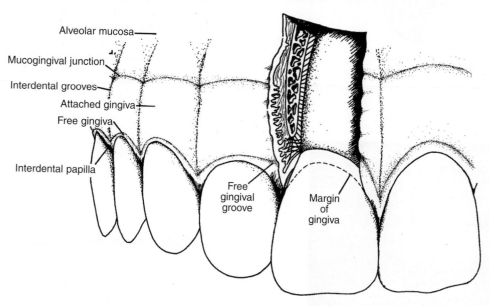

Fig. 15.**1** Diagram of the anatomy of the gingiva illustrating the location of the attached and free gingiva.

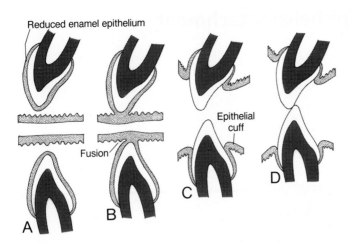

Fig. 15.**2** Development of gingiva from oral and reduced enamel organ epithelium.

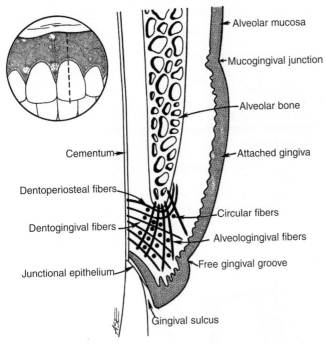

Fig. 15.**3** Diagram of histology of gingiva. Observe the fiber groups and their origins and insertions.

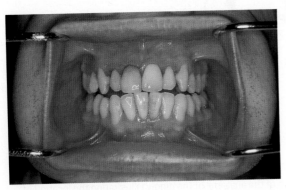

Fig. 15.**4** Appearance of normal gingiva, in older adult.

Objectives

After reading this chapter you should be able to describe the histologic structure of the gingiva in a young adult or in an aging person, discuss cellular turnover in this tissue, and describe the vascular and neural components as well as the mechanism of attachment of the gingiva to the surface of the tooth.

Development

The gingiva develops as a coalescence of oral and enamel organ epithelia (Fig. 15.**2A**). As the tooth emerges into the oral cavity, the reduced enamel organ epithelium covering the surface of the tooth fuses with the oral epithelium (Fig. 15.**2B**). With further tooth eruption, the reduced enamel epithelium separates from the primary cuticle on the surface of the enamel (Fig. 15.**15C**) The resulting cuff of epithelium and connective tissue surrounding the neck of the tooth becomes the gingiva. The reduced enamel organ epithelium continues its apical separation along the enamel surface until the tooth reaches occlusion. At that point, the gingiva covers only the cervical portion of the crown (Fig. 15.**2**). Thereafter, the epithelial attachment is limited to a zone at the cementoenamel junction.

Free Gingiva

The *free* or *marginal gingiva* can be clearly defined by four distinct boundaries: 1) *coronally*, by the gingival margin; 2) *apically*, by the free gingival groove (in the absence of this groove, the apical boundary would correspond to a line opposite the bottom of the gingival sulcus, which is usually about 1.0 to 1.5 mm apical to the free gingival margin); 3) along the *inner* margin to the tooth surface, by the gingival sulcus; and 4) on its *outer* surface, by the vestibular and oral cavities (Figs. 15.**3** and 15.**4**). The free gingival mucosa is composed of stratified squamous epithelium with a dense underlying connec-

Clinical Application

The gingival tissue and the surface of the hard palate comprise the masticatory mucosa; both are characterized by complete or partial keratinization and their function is mastication of food.

tive-tissue stroma (lamina propria) (Fig.15.**5**). The outer-surface epithelium interdigitates with the underlying connective tissue, forming long interconnected rete ridges separated by thin connective-tissue plates and papillae. This surface epithelium may be composed of keratinized, parakeratinized, or nonkeratinized epithelium (Table 15.**1**). In keratinized epithelium, there is a distinct stratum granulosum. In nonkeratinized epithelium, the cells lack the keratohyalin protein. The epithelial lining of the gingival sulcus (sulcular epithelium) differs from that of the surface epithelium in that it is thinner, lacks prominent epithelial rete ridges, and lacks signs of keratinization (Fig. 15.**6**).

Attached Gingiva

The attached gingival mucosa lies between the free gingival mucosa and the alveolar mucosa. It is separated from the former by the free gingival groove and from the latter by the mucogingival junction (Fig. 15.**3**). The mucogingival junction is the transition site from the keratinized epithelium of the attached gingiva to the nonkeratinized alveolar mucosa (Fig. 15.**1**). In a healthy mouth, the attached gingiva shows signs of stippling (orange-peel appearance) which is not found in other areas of the oral mucosa. The absence of stippling, which is brought about by edema of the tissue, can be an initial sign of pathology. A unique feature of the attached gingiva is the junctional epithelial or the epithelial attachment.

Junctional Epithelium

Junctional epithelium forms the floor of the gingival sulcus and extends apically in apposition to the surface of the enamel to form a seal between the epithelium and the tooth (Fig. 15.**5**–15.**7**). The cells of the junctional

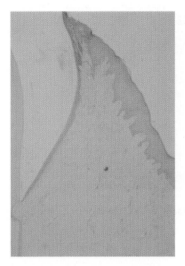

Fig. 15.**5** Histologic components of sulcular, free, and attached gingiva.

Table. 15.**1** Composition of surface epithellium of free gingiva cell

Gingival epithelium	Percent of cases	Surface nucleus present	Stratum granulosum
Keratinized	15	No	Present
Nonkeratinized	10	Yes	None
Parakeratinized	75	Partially	None

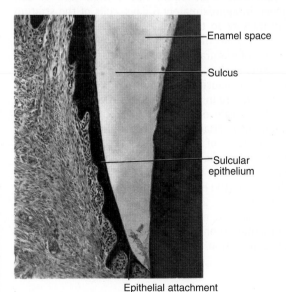

Enamel space

Sulcus

Sulcular epithelium

Epithelial attachment

Fig. 15.**6** Histology of the zone of junctional or epithelial attachment.

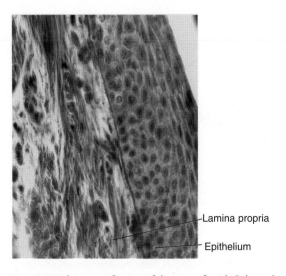

Lamina propria

Epithelium

Fig. 15.**7** Higher magnification of the zone of epithelial attachment.

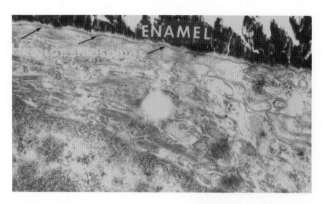

Fig. 15.**8** Ultrastructure of epithelial attachment with hemidesmosomes (arrows).

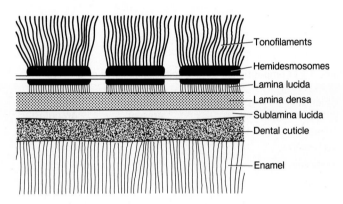

Fig. 15.**9** Diagram of the ultrastructure of attachment of hemidesmosomes to enamel.

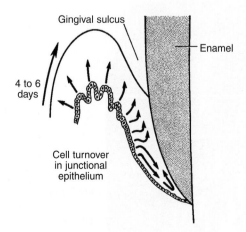

Fig. 15.**10** Epithelial cell turnover in gingiva. Note the direction of cell migration.

epithelium, or the epithelial attachment, have several identifying characteristics that distinguish them from epithelial cells in other areas of the gingiva. First, they have a smaller tonofilament-to-cytoplasmic ratio. Second, the number of mechanical adhesion sites, desmosomes between these cells, is approximately four times less in these cells than in other areas of gingival mucosa. This allows molecules of high molecular weight, as well as whole cells, to migrate into the surface of the mucosa. Finally, the organelles involved in protein synthesis and glycosylation (i. e., rough endoplasmic reticulum and Golgi apparatus) are more highly developed in these cells. The attachment of the epithelial cells to the tooth surface is an interesting and important feature of these cells. This attachment is structurally similar to the interface between epithelium and connective tissue elsewhere in the body. Epithelial attachment cells probably function much like basal epithelial cells, producing a basal lamina–like secretion or cuticular substance on the surface of the tooth. This structure may be added to by salivary glycoprotein and bacterial deposition. The junctional epithelial cells are attached to the cuticle by cell surface modifications, the hemisdesmosomes (Figs. 15.**8** and 15.**9**). A hemidesmosome consists of an attachment plaque that is approximately 20 nm thick and appears continuous with the inner part of the epithelial cell membrane. Tonofilaments insert into the hemidesmosome plaque. *Lamina lucida* and *lamina densa* regions are also seen. Cellular fibrils penetrate into the subjacent zona lucida and zona densa to facilitate attachment to the surface of the tooth (Fig. 15.**9**). This attachment is dynamic in that the epithelial cells are continuously being renewed and new desmosomes and hemidesmosomes are being formed.

Junctional Epithelium Turnover

The junctional epithelium has a high rate of cell turnover. In approximately 6 days, cells of the stratum basale migrate to the surface and are sloughed. Cells from other areas of the oral cavity have differing time schedules of maturation. During outward migration, the cells maintain their attachment to the tooth surface (Fig. 15.**10**). The responsible mechanism is probably similar to the one involved in wound healing, in which the epithelial cells migrate on the wound surface, forming and maintaining an attachment to the underlying basal lamina. Disturbance of the epithelial attachment will result in deepening of the gingival sulcus. This can be due to a number of factors: 1) effects of an inflammatory process on the cells of the epithelial attachment of the adjacent connective tissue; 2) immunologic response to bacterial antigens; and 3) mechanical irritation resulting from instrumentation or from food impaction or plaque and calculus formation.

Interdental Papilla

Those parts of the gingiva that appear between the teeth as wedge-shaped zones, extending high on the interproximal areas of the crowns on the labial and lingual surfaces, are interdental papillae (Fig. 15.**11**). This tissue fills the space created by the constricted cervical regions of adjacent crowns. *Interdental* grooves extend vertically toward the interdental papillae and correspond to the depressions between the roots of adjacent teeth.

Col

Interproximal to the vestibular and oral cavity surfaces of the interdental papilla is a concave area termed the *col* (Fig. 15.**12**). In the area of the col, the gingival epithelium is thin and nonkeratinized (Fig. 15.**13**). The morphology of the col differs between the anterior and posterior teeth. Anteriorly it is shaped like a pyramid, whereas posteriorly it is flattened. In Figure 15.**12**, the contact point between teeth and the shape of the col in both normal, inflamed and hyperemic, the col is exaggerated. The col usually exhibits signs of inflammation (Fig. 15.**14**), probably because it is difficult to keep the interproximal area clean as plaque and calculus form there. The epithelium of the col often sends numerous extensions into the underlying connective tissue (Fig. 15.**14**). With age, the vestibular and oral interdental peaks descend and at the area of the col flatten.

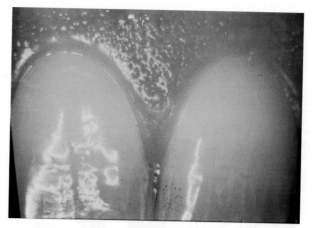

Fig. 15.**11** Clinical view of interdental papilla.

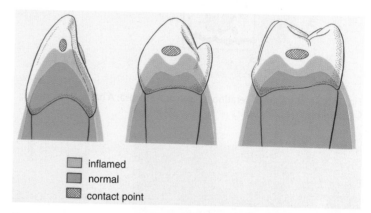

inflamed
normal
contact point

Fig. 15.**12** Diagram of positional relation of col in health and disease. Observe that the results of inflammation accentuate the col.

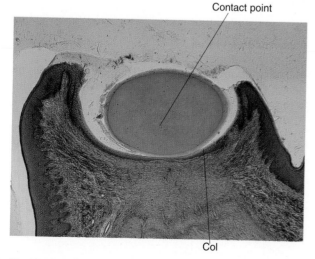

Contact point

Col

Fig. 15.**13** Epithelial lining of the col. Observe the contact point of the tooth above the col.

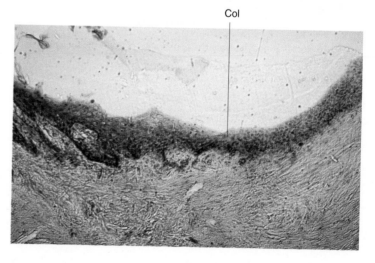

Col

Fig. 15.**14** Histology of the col as a thin layer of epithelium, with inflammatory cells and epithelial cell invasion of connective tissue.

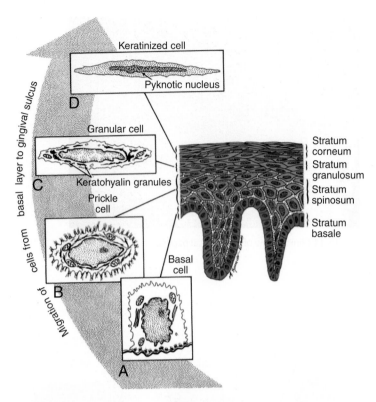

Fig. 15.**15** Maturation of keratinocytes in oral mucosa. **A** basal; **B** spinosum; **C** granulosum; **D** corneum.

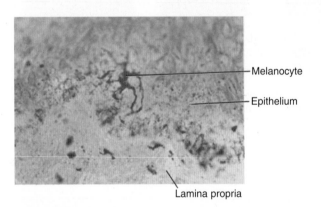

Fig. 15.**16** Nonkeratinocyte. Note the appearance of dendritic melanocyte in the stratum basale.

Keratinocytes

The keratinocyte is the predominant cell type that forms the epithelium of the gingival mucosa. In keratinized epithelium, these cells are organized into four distinct layers (Fig. 15.**15**). Just above the lamina propria is the basal cell layer (Fig. 15.**15A**). These cells are cuboidal or low columnar, and their oval nuclei usually are oriented at right angles to the plane of the epithelium–connective-tissue junction. The second layer, or stratum spinosum, is composed of four to five layers of cells (Fig. 15.**15B**). The lower cells of this layer are shaped like a polyhedron and are separated from one another by large expanses of intercellular fluid. Bridging the intercellular spaces are cytoplasmic extensions joined to each other by desmosomes. The superficial layers of the stratum spinosum contain cells that become flattened and less distinct. The third layer is the stratum granulosum (Fig. 15.**15C**). The cells of this layer contain irregular keratohyalin granules. These granules are highly characteristic of this level of the surface epithelium, but their exact origin and nature are not fully understood. The fourth and most superficial layer is the stratum corneum (Fig. 15.**15D**). Keratinized cells represent the final stage of the differentiation process. The multiple layers of these closely bound cells form a functional barrier to the passage of materials.

Intraepithelial Nonkeratinocytes

In addition to the keratinocytes, there are melanocytes, Langerhans' cells, Merkel's cells, lymphocytes, and leucocytes in the gingiva. Collectively, these cells constitute only a minor population and are localized in the basal and prickle cell layers. In routine histologic sections stained with hematoxylin and eosin, the cytoplasm of these cells appears vacuolated. Therefore, these cells are often referred to as "clear cells." They are mentioned only briefly here, as they are also described in Chapter 14.

Melanocytes

Melanocytes are highly specialized dendritic cells of neural crest origin. The function of these branched cells is to synthesize the pigment melanin, which is packaged in numerous, small, intracytoplasmic structures called melanosomes. The melanosomes are then transferred to the surrounding epithelial cells. The actual number of melanocytes does not seem to vary among individuals, although there are regional differences within the same individual. The variation in color among races is generally attributed to the functional nature of these cells (Fig. 15.**16**).

Langerhans' Cells

Langerhans' cells are similar in appearance to melanocytes. Usually, they lack melanosomes, having instead a unique rod-shaped, membrane-limited inclusion termed the Birbeck granule. Current evidence indicates that these cells may process antigens and act locally as part of the immune system (Fig. 15.**17**). These cells probably arise from the bone marrow, and they may migrate from the gingiva to regional lymph nodes.

Merkel's Cells

Merkel's Cells are located in the basal cell layer of the gingival epithelium and appear individually or in clusters. These cells appear similar to keratinocytes, possessing tonofilaments and desmosomes. Merkel's cells contain dense-cored granules and usually are associated with small, unmyelinated axons. The Merkel's cell and its associated axon function as an intraepithelial tactile receptor (Fig. 15.**18**).

Lymphocytes

Lymphocytes found in the gingival epithelium are associated with an inflammatory process. They may be found anywhere in the gingival epithelium, but most often are in the area of the junctional epithelium (Fig. 15.**19**).

Leucocytes

Leucocytes are found in the gingival epithelium, usually in the sulcular and attachment epithelium. These cells move between the epithelial cells and through its surface and become salivary corpuscles. They contribute protein and immunochemical substances to the sulcular fluid.

Fig. 15.**17** Nonkeratinocyte with Langerhans' cell. **A** Electron micrograph of rod-shaped inclusions (arrows) in cytoplasm. **B** Light micrograph of dendritic Langerhans' cell (stained with ATPase).

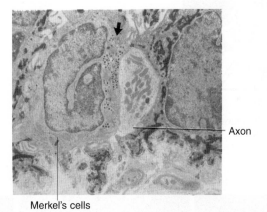

Fig. 15.**18** Merkel's cell containing dark-staining vesicles in the cytoplasm (arrow) adjacent to the nerve axon.

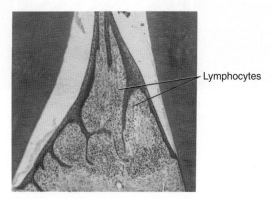

Fig. 15.**19** Inflamed gingiva with many leukocytes and lymphocytes in connective tissue.

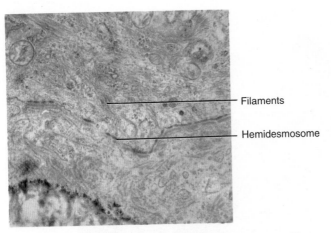

Fig. 15.**20** Ultrastructure of the junction of oral epithelium and lamina propria. The dense-staining bars in the horizontal plane are hemidesmosomes.

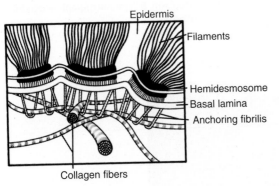

Fig. 15.**21** Diagram of hemidesmosome attaching oral mucosal cells to underlying lamina propria.

Epithelium–Lamina Propria Junction

Along the basal surface of the epithelium, the cells of the stratum basale are continuously dividing while maintaining close contact with the underlying connective tissue. Between the connective tissue and at the basal cell layer of the epithelium is a basal lamina. Hemidesmosomes of the epithelial cells attach to this lamina (Fig. 15.**20**). Hemidesmosomes are composed of an attachment plaque that possesses intracellular modifications of tonofilaments. These penetrate the plasma membrane of the cell to terminate in the basal lamina (Fig. 15.**21**), which is composed of two layers, a lamina lucida and a lamina densa. Fine collagen fibers attach to the lamina on the connective-tissue side. For further details regarding hemidesmosomes, refer to Chapter 14.

As is true throughout the body, connective tissue contributes toward maintaining the epithelium. In addition, the nature of the epithelium is largely dependent on the adjacent, underlying connective tissue. Recombination experiments have shown that epithelium transplanted to a site other than its own will soon take on characteristics of the new site. For example, if gingival epithelium is transplanted to an alveolar mucosa, loss of keratinization will occur. However, if the underlying connective tissue is transplanted with the epithelium, the original characteristics will be maintained. The interface of the epithelium of the gingiva and lamina propria is characterized by projections of the connective tissue into the overlying epithelium. Characteristics of these projections varies with age (Fig. 15.**22**). In the young adult aged 20 years, ridges of connective tissue appear (Fig. 15.**22A**). In the adult aged about 40 years, there are no ridges and individual papillae appear (Fig. 15.**22B**). In a 60 year old, the papillae decrease in number and are shorter and

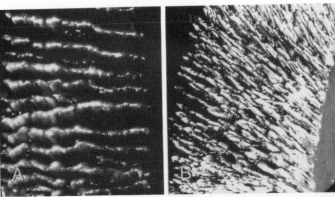

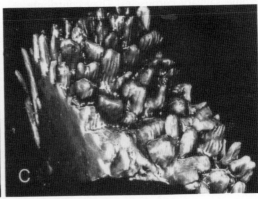

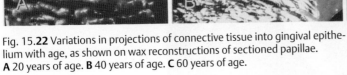

Fig. 15.**22** Variations in projections of connective tissue into gingival epithelium with age, as shown on wax reconstructions of sectioned papillae. **A** 20 years of age. **B** 40 years of age. **C** 60 years of age.

broader (Fig. 15.**22C**). Figures 15.**23A–C** illustrate the relation between the lamina propria and the epithelium at 20, 40, and 60 years in the human.

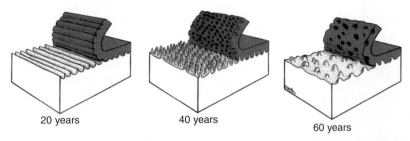

20 years   40 years   60 years

Fig. 15.**23** Diagram of interface of connective-tissue papillae and epithelium at the same age intervals as in Figure 15.22.

Lamina Propria

The lamina propria of the gingiva comprises the papillary and reticular zones, and dense bundles of collagen fibers that support the free and attached gingiva (Fig. 15.**24**). The gingiva has no submucosa. Because it has a masticatory function, its fibrous connective tissue is organized to withstand masticating forces. The fibers of the free and attached gingiva are called gingival fibers. They arise from the periosteal surface of the alveolar crest and the cervical area of the cementum, and are interspersed with fibers that course around the teeth and extend from the surface of one tooth to that of the next. The arrangement of these fibers is summarized in Table 15.**2**.

The lamina propria of the gingiva contains few elastic fibers, except those associated with the walls of the larger gingival blood vessels. This is in contrast to the lamina propria of the alveolar mucosa, which contains numerous elastic fiber bundles.

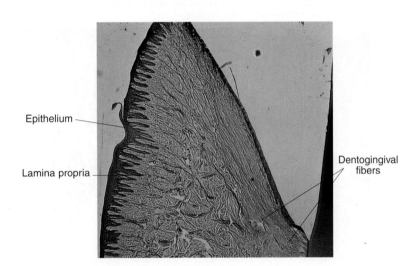

Epithelium

Lamina propria

Dentogingival fibers

Fig. 15.**24** Histology of fiber groups in gingiva.

Table. 15.**2** Gingival ligaments

Group name	Origin	Insertion
Dentogingival (free gingival)	Cervical cementum	Free and attached gingiva
Alveologingival	Alveolar crest bone	Free and attached gingiva
Circular or circumferential	Gingiva	Gingiva
Dentoperiosteal	Cervical cementum	Periosteum of outer cortical plates and cementum adjacent tooth

Clinical Application

Junctional epithelium has a higher rate of cell division than other areas of the oral mucosa. The rate of turnover of these cells is approximately six times more than that of other areas of the oral mucosa.

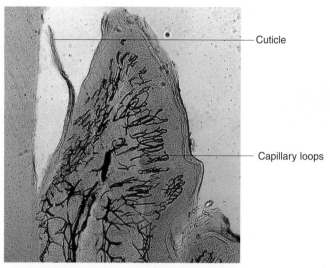

Fig. 15.**25** Blood vessels in gingiva (injected with India ink). Observe the vascular loops on connective-tissue papillae.

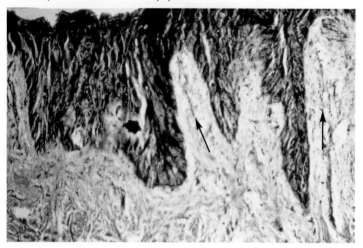

Fig. 15.**26** Nerve endings in gingival papillae. Left arrow, Meissner-type touch receptor. Right arrow, soiled temperature receptor.

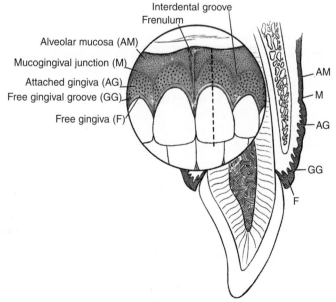

Fig. 15.**27** Summary diagram of gingival nomenclature.

Vascularity

Gingival connective tissue is highly vascular. The vessels have their origins in the periodontium and extend into the lamina propria of the gingiva. After perfusion with India ink, the well-organized capillary loops can be seen in the connective-tissue papillae (Fig. 15.**25**). In the adjacent specimen of clinically healthy gingiva, the superficial boundary of free interdental arteries arising from the alveolar arteries is shown. Histologically, the connective tissue of the papilla of the lamina propria shows loops arising from the larger vessels of the free and attached gingiva (Fig 15.**25**).

Nerves and Nerve Endings

Throughout the gingiva, nerves and nerve endings are prevalent. Receptors are seen as free endings within the papillary layer of the lamina propria. Touch endings (Meissner's corpuscles) and temperature receptors are seen as coiled terminals. Pain receptors are seen as fine fibers in the papilla. All are found in the free and attached gingiva (Fig. 15.**26**). These sensory structures are described in detail in Chapter 16.

Function

The gingiva is located around the necks of each tooth and is structured to resist the forces of mastication. Coupled with tongue and palate function, the gingiva has a *masticatory function* in supporting a bolus of food. Food is deflected from the gingiva to the tongue and is, in turn, forced between the teeth. The gingiva has a *sensory function*, as it is well innervated with pain, touch, and temperature receptors (Fig. 15.**26**). This capacity for sensitivity offers protection. Again, the gingiva acts as a compartment whose function is to protect the periodontium from the oral cavity.

Clinical Application

Ducts of the salivary glands open on all surfaces of the oral mucosa. The ones with watery secretion open on the posterior dorsum and lateral surfaces of the tongue. Those of mucous secretion open on the palatine surfaces of the mouth. All of these small glands aid in moistening and lubricating the oral mucosa, enabling speech, mastication, and swallowing.

Summary

The gingiva develops initially from the fusion of the reduced enamel epithelium and the adjacent oral mucosa. Together they form a fold of tissue around the necks of teeth, which is termed the free gingiva (Fig.15.**27**). A free gingival groove separates the free and attached gingiva . The gingiva is composed of a lamina propria with no submucosa. The lamina propria is supported by fibrous connective tissue composed of fiber groups that are: free gingival or dentogingival, alveolar gingival, circular, and dentoperiosteal. Usually, the gingival epithelium is lightly keratinized, parakeratinized, or fully keratinized. In only a few instances is it nonkeratinized. The gingiva is separated from the alveolar mucosa by the mucogingival junction, at which point any sign of keratinization disappears. The gingiva is attached to the necks of the teeth by means of an epithelial attachment. This attachment comprises a cuticular secretion of the tooth surface to which the adjacent epithelial cells have developed attachment discs, termed hemidesmosomes. These attachment sites are mobile, which allows the attachment to be maintained as the epithelial cells migrate incisally into the sulcus. The col is a valley between two interdental papillae. Its shape varies with anterior or posterior location, and its epithelium is thin and usually inflamed. The gingiva has a masticatory function and is characterized as highly vascular and well innervated.

Self-Evaluation Review

1. Describe the characteristics of the free gingiva and its boundaries.
2. Describe the characteristics of the attached gingiva and its boundaries.
3. Describe the characteristics of the interdental gingiva and its boundaries.
4. Describe the structure and function of hemidesmosomes?
5. Describe the epithelial attachment and how it may migrate.
6. What is the turnover time of the epithelial attachment?
7. Describe the development and origin of the gingiva.
8. Describe the characteristics of the col in health and disease.
9. Describe the junctional epithelium. What other names does it have?
10. Define a keratinocyte and name five nonkeratinocytes.
11. Name and describe the supporting fibers of the gingiva.
12. Describe the maturation of a keratinocyte in the mucosa.

Acknowledgements

The microphotographs in Figure 15.**22** are provided courtesy of Dr Harold Loe, DDS, Ph.D.

Suggested Readings

Barker DS The dendritic cell system in human gingival epithelium. Arch. Oral Biol. 1967;12:203–208.
Bhaskar SN, ed. Orban's Oral Histology and Embryology. St Louis, Mo: Mosby; 1990.
Dreizen S. The mouth as an indicator of internal nutritional problems. Pediatrician. 11989;116: 139–146.
Garasnza F. Glickman's clinical periodontiology. 7th ed. Philadelphia: WB Saunders; 1990.
Hill MW. The influence of aging on the skin and oral mucosa. J. Gerontol. 1984;3:35.
Kobayashi K, Rose GC, Mahan CI. Ultrastructure of the dentoepithelial junction. J. Periodont. Res. 1976;11:313–330.
Listgarten MA. Electron microscopic study of the gingivodental junction in man. Am J Anat. 1966;119:147–177.
Listgarten MA Phase contrast and electron microscope study of the junction between reduced enamel epithelium and enamelin unerupted human teeth. Arch. Oral Biol. 1966;11:999–1016.
Meeyer J, Squier CA, Gershon SJ, eds. The structure and function of oral mucosa. New York: Pergamon Press; 1984.
Schroeder HE. Ultrastructure of the junctional epithelium of the human gingiva. Helv. Odontol. Acta. 1969;13–65.
Schroeder HE, Listgarten MA. Structure of the developing epithelial attachment of human teeth. Vol 2, 2nd ed. New York: NY: S Karger; 1977.
Schroeder HE, Thelade J. Electron microscopy of normal human gingival epithelium. J. Periodont. Res. 1966;1:95–119.
Skougard MR. Cell renewal with special reference to the gingival epithelium. Adv. Oral Biol. 1970;4:251–288.
Squier CA, Waterhouse JP. The ultrastructure of the melanocyte in human gingival epithelium. Arch. Oral Biol. 1867;12:119–129.
Stern IB. Further electron microscopic observation of the epithelial attachment. Int. Asso.c Dent. Res. 1967;45:325.
Waterhouse JP, Squier CA. The Langerhans cell in human gingival epithelium. Arch. Oral Biol. 1967;12:341–348.

16 Innervation of Oral Tissues

Daniel J. Chiego, Jr. Dennis F. Turner, Donald S. Strachan

Introduction

Efferent or motor nerves carry impulses to muscles of mastication and muscles of facial expression. Efferent nerves of the autonomic nervous system are responsible for vasomotor control of the blood vessels and secretomotor control of the numerous salivary glands associated with the oral region. Sensory receptors within the mucous membrane of the oral cavity are responsible for discrimination of mechanoreception (touch, pressure, position), nociception (pain), and thermoreception (heat or cold). Sensory feedback from receptors in the gingival mucosa, palatine mucosa, and lip provides valuable information regarding the position of the tongue in the oral cavity. This information is essential for normal speech (e.g., apposition of the tongue to the teeth, palate, or lips) and mastication (e.g., shaping and positioning of the food bolus in the oral cavity before deglutition). In addition, these receptors initiate vital reflexes such as gagging and coughing. The special sense receptors for taste are also located primarily in the oral mucosa.

Objectives

After reading this chapter, you should be able to describe the organization of the peripheral nervous system and its general distribution in the oral region. You should be able to differentiate between efferent and affexent components and the functions for each of the components. You should be able to list the cranial nerves that innervate the muscles of mastication and muscles of facial expression, and to describe the nerves and functions of the autonomic nervous system to the oral region. In addition, you should be able to describe the afferent component of the peripheral nervous system involved in general sensibility of oral mucosa. Also, you should be able to describe the morphology, location, and function of the neural receptors in these tissues and have a general overview of the distribution of pain, heat, cold, and touch receptors. Regarding taste, you should be familiar with the various papillae of the tongue and the location and morphology of the taste buds. You should be able to recognize the various types of cells in a taste bud and to relate various areas of the tongue with differentiation of various taste modalities. You should be capable of cataloging the cranial nerves responsible for taste with their areas of innervation.

Classification of the Nervous System Relative to the Oral Region

The initial contents of this section includes a basic description of the nervous system. These paragraphs are intended as a review and for general background information.

The nervous system is divided into two main parts, the central and peripheral. The central nervous system is the brain and spinal cord. The peripheral nervous system includes the peripheral nerves that enter and leave the central nervous system, and the associated peripheral ganglion associated with the nerves. Nerve impulses from the central nervous system to the periphery travel on efferent nerves, and nerve impulses from the periphery to the central nervous system are carried by afferent nerves. The afferent nerves are the sensory nerves (Fig. 16.1). Efferent nerves in the oral area can be divided into two large groups: nerves to the skeletal muscle (facial and mastication), and nerves to smooth muscles and glands (autonomics). The peripheral nerves are classified by alphabetic characters modified by Greek letters (Table 16.1). The nerves to skeletal muscle are Aα fibers, which are the largest in diameter and also the fastest in the velocity of impulse conduction. Nerves to skeletal muscle end in a motor end plate that is in close relation to the cell membrane (sarcolemma) of the skeletal muscle cell (fiber). At this neuromuscular junction, acetylcholine is released from the end plate and initiates contraction of the skeletal muscle. Contraction of skeletal muscle is rapid and under the voluntary control of the individual.

The second group of efferent nerves is distributed to smooth muscles and glands. This group represents the autonomic nervous system. The name "autonomic" signifies that it is autonomous or independent from voluntary control. Smooth muscles of the oral area are primarily associated with blood vessels. The nerves to these muscles are vasomotor nerves. Smooth muscle is

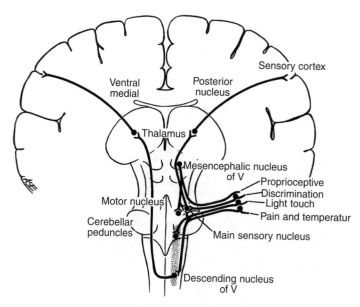

Fig. 16.1 Nuclei of cranial nerves innervating the oral region.

Table. 16.1 Cutaneous receptor organs

Class	Functional category	Morphologic category	Size of axon	Probable sensory role	Type of skin
Mechanoreceptor position (and velocity) dectors	Type I	Merkel's cell ending; touch corpuscle	Aα	Touch pressure	Hairy; glabrous (hairless)
	Type II	Ruffini's corpuscle	Aα	Touch pressure	Hairy; glabrous
Velocity detector	RA (rapidly adapting)	Meissner's corpuscle	Aα	Flutter	Glabrous
Transient detector	Pacinian (phasic, tap)	Pacinial corpuscle	Aα	Vibration, tep	Subcutaneous
Thermoreceptor	Warm	?Free endings	C	Warmth	Hairy; presumably glabrous
Nociceptor	Cold	Free endings	Aδ or C	Cooling	Hairy; glabrous
	Aδ or C high-threshold mechanoreceptor	?Free	Aδ or C	Pain from mechanical stimulation	Hairy; glabrous
	Aδ thermal	?Free	Aδ	Pain from thermal or mechanical stimulation	Hairy; glabrous
	C polymodal	?Free	C	Pain from mechanical thermal or chemical stimulation	Hairy; glabrous

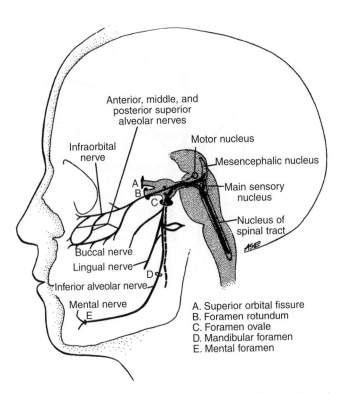

Fig. 16.**2** Trigeminal nerve: central nuclei and peripheral terminal branches to the oral region.

A. Superior orbital fissure
B. Foramen rotundum
C. Foramen ovale
D. Mandibular foramen
E. Mental foramen

arranged circumferentially around the vessel, and when the muscles contract the amount of blood flowing through the vessel is diminished. Vasocontriction in smaller arteries and arterioles play an important role in this control of blood flow. Efferent nerves to glands, also part of the autonomic nervous system, cause secretion. The term secretomotor is frequently used to describe these nerves. Autonomic nerve fibers are classified as B and C fibers and are smaller in diameter and slower in the velocity of impulse conduction (Table 16.**1**).

Efferent nerves (from the periphery to the central nervous system) of the oral cavity can be divided into three main categories: 1) Sensory nerves that correspond to the afferent nerves of the autonomic nervous system. These visceral sensory nerves are not considered to be the autonomic nervous system. However, they do provide regulatory feedback and sensory information for vasomotor and secretomotor control. 2) Afferent nerves for taste, olfaction, vision, and hearing. These are termed special afferent nerves. The nerves for taste are discussed in the last section of this chapter. 3) General afferent nerves for mechanoreception, nociception, and thermoreception (Fig. 16.**2**).

Structure and Function of Peripheral Sensory Receptors Found in Oral Mucosa

What is known about the function of somatic sensory receptors in the oral mucosa has largely been extrapolated from physiologic studies of hairy and non-hairy (glabrous) skin. To this date, only a partial correlation between structure and function has been achieved (Table 16.**1**).

The mechanoreceptors include receptors for touch, pressure, position, flutter, and vibration. They are classified as rapid acting and slow acting. The rapid-acting nerves conduct the fastest (60 to 116 m/s), are myelinated, and are the largest in diameter (10 to 16 µm). They are classified as Aa fibers, similar to the myelinated nerve fibers of skeletal muscle. Merkel's and Ruffini's corpuscles are nerve endings associated with the rapid-acting nerves. Other mechanoreceptors (Meissner's and pacinian corpuscles) are associated with afferent nerves that are slow adapting and have smaller diameter (5 to 15 µm) and slower conduction velocities (30 to 80 m/s). The nerves of the thermoreceptors and nociceptors are smaller in diameter (0.2 to 8 µm) and conduct more slowly (0.5 to 30 m/s).

Clinical Application

An injection of local anesthetic in the area of a nerve fiber bundle blocks transmission first in the small myelinated fibers, then in unmyelinated fibers, and lastly in large myelinated fibers. The small fibers (Aδ and C) are first to be blocked, resulting in loss of pain and temperature sensitivity. As the concentration of the local anesthetic increases, the conduction along large neurons is blocked, resulting in loss of touch and pressure. Recovery is in reverse order.

Proprioceptors, a type of mechanoreceptor, are sensory receptors that give information on movement and position. In dentistry, proprioceptors are important in determining the position of the mandible and bite forces. Proprioceptors are located in the periodontal ligament, in the tendons of the masseter, temporalis, and the medial pterygoid muscles. There are also proprioceptors located in the temporomandibular joint (TMJ) and the surrounding joint capsule. Studies have shown that the periodontal ligament proprioceptors are of the Ruffini type, can be rapid or slow adapting, and respond to both direction and force. The majority of the periodontal ligament proprioceptors are located in the apical one-third of the tooth socket (alveolus).

The cell bodies of the proprioceptors are located in the mesencephalic nucleus of the trigeminal nerve and are the only primary afferent nucleus in the central nervous system. Trigeminal mesencephalic neurons synapse directly with neurons in the motor nucleus of the trigeminal nerve to form monosynaptic reflexes (i.e., jaw jerk reflex). They also synapse with other nuclei within the brainstem in order to coordinate many different orofacial functions, for example swallowing, facial movement.

"Pain receptors" and "nociceptors" are terms that require definition. The term "nociceptor" is more appropriately used for these neuroreceptors, as the term "pain" generally has a broader interpretation relating to the overall subjective response of the individual. Nociceptors respond to intense mechanical stimulation, intense thermal stimuli, and noxious chemical stimulation. Nociceptors are primarily associated with unmyelinated and lightly myelinated nerve fibers.

Complete uniformity in the classification of sensory receptors has not been achieved, but with the use of ultrastructural morphology the receptors can be divided into two general categories: corpuscular receptors and free nerve endings.

Corpuscular Sensory Receptors

Corpuscular sensory receptors are characterized as having specialized cell types associated with their axon terminals: 1) Meissner's corpuscles are located high in the connective-tissue papillae. 2) Merkel's corpuscles are located at the base of epithelial rete ridges. 3) Simple coiled corpuscles are located at the base of connective-tissue papillae or in the subpapillary lamina propria.

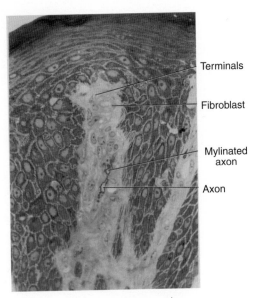

Fig. 16.**3** Meissner's tactile corpuscle.

Meissner's Corpuscles

Meissner's tactile corpuscles are located within the lamina propria, at the apex of the connective-tissue papillae, in close proximity to the overlying oral epithelium (Figs. 16.**3**–16.**5**). The corpuscle is surrounded by an incomplete capsule composed of flattened fibroblasts that lack a basal lamina, and of elastic fibers that are continuous with the general elastic network of the adjacent dermis. Most Meissner's corpuscles are innervated by two or more myelinated axons. Upon penetration of the capsule these lose their myelin sheaths and become positioned between stacks of cytoplasmic lamellae, which arose from specialized lamellar cells. The lamellar cells are separated from each other by considerable amounts of amorphous, filamentous material containing a small number of collagen fibrils. A basal lamina surrounds each lamellar cell and its cytoplasmic extensions. Numerous pinocytotic vesicles are present along the cell membranes and appear to be most abundant adjacent to the axolemma of the axon terminal. The axon terminal contains many mitochondria. Neurofilaments and neurotubules are found, but lack the uniform organization seen in the proximal parts of peripheral nerves. Meissner's corpuscles are characterized electrophysiologically as rapidly adapting mechanoreceptors functioning in tactile two-point discrimination.

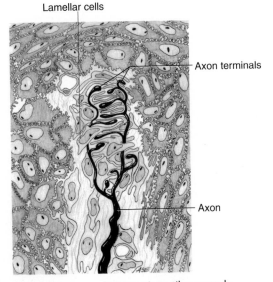

Fig. 16.**4** Diagram of Meissner's tactile corpuscle.

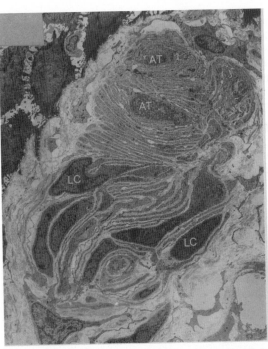

Fig. 16.**5** Meissner's tactile corpuscle is composed of flattened lamellar cells (LC) surrounding axon terminals (AT).

Merkel's Corpuscles

Merkel cells and their associated axon terminals are specialized intraepithelial complexes found individually, or in clusters, at the base of epithelial rete ridges. In semithin (1 μm) sections, clusters of Merkel's cells can be readily identified under the light microscope (Fig. 16.**6**). Merkel's cells appear to be less intensely stained than the surrounding keratinocytes (Fig. 16.**7**). The nucleus of the Merkel's cell is lobulated and often eccentrically placed, occupying proportionately less of the total cell volume than the nuclei of neighboring keratinocytes (Fig. 16.**7**). Most Merkel's cells are located at the periphery of the rete ridge, with their plasma membranes in contact with the basal lamina. A vacuolated area is often observed adjacent to the cell. This pale area corresponds to the axon terminal, seen in greater detail with the electron microscope (Fig. 16.**8**).

In the electron microscope, Merkel's cells appear to be larger and less electron-opaque than surrounding keratinocytes. They are characterized by the presence of electron-dense, membrane-bound secretary granules, cytoplasmic spikes extending between epithelial cells and into the lamina propria, and desmosomes joining the cell to the adjacent keratinocytes. The secretary granules are polarized in the cytoplasm between the nucleus and an associated intraepithelial axon terminal (Fig. 16.**8**). Membrane specializations such as thickenings are often present between the Merkel's cell and the associated axon. Myelinated fibers 2 to 4 μm in diameter supply the Merkel's corpuscle. As these fibers approach the base of the rete ridge, they lose their myelin sheath and continue as unmyelinated fibers, 0.5 to 1 μm in diameter. Merkel corpuscles have been characterized electrophysiologically as a type I, slow-adapting mechanoreceptor, functioning as a position detector. The osmophilic granules in the cytoplasm of the Merkel cell are thought to contain a neurotransmitter; however, this neurotransmitter has not yet been identified.

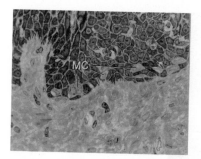

Fig. 16.**6** Merkel's (mechanoreceptor) cells (MC).

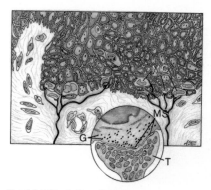

Fig. 16.**7** Merkel's cell (MC) with axon terminal. MS: membrane specialization. T: terminal. G: secretory granules.

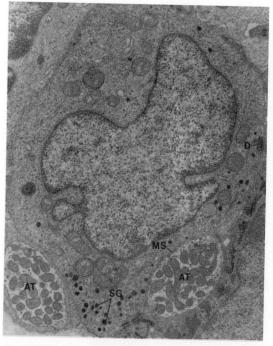

Fig. 16.**8** Merkel's cell with associated axon terminal (AT) and secretory granules (SG). Note the lobulated nucleus. MS: membrane specialization. D: desmosome.

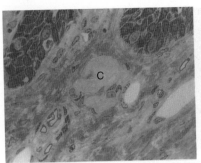

Fig. 16.9 Simple coiled corpuscle (C) adjacent to the oral epithelium.

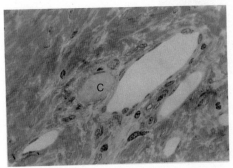

Fig. 16.10 Simple coiled corpuscle (C) adjacent to the small blood vessels in the lamina propria.

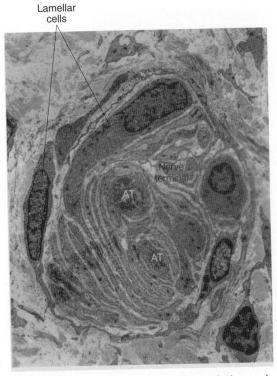

Fig. 16.11 Simple coiled corpuscle with axon (AT) wound among lamellar cells.

Simple Coiled Corpuscles

Simple coiled corpuscles are organized similar to Meissner's corpuscles. They are found at the base of connective-tissue papillae (Fig. 16.9), but are not limited to this location, often being located deeper in the lamina propria (Fig. 16.10). Since their initial discovery, they have been known by a variety of names, such as Dogiel corpuscle, Krause end-bulb, lingual corpuscle, genital corpuscle, or mucocutaneous end-organ. In contrast to Meissner's corpuscles, the simple coiled corpuscle is usually smaller and more oval in shape (Fig. 16.11). The corpuscle lacks a true capsule, and the axon terminal forms a loose coil as it winds through the lamellar cells. This results in a greater number of axon profiles when the corpuscle is sectioned for electron microscopy. The precise function of this receptor has not been determined.

Free Nerve Endings

Free nerve endings are found in abundance throughout the entire body. They may be the terminal arborization of thick or fine myelinated axons, but most often have their origin from nonmyelinated fibers. In the oral cavity free nerve endings are either intraepithelial or located in nonmyelinated fibers. In the oral cavity free nerve endings are either intraepithelial or located in the lamina

Clinical Application

Both peripheral nerve fibers and their axon terminals are extremely resistant to infection in the adjacent tissues. As long as they maintain continuity with their cell bodies, little if any pathology results. Even in severe suppurative infection, sensation is usually preserved. Histologic sections of this tissue often show intact nerve bundles surrounded by extravasated blood and pus. Thus, sensory loss in the oral cavity may be an early sign of a central-nervous-system lesion. Diseases such as multiple sclerosis, cerebrovascular accidents, and syringomyelia can produce sensory deficits in the oral cavity. Atrophy due to neurotrophic disturbances can also be manifested within the oral cavity, usually along the entire distribution of the affected nerve.

propria, just beneath the basal lamina (Figs. 16.**12**–16.**14**). Within the epithelium, the free nerve endings are found within folds of epithelial cells in the basal and prickel cell (Fig. 16.**14**). Free nerve endings within the lamina propria are characterized by abundant mitochondria in their axoplasms and partial or incomplete investment of Schwann-cell cytoplasm (Fig. 16.**13**).

Free nerve endings are generally believed to respond to more than one sensory modality. They exist in all tissues that respond to painful stimuli and are the only type of ending found in the tooth pulp, the classic model of pure nociception. In addition, they have been implicated as thermoreceptors.

Nerve Plexus

The oral mucosa contains a superficial nerve plexus just beneath the epidermis in the lamina propria, and a deep plexus within the submucosa. The deep plexus contains large nerve fibers that send smaller terminal branches toward the surface. The superficial plexus contains large and medium-size fibers, along with an abundance of sympathetic fibers.

The superficial nerve plexus allows nerve impulses from various receptors to reach a major nerve trunk via different collateral routes. Because of this arrangement, minor nerve injury does not result in sensory loss in the superficial tissues. It is also believed that this arrangement allows for more accurate localization of stimuli and discrimination between their intensities.

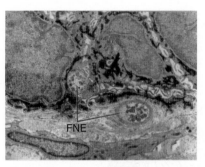

Fig. 16.**12** Free nerve ending (FNE) adjacent to the basal lamina.

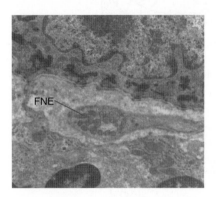

Fig. 16.**13** Free nerve ending (FNE) in connective-tissue papilla adjacent to the oral epithelium.

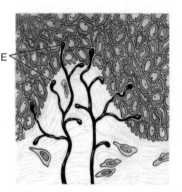

Fig. 16.**14** Diagram of intraepithelial free nerve ending (FNE). Terminals are found in the zone of stratum germinativum and connective-tissue papillae.

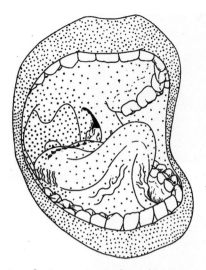

Fig. 16. **15** Location of pain receptors in the oral cavity.

Modality Distribution

Figures 16.**15** to 16.**18** illustrate the distribution of pain, heat, cold, and touch endings in the oral cavity. Pain endings are concentrated in the lips and posterior oral region. The distribution of heat and cold endings indicates that the lips are the most highly innervated. Heat receptors are concentrated in the lips. The greatest concentration of cold receptors is found in the posterior palate, tongue tip, lips, and ventral surface of the tongue. The tip of the tongue and the lips are most highly innervated by touch receptors. Table 16.**2** provides a summary of the distribution of these endings in the oral cavity.

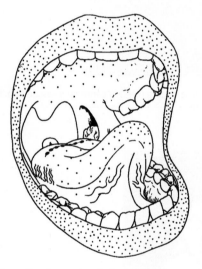

Fig. 16.**16** Location of heat receptors in the oral cavity.

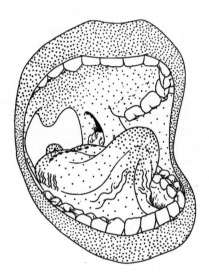

Fig. 16.**17** Location of cold receptors in the oral cavity.

Table. 16.**2** Levels of sensitivity of oral region

	Sensitivity of lips and oral mucosa		
Sensation	**Greatest**	**Moderate**	**Least**
Pain	Lips, pharynx, base of tongue, teeth	Anterior tongue, gingiva	Buccal
Heat	Lips	Anterior teeth	Ventral tongue, palate
Cold	Lips, posterior palate	Base and ventral tongue	Dorsum tongue, buccal mucosa
Touch	Lips, tip of tongue, anterior palate	Gingiva	Base tongue, buccal mucosa

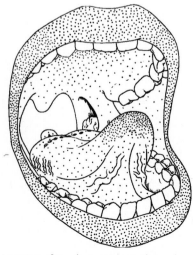

Fig. 16.**18** Location of touch receptors in the oral cavity.

Taste and Taste Receptors

Specialized sensory receptors within the oral mucosa are primarily responsible for taste. Taste reception is caused by a large number of taste receptors located on the tongue, pharynx, epiglottis, and soft palate. For a long time, it was thought that taste modalities had a corresponding location in the mouth and that these taste buds were especially sensitive to a particular taste stimulus. More recently, these differences have been shown not to be pronounced. A combination of differing taste modalities cannot explain the wide variety of taste sensations experienced by humans. Modified epithelial cells are the receptors of taste and conduct this stimulus to nerves that are in contact with these cells. The nerves then conduct impulses to the brain.

Taste-Bearing Papillae

The sense of taste is a chemical sense that is associated with specific, discrete receptor organs, the taste buds. Taste buds were recognized over 100 years ago and have been a subject of continued interest. In the human adult, taste buds number about 10 000 on the tongue, approximately 2500 on the soft palate, over 900 on the epiglottis, over 600 on the larynx and pharynx, and 250 or more on the oropharynx. Taste buds are located on the dorsum and edges of the tongue and are associated with the fungiform, circumvallate, and foliate papillae (Fig. 16.**19**). The filiform papillae bear no taste buds, although they are the most numerous of the dorsal lingual papillae.

Taste buds begin to develop and mature early in human fetal life. They appear at 7 weeks after conception and are differentiated by 14 weeks. By this time the tongue is well developed. The fifth, seventh, and ninth cranial nerves are also located in this area underlying the mucosa. This relationship is important to the development of taste buds because an unknown neurotrophic substance is probably responsible for differentiation and maintenance of taste buds.

Fungiform Papillae

Fungiform papillae are mushroom-shaped papillae, about 0.5 to 1 mm in diameter, and are larger at their free surface than at their base. They project slightly above the surface of the tongue (Fig. 16.**20**). In 40% of these rounded papillae, taste buds are located on the epithelium of the convex dorsal surface (Figs. 16.**21** and 16.**22**). In approximately half of the 40%, one to three taste buds are found, and in the remainder four or more are found. Because the fungiform papillae project slightly above the surrounding filiform papillae, tasteable substances have easy access to these receptors. Taste buds of the fungiform papillae appear to be somewhat different from the circumvallate and foliate. The three cell types present in the other papilla are not clearly recognizable in the fungiform. This may be because the innervation is

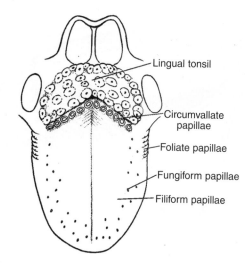

Fig. 16.**19** Tongue with site of taste buds.

- Lingual tonsil
- Circumvallate papillae
- Foliate papillae
- Fungiform papillae
- Filiform papillae

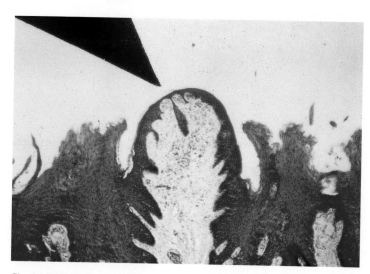

Fig. 16.**20** Fungiform papilla with taste bud (arrow).

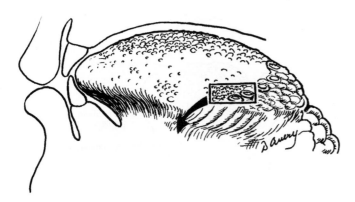

Fig. 16.**21** Circumvallate papilla.

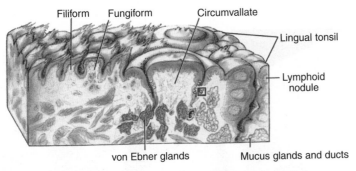

Fig. 16.**22** Circumvallate papilla with taste buds and serous glands (von Ebner).

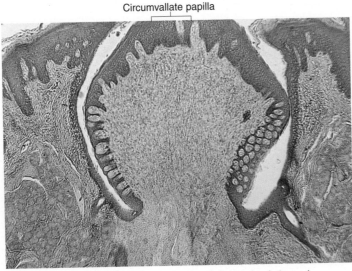

Fig. 16.**23** Circumvallate papilla with ducts of serous glands (arrow).

from the seventh nerve and the others are from the ninth. (Remember this when you read the description of the taste buds later in this chapter.) Fungiform papillae are located mainly on the tip and along the sides of the tongue. The threshold for sweet, salty, and sour modalities is the least in these areas.

Circumvallate Papillae

As described earlier, the circumvallate papillae are named for their shape, as each round papilla is surrounded by a trench and a wall (vallum): thus the term circumvallate (Figs. 16.**21** and 16.**22**). In humans, a row of eight to 12 circumvallate papillae, each 2 to 4 mm in diameter, is located at the junction of the body (anterior two-thirds) and base (posterior one-third) of the tongue. Approximately 250 taste buds are contained in the wall of each papilla (Fig. 16.**23**). Therefore, approximately 2500 taste buds occur in this location. No taste buds appear on the dorsal aspect of the papilla: only in the walls facing the trench. Beneath these papillae are located the serous glands (of von Ebner), which produce a serous fluid. This fluid functions to flush out the trenches around the papillae so that new tastes may be perceived. In Figures 16.**22** and 16.**23**, observe the ducts that open from these glands into the floor of the trenches. A variety of taste sensations, such as salty, sour, bitter, and sweet, are perceived by these taste cells.

Foliate Papillae

Foliate papillae are leaf–like, consist of eight to 12 clefts, and are located along the lateral posterior borders of the tongue (Fig. 16.**19**). The taste buds of these papillae are similar to those of the circumvallate papillae, as both walls of the clefts (Fig. 16.**24**), and number approximately 1280 taste buds per cleft or 2560 per papilla (Figs. 16.**21** and 16.**24**). They are most sensitive to the sour, salty, and bitter modalities. Like the trenches of the circumvallate papilla, the trenches of the foliate papilla have ducts of underlying serous glands opening into them.

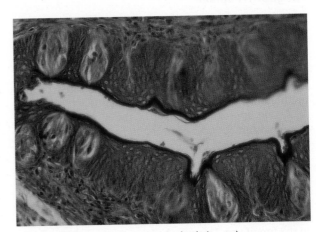

Fig. 16.**24** Foliate papilla with taste buds (arrow).

Taste-Bud Structure

Taste buds are goblet-shaped clusters of cells that are oriented at right angles to the surface of the epithelium (Fig. 16.**25**). Each barrel-shaped taste bud has a small pore that opens into the oral cavity, through which the tasteable substances may contact the the bud cells (Fig. 16.**24**). Taste buds are relatively constant in size, measuring between 60 to 80 µm in length and 35 to 45 µm at their maximum diameter. Taste cells extend from the basal lamina in contact with the connective tissue to the free surface of the epithelium, where the taste pore is surrounded by as few flattened epithelial cells. The cells of the taste bud are modified epithelial cells that function as taste receptors. Because they transmit to nerve endings, these receptors are considered to be neuroepithelial cells. Under the light microscope, taste buds appear to contain two types of cells: thick, light-staining cells and thin, dark-staining cells (Fig. 16.**25**). Some investigators believe one cell type comprises the functional receptor cells whereas accompanying cell types are support cells. Taste cells have been found not to divide, and each type is renewed by differentiation from the more peripheral or basal cells in the taste bud or the surrounding epithelium. Thus, each cell type is a distinct line of cells with no transition between lines. In regenerating, early forms of each type appear at about the same time. The approximate numbers of taste buds in human circumvallate papillae have been determined from birth to old age (Table 16.**3**). The number of taste buds in each circumvallate papilla appears to be relatively constant throughout life. There may be a slight decrease in number in old age, although other investigators note negligible loss in older, healthy individuals. Therefore, even in older individuals, taste loss may be minimal.

When taste buds are examined under the electron microscope, taste-bud structure is seen to consist of several types of stave-shaped cells (Figs. 16.**26** and 16.**27**).

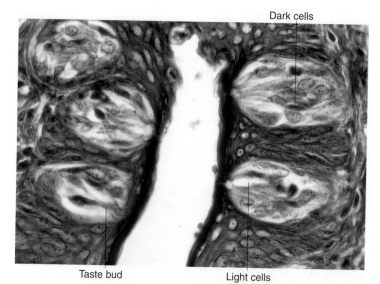

Fig. 16.**25** Taste buds.

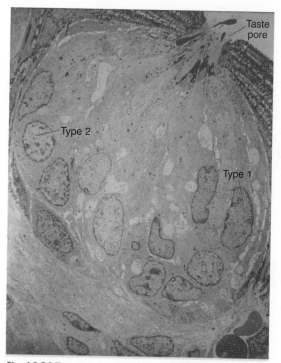

Fig. 16.**26** Transmission electron micrograph of a taste bud.

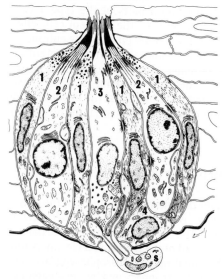

Fig. 16.**27** Diagram of a taste bud. Type 1 dark cells represent 60% of cells; type 2 light cells, 30%; type 3, 7%; and type 4, basal cell.

Table. 16.**3** Number of taste buds in human circumvallate papilla from birth to old age

Age	Mean no. of taste buds per papilla and trench wall
0-11 m	251
1-3 y	260
4-20 y	326
30-45 y	242
50-70 y	268
74-85 y	101

Clinical Application

Trigeminal neuralgia or tic douloureux is one of the most painful conditions associated with the head and neck. Although the cause of this disease is not totally understood, it is thought to be due to vasospasms or compromises to the blood supply of the trigeminal ganglion. Another hypothesis is that following abnormal nerve healing, trigger zones are created at tooth-extraction sites. The severe pain associated with this disease usually originates along the distribution of the specific sensory nerve to the area.

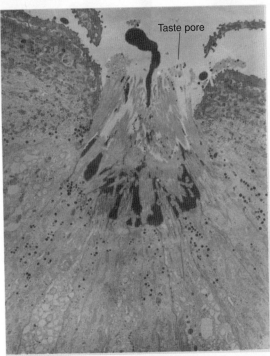

Fig. 16.28 Taste pore. Epithelial cells surround the pore. Note microvilli of type 1 and 2 cells and dense substance (below) in type 1 cell and between cells (above).

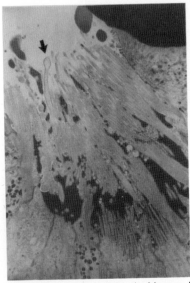

Fig. 16.29 Taste pore. Note the blunt ending of the type 3 cell (arrow). Observe the microvilli of type 1 and 2 cells surrounding it.

Type I dark cells represent 60% of all cells in the bud. They appear to have an electron-dense cytoplasm and their apical cytoplasm contains dark granules.

These cells terminate in microvilli consisting of 30 to 40 slender processes that enter the outer taste pore (Fig. 16.27). Type 2 cells have a lighter cytoplasm, with clear apical ends and with shorter, less numerous microvilli that terminate in the inner pore (Figs. 16.27 and 16.28). The latter type cells represent about 30% of the total cells in the bud. Type 3 cells represent approximately 7% of the taste cells and are similar to type 2 cells in appearance. Type 3 cells do not terminate in microvilli, as do types 1 and 2, but have a blunt, rounded tip that ends in the outer taste pore (Figs. 16.27 and 16.28). Type 4 cells are the basal cell located in the base of the bud (Fig. 16.27). Cell types 1, 2, and 3 reach from the base of the bud to the pore. Type 1 cells separate the other two types and are extensively in contact with each other (Fig. 16.27). Taste cells or gemma cells are generally lighter than the surrounding perigemmal epithelial cells, which are notable for their content of dense fibrils (Fig. 16.28). The nuclei of the taste cells are confined to the lower third or middle of the type 1, 2, and 3 cells. At the base, the taste bud is in contact with a basement lamina, which is in contact with the connective tissue. The taste bud opens centrally to the underlying tissue by a basal pore (Fig. 16.27).

The outer pore on the oral surface is an opening in the flattened keratinized cells. The details of a taste pore and its inner pit are seen in Figures 16.27 and 16.28. The epithelial cells surround and form the outer pore (Fig. 16.28), into the surface of which the microvilli of the dark cells (type 1) extend. The inner taste pore is a ring. Its walls are formed by the apices of the type 1 cells and the floor by the apices of the type 2 cells (Figs. 16.27–16.29). Type 3 blunt-ending cells extend through the inner pore to a position close to the surface of the outer pore (Fig. 16.29). The pit and inner pore are filled with a dense substance that appears to be similar to the granules seen in the apical parts of the type 1 cells. Junctional complexes between the adjacent cells effectively seal the floor of the inner pit from the entrance of oral fluids and tasteable substances into the interior of the taste bud. Tasteable substances therefore absorb onto the surface of microvilli membranes, which causes depolarization of the taste-bud cells. The depolarization causes generation of an action potential in the afferent nerve fibers.

Taste Receptor Nerve Supply

Taste reception for the anterior two-thirds of the tongue (fungiform papillae) is carried by the facial nerve (chorda tympani fibers). The circumvallate and foliate papillae and the posterior third of the tongue receive innervation from the ninth cranial nerve (glossopharyngeal). Taste buds in the soft palate are innervated by the greater petrosal nerve, a branch of the seventh cranial nerve. Those in the walls of the pharynx and epiglottis relay their taste impulses by way of the 10th cranial nerve (vagus) (Fig. 16.**30**). All taste fibers from these three cranial nerves converge in the tractus solitarius in the brainstem (Fig. 16.**30**). Gustatory nerves are responsive to the four basic taste modalities, to some degree but there are basic differences in levels of sensitivity. The lateral parts of the body of the tongue comprise a receptive zone of the seventh nerve. The more anterior part of this zone is sensitive to sweetness and saltiness, and the posterior portion to sourness.

Nerve fibers to the taste cells arise from nerve plexus in the underlying connective tissue and enter the taste bud through the basal pore as shown in Figure 16.**31**. One nerve fiber may supply four or five papillae, or many nerve fibers may supply a single papillae (Fig. 16.**31**). This may explain some of the overlap in levels of sensitivity to various tastes. The total number of nerve fibers found in a taste bud far exceeds the number of nerves entering a taste bud. This means that there is a high degree of branching of the terminal portion of the taste-receptor fibers (Fig. 16.**32**). Some axons are noted to contact type 1 cells in the basal region, whereas others spiral around the taste cells into the apical regions of the bud. No typical synapses are seen with the nerves and types 1 and 2 cells, and this is called a diffuse relationship (Fig. 16.**33**). A chemical synapse is seen with type 3 cells, however, and this is known as a direct relationship (Fig. 16.**33**). Observe in Figure 16.**33** the light or dark vesicles adjacent to the nerve ending (arrow), indicating the presence of neurotransmitter substance. Thus, the type 3 cell may be the taste receptor cell, or there may be two types of pathways, one that relates to type 1 and 2 (diffuse) cells and one that is a direct chemical pathway in type 3 cells.

Although there is evidence of taste-cell turnover, the nerve fibers in the taste bud are permanent. It is unlikely that there is a continual shifting of the taste cells during which their relation with the nerves is maintained.

Nerves are important to the maintenance of the taste cells. Resection of nerves to the taste buds in experimental animals results in degeneration and loss of taste cells. This occurs rapidly, with disorganization of cells seen after 2 days, and with the disappearance of most taste buds by 7 days. A few taste cells persist for longer periods, up to 14 days. After the nerve supply is re-established to the area, taste cells reappear and function

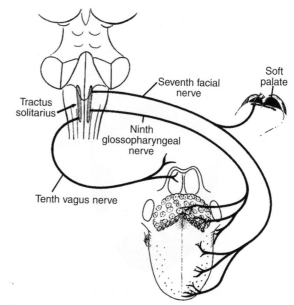

Fig. 16.**30** Nerves from anterior and posterior tongue, epiglottis, and soft palate lead to the tractus solitarius in the braistem.

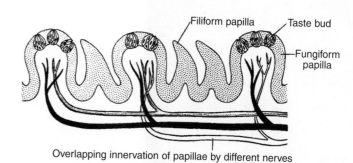

Fig. 16.**31** Innervation of taste buds. One nerve supplies several papillae. A second nerve may supply the same papillae.

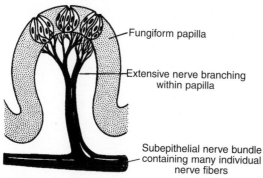

Fig. 16.**32** Branching of nerve fibers in fungiform papilla.

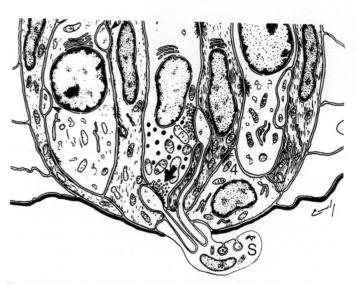

Fig. 16.**33** Nerve and taste cell relation. Large arrow: chemical synapse. Small arrow: diffuse relations. 4: basal cell. S: Schwann cell.

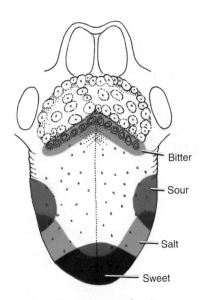

Fig. 16.**34** Location of taste perception in oral cavity.

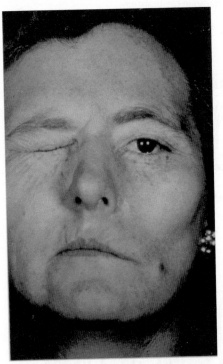

Fig. 16.**35** Appearance of patient with Bell's palsy.

returns. The pattern of cell renewal suggested by these studies is that new epithelial cells originate from the lateral boundaries of the bud. As differentiation occurs, the three main cell types form in the central regions.

Taste Receptor Function

Classically, four taste modalities have been recorded: sweet, salty, sour, and bitter. They are perceived to some extent in different localities on the tongue and oropharynx (Fig. 16.**34**). Concentrations are a factor, as at low levels bitter taste has a slightly lower threshold on the front of the tongue. At higher concentrations, a bitter stimulus is more notable at the posterior of the tongue. Perception of water taste is believed to be due to a process of adaptation, and electric taste is recognized when one touches two dissimilar metals to the tongue. No separate receptors have been located for any of the four basic taste modalities, or water or electric.

Mixing the four basic modalities cannot account for every flavor we are capable of experiencing. Factors such as temperature and odor also contribute to flavor determination. All taste buds appear to be able to detect subtleties in taste, such as the difference between citric and acetic acid or between lactose and fructose. This illustrates a discriminatory ability within taste cells, as they can identify substances even when they are mixed. Investigations have shown that taste buds possess a wide spectrum of enzymes. As tasteable substances absorb on the microvilli membranes, they may function in depolarization of the taste cell, which, in turn, generates the action potential in the close-lying nerves.

Clinical Application

Patients with Bell's palsy, which results in paralysis of the seventh cranial nerve, are sometimes encountered in the dental office (Fig. 16.35). Various causes of this condition include an injection, trauma and iatrogenically induced lesions, and anesthesia, all of which can be disconcerting to the patient. Slurred speech, drooping facial musculature, and reduced ability to eat or drink are some of the signs of this disease. Fortunately for the patient, the effects of Bell's palsy is usually limited from a few weeks to 2 months.

Summary

The oral mucosa is richly innervated with sensory nerve endings and receptors that provide a significant role in the perception of pain (nociceptors), temperature (thermoreceptors), and touch (mechanoreceptors) (Fig. 16.**37**). A substantial number of receptopathetic nerves also contribute to vascular tone and possibly to the perception of pain. The cranial nerves supplying the oral cavity originate from the trigeminal facial glossopharyngeal and vagus nerves. Mechanoreceptors for touch and pressure include Meissner's corpuscles, Merkel's corpuscles, and simple coiled corpuscles. Meissner's corpuscles adapt rapidly whereas Merkel's corpuscles adapt slowly. Free nerve endings are characterized as thermoreceptors and nociceptors. Superficial and deep nerve plexuses also are located in the oral mucosa. They provide collateral pathways for the innervation of sensory receptors. Table 16.**2** provides a summary for various sensation types in the oral cavity.

Taste buds are small, ovoid neuroepithelial structures located primarily on the dorsal and lateral surfaces of the tongue and oropharynx. They are located in fungiform, circumvallate, and foliate papillae and function in tasting sweet, salt, sour, and bitter tastes. Taste buds are goblet-shaped clusters of four types of cells. Type 1 (dark) cells are long and thin and represent the majority of the taste cells. Type 2 cells contain no dark granules and represent about 30% of the cells, and type 3 cells represent about 7% of the taste cells and exhibit chemical synapses with the nerve endings. Type 4 are basal cells whose function is not understood. Type 3 cells show evidence of neural reception of taste. There are about 14 000 taste buds in the human oropharynx. It is believed that the sense of smell makes an important contribution to taste.

Clinical Application

Trigeminal neuralgia or tic douloureux is one of the most painful conditions associated with the head and neck. Although the cause of this disease is not totally understood, it is thought to be due to a relatively poor blood supply to the trigeminal ganglion. Another hypothesis is that following abnormal nerve healing, trigger zones are created at tooth extraction sites. The severe pain associated with this disease usually originates along the distribution of the specific sensory nerve to the area. Herpes simplex 1 and herpes zoster (varicella zoster) are two diseases that may be manifested in the oral mucous membranes (Fig. 16.**36**). These viruses enter the body either through direct sexual contact or by abrasions of the skin or mucous membrane. The virus then migrates, via a sensory nerve, to the sensory ganglion and eventually resides in the trigeminal ganglion. During times of stress or debilitation, the virus travels anterogradely to the nerve terminal to infect adjacent epithelial cells, with resultant formation of multiple painful vesicles that rupture and then heal usually in 9 to 14 days. Both viruses are found over part or all of the distribution of the sensory divisions of the trigeminal nerve.

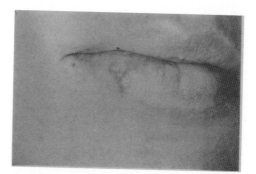

Fig. 16.**36** Appearance of herpes simplex 1 lesion.

Self-Evaluation Review

1. List the types of nerve endings found in the oral mucosa. Where are they located?
2. Describe the general somatic afferent innervation of the oral mucosa.
3. What functions are assigned to free nerve endings?
4. Briefly characterize corpuscular receptors.
5. What plexus has an abundance of autonomic fibers?
6. Discuss the location and number of taste buds in the adult. Do these change in number during life?
7. Describe the several kinds of cells of the taste bud.
8. What nerves carry taste impulses from the oral cavity?
9. What happens if you resect a nerve to a taste bud?
10. Locate the greatest number of pain, heat, cold, and touch receptors in the oral cavity.

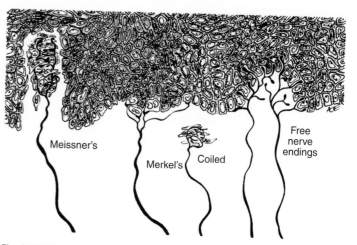

Fig. 16.**37** Summary diagram of appearance of various nerve endings in oral mucosa.

Acknowledgements

I wish to acknowledge the contribution of Professor Raymond G Murray, Department of Anatomy, University of Indiana, School of Medicine, who read and assisted with the section on taste for the first edition, and contributed Figures 16.26–6.29 and Figure 16.**33**. I further wish to acknowledge the contributions of Professor Robert M Bradley, DDS, who reviewed the first and third editing of the text on taste and contributed Figures 16.**31** and 16.**32**.

Suggested Readings

Alvarez Arenal A, Fodriguez Gonzalez MA,Villa Virgil A, et al. Lingual neurons: Localization, morphology and possible functional significance. Advances en Odontoestomatologia. 1989;5(3):113–116.

Barr ML, Kierman JA. The Human Nervous System An Anatomical Viewpoint. 6th ed. Philadelphia, Pa: Lippincott; 1993:35–45.

Bradley RM. Basic Oral Physiology. Chicago, III: Yearbook; 1981.

Dubner R, Sessle BJ, Storey AT. The Neural Basis of Oral and Facial Function. New York, NY.: Plenum Press; 1978.

Jacobson EB, Dinstad I, Heyeraas KJ. Nerve fibers immunoreactive to calcitonin gene-related peptide, substance P, neuropeptide Y and dopamine beta-hydroxylase in innervated and deneverated oral tissues in ferrets. Acta Odontol. Scand. 1998;556(4):220–228.

Kruger L, Mantyh P. Gustatory and related chemosensory systems. In: Bjorklund A, Hokfelt T, Swanson LW, eds. Handbook of Chemical Neuroanatomy. Vol. 7. Integrated systems of the CN.S., Part II. Amsterdam: Elsevier; 1989.

Masonobe T, Tankere F, Lamas G, et al. Reflexes Elicited from Cutaneous and Mucosal Trigeminal Afferents in Normal Human Subjects. Brain Res. 1998;810(1–2):220-228.

Mori H, Ishida-Yamamoto A, Senba E, Ueda Y, Tohyama M. Calcitonin gene-related peptide containing neurons innervating both pulp and buccal mucosa in the rat: an immunohistochemical analysis. J. Chem. Neuroanat. 1990;3(3):155–163.

Oakley B. Neuronal-epithelial interactions in mammalian gustatory epithelium. In: Regeneration of Vertebrate Sensory Receptor Cells. Chichester: Wiley; 1991:277–287.

Palay SL. The general architecture of sensory neuroepithelia. In: Regeneration of Vertebrate Sensory Receptor Cells. Chichester: Wiley; 1991:3–24.

Rustioni A, Weinberg RJ. The somotosensory system. In: Bjorklund A, Hokfelt T, Swanson LW, eds. Handbook of Chemical Neuroanatomy. Vol. 7. Integrated systems of the CN.S., Part II. Amsterdam: Elsevier; 1989.

Tachibana T, Sakakura Y, Ishizekl K, Lida Sawa T. An Experimental study of the influence of sensory nerves on Merkel cell differentiation in the labial mucosa of the rabbits. Archivum Histogicum-Japonicum-Nippon Soshik igaku Kiroku. 1983;46(4):469–477.

Tuisku F, Hildebrand C. Combined Retrograde Tracing and Immunohistochemistry of Trigeminal Ganglion Neurons Projecting to Gingiva or Tooth Pulps in Lower jaw of the Cichilid Tilaipia Mariae. J. Neurocytol. 1997;26(1):33–40.

SECTION V
Structure of the Glands of the Oral Cavity and Their Products

17 Development, Structure, and Function of the Salivary Glands

Robert M. Klein

Introduction

The human salivary glands are important organs of the oral cavity that produce saliva, an essential fluid required for normal speech, taste, mastication, swallowing, and digestion. Saliva functions in the maintenance of oral health through its antimicrobial, cleansing, lubricating, and buffering functions as well as its role in digestion. While the functions of saliva will be discussed in Chapter 18, the purpose of this chapter is to discuss the development, structure, and function of the major and minor salivary glands in health and disease. From an educational point of view, the salivary glands provide an opportunity to review basic developmental and cell biologic concepts. The salivary glands are an excellent model for the developmental process of branching that forms the infrastructure of these glands. The chapter also reviews the secretory pathway from reading of the genetic material in the nucleus to release of secretory product, since the proteins found in the saliva represent an ideal model of packaging of materials for secretion. Regulatory pathways, including signal transduction mechanisms, are discussed in the chapter as part of the overall description of secretion. Finally, some of the diseases that affect the salivary glands are discussed briefly to provide a clinical framework for the oral biology of salivary glands discussed in this chapter.

Objectives

After reading this chapter you should be able to describe the embryologic development of the salivary glands, list the six developmental stages, and describe how the ECM influences the developmental processes of morphogenesis and differentiation. You should also be able to describe the developmental regulation of salivary gland position, branching, and cytodifferentiation. In addition, you should be able to classify the salivary glands according to morphologic and functional criteria as well as describe the histology (light microscopy and ultrastructure) of the salivary glands, including the acinar and duct components. For the section dealing with saliva formation, you should be able to describe primary saliva formation and its modification by the duct system, as well as list the transport systems used by acinar and duct cells to form the saliva. The cell biology of the regulation of the acinar cell is discussed in this chapter. You should be able to describe the secretory pathways (regulated and constitutive) within an acinar cell, including transcription, translation, and post-translational events in the endoplasmic reticulum, Golgi apparatus, and secretory vesicles. Moreover, you should be able to describe the cell biologic events involved in the development of secretory immunity (the synthesis of immunoglobulin A [IgA] and secretory component) and G protein regulation of cyclic AMP- and Ca^{++}-mediated signal transduction pathways. Finally, you should be able to: describe the innervation of the salivary glands and the influence of the parasympathetic and sympathetic nervous systems on the synthesis and secretion of saliva; describe the pharmacology of salivary gland secretion, including the action of α- and β-receptors, and give examples of the pathologic alterations and aging changes that occur in the salivary glands.

Development of the Salivary Glands

General Developmental Processes

Epithelial–Mesenchymal Interactions
The development of glandular tissue in mammals involves interactions of the epithelium with the underlying mesenchyme to form the functional part of the gland. These epithelial–mesenchymal interactions are defined by developmental biologists as proximate tissue interactions—also known as secondary induction—in which the presence of mesenchyme in close proximity to the epithelium is required for the normal development of the epithelium. For example, epithelial–mesenchymal interactions regulate both the initiation and growth of the glandular tissue and the eventual cytodifferentiation of cells within the salivary glands. The mesenchyme, therefore, is required for normal development as well as formation of the supporting part of the adult gland.

Mesenchyme

Extracellular matrix (ECM) and basal lamina.
Mesenchyme is composed of undifferentiated pluripotential connective-tissue cells (e.g., fibroblasts, mast cells, and macrophages) and ECM. The ECM consists of the glycosaminoglycans (GAGs) and proteoglycans that give a gel–like characteristic to the ECM. The GAGs (e.g., chondroitin sulfate, keratan sulfate) are bound to a core protein to form proteoglycan subunits. The subunits are noncovalently bound to hyaluronic acid (another GAG) to form the bristle brush–like structure of the proteoglycan aggregate found in the ECM. The proteoglycans carry out a number of important functions in the ECM. They form the hydrated ground substance, but also function in filtration (e.g., the renal glomerular basement membrane), and bind signaling molecules such as growth factors in close proximity to their target cells. The collagens

comprise the fibrous component that establishes the tensile strength of the ECM. The adhesive properties of the ECM can be attributed primarily to two glycoproteins: laminin and fibronectin that are found in the basal lamina under epithelia and the surrounding ECM respectively.

The basal lamina is a supramolecular mat underlying the epithelium; it is composed of type IV collagen, glycoproteins such as laminin, nidogen/entactin, and proteoglycans. Laminin and entactin are glycoproteins that interact with each other and specifically with other components of the ECM through their receptors, a family of transmembrane linker proteins, known as the integrins. The integrins are critical molecules in the development and function of organs because they are the means of linkage and communication between cells and the ECM. They allow communication across the plasma membrane from the inside to the outside of the cell. One of the most important integrins is the fibronectin receptor found as a transmembrane glycoprotein. It has connections to both the cytoskeleton of the cell and the ECM through specific regions, or domains, which allow the cell to communicate from its intracellular environment (cytoskeleton) to its extracellular environment (fibronectin). Integrins such as fibronectin receptor and laminin receptor allow cell matrix interactions while the intracellular adhesion molecules (ICAMs) facilitate cell–cell communication by linking the ECM to the cytoskeleton within the cell cytoplasm. This linkage is crucial for changes in cell shape, motility, migration, proliferation, and differentiation all of which occur during salivary gland development.

The basal lamina is secreted by the epithelium; it serves supportive and filtering functions and also regulates migration, polarity, and differentiation of epithelial cells. The surrounding ECM is synthesized by connective-tissue cells and contains ECM molecules such as collagen types I and III, the glycoproteins fibronectin and tenascin, and GAGs like chondroitin sulfate which are assembled into proteoglycans. The components of the basal lamina and surrounding ECM therefore differ in the types of glycoproteins and proteoglycans present.

Influence of the ECM on Development. The ECM provides regulatory cues for cell proliferation, cell differentiation, and morphogenesis, the major developmental processes required for the formation of adult salivary gland structure. Cell proliferation is the increase in number of cells that occurs during development as organs enlarge and also in cell replacement systems (e.g., gastrointestinal epithelium) throughout life. Proliferating cells enter the cell cycle, replicate their DNA and subsequently undergo cytokinesis to form two progeny (i. e., daughter cells). These cells may either undergo specialization or remain as part of a dividing or stem cell population that continues to proliferate. Differentiation describes those processes responsible for the development of cell specificity and diversity as observed at the morphologic or molecular level. Differentiated cells express a specific portion of the genome that is characteristic of that particular cell type. Morphogenesis describes those developmental processes that are responsible for the formation of the shape and form of an organ. Morphogenesis is a developmental process that requires several other developmental processes such as cell proliferation and migration. Glandular branching, as occurs in the developing salivary glands, is one of the best examples of a morphogenetic process. Morphogenesis and differentiation are independent, yet concurrent processes required for the development of adult architecture and specificity of cell types, respectively.

General Developmental Pattern of the Salivary Glands

All salivary glands follow a similar developmental pattern. The functional glandular tissue (parenchyma) develops as an epithelial outgrowth (glandular bud) of the buccal epithelium that invades the underlying mesenchyme. The connective-tissue stroma (capsule and septa) and blood vessels form from the mesenchyme. The mesenchyme is composed of cells derived from neural crest and is essential for the normal differentiation of the salivary glands. However, as mentioned previously, it is the ECM components, synthesized by mesenchymal connective-tissue cells, which provide important signals that direct the morphogenesis and differentiation of the glandular bud.

Bud Formation and Gland Origin

As the epithelial bud forms during development, those portions of the bud closest to the stomodeum (primitive oral cavity) eventually differentiate into the main excretory duct of the gland, while the most distal portions arborize to form the terminal portions of the duct system, the secretory end pieces or acini. The origin of the epithelial buds is believed to be ectodermal in the parotid and minor salivary glands and endodermal in the submandibular and sublingual glands. The breakdown of the oropharyngeal (buccopharyngeal) membrane during the fourth week of development, however, permits the intermingling of stomodeal ectoderm and cranial foregut endoderm, which complicates the identification of specific germ layer origin of the salivary glands.

The parotid glands originate near the corners of the stomodeum by the sixth week of prenatal life. The submandibular glands arise from the floor of the mouth at the end of the sixth or the beginning of the seventh week in utero. The sublingual glands form lateral to the submandibular primordia at about the eighth week. The sites of origin of the major salivary glands are shown in Figure 17.**1**, which is a composite diagram representing multiple serial sections. All minor salivary glands form from the epithelium, but do not begin to develop until the twelfth prenatal week.

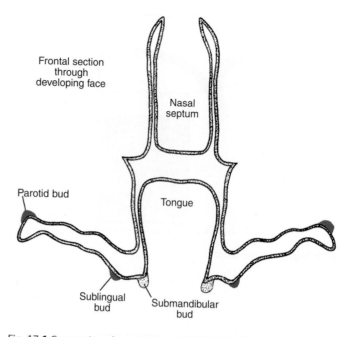

Fig. 17.**1** Composite schematic diagram of the origin of the salivary glands from multiple serial sections (frontal view). The parotid glands originate near the corners of the stomodeum (developing oral cavity), the submandibular glands arise from the floor of the mouth, and the sublingual glands originate lateral to the submandibular primordia.

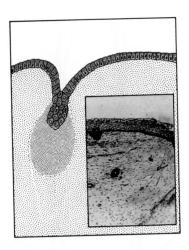

Fig. 17.**2** Stage I, bud formation.

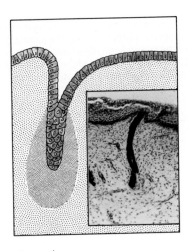

Fig. 17.**3** Stage II, cord growth.

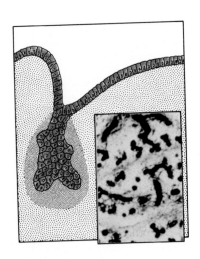

Fig. 17.**4** Stage III, branching of the cords.

Stages of Development

Salivary gland development may be divided into six stages.

Stage I. Formation: induction of oral epithelium by underlying mesenchyme. The mesenchyme underlying the buccal epithelium induces proliferation in the epithelium, which results in tissue thickening and formation of the epithelial bud (Fig. 17.**2**). The growing bud is separated from the condensation of mesenchyme by a basal lamina that is secreted by the epithelium. Although the site and the time of development differ slightly for the three major salivary glands, the processes involved in development are similar.

Stage II. Formation and growth of the epithelial cord. A solid cord of cells forms the epithelial bud by cell proliferation (Fig. 17.**3**). Condensation and proliferation occur in the surrounding mesenchyme that is closely associated with the epithelial cord. The basal lamina, although not visible at the magnification used for Figure 17.**3**, is found between the cord and the mesenchyme. It is composed of GAGs, collagen, and glycoproteins. The basal lamina, as well as the surrounding mesenchyme, influences morphogenesis and differentiation of the salivary glands throughout their development. The functions of the basal lamina and ECM will be discussed in more detail in the sections of this chapter dealing with the developmental processes involved in the ontogeny of the salivary glands.

Stage III. Initiation of branching in terminal parts of the epithelial cord and continuation of glandular differentiation. The epithelial cord proliferates rapidly and branches into terminal bulbs (presumptive acini). The growth in length of the solid epithelial cords and the differentiation of the berry–like terminal bulbs are shown in Figure 17.**4**.

Stage IV. Repetitive branching of the epithelial cord and lobule formation. The branching continues at the terminal portions of the cord, forming an extensive tree–like system of bulbs. This branching process is evident in Figure 17.**5**, which shows a section from a developing human salivary gland. As branching occurs, connective tissue differentiates around the branches,

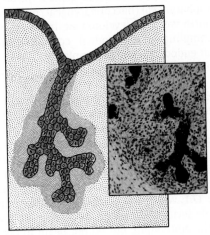

Fig. 17.**5** Stage IV, lobule formation.

eventually producing extensive lobulation. The glandular capsule forms from mesenchyme and surrounds the entire glandular parenchyma.

Stage V. Canalization of presumptive ducts. Canalization of the epithelial cord, with formation of a hollow tube or duct, usually occurs by the sixth month in all three major salivary glands (Fig. 17.**6**). Lumens appear first in the proximal (oral, terminal) and distal portions of the main excretory duct and in the branch ducts, then in the mid-portion of the main duct, and lastly in the acini, all of which precede the formation of the secretory granules. Lumen development occurs as a result of the formation of tight junctions (zonulae occludens) among the cells surrounding what was initially a simpler intercellular space. Extensive branching of the duct structure and growth of connective-tissue septa continue at this stage of development (Fig. 17.**6**).

Stage VI. Cytodifferentiation. The final morphologic stage of salivary gland development is the cytodifferentiation of the functional acini and intercalated ducts. During this period, mitotic activity shifts from the entire epithelial cord to the terminal bulb portions. Cells of the bulb region are the stem cells that undergo cell proliferation and subsequent differentiation into acinar cells as well as duct cells (Figs. 17.**7A** and **B**). Myoepithelial cells also arise from epithelial stem cells in the terminal bulbs of the developing duct system and develop in concert with acinar cytodifferentiation. Maturation of the acinar cells occurs in specific stages classified according to the morphology of secretory granules and cellular organelles. Acinar development differs for serous and mucous cells. Therefore, the parotid, submandibular, and sublingual salivary glands show variation in cytodifferentiation patterns. Terminal bulb cells eventually differentiate into the intercalated duct cells of the adult glands and serve as a stem cell for acinar, myoepithelial, and ductal cells (Fig. 17.**7B**). Secretagogue stimulus-secretion coupling mechanisms and innervation of the gland continue to mature following cytodifferentiation.

Processes Involved in Salivary Gland Development

General

Development of the salivary glands is influenced by intrinsic and extrinsic factors that regulate the processes of cell proliferation, differentiation, and morphogenesis. The intrinsic factors are defined as the preprogrammed pattern of gene expression specific for each cell type. Following this preprogrammed script, with genes turned on and turned off at appropriate times, leads to the normal development and growth of tissues and organs and the differentiation of cells. Extrinsic factors are signals provided by cell–cell and cell–matrix interactions as well as by cytokines, hormones, and growth factors in the extracellular milieu. The extrinsic factors define boundaries between groups of cells during development.

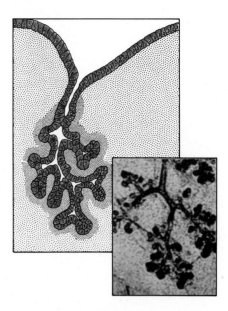

Fig. 17.**6** Stage V, canalization of cords to form ducts.

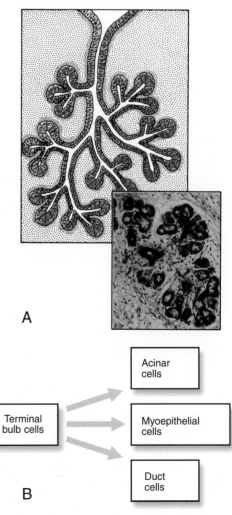

A

B

Fig. 17.**7 A** Stage VI, cytodifferentiation. **B** Schematic diagram illustrating the origin of myoepithelial, acinar, and ductal cells from the terminal bulb cells, which function as stem cells during development, adulthood, and following injury.

The fruit fly (Drosophila) has been used as a model of embryonic development. In that system, there is a shift during development between three categories of genes. Maternal genes are expressed during oogenesis by the mother and act during oocyte maturation. Maternal genes define broad regions within the egg. They regulate the expression of segmentation genes that determine the number and/or polarity of segments. The segmentation genes effectively define smaller regions of the embryo. The last group of genes are the homeotic genes that regulate the development of one body part compared to another. A regulatory cascade determines the pattern of gene and transcription factor expression during formation of specific organs such as the salivary glands. Homologous genes to those identified in Drosophila are being identified in mammalian development with remarkable conservation of structure and regulatory functions.

Positioning of the Glands

Little is known about the regulation of salivary gland position in vertebrates. Much of the information about organ positioning during development has been obtained from studies of Drosophila. In Drosophila polarity is established initially along an anterior→posterior (head→tail) axis that establishes the segmentation of the embryo. Further development within each segment establishes a dorsal→ventral (back→abdomen) gradient that is translated into specialized structures in each segment of the larva and eventually the adult segmented fly. The formation of specialized structures in each segment (e.g., the formation of salivary glands) is regulated by homeotic genes. These genes contain a homeobox domain that is a 60-amino acid, DNA-binding domain. In Drosophila, the gene Sex combs reduced (Scr) is a homeotic gene that encodes a transcription factor responsible for the location of the salivary glands. Scr is uniformly transcribed in the cells of the posterior head segment where the Drosophila salivary glands will develop. In transgenic flies, overexpression of Scr results in salivary gland development at ectopic sites. In knockout flies, where Scr is not expressed, the salivary glands fail to form. Protein products of other genes establish the limits of salivary gland development by inhibiting the expression of Scr. The dorsal and ventral boundaries of salivary-gland formation in Drosophila are established by genes homologous to mammalian genes, such as bone morphogenetic protein-4 (BMP-4).

The relationship of Scr and Drosophila salivary gland development to mammalian salivary gland morphogenesis remains unclear. The correct patterning of vertebrate embryos is based upon the appropriate expression of Hox genes. The expression and restriction of Hox genes are responsible for the differentiation of cells along the anterior–posterior axis of all metazoans. Hox gene expression occurs in the vertebrate nervous system and its derivatives, including the neural crest cells. The neural crest is instrumental in the formation of the salivary glands, teeth, and the overall craniofacial morphology through the formation and differentiation of the branchial arches. Scr, the gene that regulates salivary gland positioning in Drosophila is homologous to one of the Hox genes, but the role of its homologue in mammalian salivary gland development remains unclear. In other branching organs such as the lung, branching morphogenesis, cell–cell and cell–matrix communication, cell fate, and cell differentiation appear to be regulated by the Hox genes.

The homology between the genes that restrict Drosophila salivary gland position and mammalian genes is also of current research interest. BMP-4 is known to regulate downstream events in other differentiating mammalian organs such as the teeth. The teeth are formed and differentiate through reciprocal signaling between the epithelium and mesenchyme in a similar fashion to salivary gland development. It is likely that genes such as BMP-4 that limit the "permissibility" of Scr expression in Drosophila also are involved in the cascade of gene expression that regulates epithelial–mesenchymal interactions involved in branching and other morphogenetic events.

Branching of the Epithelial Cord

Branching is the primary morphogenetic process in salivary gland development. It has been studied extensively by analysis of salivary gland rudiments grown in a culture dish (in vitro). Cleft formation in distal buds initiates the branching process that is followed by epithelial proliferation (Fig. 17.**8**). Collagen type III accumulates at cleft points and appears to be critical for branching to occur (Fig. 17.**8B**). Types I and IV collagen appear to be more important for the maintenance and support of established branches (Fig. 17.**8C**). There is an increased

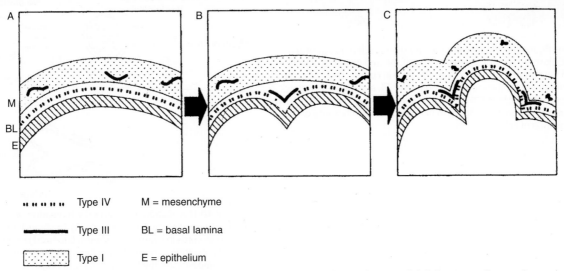

·· ·· ·· ·· Type IV	M = mesenchyme
—— Type III	BL = basal lamina
[:::::::] Type I	E = epithelium

Fig. 17.**8** Schematic drawing of cleft formation during salivary gland branching. **A**, **B**, and **C** are sequential steps during branching morphogenesis. The interaction of the mesenchyme, epithelium, and basal lamina as well as the location of collagen types I, III, and IV during development are illustrated. The removal of GAGs occurs on the basal surface of the epithelium and results in disruption of the basal lamina during cleft formation, as shown in **B**.

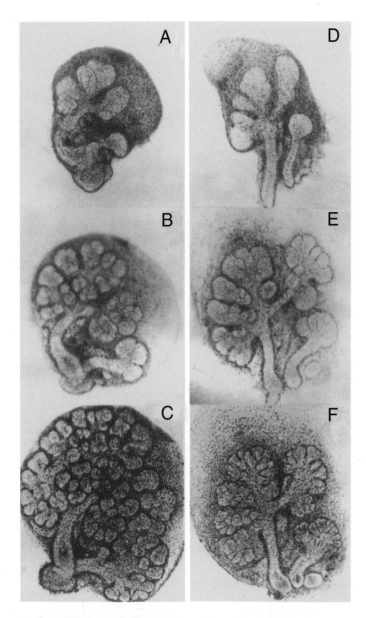

Fig. 17.**9** This figure illustrates living salivary gland rudiments in organ culture. **A–C** illustrate control rudiments after 0, 24, and 48 hours of culture. The size and number of lobules increase with time in culture. **D–F** show the effects of tunicamycin at the same time points (0, 24, and 48 hours respectively). Tunicamycin blocks N-linked glycosylation resulting in normal branching and lobule formation, but smaller, miniature lobes form because of the resulting inhibition of cell proliferation.

ratio of collagen type I: type III during in vitro branching, consistent with this concept that type I leads to stabilization while type III is more involved in active branching. More recent studies also indicate that proteoglycan biosynthesis and deposition are required for branching, but not growth of the rudiments. Chondroitin sulfates are the predominant GAGs in the basal lamina of actively branching young rudiments and appear to increase during stabilization.

The independence of epithelial expansion and branching has been demonstrated by use of tunicamycin with salivary gland rudiments in vitro. Tunicamycin inhibits N-linked glycosylation resulting in dramatically decreased protein accumulation and cell proliferation (i.e., epithelial expansion), but epithelial branching is unaffected. In the accompanying figures, control cultures are shown in Figures 17.**9A–C** and tunicamycin cultures are shown in Figures 17.**9 D–F**. After tunicamycin treatment branching occurs and lobules form normally, with inhibited cell proliferation, resulting in a smaller rudiment with miniature lobes. In contrast, the size and number of lobules increase in control cultures.

Branching and proliferation must be coordinated processes for normal development of the salivary glands to occur. Mitotic activity is normally localized in the most peripheral regions of the bud (Fig. 17.**10A**). Treatment with hyaluronidase disrupts the basal lamina

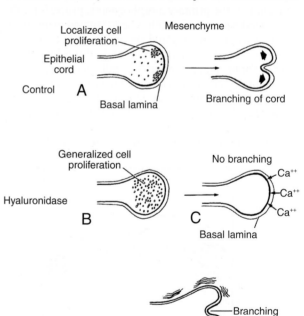

Fig. 17.**10** This diagram illustrates the regulation of branching during salivary-gland development. **(A)** The branching of salivary gland cell cords in controls are shown. Localized cell proliferation occurs, resulting in normal branching. **(B)** The effects of hyaluronidase alter the basal lamina resulting in the generalized cell proliferation and the absence of branching. The alterations of the basal lamina may result in disruption of ion fluxes that affect cell proliferation and other developmental processes **(C)**. **(D)** The normal branch point is shown resulting from appropriate cell proliferation, collagen synthesis, and collagenolytic activity.

interfering with the signal required for cleft formation. Destabilization of the basal lamina therefore inhibits cleft development, but also affects subsequent events such as cell proliferation. For example, in the absence of a normal basal lamina there is an absence of branching, and uniform cell proliferation replaces localized mitotic activity (Fig. 17.**10B**). The basal lamina is, therefore, implicated in the stabilization of the epithelium and the initiation and maintenance of lobular morphology.

The basal lamina may regulate morphogenetic changes directly or by selective filtration or channeling of materials to the epithelium. For example, the regulation of the flow of ions such as Ca^{++} (Fig. 17.**10C**) to the epithelium may alter the function of microtubules and microfilaments in cellular proliferation, migration, and arrangement. Synthesis of collagen (collagenogenic) and selective collagen breakdown (collagenolysis) play a critical role in salivary gland development. For example, collagen synthesis by the mesenchyme provides structural stabilization after branching has occurred (Fig. 17.**10D**). The stabilization appears to be provided by types I and IV collagen (Fig. 17.**8B** and **C**) that are associated with maintenance and support of the branched organization of the adult gland. In addition, collagenolytic activity in the epithelium and mesenchyme may allow for selective breakdown of the basal lamina and communication between the epithelium, basal lamina, and surrounding mesenchyme at key stages of development.

Cytodifferentiation

The interaction of the epithelium and mesenchyme is best studied in a culture dish (in vitro) where epithelium can be grown in the presence of selected components of the basal lamina and specific growth factors. Salivary gland rudiments branch in vitro in the absence of mesenchymal cells, but in the presence of other factors. A developing salivary gland epithelial rudiment is shown in Figure 17.**11A** with three clefts present at the beginning of culture. The epithelium is grown in serum with the use of an artificial matrix known as Matrigel, composed primarily of laminin, type IV collagen, heparan sulfate, entactin, and nidogen. Using this system, it has been observed that different growth factors appear to regulate distinct parts of morphogenetic process. Fibroblast growth factor (FGF) has been shown to alter stalk elongation (Figs. 17.**11C** and D), while epidermal growth factor (EGF) regulates branching (Fig. 17.**11B**) in this in vitro system. The combination of FGF and EGF (Figs. 17.**11E** and **F**) results in a morphology similar to that observed in the developing salivary gland in vivo. ECM molecules regulate the presentation and distribution of growth factors to the epithelium at appropriate times during in vivo morphogenesis. Therefore, the ECM in concert with specific growth factors appears to regulate the complex processes involved in branching morphogenesis.

The initiation of cytodifferentiation of salivary gland acinar cells is believed to be dependent on prepro-

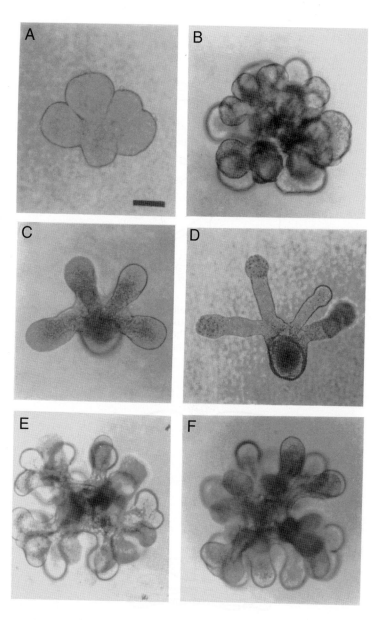

Fig. 17.**11** Submandibular gland rudiment in culture. **A** Epithelial explant with three clefts at the beginning of culture. **B** Epithelial explant grown in 10ng/ml of EGF for 2 days. Remarkable branching morphogenesis occurs with little stalk elongation following EGF. **C** and **D** show epithelial explants grown for 2 days in FGF at low and high doses, respectively. No new lobules form, but stalks extend at the base of pre-existing clefts at the higher dose **(D)**. **E** and **F** are photomicrographs of epithelial explants grown for 2 days in EGF and FGF. They differ only in the concentration of FGF. In both cases, there is lobule and stalk formation, as EGF and FGF appear to act synergistically to simulate development observed in vivo.

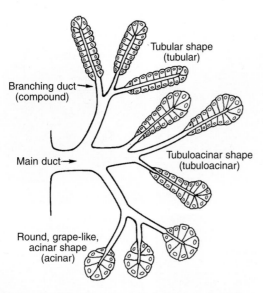

Fig. 17.**12** Diagram of the structure of a tubuloacinar gland. The end pieces are acinar (serous), tubular (mucous), or tubuloacinar (mixed, containing both serous and mucous components). The term "acinar" has become the accepted term for all end pieces despite the differences in acinar, tubular, and tubuloacinar morphology.

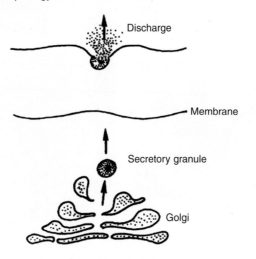

Fig. 17.**13** Diagram illustrating the merocrine secretory process in which the cell and its apical membrane remain intact during the secretory process. Secretory contents of the granules are released and membrane is recycled.

Table 17.**1** Minor salivary glands*

Name	Location	Type of secretion
Labial (superior and inferior)	Lips	Mixed (predominantly mucous)
Buccal	Cheek	Mixed (predominantly mucous)
Glossopalatine	Anterior faucial pillar Glossopalatine fold	Pure mucous
Palatine	Hard palate Soft palate Uvula	Pure mucous
Lingual (tongue)	Anterior	Mixed (predominantly mucous)
	Circumvallate papillae (von Ebner's glands)	Pure serous
	Posterior	Pure mucous

*Contribution to saliva 5—10%

grammed development occurring in early stages of morphogenesis. There is evidence, however, that secretory cell differentiation may proceed independently of mesenchymal factors. A period of in situ epithelial–mesenchymal contact is required for cytodifferentiation, and once this contact has taken place, exocrine cell differentiation occurs without continued presence of mesenchyme. Therefore, it appears that there is a "partial coupling" of the independently controlled processes of gland morphogenesis and cytodifferentiation. Full differentiation of functional secretory components is apparent at birth, but is not complete until the onset of a solid diet and the presence of masticatory stimuli.

This postnatal developmental process includes: 1) The maturation of stimulus-secretion coupling that links secretagogue-membrane receptors to signal transduction pathways within the cell and controls acinar cell secretion; and 2) the establishment of neural connections from the autonomic nervous system, the primary regulator of salivary gland function. The regulatory function of the autonomic nervous system will be discussed later in the chapter.

Classification of the Salivary Glands

The glands of the body may be classified into two general types: 1) Exocrine—those glands with a duct system to transport secretion from the glands; and 2) endocrine—those ductless glands dependent on blood supply for delivery of their secretory product(s). Salivary glands are classified as exocrine glands, but these glands are associated with a number of biologically active substances (e.g., nerve growth factor and epidermal growth factor) that may be secreted by an endocrine mechanism. The salivary glands are classified as compound tubuloacinar glands, which indicates the presence of a branched duct system and secretory units with both tubular and acinar portions (Fig. 17.**12**).

The glands of the body are also classified according to the method of secretory production. The salivary glands are merocrine glands. The term merocrine is derived from the Greek words "meros," meaning part, and "krino," meaning to separate. The classification of these glands as "partially secreting" is not completely correct, however. Salivary glands are repeatedly functional, since secretory release occurs through a process of fusion of membranous secretory vesicles (granules) with the apical plasma (cell) membrane known as exocytosis (ex = out of, osis = process). The process of storage of secretory product in membrane-bound vesicles coupled with the insertion of vesicular membrane into the apical membrane (Fig. 17.**13**) of the cell preserves the vesicular contents and conserves cell membrane. The vesicular membrane that is added to the apical membrane is later recycled through endocytosis for reutilization in the formation of new secretory vesicles.

The salivary glands of mammalian species may be divided into major and minor salivary glands. The major salivary glands produce most of the 0.5 to 0.75L of saliva produced daily. These three glands are located apart from the oral cavity with which they communicate by large excretory ducts. There are three pairs of major salivary glands: the parotid, the submandibular (formerly submaxillary), and the sublingual glands. The minor salivary glands are found in the oral cavity and are named according to their location: buccal, labial, lingual, palatine, and glossopalatine. The names of the glands are based on their location, with the exception of those named as eponyms (i.e., Von Ebner's glands). Thus, the parotid is "around the ear," sublingual is "under the tongue," submandibular is "under the mandible," buccal are in the buccal mucosa, and palatal are in the mucosa of the palate. Additionally, the salivary glands may be classified by types of secretion: serous, mucous, and mixed. Mucous secretion produces mucins, which act as a lubricant to aid in mastication, deglutition, and digestion. Serous secretion contains water, enzymes (primarily salivary amylase and some maltase), a variety of salts, and organic ions. The parotid gland is an example of a purely serous secreting gland, the palatine glands are purely mucous, and the submandibular and sublingual glands are mixed-type glands (Tables 17.**1** and 17.**2**).

The serous component of the saliva aids in mastication and the removal of debris from the oral cavity; however, its digestive potential in the breakdown of carbohydrates has been debated because of the short period of

Table 17.**2** Major salivary glands

Gland	Size	Location	Capsule	Type of secretion	Approximate contribution to saliva (%)	Striated ducts
Parotid	Largest	Anterior to ear	Extensive	Purely serous in adult, predominantly serous in newborn	25	Long
Submandibular	Intermediate	Beneath the mandible near the angle	Extensive	Predominantly serous	60	Longer than in parotid
Sublingual	Smallest	Anterior floor of the mouth	Minimal	Predominantly mucous	5	Very short

Intercalated ducts	Sympathetic innervation (vasomotor)	Parasympathetic innervation (secretomotor)		Blood Supply	
		Preganglionic	Postganglionic	Arterial	Venous
Long and narrow	Postganglionics via superior cervical ganglion (SCG)	Inferior salivatory nucleus→ninth nerve	Otic ganglion→ auriculo-temporal nerve→gland	Branches of external carotid artery	Veins generally follow the course of the arteries
Shorter than in parotid	Postganglionics via SCG	Superior salivatory nucleus→chorda tympani of seventh nerve	Submandibular ganglion→gland	Branches of facial and lingual artery	Same as for parotid gland
Inconspicuous	Postganglionics via SCG	Superior salivatory nucleus→chorda tympani of seventh nerve	Submandibular ganglion→gland	Sublingual and submental artery	Same as for parotid gland

time between chewing and the entrance of foods into the esophagus and stomach. However, there is strong evidence for a digestive role for saliva. Following a meal, the pH in the stomach remains in a range (6.7–7.5) that allows activity of amylase, DNAse, and other enzymes. In humans, the gastric acidity/juice penetrates the large bolus of food slowly enough to allow ample time for activity of amylase and lipase (another enzymatic component of saliva that breaks down fats). These phenomena have the effect of aiding the overall digestive process by: 1) breaking down globs of food to starch/sucrose/lipid 2) facilitating access to the inner portions of the bolus by gastric and intestinal juices, and 3) aiding in the clearance and swallowing of food stuck to the teeth and oral mucosa.

The Major Salivary Glands

The locations of the major salivary glands in an adult human are shown in Figure 17.**14**. The parotid, which is the largest gland, is located anterior to the external acoustic meatus and mastoid process, inferior to the zygomatic arch, lateral and posterior to the ramus of the mandible, and on the surface of the masseter muscle. Anatomically, the parotid gland is closely associated with the facial nerve, external carotid artery, superficial temporal and maxillary veins, and numerous cervical lymph nodes. The relation of the gland to the facial nerve begins early in fetal development (Fig. 17.**15** shows anatomic relations at about 10 weeks of prenatal age).

The parotid (Stensen's) duct extends from the lateral surface of the gland, anteriorly, across the masseter muscle and the buccal fat pad. At the anterior border of the masseter, it bends medially at a sharp angle, piercing the fat pad and buccinator muscle to open into the oral cavity in a papilla opposite the crown of the second maxillary molar tooth. The epithelium of the duct becomes continuous with the mucous membrane of the mouth.

The submandibular gland is located medial to, and under partial cover of, the mandible. It is closely associated with the mylohyoid and medial pterygoid muscles, sub-

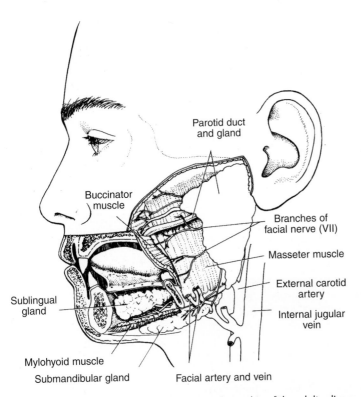

Fig. 17.**14** Diagram illustrating the anatomic relationship of the adult salivary glands and associated head and neck structures.

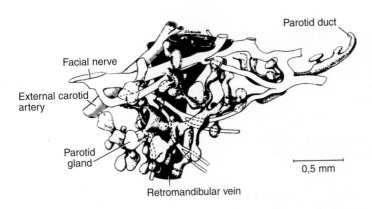

Fig. 17.**15** Relation of the branches of the facial nerve to the developing human fetal parotid gland.

mandibular lymph nodes, and facial arteries and veins. The submandibular (Wharton's) duct extends anteriorly, in the floor of the mouth, to open into the oral cavity at the sublingual papilla at the side of the frenulum of the tongue.

The sublingual is the smallest of the major salivary glands and is located beneath the mucous membrane of the floor of the mouth. Although the parotid and submandibular glands are encased in an extensive connective-tissue capsule, the sublingual gland lacks a distinct capsule. Compared with the parotid and the submandibular, the sublingual consists of a large portion and collection of small glands rather than a single, clearly delineated gland. The main excretory duct of the sublingual gland (Bartholin's) may join the submandibular duct or open into the oral cavity with a separate sublingual papilla. Numerous smaller sublingual ducts (Ducts of Rivinus) may join the submandibular duct or open separately into the floor of the mouth.

General Structural Plan of the Salivary Glands

The general arrangement of the glands is similar to the arrangement of grapes on a vine (Fig. 17.**16**), with the stems representing the branching duct system of the compound glands and the grapes representing acini composed of five to seven secretory acinar cells. Figure 17.**17** illustrates the general structural plan of a compound tubuloacinar gland. There are three types of secretory end-pieces: serous, mucous, and mixed (both serous and mucous). There also are several types of ducts: intercalated and striated ducts, which are described as intralobular (within a lobule), and interlobular (excretory) ducts (between lobules). Surrounding and supporting the duct and secretory system is a capsule of connective tissue (more extensive in the parotid and submandibular glands) that extends into the glands as septa dividing the parenchyma into lobes and lobules. The connective tissue is essential both as a framework for support of the glands and as a conduit for nerves (primarily autonomic), blood vessels, and lymphatics. The

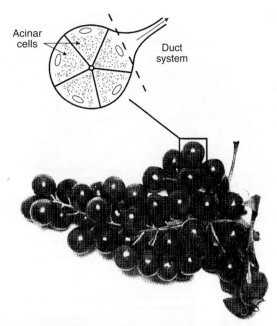

Fig. 17.**16** The structure of an acinar-exocrine gland. Photograph of grapes on a vine. This arrangement is analogous to the acinar structure found in the salivary glands. The grapes represent acini, each composed of five to seven acinar cells (see inset). The secretion of the acinar cells is released into the duct system (represented by the vine). The vine extends from the acini to the oral cavity, where the salivary secretions are released into the oral cavity as saliva to aid in digestion. The connective tissue of the gland capsule and septa surrounds and divides the gland into separate lobules. Myoepithelial cells surround the acini and squeeze the secretion out of the acinus following neural stimulation.

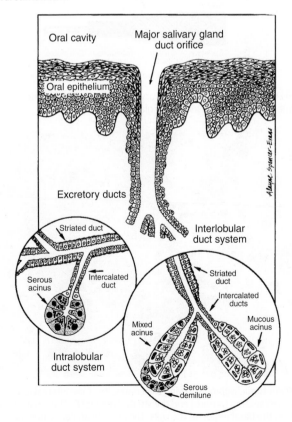

Fig. 17.**17** Histologic plan of a compound tubuloacinar gland (e.g., the major salivary glands) including the duct system leading to the oral cavity.

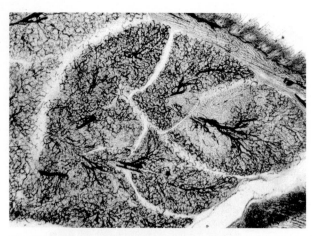

Fig. 17.**18** Photomicrograph illustrating the histology of a salivary-gland lobule following microvascular injection of dye to illustrate the distribution of blood vessels.

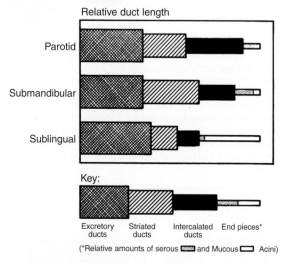

Fig. 17.**19** Diagram comparing the salivary-gland duct system in the human parotid, submandibular, and sublingual glands.

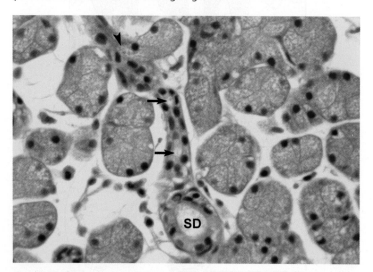

Fig. 17.**20** Photomicrograph showing the continuity of the intercalated duct shown in cross section (arrows) and the striated duct (SD). The striations are not visible in the basal region of the cells. The arrowhead delineates the point at which the intercalated duct (in longitudinal section) can be observed draining an acinus.

pattern and extent of the vascular supply of the salivary glands is demonstrated in Figure 17.**18**, which shows rat parotid gland injected with a dye such as India ink. The injection reveals how the larger vessels enter each lobe at one point and branch to supply each lobule. The duct system of the salivary glands drains the lobules and lobes in a similar manner.

Duct System

The duct system differs in each of the major salivary glands (see Table 17.**1**). Figure 17.**19** illustrates the differences in the ductal distribution between the parotid, submandibular, and sublingual glands. The duct system has two main structural parts: the intralobular and the interlobular portions. Intralobular ducts are of two types: intercalated and striated (secretory). The other portion of the duct system is termed the excretory ducts. In Figure 17.**19**, the excretory ducts are indicated by cross-hatched areas, striated ducts by the striped areas, and intercalated ducts by darkly shaded areas. The secretory portions or end pieces are either mucous (unshaded), serous (spotted), or mixed. The intercalated ducts are longest in the parotid, intermediate in the submandibular, and shortest in the sublingual glands. The sublingual glands have the fewest number of intralobular ducts, since both striated and intercalated ducts are very short.

Histology and Function of the Duct System

Intercalated ducts are the first (most distal) element of the intralobular duct system, are lined by a low cuboidal epithelium (Figs. 17.**20** and 17.**21**), and drain the secretory end pieces (acini). The intercalated duct cells contain a few secretory granules, some rough endoplasmic reticulum (RER), mitochondria, and a round or oval centrally placed nucleus (Fig. 17.**21**). Striated ducts are the next largest intralobular type and are located between the intercalated ducts and the excretory ducts. The striated

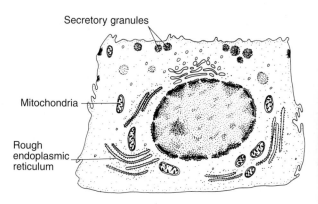

Fig. 17.**21** Diagram illustrating the ultrastructure of an intercalated duct cell.

ducts (also known as the secretory or salivary ducts) are the most specialized of salivary gland ducts and carry out most of the ionic transport functions that occur along the route of the saliva from the acinar lumen to the oral cavity. They are lined by tall, columnar epithelial cells with a distinctly eosinophilic cytoplasm and spherical, centrally or eccentrically placed nuclei (Figs. 17.**22** and 17.**23**). The term "striated" refers to the light microscopic appearance of the basal cytoplasm (Fig. 17.**23**) that has well-developed striations perpendicular to the base of the cells. This appearance results from infoldings of the basal plasma membrane that produce cytoplasmic rows containing numerous mitochondria (Figs. 17.**22** and 17.**24**). In Figure 17.**24**, the striated duct cells are shown surrounding the lumen. Sodium reabsorption and potassium excretion occur within these cells, which are affected by changes in levels of adrenal cortical steroid hormones, mainly aldosterone. Therefore, the striated ducts are similar, functionally and histologically, to cells of the renal distal tubule. Sodium reabsorption by these cells changes the saliva from an isotonic to a hypotonic osmolarity, although the excretory duct system is also involved in this process.

The other ducts of the glands travel through the connective-tissue septa between lobules and form the excretory ducts or the interlobular portion of the duct

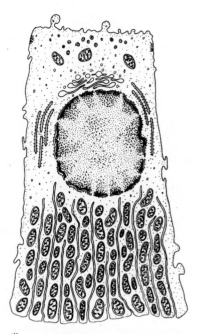

Fig. 17.**22** Diagram illustrating the ultrastructure of a striated duct cell. Observe the infolding of the basal plasma membrane and numerous mitochondria located in the infoldings.

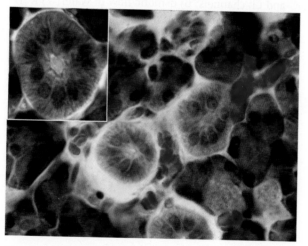

Fig. 17.**23** A light microscopic photomicrograph of three striated ducts with prominent striations. A higher magnification view of one striated duct is shown in the inset.

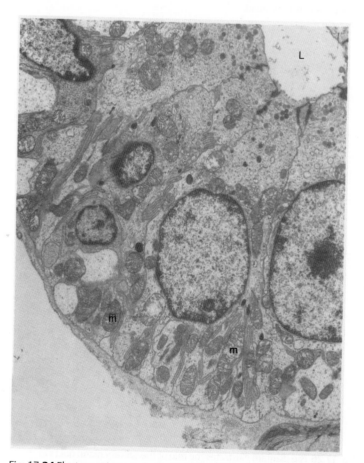

Fig. 17.**24** Electron micrograph showing the relationship of striated duct cells surrounding the central lumen (L) of the duct (upper right in the electron micrograph) and the presence of numerous mitochondria (m) in the striated duct cells.

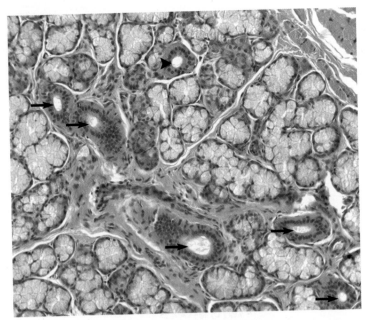

Fig. 17.**25** The histology of several interlobular (excretory) ducts (arrows), surrounded by interlobular connective tissue, is shown in the photomicrograph. The epithelium of interlobular ducts is predominantly stratified columnar. Occasional ducts may possess a pseudostratified epithelium. A duct that is transitional between intralobular (striated) and interlobular is labeled with an arrowhead.

system. The portions between the lobules join larger ducts, that then join interlobar portions (between the lobes), with the main excretory duct emptying into the oral cavity. As the excretory ducts become larger, the epithelium lining of these ducts changes from simple columnar to pseudostratified (Fig. 17.**25**) or stratified, columnar epithelium. At or near the entrance to the oral cavity, the main excretory ducts become lined with stratified squamous epithelium continuous with the buccal epithelium (Fig. 17.**17**).

Saliva Formation: Ionic Transport

Saliva is formed in a two-stage process. The first stage is the production of the primary secretion by the acinar cells. The ducts carry out the second stage in which the isotonic primary secretion is modified into the hypotonic saliva that enters the oral cavity. A number of different systems are involved in ionic transport across the basolateral and luminal surfaces of acinar and duct cells. According to current knowledge these systems appear to include: 1) a Na^+/K^+ -ATPase; 2) $Na^+/K^+/Cl^-$ co-transport system; 3) bicarbonate secretion driven by a Na^+/H^+ exchanger; 4) chloride secretion driven by parallel Na^+/H^+ and Cl^-/HCO_3^- exchangers; 5) Ca^{++} -regulated K^+ and Cl^- channels; 6) osmotic flow of water; 7) K^+/H^+ exchangers; and 8) paracellular transport of Na^+ and water. These transport systems are active in acinar cells as well as intralobular, interlobular, and/or excretory portions of the duct system. The primary saliva formed and released from acinar cells is isotonic and is modified by duct cells to form the hypotonic solution by the removal and addition of specific ions (Fig. 17.**26**). Considerable research has been carried out on the ionic transport systems that function in the salivary glands.

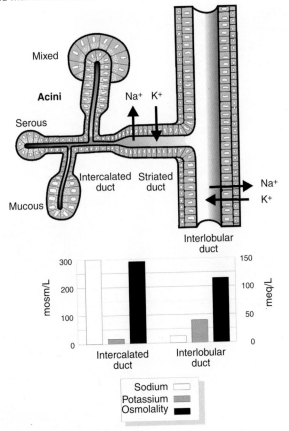

Fig. 17.**26** The diagram illustrates the role of the salivary gland ducts in resorbing Na^+ and excreting K^+. The changes in osmolarity and milliequivalents of Na^+ and K^+ as saliva passes from the intercalated to the interlobular ducts is indicated in the bar graphs. The striated ducts are the primary site of ionic transport.

Figure 17.**27** shows the current view of acinar ionic transport systems that account for the secretion of primary saliva by acinar cells.

On the basolateral membrane, the Na⁺/K⁺-ATPase exchanges 3Na⁺ in an outward direction toward the interstitium with 2K⁺ moving inward. The result is the maintenance of high intracellular K⁺ and low intracellular Na⁺. The Na⁺/K⁺-ATPase generated, inward-directed Na⁺ gradient drives the Na⁺/K⁺/Cl⁻ co-transporter. This co-transporter is essential for the transport of Cl⁻ into the acinar cell. Na⁺/H⁺ and Cl⁻/HCO₃⁻ exchangers allow transport of HCO₃⁻ and protons (H⁺) while Cl⁻ and Na⁺ are taken up by the acinar cell. On the luminal surface, chloride channels allow for rapid efflux of Cl⁻ following cellular stimulation. Activation of acetylcholine receptors (Fig. 17.**27**) following parasympathetic nerve stimulation results in increased intracellular calcium [Ca⁺⁺]i that drives the apical Cl⁻ channel. Elevated [Ca⁺⁺]i also activates the Ca⁺⁺-activated K⁺ channel on the basolateral surface to preserve the membrane potential.

Stage two of the salivary secretion process is the modification of the primary saliva by the duct system. The function of the duct system in modifying the primary isotonic saliva produced by acinar cells to the hypotonic saliva released into the oral cavity is shown in Figures 17.**26** and 17.**28**.

The duct cells function to reabsorb Na⁺ and Cl⁻ and secrete K⁺ and HCO₃⁻ without water reabsorption, resulting in a hypotonic saliva. The basolateral membrane of duct cells possesses high Na⁺-K⁺ ATPase activity and a Na⁺/H⁺-exchanger as well as Cl⁻ and K⁺ channels. The apical (luminal) surface possesses Na⁺ and Cl⁻ channels as well as Na⁺/H⁺, Cl⁻/HCO₃⁻, and H⁺/K⁺ exchangers. A genetic mutation in the cystic fibrosis (CF) gene alters Cl⁻ and other channels in the salivary glands and leads to the array of symptoms found in CF (see Clinical Applications on CF).

During salivary secretion there is a rapid movement of water following stimulation. Since acinar cells shrink dramatically following stimulated secretion, it appears that most of the water moves by osmosis in response to Na⁺ in the primary saliva. There is also evidence for paracellular or transcellular movement of water. Aquaporins are a family of small (30kDa), homologous integral membrane proteins that function as highly selective water channels in fluid-transporting epithelia. Aquaporins 1 and 5 (AQP 1, AQP 5) are the predominant aquaporins in the human salivary glands. AQPs are localized primarily in serous acini on the apical membranes of acinar cells, including the intercellular canaliculi discussed in the next section of this chapter (Fig. 17.**29**). AQPs are sensitive to secretagogues. For example, treatment of parotid acinar cells with epinephrine results in trafficking of AQP 5 from intracellular membranes to the apical plasma membrane by a calcium-mediated mechanism. AQPs are the focus of considerable research to develop gene therapy for the transfer of human AQPs to salivary glands of patients with reduced salivary function and dry mouth (xerostomia).

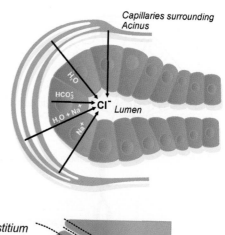

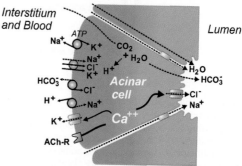

Fig. 17.**27** The diagram illustrates the pumps, exchangers, and channels involved in acinar cell production of the primary saliva. Parasympathetic endings release acetylcholine; this binds to the acetylcholine-receptor causing an increase in intracellular Ca++ that stimulates secretion and channel activity. Dotted arrows indicate passive transport and solid arrows indicate active transport. Process involved in ductal ion transport are shown in Figure 17.**28**.

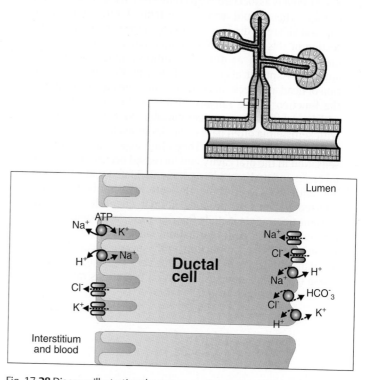

Fig. 17.**28** Diagram illustrating the pumps, exchangers, and channels involved in duct transport activity in the salivary glands. The diagram is a composite of mechanisms that are believed to occur in striated and interlobular ducts. The dotted arrows indicate passive transport, the solid arrows active transport.

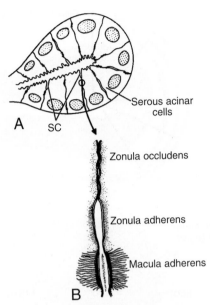

Fig. 17.**29 A** Diagram of the arrangement of secretory canaliculi (SC), acinar cells, and junctional complexes. **B** Diagram of a typical junctional complex composed of a triad of zonula occludens (tight junction), zonula adherens, and macula adherens (desmosome). It should be noted that junctional complexes consisting only of tight junctions lacking zonulae adherentes and desmosomes have been frequently observed between salivary gland acinar cells.

Histology and Function of the Secreting Units (Acini)

The salivary gland acini are of three types: serous, mucous, or mixed. The proportion of the three types of acini differs in the three major and the minor salivary glands. The morphology of the serous acinus will be discussed first. The serous acinar cell is an ideal example of protein produced for export, so the secretory pathway with a focus on the salivary proteins will be discussed in the next section of this chapter. The morphology and cell biology of the mucous acinar cell will be discussed in the last part of this section on the structure and function of acini.

Serous Cells

Serous cells are similar to pancreatic acinar cells; they are shaped like a pyramid, with basal nuclei and numerous secretory granules in the apical cytoplasm. In cross section, the serous cells of each acinus surround a small, central lumen that usually is not visible at the light microscopic level. The lateral surface between adjacent serous acinar cells demonstrates a junctional complex (Fig. 17.**29A**). The appearance of a typical junctional complex with a zonula occludens (tight junction), a zonula adherens (intermediate junction), and a macula adherens (desmosome) is shown in Figure 17.**29B**.

Clinical Application

Xerostomia is associated with connective-tissue diseases, for example rheumatoid arthritis, systemic lupus erythematosus, and Sjögren's disease (discussed in the connective-tissue section of this chapter). Xerostomia may also be caused by medications such as diuretics, antihistamines, or tricyclic antidepressants. It also occurs following therapeutic radiation of head and neck cancers. The radiation adversely affects the function of the salivary glands leading to xerostomia, which includes many uncomfortable symptoms. Patients with xerostomia often have difficulty in swallowing food and speaking for long periods. They often experience a burning sensation in the oral cavity and increased occurrence of dental caries and oral candidiasis. It is anticipated that gene therapy with APQs will eventually cure xerostomia and allow affected patients to produce normal quantities of saliva. Current treatments include fluoride rinses and topical applications to inhibit caries formation, saliva substitutes, stimulation of salivary production with sugarless candies, and avoidance of drinks or foods with a very high sugar content. These treatments obviously focus on symptoms rather than the cause of the xerostomia.

Modifications of the junctional complex occur in relation to the lateral intercellular spaces and secretory canaliculi. The secretory canaliculi are found between adjacent serous cells and between serous cells (serous demilune) that cap a mixed acinus. In this situation they are responsible for transporting serous secretions to the mucous acinar lumen. The secretory canaliculi (capillaries) radiate from the lumen intercellularly in a serpentine pattern and may extend almost to the basal lamina surrounding the acinus (Fig. 17.**29**). A junctional complex may be found near the surface or between a secretory canaliculus and the intercellular space. Junctional complexes are also found between adjacent duct cells. In Figure 17.**30**, note the desmosomes (d) located along lateral surfaces of cells surrounding the lumen of an intercalated duct.

A basal lamina is secreted by epithelial cells during development and is found underlying both acinar and ductal cells. It is composed of GAGs, collagen, and glycoproteins and forms a structural scaffolding for the acini. At the electron microscopic level, serous cells have abundant RER, secretory granules, and a Golgi apparatus (Figs. 17.**31** and 17.**33**). In rodent species that lend themselves to intensive morphologic and functional studies, considerable diversity has been found among acinar cells. A similar diversity has been established at the morphologic level in human salivary gland acinar cells.

Clinical Application

CF, is a common genetic disease among Caucasian children (1 in 2 000 births), is characterized by a general dysfunction of the salivary and other exocrine glands and eventually results in pulmonary, digestive, and nutritional difficulties. The most obvious characteristic of salivary glands from children with cystic fibrosis is accumulation of glycoproteinaceous (PAS-positive) material in acinar cells and ducts leading eventually to obstruction of the ducts. CF is caused by mutations in the gene that encodes the CF transmembrane conductance regulator (CFTR). CFTR is a cyclic AMP-regulated chloride channel, central to chloride and bicarbonate secretion in the salivary glands as well as other organs in the gastrointestinal and respiratory systems. The CFTR protein also functions as a regulator of other channels in addition to its function as a cAMP-regulated Cl- channel. The gene for CFTR has been localized at the CF locus assigned to the long arm of chromosome 7 band q31, and a number of mutations have also been identified. Human gene therapy with aerosols containing normal CFTR has been used in clinical trials to attempt to reverse the abnormal functioning of cells in the airways of patients suffering from CF. The gene therapy clinical trials have been disappointing so far. Problems include low levels of transfection, short-lived expression, and immune response to the vectors. It appears that effective gene therapy may be years away from fruition. More promising for the near future is the pharmaceutical approach using drugs which aid folding of the mutant ΔF_{508} protein gene product allowing functional CFTR to reach the plasma membrane.

Fig. 17.**30** Ultrastructure of an intercalated duct showing the arrangement of individual intercalated duct cells around the lumen (L) of the duct. Desmosomes (d) between the duct cells are labeled near the duct lumen.

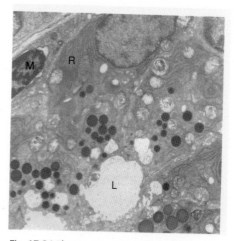

Fig. 17.**31** Electron micrograph of a serous acinus. L: lumen. R: the rough endoplasmic reticulum. m: a myoepithelial cell.

The Secretory Pathway

The salivary glands primarily produce amylase and mucous for export. Serous acinar cells synthesize amylase while mucous acinar cells synthesize mucus. Both of these products are synthesized by classical exocrine pathways. Acinar cells also produce an array of membrane proteins and lipids as well as other molecules destined for release. The next section will review the basics of transcription, translation, post-translational modifications, and transport through the membrane-surrounded portions of the secretory pathway (RER, Golgi apparatus, and secretory vesicles) with a focus on the serous salivary gland acinar cell. Transcription and translation are the fundamental steps in the transfer of genetic information from DNA→RNA→protein.

Transcription [DNA-Directed Synthesis of Messenger RNA (mRNA)]

The genetic information for all cells is encoded in the DNA. The first step in secretion is the transcription of the DNA into specific messenger RNAs (mRNAs). Genes are transcribed in the nucleus. In the case of amylase, there is considerable information about the gene in humans. α-amylase is produced by two major tissues in humans: the salivary glands and the pancreas. There are two forms of human α-amylase, a pancreatic-specific gene and a salivary gland-specific gene. The α-amylase found in the salivary glands is a recent development in evolution that arose from the pancreatic amylase gene. The salivary gland specificity appears to have developed by insertion of a retrovirus upstream of the amylase gene. A human parotid specific enhancer has been identified within the retroviral region. The full-length salivary amylase cDNA contains 215 base pairs of 5'-untranslated region, 1536 base pairs of coding sequences, and 33 base pairs of 3'-untranslated region. The predicted protein product derived from the cDNA contains 511 amino acids. The human amylase gene is found on chromosome band Ip21. There are actually three human α-amylase genes designated as AMY1A, AMY1B, and AMY1C. There is a diversity of gene expression found in human populations and between the major and minor salivary glands.

Transcription begins with the binding of RNA polymerase to specific DNA sequences near the amylase gene called the promoter DNA elements. Ribonucleotides are sequentially added to each other to form the messenger RNA (mRNA) chain from the 5' to the 3' end. This process is regulated by factors that bind to DNA (DNA-binding proteins), changing the conformational arrangement of the DNA, or binds polymerases leading to further recruitment of polymerases. In the case of human α-amylase, transcription is initiated from a non-translated exon within a γ-actin pseudogene located upstream of the amylase genes.

RNA processing is a key step in the secretory pathway in

which the primary transcript is modified to form the mature transcript. The mature transcript differs from the primary transcript in the addition of a 5' cap, addition of a polyadenosine (poly A) tail, and removal of the intron segments that constitute the non-coding or non-information-containing segments of the primary transcript. In the case of the human salivary α-amylase, there are 11 exons and 10 introns in the 10kb length gene.

Translation and Function of the Endoplasmic Reticulum

The second step in genetic expression is the translation of the messenger RNAs to form protein. Following transcription and the processing/maturation of the primary transcript, mRNAs exit the nucleus through the nuclear pores and travel to the cytoplasm where translation of the genetic message occurs. Translation requires the presence of all three forms of RNA. It is directed by the code encrypted within the mRNA that is translated into protein. In this process, a chain of codons is "translated" into a chain of amino acids. Each amino acid is transferred to the ribosome by a transfer RNA (tRNA) while ribosomal RNA (rRNA) is an important component of the ribosomal complex.

Translation for secretory proteins such as amylase occurs on ribosomes in association with the RER. The salivary glands produce an array of other proteins, including statherins, cystatins, agglutinin, proline-rich proteins, and histatins, also destined for release into the saliva. Proteins destined for organelles are synthesized on isolated or "free" polysomes not associated with the endoplasmic reticulum (ER) membrane. The translation rate of protein is dependent upon the rate of transcription and the degradation of mRNAs in the cytoplasm.

The critical event in the secretion of a protein is the translocation of the nascent peptide from the cytosolic to the cisternal space of the RER. The key player in translocation is the signal recognition particle (SRP) that binds to the ribosome and the signal peptide. As the peptide is being synthesized, it is simultaneously inserted into the ER lumen following cleavage by a specific peptidase.

Secretory proteins, such as amylase, are translocated across the RER to the cisternal space under the direction of a presequence in accordance with the signal hypothesis. The presequence is cleaved cotranslationally from the newly synthesized molecule. Following translation of the mRNA, the newly synthesized secretory protein follows a pathway from the RER to the surface of the cell. This intracellular transport pathway for secretory proteins within an acinar cell is best illustrated by a classical pulse-chase experiment in which isolated salivary gland acini are labeled with a radioactive amino acid such as leucine (i.e., ^{3}H-leucine). Proteins synthesized in the presence of ^{3}H-leucine are radiolabeled and may be visualized by a photographic technique using a photosensitive film coupled with electron microscopy. This technique is known as electron microscopic autoradiography, in which radioactive silver grains produced by radioactive decay can be quantitated in each intracellular compartment. Figure 17.**32A** indicates the time-dependent distribution of grains in each subcellular

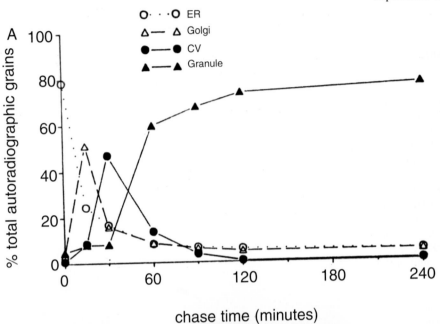

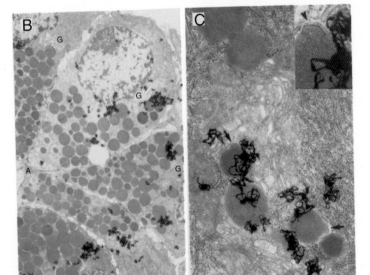

Fig. 17.**32** Electron microscopic analysis of parotid acinar cells pulse-labeled with ³H-leucine. **A** Quantitative results obtained at each time period following the pulse chase. Autoradiographic grains present over specific subcellular compartments are expressed as a percentage of total grains counted at each time interval following the pulse chase. **B** Representative low-power view of an acinar profile at 60 minutes following chase. An acinar lumen (A) and several Golgi regions (G) are marked. Note the labeling of immature granules in the Golgi regions. **C** Higher magnification showing heavy labeling of immature granules near the Golgi apparatus at 60 minutes following chase. Note the relative absence of Golgi labeling at this chase time and that heavily labeled immature granules possess coated membrane evaginations (arrows). The inset highlights the coat (arrowhead) of the granule located at the center of the field in **(C)** Bars: **(B)** 2.0 μm: **(C)** 0.5 μm.

compartment following a short exposure to ^{3}H-leucine. Labeling after 60 minutes is shown in Figure 17.**32B**. An acinar lumen (A) and several regions containing Golgi (G) are labeled. Autoradiographic grains are present over immature granules present in the Golgi regions. These granules often possess coated membrane evaginations that have been associated with secretory sorting processes. For example, proteins may be sorted into vesicles for constitutive release from the cell. The inset in Figure 17.**32C** shows the coat (arrowhead) of the granule located in the center of the field in C. The coating is clathrin, the same coating molecule involved in recycling of membrane from the plasma membrane (endocytosis).

Specific processes occur in each intracellular compartment during the maturation of secretory proteins within acinar cells. Several processes occur within the RER including initiation of: 1) folding; 2) glycosylation; and 3) processing of sugar molecules on the maturing secretory proteins. Glycosylation in the endoplasmic reticulum occurs by block glycosylation of proteins. Dolichol, a membrane-bound lipid located on the luminal side of the ER is transferred to the nascent peptide. Transfer is followed by trimming and processing that begins in the ER and continues in the Golgi apparatus.

The Golgi Apparatus

Membranous transport vesicles (Fig. 17.**33**) provide the mechanism for RER to Golgi transport. These vesicles move to the Golgi apparatus where the protein synthesized by the RER is further modified (e.g., glycosylation) and packaging of secretory granules is completed (Figs. 17.**33** and 17.**34**). Vesicles bud from the ER and carry synthesized proteins to the Golgi apparatus. The Golgi apparatus may be considered as a flattened stack of cisternal compartments responsible for the post-translational modification and sorting of newly synthesized proteins and lipids. The Golgi compartments are in order: 1) cis-Golgi-network (CGN); 2) cis; 3) medial; 4) trans; and 5) trans-Golgi network (TGN). Each compartment is involved in specific steps in protein synthesis (Fig. 17.**34**).

Secretory Vesicles (Granules)

The secretory vesicle or granule is the vehicle for movement of secretory proteins from the Golgi to the cell membrane. Secretory vesicles bud from the TGN and move toward the plasma membrane. Fusion of these vesicles with the cell membrane is believed to be regulated by the same processes that regulate docking and fusion of synaptic vesicles with the presynaptic plasma membrane at the synapse. The process involves the recognition of the appropriate plasma and vesicle membrane receptors and penetration of the vesicle through the membrane cytoskeleton. The process is known as the SNARE hypothesis and postulates that cytosolic proteins mediate vesicle docking through binding with their receptors on plasma and vesicle membranes. Cytosolic

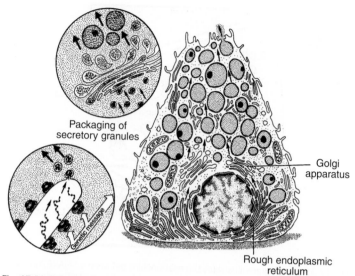

Packaging of secretory granules

Golgi apparatus

Rough endoplasmic reticulum

Fig. 17.**33** Diagram illustrating the subcellular organelles involved in the secretory pathway in salivary gland acinar cells and their functions. Lower circle (inset) shows the rough endoplasmic reticulum (RER) with the translocation of proteins from the cytosol to the cisternal space. Transport vesicles from the RER arrive at the Golgi (upper circle, inset). Vesicles from the RER arrive at the *cis* face and pass through the stacks (cisternae) of the Golgi apparatus. Budding vesicles exit from the *trans* face on their way to the membrane or lysosomes. The Golgi is responsible for intracellular sorting of proteins, as well as glycosylation and sulfation reactions.

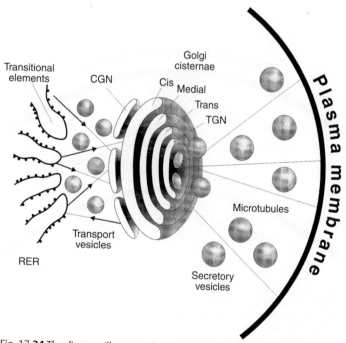

Transitional elements

CGN

Golgi cisternae

Cis

Medial

Trans

TGN

Plasma membrane

Microtubules

Transport vesicles

RER

Secretory vesicles

Fig. 17.**34** The diagram illustrates the compartments of the Golgi apparatus. Each compartment is associated with specific protein modifications and contains the enzymes required for those modifications.

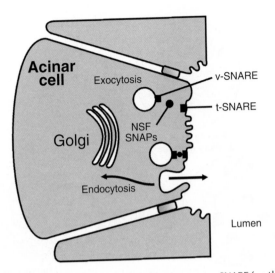

Fig. 17.**35** The diagram illustrates the relationships between v-SNARE (on the vesicle membrane), t-SNARE (on the target membrane), and NSF and SNAPs that facilitate recognition and docking of the vesicle with the cytoplasmic face of the cell membrane. SNARE is the abbreviation for <u>SNAP</u> <u>re</u>ceptor.

factors include NSF (N-ethylmaleimide-sensitive fusion protein), the SNAPs (soluble NSF attachment proteins), and the SNAP receptors that are cutely called SNAREs. There are two types of SNAREs: v-SNAREs associated with the vesicle/granule membrane and t-SNAREs present on the granule target, the plasma membrane (Fig. 17.**35**). Rab, a monomeric guanosine triphosphatase (GTPase), is also found on the vesicular membrane in its Rab-GTP configuration (Fig. 17.**36**). When a v-SNARE recognizes the appropriate t-SNARE, the Rab-GTP hydrolyzes to Rab-GDP. The GDP configuration of Rab dissociates from the target membrane facilitating recycling to the membrane of origin. Docking is followed by membrane fusion. This process is not well understood, but requires a fusion protein (fusigen has been identified in mammalian cells) that destabilizes hydrophilic forces at the interface between the vesicular and target membranes.

The majority of salivary secretory proteins are released by fusion of the granule with the cell membrane, that is, exocytosis under the regulation of acinar cell secretagogues. This process is known as regulated secretion in contrast to the secretagogue-independent mechanism of continual vesicular shuttling known as constitutive secretion (Fig. 17.**37**). Vesicles in acinar cells are responsible for transport of membrane proteins to the apical or basolateral surfaces of these highly polarized cells. Vesicles also contain secretory proteins destined for release in the absence of secretagogue (Fig. 17.**37**).

Fig. 17.**36** This diagram illustrates the relationship of v-SNARE, t-SNARE, SNAP, and Rab-GTP at the presynaptic nerve terminal. The same molecules are believed to be involved in vesicular docking in salivary gland acinar cells. SNAREs on the vesicular (v) and target (t) membranes initiate docking by a Ca++–dependent mechanism. Docking is secured by Rab-GTP. Fusion of the two membranes is initiated through the action of NSF/SNAP and a fusigen.

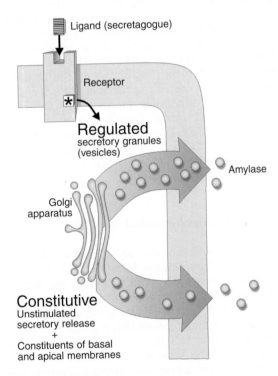

Fig. 17.**37** The diagram illustrates the regulated and constitutive pathways in a salivary gland acinar cell. The regulated pathway is stimulated by a secretagogue binding to a cell surface receptor. Constitutive secretion does not require a ligand. The asterisk (*) indicates the conformational change that occurs after ligand binding.

Lysosomal activity is also involved in the secretory process. Mannose-6-phosphate is attached to lysosomal enzymes during maturation and becomes the signal that directs these enzymes from the Golgi to lysosomes. Lysosomes contain acid hydrolases that are required for intracellular degradation. For example, after response to a secretagogue, the acinar cell produces an abundance of protein that must be degraded. A similar process, called crinophagy in classical histology books, occurs after prolonged absence of secretagogue. In the absence of secretagogue lysosomal vesicles fuse with secretory granules, causing breakdown of excess granules. In addition to crinophagy, lysosomes are required for processing of endocytosed material and for autophagy of "worn-out" intracellular organelles.

The ultrastructural features of a serous acinus are shown in Figure 17.**31**. Granules ready for release are observed near the lumen. Serous cells in the salivary glands are responsible for the production of salivary α-amylase (α-1,4-glucan-4-glucanohydrolase, EC 3.2.1.1). This enzyme catalyzes the hydrolytic breakdown (hydrolysis) of α-1,4-glycosidic bonds typical of complex carbohydrates. Carbohydrates that are taken into the oral cavity as part of the diet are large polymeric structures that are hydrolyzed to form the disaccharide maltose, which is cleaved to form two molecules of glucose by the enzyme, maltase. Amylase thus carries out the critical step in providing glucose, the primary source of energy and carbon for cellular function. Some authors have classified human serous cells as seromucous, since periodic-acid-Schiff (PAS) stains the cells positively for glycoprotein. The traditional nomenclature of serous acinar cells is used in this chapter, however.

Mucous Cells

Mucous cells are triangular or pyramidal and contain numerous granules containing mucins. The secretory pathway is similar to that of the serous acinar cell. However, the Golgi apparatus contains unusually prominent vesicles on the trans-side of the Golgi apparatus. Radiolabeled sulfate ($^{35}SO_4^=$) is rapidly incorporated into the Golgi apparatus during the synthesis of polysaccharide-rich mucins that are released into the saliva. There is evidence for asynchronous release of mucous within acini and selective regulation of release by the parasympathetic nervous system, but these data are equivocal since mucus secretion has been studied to a lesser extent than serous acinar cell secretion. The appearance of mucous cells depends on the secretory phase of the cells (Fig. 17.**38**). They are reduced in size after release of mucin. Mucous cells require special stains, such as PAS or mucicarmine, to demonstrate the presence of mucin granules. In normal hematoxylin and eosin (H and E) preparations, these cells generally have a washed-out cytoplasm because organic solvents remove mucin. These cells typically are observed to possess a flattened basal nucleus (Figs. 17.**38** and 17.**39**).

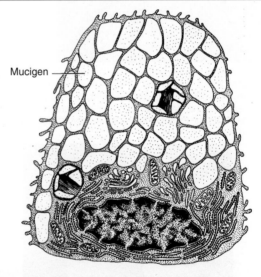

Mucigen

Fig. 17.**38** Diagram of the ultrastructure of a mucous acinar cell.

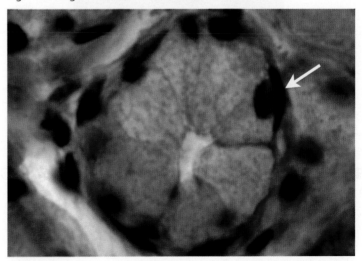

Fig. 17.**39** Light micrograph showing the structure of a mucous acinus. A myoepithelial cell is labeled with an arrow.

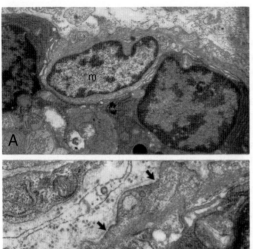

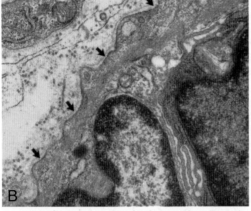

Fig. 17.**40** Electron micrographs showing the relationship between the myoepithelial cell and an acinus. **A** Ultrastructure (low magnification) of a myoepithelial cell (m) encompassing an acinar cell (a). **B** Ultrastructure (higher magnification) of a myoepithelial cell. The cytoplasm contains parallel microfilaments (f). Arrowheads delineate the extent of the basal lamina surrounding the myoepithelial cell and acinus.

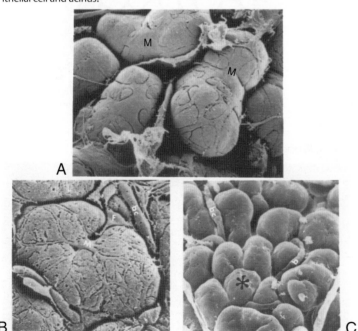

Fig. 17.**42** Scanning electron micrograph showing the relationship of myoepithelial cells to the acini. There are differences in myoepithelial-cell morphology in different salivary glands and between species. **A** The terminal portion of a sublingual acinus. The myoepithelial cells (M) cover a large part of the acinus (F: fibroblast–like cells). **B** The terminal portion of a submandibular acinus. M: myoepithelial cells. bc: blood capillary. **C** The terminal portions of the parotid gland are shown (*); note the absence of myoepithelial cells. The parotid gland in humans contains large numbers of myoepithelial cells in contrast to the absence of myoepithelial cells seen in this scanning electron micrograph from the rodent parotid gland.

Myoepithelial Cells

Basket or omit basal myoepithelial cells are branched stellate cells that lie between the basal lamina and the acinar cells (Figs. 17.**39** and 17.**40A** and **B**). The myoepithelial cells have long processes that encompass the acinus and intercalated duct (Fig. 17.**41**). In light microscopy (Fig. 17.**39**), only the nuclei of the cells usually are visible, but ultrastructurally these cells have parallel microfilamentous arrangements similar to those demonstrated in smooth muscle cells (Figs. 17.**40A** and **B**). Scanning electron micrographs of myoepithelial cells are shown in Figure 17.**42A** with myoepithelial cell processes surrounding the terminal portions of the acini of the sublingual gland (Fig. 17.**42A**) and submandibular gland (Fig. 17.**42B**). There are morphologic differences in myoepithelial cells between the salivary glands and between species. Note the absence of myoepithelial cells around terminal acini in the rat parotid gland (Fig. 17.**42C**), where the myoepithelial cells are located around the intercalated ducts. This is unlike the human parotid gland, which has the conventional distribution of myoepithelial cells. It is also important to note that the pancreas, in comparison to the salivary glands, totally lacks myoepithelial cells. Myoepithelial cell processes wrap around portions of the duct system and serve to squeeze secretion from the acinus and the associated duct system. The parasympathetic and sympathetic nervous systems have a synergistic effect on myoepithelial cells, resulting in stimulation of contraction. Contraction of the myoepithelial cells facilitates the movement of secretory products from the acinus toward the oral cavity. The myoepithelial cells also provide isometric force and support for the glandular parenchyma during the sustained secretory response. There is a general correlation between the thickness of myoepithelial cell processes and the viscosity of the secretory product—they are thickest, for example, on mucous acini. This correlates with their contraction and luminal reinforcement/compression roles in the movement of secretions out of the acini and intercalated ducts and into the larger ducts.

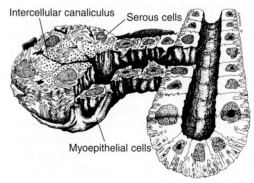

Fig. 17.**41** Diagram illustrating the relationship of myoepithelial cells, acinar cells, and the intercalated and striated ducts.

Histologic Structure of the Acinus

The acinus or secretory portion (end piece) of the gland varies from a purely serous or a purely mucous type to a mixed type containing both serous and mucous cells (Fig. 17.**43**). Serous and mucous acini differ in shape and size, with mucous acini having a more tubular shape. Mixed acini have mucous and serous cells in different positions within the secretory end piece. The mucous cells are closest to the intercalated ducts, with the serous cells forming demilunes capping over the blind ends of the mucous acini (Fig. 17.**43**). The serous cells are not separated from the lumen of the acinus, but are connected to it by secretory (intercellular) canaliculi that pass between the mucous cells. All acini are surrounded by a basal lamina that structurally supports them. Myoepithelial cells are located between the acinar cells and the basal lamina (Figs. 17.**39** and 17.**40A** and **B**).

Function of Connective-Tissue Cells

The connective tissue that forms the capsule and septa (stroma) of the salivary glands and surrounds ducts and acini contains plasma cells, fibroblasts, macrophages, and lymphocytes. However, the connective tissue is not merely a structural support. The connective tissue assists in the maintenance of homeostasis in the oral cavity and in inflammatory processes associated with pathology and disease.

Secretory Immunity: The Synthesis and Secretion of Immunoglobulin A

Bone-marrow-derived, B lymphocytes differentiate into immunoglobulin-producing plasma cells (Fig. 17.**44**) in the connective tissue of the salivary glands. The primary immunoglobulin produced is secretory immunoglobulin (IgA). IgAs are an essential part of the mucosal immune system and are secreted into the oral cavity for defense against bacterial, viral, and other pathogens. IgAs are not

Clinical Application

The connective tissue of the salivary glands is affected in diseases such as rheumatoid arthritis and systemic lupus erythematosus as well as Sjögren's syndrome. Sjögren's syndrome may occur as a primary disorder or as a consequence of other rheumatic diseases. It is characterized by an extensive lymphocytic infiltration of T and B lymphocytes. B lymphocyte hyperactivity leads to production of high titers of autoantibodies with the assistance of many helper T lymphocytes that infiltrate the salivary glands and assist in the differentiation of B lymphocytes into plasma cells and memory B cells. Sjögren's syndrome patients suffer from xerostomia as the disease progresses and salivary function is greatly reduced.

The salivary glands are also involved in antibody production under normal circumstances, especially the production of secretory immunoglobulin (IgA). Plasma cells and acinar cells combine in a cooperative relationship to produce the molecules that establish secretory immunity and mucosal defense of the oral cavity.

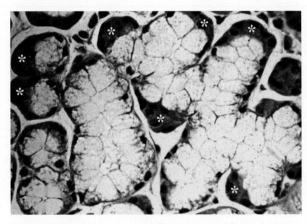

Fig. 17.**43** The photomicrograph illustrates several mixed acini. Each serous demilune is labeled with an asterisk (*).

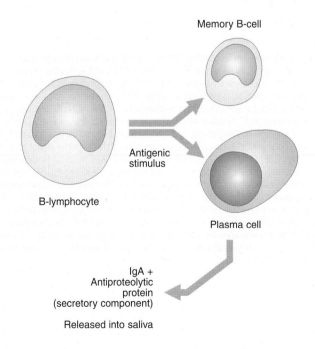

Fig. 17.**44** Diagram illustrating the formation of IgA by plasma cells (derived from B lymphocytes). Secretory component is synthesized by acinar and duct cells and is added to IgA. The mechanism is shown in detail in Figure 17.45.

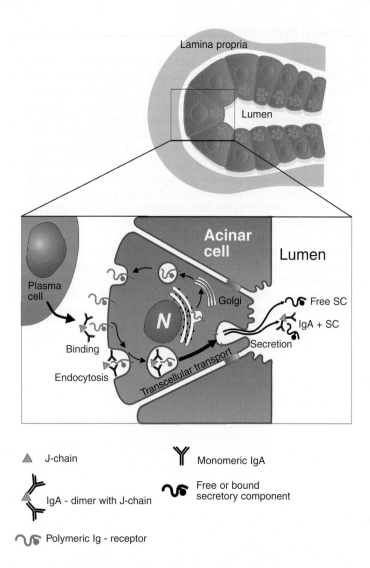

△ J-chain

Y Monomeric IgA

IgA - dimer with J-chain

Free or bound secretory component

Polymeric Ig - receptor

Fig. 17.**45** Diagram illustrating the formation of IgA and secretory component (SC). SC essentially serves as the receptor for IgA and is also the protective part of the IgA-SC complex. IgA is synthesized and secreted by plasma cells. Transmembrane SC is synthesized in the RER of the acinar cell and is glycosylated in the Golgi apparatus. It is phosphorylated in the TGN of the Golgi apparatus, forming pIgR, which is inserted as a transmembrane receptor on the basolateral surface. Binding of IgA to pIgR results in a ligand complex that undergoes endocytosis. Transcytosis is accomplished through the endosome system with release of the SC-IgA complex (pIgR-IgA) as well as some free excess SC at the luminal surface. Free SC is believed to play a role in secretory immunity by inhibiting adhesion of Gram-negative bacteria. The free and bound secretory component differ from the pIgR (polymeric Ig receptor) in that a piece of the receptor is retained in the luminal membrane upon release of SC or SC + IgA. Therefore, the receptor is sometimes referred to as a "sacrificial receptor." Although it is shown in an acinar cell, ductal cells probably synthesize much of the secretory component because of the more abundant connective tissue around the larger ducts.

released by themselves, but in a bound form coupled to a protein (secretory component) that prevents proteolysis during transport and particularly in the proteolytic environment of the oral cavity.

The production of IgA and its release into the oral cavity represents an important example of transcytosis. In transcytosis, uptake by endocytosis at one surface is followed by transport across the cell with release by exocytosis at the opposite surface. Synthesis of IgA occurs in subepithelial plasma cells in the connective tissue (lamina propria) surrounding the acinus and ducts (Figs. 17.**44** and 17.**45**). IgA forms a dimer of two IgA molecules and includes an additional immunoglobulin segment called the J-chain. The dimeric (polymeric) IgA binds to a receptor on the cell surface called the polymeric immunoglobulin receptor (pIg-receptor), that is the membrane-bound form of secretory component (Fig. 17.**45**). The pIg-receptor (membrane-bound secretory component), like all transmembrane and secretory proteins, is formed on the RER and undergoes modifications such as glycosylation and phosphorylation in the RER and Golgi. It is subsequently inserted in the basal plasma membrane where the receptor is available for uptake of dimeric IgA. The binding of IgA to the membrane-bound secretory component results in uptake of the complex by endocytosis. Vesicles containing the complex traverse the acinar or duct cell. Bound secretory component-IgA complex and a little free secretory component are released at the apical surface of the acinar or duct cell into the lumen. This exocytotic release occurs in conjunction with retention of a transmembrane piece of the pIg receptor that stays in the membrane (Fig. 17.**45**). The remainder of the pIg-receptor is released as sIgA and is therefore known as a "sacrificial receptor". In this system, membrane-bound secretory component forms the receptor for dimeric IgA, functions as a carrier molecule for transport across the cell cytoplasm, and protects IgA from degradation in the oral cavity. This process also occurs in ductal cells, particularly interlobular ducts that are surrounded by extensive connective tissue.

Innervation of the Salivary Glands

Salivary gland secretion is regulated primarily by sympathetic and parasympathetic autonomic nerves (Fig. 17.**46**). In general, β-adrenergic stimulation of the salivary glands results in an organic secretion (i.e., via exocytosis), while parasympathetic stimulation is largely watery. Sympathetic fibers arise from the thoracolumbar region of the spinal cord, synapse primarily in the superior cervical ganglia, and travel with blood vessels to reach the salivary glands. These fibers are of two types: vascular (primarily vasoconstrictive) and secretory-type sympathetics. Parasympathetic fibers originate in the superior and inferior salivatory nuclei of the brainstem and synapse in a ganglion in close proximity to the glands (Table 17.**1** and Fig. 17.**46**). In the parotid gland, preganglionic fibers travel with the glossopharyngeal (ninth cranial) nerve to the otic ganglion; from the ganglion, postganglionic fibers travel with the auriculotemporal nerve to the gland. The parasympathetic innervation of the sublingual and submandibular glands originates in the superior salivatory nucleus. The pathway involves the facial nerve (VII) via the chorda tympani (preganglionic) to the submandibular ganglion. After synapsing, the postganglionic fibers innervate the glands. There is some evidence that individual acinar, myoepithelial, and duct cells may receive a dual autonomic innervation. The main impetus for granule release by exocytosis in acinar cells is norepinephrine released from sympathetic postganglionic fibers in the gland. The associated increases in cyclic AMP result in subsequently elevated levels of protein synthesis. The norepinephrine binds to specific adrenoreceptors (adrenergic receptors) on the basolateral surface of the acinar cells and results in elevation of intracellular cyclic AMP, as shown in Fig. 17.**47**. Parasympathetic stimulation primarily regulates fluid secretion through elevation of cytosolic-free, intracellular calcium $[Ca^{++}]_i$ (Fig. 17.**49**). The elevated $[Ca^{++}]_i$ stimulates AQP trafficking to the apical plasma membrane and rapid water movement. Parasympathetic stimulation causes an immediate increase in protein synthesis and secretion, although the secretory mechanism appears to involve non-storage granule vesicular secretion. The sympathetic and parasympathetic nerves also control blood flow through the salivary glands, which is a major factor in regulation of salivary flow rates. The parasympathetic nerves produce vasodilatation and increased production of saliva. The sympathetic nerve influence varies with the pattern of sympathetic activity. Unfortunately, few studies have attempted to investigate the effects on secretion of stimulation of both branches of the autonomic nervous system at physiologic levels as occurs in the animal. There is also evidence that non-cholinergic, non-adrenergic fibers (e.g., vasoactive intestinal peptide [VIP]) are involved in the regulation of salivary gland function through control of blood flow and production of saliva.

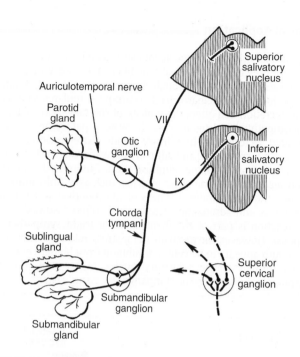

Fig. 17.**46**. Diagram illustrating the parasympathetic and sympathetic innervation of the salivary glands.

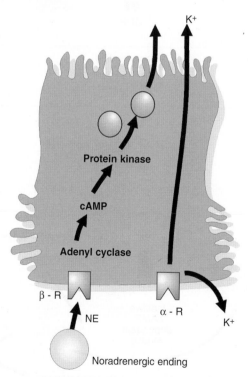

Fig. 17.**47** Diagram illustrating the effects of α- and β-adrenergic stimulation on acinar cell activity. β-R and α-R represent receptors for beta and alpha receptors respectively.

Clinical Application

Parasympathetic cholinergic agents such as pilocarpine stimulate both preganglionic sympathetic fibers and parasympathetics. These drugs function through cholinergic receptors that may also be located on acinar cells. Pilocarpine stimulates salivary gland secretion and alters the tonicity of the saliva. Atropine, a parasympatholytic drug, inhibits the watery, parasympathetic-mediated secretion of the salivary glands. Extreme dryness of the mouth (xerostomia) and difficulty in swallowing and talking may result from atropine administration. Diminished salivary gland secretion is a side effect of drugs such as antihistamines, opiates, and barbiturates. Dryness of the mouth is associated with stress and adrenaline secretion. It is often assumed that this reaction is part of the flight, fight, or fright sympathetic response. However, the mechanism for stress-related dryness of the mouth appears to be central inhibition from higher centers, which influences the salivatory nuclei, rather than direct peripheral inhibition by the sympathetic nervous system.

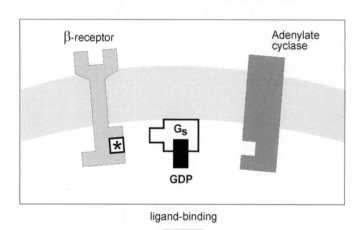

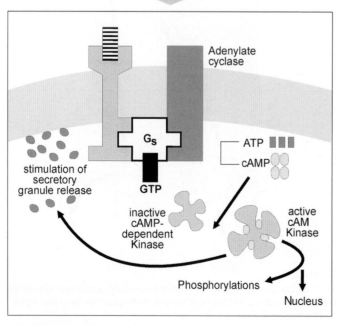

Fig. 17.**48** Diagram illustrating the β-receptor-activated cyclic AMP-dependent regulatory process. An asterisk (*) indicates the conformational change that occurs after ligand binding, exposing the G$_S$-binding site.

Pharmacology of the Salivary Glands

The extensive autonomic innervation of the salivary glands establishes a sensitivity to autonomic pharmacologic agents. Postganglionic sympathetic nerves release the neurotransmitter norepinephrine. Preganglionic sympathetic and preganglionic and postganglionic parasympathetic nerves release acetylcholine. Sympathetic noradrenergic endings are influenced by pharmacologic adrenergic agonists and antagonists and may be classified into two subclasses of receptors: alpha (α) and beta (β) (Fig. 17.**47**). Isoproterenol is a β-adrenergic agonist that stimulates secretion in the salivary glands by binding to receptors on acinar cell plasma membranes. β-receptors function through the intracellular second messenger, cyclic AMP. Stimulation of α-receptors induces the release of K$^+$ ions across the plasma membrane at both apical and basal surfaces, as well as calcium-mediated water movement through the AQPs.

Regulation of Secretion

The secretory process can be separated into two parts: secretion of fluid and electrolytes, and secretion of proteins by exocytosis. Exocytotic processes appear to be regulated through the action of β-receptors while α- and muscarinic receptors may affect exocytosis in addition to their function in regulation of fluid and ion secretion. β-receptors act through a cyclic AMP pathway while α-, muscarinic, and other neurotransmitter receptors function primarily through calcium-mediated pathways involving the phosphoinositide cycle.

Beta(β)-Adrenergic Receptors and Cyclic AMP

Isoproterenol, as well as naturally occurring catecholamines, bind to beta (β) receptors. These receptors are single polypeptide chain transmembrane glycoproteins that transverse the lipid bilayer of the plasma membrane more than once (i.e., multipass structure). In fact, they have a precise orientation with a distinct seven-pass structure, characteristic of receptor proteins linked to GTP-binding regulatory proteins (i.e., G proteins). There is a large family of receptor proteins that facilitate guanosine-triiphosphate (GTP)-binding required for the activation of the receptor-G protein complex. One of these G proteins is stimulatory (i.e. G$_S$) and in the inactive state is bound to GDP (Fig. 17.**48**). When isoproterenol binds to the β-receptor a G$_S$-binding site is exposed and the G$_S$-protein binds to the , receptor (Fig. 17.**48**). The resulting complex is capable of binding GTP in exchange for GDP activating the G protein. A subunit of the activated G$_S$-protein activates adenylate cyclase. The G-protein system allows for amplification of the receptor-signal transduction response at two levels during ligand-receptor binding: 1) the production of numerous activated G$_S$-molecules; and 2) prolongation of the activation of adenylate cyclase. Activation ends when the G protein hydrolyzes GTP to GDP and another cycle can begin. Adenylate cyclase is the enzyme that catalyzes the conversion of adenosine triphosphate (ATP) to the intracellular second messenger, cyclic AMP. This messenger regulates many aspects of intracellular metabolism and function, including secretion, through the phosphorylating action of cyclic AMP-dependent protein kinase (A-kinase). The resulting protein phosphorylation stimulates exocytosis (e.g., to release amylase-containing secretory granules), but also leads to activation of nuclear regulatory factors and induction of gene expression (e.g., increased transcription of the amylase gene) (Fig. 17.**48**).

Calcium and the Phosphoinositide Cycle

Stimulation of acinar cells by muscarinic cholinergic, α-adrenergic (specifically the α_1-subtype), and some peptide neurotransmitters results in an elevation of intracellular calcium. Binding of ligands to these specific receptors activates another G protein known as G_q that serves to activate phospholipase C (Fig. 17.**49**). Activation of phospholipase C is the key step in the phosphoinositide pathway and catalyzes the formation of diacylglycerol (DAG) and inositol triphosphate (IP_3) from the substrate phosphatidylinositol 4,5-bisphosphate (PIP_2). DAG activates protein kinase C that in turn phosphorylates cytosolic proteins, but may also increase specific gene transcription (Fig. 17.**49**). IP_3 binds to receptors on intracellular membranes, resulting in mobilization of intracellular calcium by opening of gated Ca^{++} channels. As mentioned earlier in the section on water transport, calcium also rapidly mediates the trafficking of AQPs from intracellular membranes to the apical plasma membrane following stimulation with epinephrine that acts primarily through α_1-receptors.

Other Pathways and Interactions of Pathways

Muscarinic and a specific subtype of α-receptor (α_2) also inactivate adenylate cyclase through the inhibitory G-protein known as G_i. These receptors are linked to adenylate cyclase by an inhibitory G-protein, which subsequently binds GTP rather than the GDP that is bound in the inactive state. In addition, there is interaction between the cyclic AMP and the calcium pathways. For example, the A-kinase that is dependent on cyclic AMP elevation may phosphorylate Ca^{++}-channel proteins in intracellular membranes, or the plasma membrane, changing calcium fluxes within the cell or between the cell and its environment.

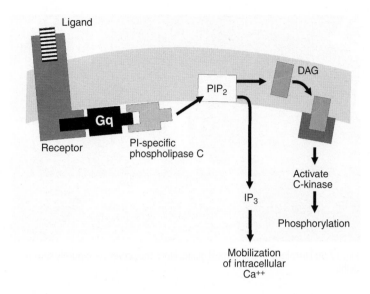

Fig. 17.**49** Diagram illustrating the phosphoinositide cycle and calcium ion-mediated signal transduction mechanisms.

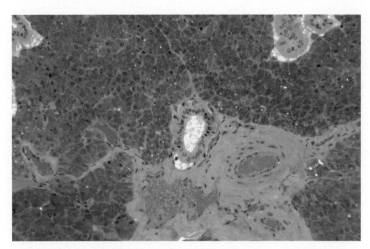

Fig. 17.**50** Histology of the parotid gland. Note the presence of purely serous acini.

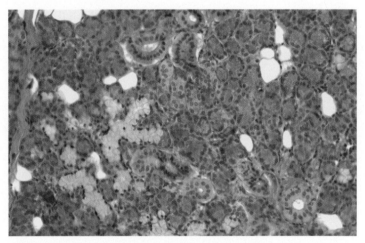

Fig. 17.**51** Histology of the submandibular gland. Note the presence of both serous and mucous acini, with a predominance of serous acinar cells.

Growth Factors and Peptides Secreted by the Salivary Glands

Two major growth factors have been isolated from the rodent salivary glands. Nerve growth factor (NGF) stimulates the growth of sympathetic ganglion cells, while epidermal growth factor (EGF) influences tooth eruption, epidermal keratinization, and cell proliferation and differentiation throughout the body. These growth factors are localized in specialized duct cells known as the granular convoluted tubules of the submandibular gland in rodents. EGF is found in human salivary glands, but predominantly in the intercalated ducts of the parotid gland. Granular convoluted tubule cells do not exist in the human submandibular glands. EGF is absorbed from the saliva by cells lining the oral cavity, esophagus, stomach, and small intestine. In the stomach, EGF appears to provide protection against ulceration and promotes healing of ulcers. The EGF levels in human saliva are approximately 1/1 000 those found in rat or mouse saliva. The presence of so much EGF in male rodent salivary glands has been teleologically associated with preening and a beneficial effect on skin wounds and normal epidermal cell turnover. Nonetheless, human salivary EGF may also be significantly active, via more or more active EGF receptors for EGF on the target cells. NGF and its transcripts have not been identified in human salivary glands. Atrial natriuretic peptide, renin, and other factors have been found in several species, while glucagon–like protein has been found in the human submandibular gland. Atrial natriuretic peptide is a protein first identified in the atria of the heart, which has an important function in electrolyte balance. Since ANP has been localized in the salivary glands it could regulate fluid balance in these organs that produce fluid equal to 20% of the plasma volume on a daily basis.

Distinguishing Characteristics of the Major Salivary Glands

Parotid Gland

The parotid gland is a purely serous gland in humans. The interlobular connective tissue contains a large number of fat cells that increase with age (Fig. 17.**50**). Fat cells may be distinguished from mucous cells by their totally vacuolated appearance and lack of mucigen. In the parotid gland, serous cells stain deeply with H and E, and intralobular ducts are prominent (Fig. 17.**50**, Table 17.**1**).

Submandibular Gland

The submandibular gland is a mixed-type of gland (in humans the majority of acini are serous). The ductal-arrangement of this gland is similar to that of the parotid gland, but with more striated ducts and fewer intercalated ducts. Acini are either purely serous or are mixed tubules comprising smaller serous and larger mucous cells (Fig. 17.**51**). Serous demilunes are evident. In some species, striated duct cells are modified in structure and are called granular convoluted tubule cells. In rodents, these specialized ducts store and secrete hormones and other pharmacologically active substances, such as NGF, renin, and EGF. Granular convoluted tubule cells do not exist in the human salivary glands.

Sublingual Gland

Most of the acini in this gland are mucous-secreting. There are few purely serous acini in humans (Fig. 17.**52**). There are, however, a few mixed acini with serous demilunes. Both segments of the intralobular duct system are poorly developed, and intercalated ducts are virtually absent. There is an absence of striations in the columnar cells lining the intralobular ducts that resorb sodium from the saliva. The absence of striations would imply that the resorption machinery is absent from the sublingual gland duct system. In fact, sublingual saliva has a much higher concentration of sodium than the other major salivary glands.

Distinguishing Characteristics of the Minor Salivary Glands

The minor salivary glands are located throughout the oral cavity in the lips, cheeks, hard and soft palate, tongue, and sublingual sulcus or floor of the mouth. They are unencapsulated and are named according to their location (i.e., labial, buccal, glossopalatine, palatine, and lingual). There are serous, mucous, and mixed-type minor salivary glands, as indicated in Figure 17.**53** and Table 17.**2**. These glands produce enzymatic and mucous secretions that are similar to those of the major salivary glands. Their secretory activity appears to be continuous rather than in response to specific stimuli. The minor salivary glands produce only about 10% of total salivary secretion, but approximately 70% of mucous secretion. The secretory products of the minor salivary glands empty into the oral cavity through numerous small ducts. In Figure 17.**54**, an interlobular (excretory duct, D) drains the predominantly mucous acini of a labial salivary gland. The minor salivary glands are polystomatic (multiple main excretory ducts), as compared to the parotid and submandibular glands that are monostomatic (one main excretory duct). The ducts of the minor salivary glands, particularly those in the region of the lips, tend to form cysts (mucoceles, see Clinical Application).

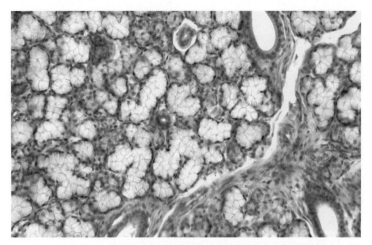

Fig. 17.**52** Histology of the sublingual gland. Note the presence of both serous and mucous acini, with a predominance of mucous acinar cells.

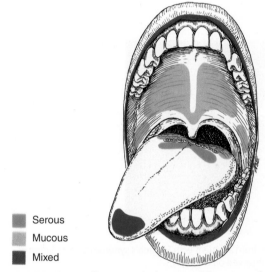

Serous

Mucous

Mixed

Fig. 17.**53** Diagram illustrating the location of the minor salivary glands.

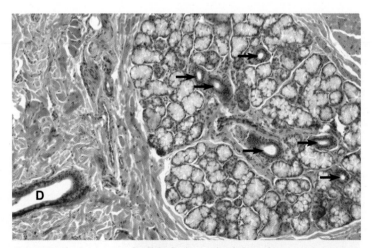

Fig. 17.**54** Photomicrograph of labial salivary glands (mostly mucous). A group of intralobular and smaller interlobular ducts are labeled with arrows. The smaller ducts drain into the larger interlobular (excretory) duct (D), which reaches the oral cavity.

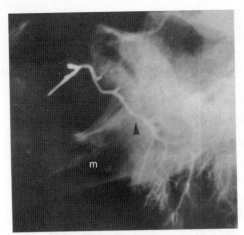

Fig. 17.**55** Normal sialogram of the human parotid gland.

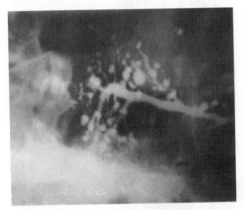

Fig. 17.**56** Sialogram from a patient with Sjogren's syndrome. Sacculation of the parotid duct is observed on the X-ray.

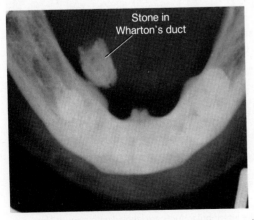

Fig. 17.**57** Occlusal film showing a patient with a stone (calculus) in the submandibular (Wharton's) duct.

Clinical Application

Mucoceles are retention cysts of the minor salivary gland ducts and contain mucus. They may be found throughout the oral cavity wherever minor salivary gland ducts open, but are most common on the lower lip. Mucoceles probably arise following irritation or mechanical trauma to the salivary gland ducts, which results in rupture or sometimes obstruction of the duct. The seepage of mucus into the surrounding connective tissue (lamina propria and submucosa) leads to inflammation and the formation of granulation tissue.

Clinical Application

The use of sialography to assess salivary gland function and dysfunction. A few diseases that alter the structure and function of the salivary glands are diagnosed by the use of an important X-ray technique, sialography. In sialography, a radiopaque substance is injected into the main salivary duct system before an X-ray is taken. Figure 17.**55** shows a normal sialogram with the duct and mandible labeled. Sialography is useful in the diagnosis of patients with tumors, Sjögren's syndrome, and salivary calculi.

Clinical Application

Sjögren's syndrome. Sjögren's syndrome is an autoimmune disease resulting in exocrine dysfunction, which was discussed in the connective-tissue section of this chapter. The syndrome is characterized by the absence or diminution of saliva and/or tears. The submandibular, parotid, palatine, and labial glands are the most frequently affected by the disease, which is manifested by extensive lymphoid infiltration and atrophy of the ductal, acinar, and myoepithelial cells. Proliferation of lymphoepithelial elements results in narrowing of the duct, with localized dilations proximal to the zones of narrowing. Sacculation of the parotid duct and the excretory ducts is shown in Figure 17.**56**, a lateral sialogram from a patient with Sjögren's syndrome.

Clinical Application

Salivary stones (sialolithiasis). Salivary duct stones occur most commonly in the submandibular duct and less commonly in the parotid duct. When such stones are small, they may have only a minor influence on gland function; larger stones, however, may obstruct the duct and produce large back-pressures on the gland, which induces sialoadenitis (inflammation), pain, and swelling with destruction of the parenchyma in severe cases. Calcium phosphate in the form of hydroxyapatite is the primary mineral component. Microorganisms are found within the calculi and are probably involved in the formation and growth of these structures. Figure 17.**57** demonstrates a large laminated stone at the orifice of Wharton's duct.

Clinical Application

Effects of aging on the salivary glands. Aging has an effect on the structure of the salivary glands. With age there is generally a decrease in salivary flow. The parotid, submandibular, and minor salivary glands all have histologic changes with age that include: 1) Acinar atrophy accompanied by fibrosis; 2) Replacement of the secretory tissue with adipose tissue; 3) Structural alterations in the ducts including intraductal deposits; 4) The appearance of oncocytes, enlarged, inactive secretory cells with pycnotic nuclei, which seem to arise from the acini. These changes occur independently of disease processes.

Clinical Application

Diseases and the salivary glands: diabetes and alcoholism. Endocrine diseases such as diabetes mellitus and disorders such as alcoholism result in sialadenosis (non-inflammatory and non-neoplastic disorders of the salivary glands) and sialadenitis (inflammation of the salivary glands) respectively. The result in both cases is a decrease in salivary flow rate. Neurologic diseases that affect the autonomic nervous system may alter the rate of salivation.

Clinical Application

Salivary gland neoplasms: The most common form of neoplasm of the salivary glands is the pleomorphic adenoma, which is a benign, slow-growing, and firm tumor most often located in the parotid, palatine, or buccal glands. The more common salivary gland malignant neoplasms include mucoepidermoid carcinoma, adenoid cystic carcinoma, and adenocarcinoma. These malignancies tend to be highly invasive, often causing ulceration and affecting nerves (recall the close relationship of the parotid gland to the facial nerve [Fig. 17.**15**]), leading to facial paralysis or numbness.

Clinical Application

Salivary flow rate is inversely related to the incidence of dental caries. Salivary factors influence the onset of periodontal disease and calculus formation. For example, increased plaque and calculus occur on the surface of the teeth opposite the openings of the main salivary gland excretory ducts. (Plaque formation and factors related to periodontal disease are discussed in Chapter 18.)

Summary

The human salivary glands are important organs of the oral cavity that produce saliva, an essential fluid required for normal speech, taste, mastication, swallowing, and digestion. In addition to its function in digestion, saliva maintains oral health through its antimicrobial, cleansing, lubricating, and buffering functions.

The three major salivary glands are the parotid, submandibular, and sublingual. In addition, there are numerous minor salivary glands in the cheeks, tongue, palate, lips, and other sites in the oral cavity that contribute to saliva production.

The salivary glands develop following a pattern of epithelial–mesenchymal interactions between the outgrowths of the oral (buccal) epithelium and the underlying mesenchyme. Salivary gland development requires the processes of differentiation, proliferation, and morphogenesis. The growth (proliferation of cells), cytodifferentiation (development of specific cellular phenotypes), and morphogenesis (development of shape and form) of the gland depend on both intrinsic and extrinsic factors. The programmed pattern of cell-specific gene expression is the genetic script established early in development, while extrinsic factors include cell–cell and cell–matrix interactions and growth factors. Accumulating evidence indicates that the positioning of the glands and the branching process is regulated by genes homologous to those regulating segmental differentiation in Drosophila (homeotic genes).

Interactions between cells as well as between cells and the ECM influence each of the steps in salivary-gland development. The glands develop in six stages: 1) Induction of bud formation from the oral epithelium by the underlying mesenchyme; 2) Formation and growth of the epithelial cord; 3) Initiation of branching in terminal parts of the cord; 4) Lobule formation through repetitive branching of the epithelial cord; 5) Canalization of the cords to form ducts; 6) Cytodifferentiation.

Branching is the primary morphogenetic process during salivary gland development. Branching begins with cleft formation followed by coordinated cell proliferation; however, branching and growth remain independent events. An intact basal lamina and the presence of mesenchyme are required for normal branching. Collagen synthesis stabilizes and maintains the branch points. Specific growth factors presented by ECM proteins appear to regulate events such as branching and lobule elongation.

The salivary glands are classified as: 1) Exocrine (having a duct system); 2) Compound tubuloacinar (a branched duct system with both tubular and acinar end pieces); 3) Merocrine (repeatedly functional) since cytoplasmic contents and cell membrane are conserved during secretion.

The salivary glands are classified as major and minor with serous, mucous, and mixed types of secretion. Three pairs of major salivary glands secrete into the oral cavity: parotid, submandibular, and sublingual glands. The major salivary glands produce most of the saliva, although the minor glands contribute their secretions to the 0.5 to 0.75L of saliva produced daily. The parotid ("around the ear") glands are the largest salivary glands and in humans secrete primarily an enzyme-rich serous secretion. The submandibular ("under the mandible") glands are mixed glands, mostly serous, that are located beneath the angle of the mandible. The sublingual ("under the tongue") glands are located beneath the floor of the oral cavity and are of the mixed type, albeit primarily mucous secretion.

Saliva is produced in a two-step process. Step one is the production of the primary saliva by the acinar cells. This original secretion is isotonic and is modified by the duct system into the hypotonic secretion released into the oral cavity. The duct system of the salivary glands consists of intralobular and interlobular portions. The intralobular portions include the intercalated ducts draining the acini and the striated (or secretory) ducts. Striated ducts are responsible for most of the sodium and potassium exchange (sodium reabsorption and potassium excretion) and they are believed to function in a manner similar to that of cells of the distal renal tubule. Their appearance resembles that of the distal renal tubule with basal infoldings of the plasma membrane stocked with numerous mitochondria that provide energy for active transport. Ductal and acinar cells use a variety of pumps, channels, and exchangers to carry out the important process of ionic transport to and from the saliva as it passes from the acini to the oral cavity. The aquaporins (AQPs) are a family of transmembrane proteins that facilitate the extensive water transport required for formation of saliva. Replacement of the gene for AQP is currently being investigated as an eventual means of treating patients who produce inadequate amounts of saliva leading to xerostomia.

The intercalated ducts are longest in the parotid gland, and the striated ducts are longest in the submandibular gland. The secretory ducts empty into the interlobular (excretory) ducts; these ultimately unite to form the main excretory duct, which subsequently opens into the oral cavity.

The secretory portions of the glands are called acini and contain serous or mucous cells, or both. Serous cells primarily secrete salivary amylase. The mucous cells secrete mucins. Myoepithelial cells, which appear to be of epithelial origin, wrap around the acinus and serve a contractile function, squeezing secretory material from the acinar cells, but also maintaining the cytoarchitecture of the acinus during secretion.

Secretion has been studied extensively in the serous

cells of the salivary glands. Release of amylase occurs primarily by a regulated secretory pathway in response to the binding of a secretagogue to cell surface receptors. Constitutive secretion utilizes vesicular shuttling to maintain basal (unstimulated) protein secretion and to transport membrane components to the apical and basolateral membranes. Specific processes occur in each intracellular compartment. The RER is the site of synthesis and initiation of folding, glycosylation, and processing of the sugars attached to proteins. In the Golgi apparatus further glycosylation as well as packaging and concentration of secretory products occurs. Secretory granules (vesicles) in the regulated pathway carry amylase to the cell surface where exocytosis occurs as the secretory granule fuses with the cell membrane.

Secretion is regulated by several intracellular systems. β-adrenergic drugs bind to β-receptors, stimulating a cascade of events involving stimulatory G-protein (G_s) and cyclic AMP. For example, when isoproterenol binds to the β-receptor, a G_s-binding site is exposed intracellularly and G_s-protein binds to the β-receptor. This complex binds GTP and activates cAMP, the well-defined second messenger that regulates metabolic events through phosphorylation and more indirectly through nuclear events. Intracellular calcium also regulates secretion through interaction with another G protein called G_q. This G protein activates the phospholipase C that catalyzes the formation of diacylglycerol (DAG) and inositol triphosphate (IP_3). Diacylglycerol activates C-kinase leading to increased cytosolic protein phosphorylation and gene transcription, while inositol triphosphate opens intracellular calcium channels. Another G protein (G_i) mediates signal transduction during muscarinic and α-receptor stimulation. This inhibitory G protein inactivates adenylate cyclase. These intracellular systems do not exist independently, but interact to regulate secretory events.

The salivary glands are also involved in the development of secretory immunity. The plasma cells in salivary gland connective tissue produce secretory immunoglobulin (IgA). Acinar and duct cells synthesize secretory component, which functions as a transmembrane receptor for dimeric IgA, a carrier for transcytosis across the acinar or duct cell, and a protective molecule that is attached to IgA upon release into the lumen.

The salivary glands receive an elaborate autonomic innervation from both sympathetic and parasympathetic nerves and they are sensitive to autonomic pharmacologic agents. β-adrenergic stimulation of the salivary glands results in an organic secretion (i.e., via exocytosis), while parasympathetic stimulation is largely watery. As well as having other normal functions, the salivary glands function in digestion and immune responses. These important organs of the oral cavity are affected in a number of pathologic conditions, such as Sjögren's syndrome, salivary calculi, mucoceles, and CF, and are significantly altered during the normal aging process.

Self-Evaluation Review

1. Describe the six stages in the development of the salivary glands. How do the ECM and basal lamina influence salivary gland morphogenesis and cytodifferentiation? What are the homeotic genes?

2. How are the salivary glands classified, on the basis of secretion or structure? Where are the major and minor salivary glands located? How do the three major salivary glands differ in histologic appearance (serous, mucous, or mixed type)?

3. Define the following terms: parenchyma, stroma, exocytosis, demilunes, and intercellular (secretory) canaliculi.

4. Describe the steps in the secretory pathway, beginning with nuclear events and progressing through the release of secretion. What is the primary secretion? How is it modified by the duct system? List the ionic transport systems that are used by the acinar and ductal cells to produce saliva. What are the aquaporins (AQPs)? How can they be used for treatment of humans with salivary secretory problems? Compare and contrast constitutive and regulated secretion.

5. Define transcription, translation, introns, exons, primary transcript, and the signal hypothesis.

6. Describe the appearance of the serous, mucous, and mixed acinar cells at the light and electron microscopic levels. Describe the light microscopic appearance of the intercalated, striated, and excretory ducts. Describe the functions of myoepithelial cells. Where are they located?

7. Describe the function of cyclic AMP, G proteins, the phosphoinositide cycle, and calcium in the regulation of acinar cell secretion.

8. Describe the synthesis of IgA and secretory component and the cells involved. What is the function of secretory component?

9. Describe the parasympathetic and sympathetic nerve distribution to the salivary glands and the regulatory role of the autonomic innervation.

10. Define xerostomia, sialography, salivary calculi, Sjögren's syndrome, and mucoceles.

11. What is the cause of CF? What is the cellular/molecular defect that results in the symptoms seen in CF?

Acknowledgements

Figure 17.**9** is reproduced with permission of the author and publisher from: Spooner BS, Bassett KE, Spooner BS Jr. Embryonic salivary gland epithelial branching activity is experimentally independent of epithelial expansion activity. Developmental Biology. 133:569,1989 (Academic Press Inc.).

Figure 17.**11** is reproduced with permission of the author and publisher from: Morita K, Nogawa H. Developmental Dynamics. 215:148–154, 1999 (Wiley-Liss, Inc.).

Figure 17.**15** is reproduced with permission of the author and publisher from: Gasser R. The early development of the parotid gland around the facial nerve and its branches in man. Anatomic Record. 167:63, 1970 (Alan R Liss, Inc.).

Figure 17.**32** is reproduced with the permission of Zastrow MV and Castle JD. Protein sorting among two distinct export pathways occurs from the content of maturing exocrine storage granules. Journal of Cell Biology. 105:2675, 1987 (The Rockefeller University Press).

Figure 17.**42** is reproduced with permission of the author and publisher from: Nagato T, Yoshida H, Yoshida A, Uehara Y. A scanning electron microscope study of myoepithelial cells in exocrine glands. Cell and Tissue Research. 209:1, 1980 (Springer Verlag).

Figure 17.**41** is reproduced with permission of the author and publisher from: Tandler B. Salivary glands and the secretory process. In: Textbook of Oral Biology. JH Shaw et al, eds. Philadelphia: WB Saunders Co; 1978.

Figures 17.**55**, 17.**56**, and 17.**57**, two sialograms and one X-ray, are copied (with permission) from the Diagnostic Radiologic Health Sciences Learning Laboratory, as developed by the Radiologic Health Sciences Education Project, University of California–San Francisco, under contract with the Bureau of Radiologic Health, the Food and Drug Administration, and in cooperation with the American College of Radiology. (Additional information is available from the American College of Radiology, 560 Lennon Lane, Walnut Creek, California 94598.)

Figures 17.**16**, 17.**34**, and 17.**36** are provided courtesy of Drs McKenzie and Klein from their text, Basic Concepts in Cell Biology and Histology (McGraw-Hill Book Company, 2000); with permission of McGraw-Hill Book Company.

The author thanks the late Karl A Youngstrom, MD PhD, for his assistance with the reproduction of the sialograms and X-rays, Barbara Fegley and the late William Bopp for electron microscopic technical assistance. I am grateful to Drs Bernard Tandler, Raymond F Gasser, J David Castle, Kuniharu Morita, Brian Spooner, and Hiroyuki Nogawa, and the American College of Radiology for their contribution of figures. Drs William D Ball, Robert C. De Lisle, Robert S Redman, and Brian Spooner are acknowledged for their painstaking critique and suggestions for updating this chapter. Electron microscopy was provided by the University of Kansas Medical Center Electron Microscopy Research Service Laboratory. The electron microscopy was funded in part by grants from the National Institute of Dental and Craniofacial Research. The author also acknowledges the new artwork in this (3rd) edition drawn by Larry Howell and the invaluable graphics assistance of Eileen Roach.

Suggested Readings

Alberts B, Bray D, Lewis J, Raff M, Roberts K, Watson, JD. Molecular Biology of the Cell. 3rd ed. New York, NY: Garland Publishing; 1989.

Ambudkar, IS. Regulation of calcium in salivary gland secretion. Crit. Rev. Oral Biol. Med. 2000;11:4–25.

Banerjee SD, Cohn RH, Bernfield MR. Basal lamina of embryonic salivary epithelia. Production by the epithelium and role in maintaining lobular morphology. J. Cell Biol. 1977;73:445–463.

Baum, BJ, Ambudkar IS, Horn VJ. Neurotransmitter control of calcium mobilization. In: Dobrosielski-Vergona K, ed. Biology of the Salivary Glands. Boca Raton, FL: CRC Press; 1993:105–127.

Bradley RM. Salivary Secretion. In: Getchell TV et al., eds. Smell and Taste in Health and Disease. New York, NY: Raven Press; 1991:127–144.

Castle D. Cell biology of salivary protein secretion. In: Dobrosielski-Vergona K, ed. Biology of the Salivary Glands. Boca Raton, FL: CRC Press; 1993;81–104.

Cook DI, Van Lennep EW, Roberts ML, Young JA. Secretion by the major salivary glands. In: Johnson LR, ed. Physiology of the Gastrointestinal Tract. New York, NY: Raven Press; 1994:1061–1117.

Cutler LS. The dependent and independent relationships between cytodifferentiation and morphogenesis in developing salivary gland secretory cells. Anat. Rec. 1980;196:341–347.

Denny PC, Ball WD, Redman RS. Salivary glands: A paradigm for diversity of gland development. Crit. Rev. Oral Biol. Med. 1997;8:51–75.

Field A, Scott J. Changes in the structure of salivary glands with age. In: Dobrosielski-Vergona K, ed. Biology of the Salivary Glands. Boca Raton, FL: CRC Press; 1993:397–439.

Garrett JR. The proper role of nerves in salivary secretion: A review. J. Dent. Res. 1987;66:387–397.

Garrett JR, Ekstrom J, Anderson LC, eds. Glandular Mechanisms of Salivary Secretion. New York, NY: S Karger; 1998.

Gasser RF. The early development of the parotid gland around the facial nerve and its branches in man. Anat. Rec. 1970;167:63–78.

Guggenheim B, Shapiro S, eds. Oral Biology at the Turn of the Century: Misconceptions, Truth, Challenges and Prospects. New York, NY: S Karger; 1999.

Kukuruzinska MA, Tabak LA, eds. Salivary Gland Biogenesis and Function. New York: New York Acad Sci. (Ann NY Acad Sci. V842);1998.

Lawson KA. The role of mesenchyme in the morphogenesis and functional differentiation of rat salivary epithelium. J. Embryol. Exp. Morphol. 1972;27:497–513.

McKenzie JC, Klein RM. Basic Concepts in Cell Biology and Histology. New York, NY: McGraw-Hill; 2000.

Malamud D, Tabak L, eds. Saliva as a Diagnostic Fluid. New York, NY: New York Acad Sci. (Ann NY Acad Sci. V694); 1993.

Nakanishi Y, Nogawa H, Hashimoto Y, Kishi JI, Hayakawa T. Accumulation of collagen III at the cleft points of developing mouse submandibular epithelium. Development. 1988;104:51–59.

Palade GE. Intracellular aspects of the process of protein synthesis. Science. 1975;189:347–358.

Quissell DO. Stimulus-exocytosis coupling mechanism in salivary gland cells. In: Dobrosielski-Vergona K, ed. Biology of the Salivary Glands. Boca Raton, FL: CRC Press; 1993:105–127.

Schramm M, Selinger Z. The function of α-, β-adrenergic receptors and a cholinergic receptor in the secretory cell of rat parotid gland. In: Ceccarelli B, Cleminti F, Meldolesi J, eds. Advances in Cytopharmacology. New York, NY: Raven Press; 1974:29–32.

Shear M. The structure and function of myoepithelial cells in salivary glands. Arch. Oral Biol. 1966;11:769–780.

Spooner BS, Wessells NK. An analysis of salivary gland morphogenesis: role of cytoplasmic microfilaments and microtubules. Dev. Biol. 1972;27:38–54.

Tandler B. Ultrastructure of the human submaxillary gland. I. Architecture and histologic relationships of the secretory cells. Am. J. Anat. 1962;111:287–307.

Tandler B. Salivary glands and the secretory process. In: Shaw JH, Sweeney EA, Cappuccino CC, Meller SM, eds. Textbook of Oral Biology. Philadelphia, PA: WB Saunders; 1978:547–592.

Turner RJ. Mechanisms of fluid secretion by salivary glands. Ann NY Acad Sci. 1993;694:24–35.

Work WO, Johns ME. Symposium on salivary gland diseases. Otolaryngol. Clin. North Am. 1977;10:259–463.

Young JA, Van Lennep EW. The Morphology of Salivary Glands. New York, NY: Academic Press; 1978.

18 Histology of Saliva, Pellicle, Plaque, and Calculus

James K. Avery

Introduction

Salivary glands daily secrete approximately 7500mL of saliva. It is a complex secretion and has two major functions: to keep the oral tissues moist and to provide protection from caries. The latter function is accomplished by constant deposition of salivary mucoprotein on the tooth surface. This will result in the gradual formation of the acquired tooth covering termed the pellicle (also termed the cuticle). The *acquired pellicle* is a structureless, nonmineralized layer, initially less than 1 μm thick, which forms rapidly on the polished tooth surface when it is contacted by saliva. Soon micro-organisms may appear on or within the pellicle and begin proliferating. Within 24 hours, in a protected site and without cleansing, a soft observable deposit termed plaque appears. Plaque may lead to either mineralized calculus or caries, which are important in the consideration of oral histology. These structures are on or in the teeth of most individuals. Thus in the absence of adequate oral hygiene, saliva may transcend its protective function and serve as a medium for micro-organisms that contribute to caries or periodontal disease. Saliva is 90% water; the remaining 10% is composed of small amounts of other numerous substances. Amylase, which acts on carbohydrates and produces glucose and maltose, is found in saliva. A lipolytic enzyme produced by the lingual glands hydrolyzes triglycerides to diglycerides and fatty acids. Digestion, to a limited extent, thus begins in the oral cavity. In addition, at least four salivary proteins inhibit the growth and the secretion of peroxidase by oral bacteria. Thiocyanate and iodine in saliva are bactericidal, and lysosome hydrolyzes bacterial cell walls. Salivary IgA inhibits adherence of micro-organisms to oral tissues.

Objectives

After reading this chapter, you should be able to describe the composition and histology of saliva. You should also be able to discuss the formation and histology of the pellicle, plaque, and calculus.

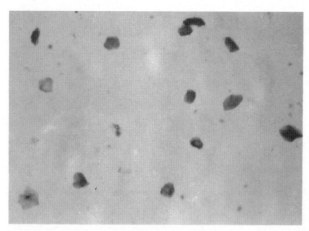

Fig. 18.**1** Salivary smear showing epithelial cells.

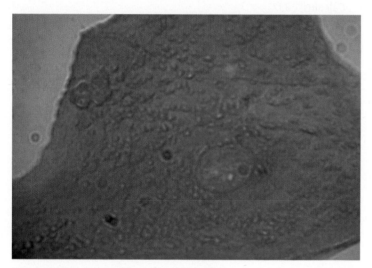

Fig. 18.**2** Bacteria on surface of epithelial cell.

Saliva

Desquamated epithelial cells are the most common cellular elements, other than bacteria, found in saliva. These cells are sloughed into the saliva and can be found in any salivary smear (Fig. 18.**1**). They are large, flat, and polygonal. They can be found floating free in the saliva and, on swabbing of the mucosa, are found in large numbers. Because most of the oral mucosa is nonkeratinized, the majority of observed epithelial cells are nucleated. The nucleated cells, when viewed microscopically, reveal sex differences. The presence of a large chromatin granule adjacent to the nuclear membrane indicates the nucleus of a female. A view of an epithelial cell at a higher magnification than that seen in Figure 18.1 reveals the centrally located nucleus and numerous bacteria adhering to the surface of the cell (Fig. 18.**2**).

Saliva also contains lymphocytes and polymorphonuclear leukocytes. When these are in the oral cavity, they are termed *salivary corpuscles*. The number of salivary corpuscles in saliva is dependant on the state of oral health. Elevated levels of lymphocytes in saliva are observed if the tonsils are infected. Higher levels of leukocytes and lymphocytes originate from the gingival crevice as a result of infected pockets around the teeth. Figure 18.**3** is a view of inflamed gingiva with numerous leukocytes, lymphocytes, and plasma cells. A gingival pocket with plaque, bacteria, and inflammatory cells is seen in Figure 18.**4**, with the epithelium on the left and root cementum and dentin on the extreme right. Leukocytes as well as densely stained plaque are seen on the right. Some lymphocytes wander away from the germinal centers of the tonsils, especially if the tonsils are infected. They migrate out of the tonsillar crypts into the pharyngeal and oral cavities to become *salivary corpuscles*. Lymphocytes may function in antibody–antigen relationship and may also function as macrophages, as

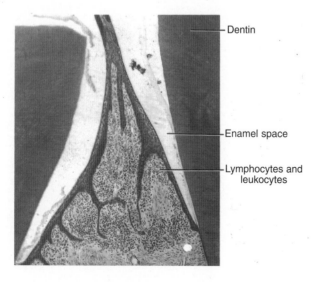

Dentin

Enamel space

Lymphocytes and leukocytes

Fig. 18.**3** Gingivitis resulting in leukocytes and lymphocytes in saliva.

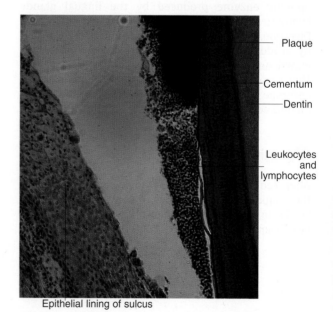

Plaque

Cementum

Dentin

Leukocytes and lymphocytes

Epithelial lining of sulcus

Fig. 18.**4** Plaque and bacteria in gingival crevice.

seen in Figure 18.**5**. Note the engulfed coccal bacteria in this salivary lymphocyte.

Analysis of a salivary smear will likely yield, in addition to desquamated epithelial cells and salivary corpuscles, clumps of mucin to which bacteria are attached (Fig. 18.**6**). Secretory glycoproteins of mucins represent the main organic substance of saliva and may be readily seen if the salivary smear is stained.

Pellicle

The structures that cover the tooth surface may be either *developmental* or *acquired*. The *developmental cuticles* include the *primary acellular cuticle* or dental cuticle, formed as the final secretory product of ameloblasts, and the *secondary cellular cuticle*, formed from remnants of the reduced enamel epithelium. The term "cellular" is misleading in that cellular outlines are lost as the secondary cuticle becomes keratinized. Both developmental cuticles are lost, or worn away almost entirely, as a result of mastication. Some reduced enamel epithelium initially remains in the depths of the gingival crevice and is eventually "turned over" as the basal epithelium cells proliferate throughout life. A third developmental tooth covering is the *coronal cement* found as thin patches of acellular cementum in the cervical area of the crown.

The *acquired coverings* of the tooth surface include the cuticle, preferably termed the *pellicle*, which is thin, structureless membrane that forms as a result of salivary mucoproteins and sialoproteins bathing the tooth surface (Fig. 18.**7**). The presence of a deep, narrow, central fissure in the occlusal surface allows the salivary proteins to accumulate in its depth. The inability of a toothbrush to clean such a fissure properly results in an area such as is seen in Figure 18.**8**. Although an acquired pel-

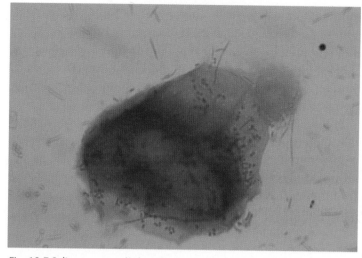

Fig. 18.**5** Salivary corpuscle: lymphocyte with bacteria on its surface (arrow).

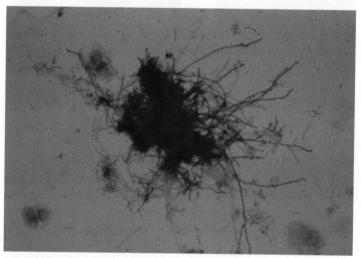

Fig. 18.**6** Clumps of mucin in saliva.

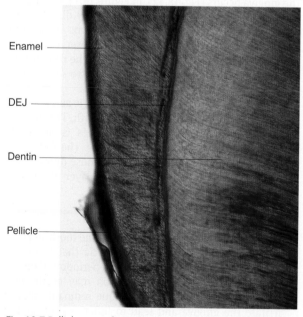

Enamel

DEJ

Dentin

Pellicle

Fig. 18.**7** Pellicle on surface of enamel. DEJ: dentinoenamel junction.

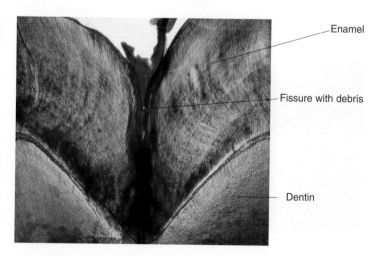

Enamel

Fissure with debris

Dentin

Fig. 18.**8** Plaque in central fissure of enamel.

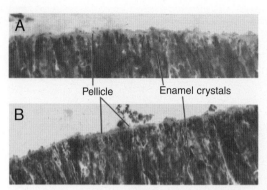

Fig. 18.**9 A** Transmission electron micrograph of bacteria-free acquired pellicle on surface of enamel. **B** Ultrastructure of bacteria-free acquired pellicle on enamel surface.

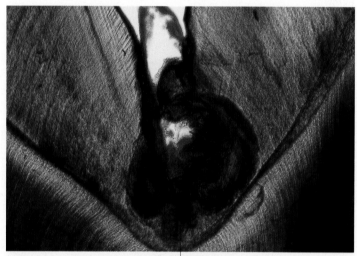

Plaque in central fissure

Fig. 18.**10** Plaque and early caries in central fissure of human molar.

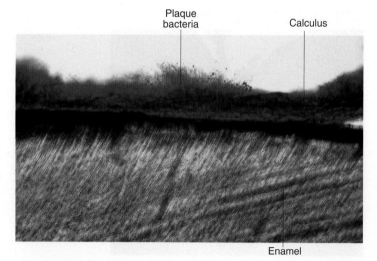

Plaque bacteria   Calculus

Enamel

Fig. 18.**11** Plaque bacteria on surface of thin layer of calculus on cervical enamel.

licle covers the tooth surface, it will penetrate in any convenient discrepancy on the tooth surface, such as a crack, overhanging filling, or a lamella.

At an ultrastructural level, the acquired pellicle has a fine granular appearance and is approximately 500 Å in thickness. It may be devoid of micro-organisms. The tooth surface seen in Figures 18.**9A** and **B**, happens to be bacteria-free. The thin pellicle is seen overlying the densely packed crystals of enamel apatite, which have their long axes perpendicular to the enamel surface. This area is described as the prismless zone of enamel.

Plaque

The central fissure in a premolar or molar is a site for accumulation of oral micro-organisms that readily colonize it. They attach to any convenient mucins and take advantage of any food debris. These micro-organisms rapidly form into a thick plaque and attack the enamel surface (Fig. 18.**10**). In Figure 18.**10**, the developing cavity is limited to the enamel but will probably soon expand along the dentinoenamel junction (DEJ) to penetrate the dentinal tubules.

The cervical area of the tooth is another region susceptible to plaque development and subsequent destruction of the tooth surface. In Figure 18.**11**, the filamentous bacteria of the plaque are seen on the cervical enamel surface. Beneath the plaque is a thin deposit of calculus. Instead of caries destroying the surface of the tooth shown in this figure, the pH was sufficiently alkaline to result in the deposit of minerals on the cytoskeleton of bacteria, and calculus was formed. Mineralization rather than demineralization has occurred.

When plaque development takes place in a gingival sulcus, the bacteria increase in number and, with the addition of the calculus as an irritant, inflammation of the gingiva occurs (Fig. 18.**12**). In Figure 18.**12**, calculus is seen overlying the enamel space (enamel dissolved in tissue preparation), and cells and organisms are seen in the plaque at the depth of the pocket. Observe that the epithelial attachment is on the surface of the cementum, not the enamel. Inflammatory cells are also seen in the lamina propria underlying the epithelium.

The plaque or microbial flora is not static and is closely related to the state of periodontal health. The flora in the supragingival and subgingival zones is different, depending on the extent of the disease. The following brief description summarizes some of these differences. In patients with *normal* tissues, a thin layer of coccoid

Clinical Application

The destructive events occurring on the tooth's surface lead from deposition of bacteria that form a plaque to the condition of caries or periodontal disease. If acidic, enamel dissolution may occur; if basic, calculus may form in plaque remnants that irritate the gingiva and lead to inflammation and tissue necrosis.

bacteria may appear on the pellicle. In patients with *gingivitis*, more filamentous bacteria with a corncob appearance have been reported supragingivally. In addition, greater numbers of Gram-negative bacteria, flagellated cells, and spirochetes can be found in the sulcus. In patients with periodontitis, as in patients with gingivitis, more filamentous bacteria with a corncob appearance have been reported supragingivally. In addition, a greater number of Gram-negative bacteria, flagellated cells, and spirochetes adhere to the root surface subgingivally. Periodontosis patients exhibit predominantly (although sparsely) Gram-negative bacteria. These patients also exhibit a unique lobulated cuticular deposit that appears electron dense.

A transmission electron micrograph (Fig.18.**13**) reveals the appearance of 7-day-old dental plaque. At the bottom of the field is the surface of the enamel covered with a thin, dark-staining pellicle. Above this line is the feltwork of plaque micro-organisms. Filamentous bacteria are seen at the top of the micrograph. When the deeper portion of the 7-day-old plaque is studied at higher magnification with transmission electron microscopy, the identity of the bacteria on the enamel surface can be seen (Fig. 18.**14**). The clear space at the bottom of the field represents the demineralized surface enamel. Overlying it is a thin, electron-dense pellicle. The deepest part of the plaque consists of a condensed microbial layer that appears as a darkly stained band resting on the pellicle. Above this layer is a superficial layer of coccoid and filamentous micro-organisms. The light areas in the plaque contain cell remnants, mucopolysaccharide substances, and glycoproteins. In this zone, active acid production by the cocci occurs, resulting in surface etching and dental caries.

A higher magnification of the condensed microbial layer of plaque, on an enamel surface, is seen in Figure 18.**15**. Below is enamel with the thin black pellicle on its surface. At this high magnification, a pellicle is seen to be discontinuous. The remainder of the field shows the condensed microbial layer consisting of coccoid micro-

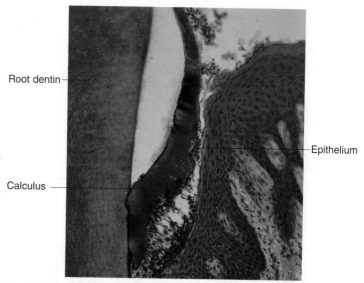

Fig. 18.**12** Gingival sulcus with calculus, plaque, and bacteria. Enamel was removed in tissue preparation, producing enamel space.

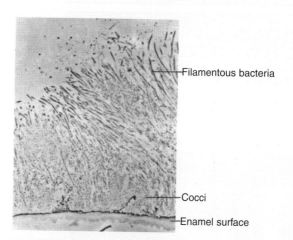

Fig. 18.**13** Transmission electron micrograph of plaque bacteria on enamel surface after 7 days.

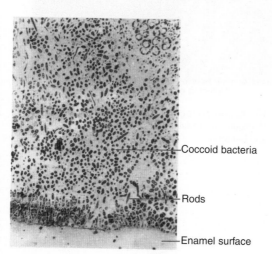

Fig. 18.**14** Electron micrograph of bacteria on enamel surface seen in Figure 18.13, with coccoid and rods noted.

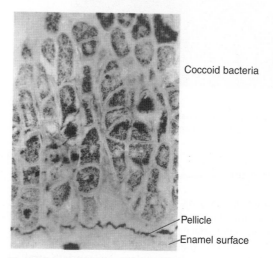

Fig. 18.**15** Ultrastructure of condensed bacterial layer on enamel surface denotes the region of active cell division.

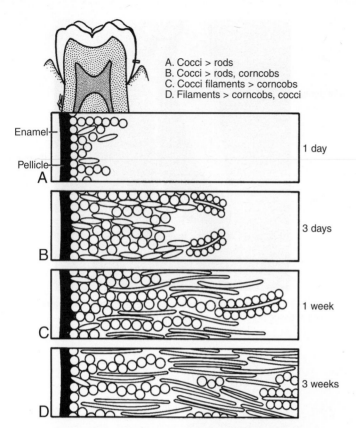

A. Cocci > rods
B. Cocci > rods, corncobs
C. Cocci filaments > corncobs
D. Filaments > corncobs, cocci

Fig. 18.**16** Changes in composition of plaque with time. On day 1, cocci and rods can be seen; after 1 week, filamentous bacteria appear.

organisms, which appear to be dividing in a plane perpendicular to the enamel surface. Polysaccharides are located between the bacteria. Ribosomes can also be observed in a few bacteria.

Numerous dental investigators have shown that the composition of plaque changes with time (Fig.18.**16**). Initially, cocci and rods appear, and after a week filamentous organisms are seen. The composition of the plaque is dependent on the extent of gingival disease and its location supragingivally or subgingivally.

As seen in Figures 18.**9A** and **B**, the outermost area of enamel in the teeth of most patients is composed of a prismless zone about 30 µm thick. In this zone, the c-axis or long axis of the apatite crystals is situated almost perpendicular to the tooth surface. The initial carious lesion involves this zone, as plaque bacteria cause dissolution of some of these crystals. This dissolution is illustrated in Figure 18.**17**; a brown spot is seen on the left, and normal tooth structure is seen on the right. Situated between the overlying bacteria of the plaque and the enamel surface is an amorphous-appearing pellicle. Enamel crystal dissolution is seen in the superficial zone on the left. Another case of a superficial lesion in the enamel of an adult human is seen in Figure 18.**18**. In this figure, a small penetrating defect filled with organic materials is observed. Remains of an organic pellicle overlying a surface zone of altered enamel can also be seen.

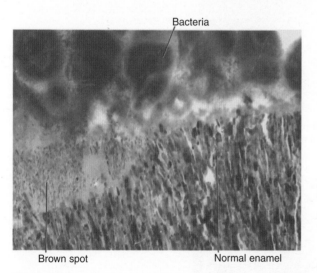

Fig. 18.**17** Electron micrograph of initial carious lesion on enamel surface, with enamel crystal dissolution (left) under bacteria.

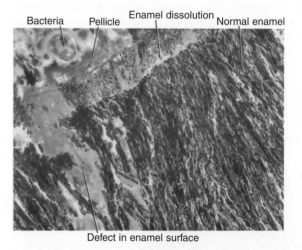

Fig. 18.**18** Electron micrograph of penetrating defect in enamel filled with organic material and of enamel dissolution under pellicle and bacteria.

Clinical Application

Plaque bacteria ferment sugars to lactic acid, which will then destroy the mineralized enamel. Destruction of the protective pellicle and the enamel surface is a progressive process. A disclosing agent can expose plaque bacteria to facilitate its removal but plaque will re-form unless appropriate oral hygiene is practiced.

Calculus

The formation of calculus begins by a process opposite to that of tooth surface dissolution. The beginning of inorganic crystallization of the tooth surface occurs in the inner organic layer of the pellicle and the overlying bacteria of the dental plaque (Fig. 18.**19**). Dense granular particles that appear smaller than enamel apatite crystals are around and in the bacterial matrix. Calcification then spreads between the bacteria into the adjacent plaque. Calcification first takes place in the cell walls, and then the cores of the bacteria calcify to produce calculus. The surface of the tooth then becomes covered with a continuous layer of apatite crystals. This layer gradually thickens as further deposition occurs.

Figure 18.**20** illustrates the appearance of calculus formed in root dentin. Dentinal tubules containing large atypical mineral crystal can be seen (lower left). This indicates that demineralization related to the carious process was reversed and precipitation of mineral had occurred. At the top of the electron micrograph, calcified bacteria and matrix can be seen.

As is seen in Figure 18.**21**, there is close adaption of calculus to the irregular surface of root dentin. The adaption seen in this figure was a result of scaling of the root surface. The calcified bacteria appear as circular profiles. Observe how much smaller the hydroxyapatite crystals are in the calculus compared with the underlying dentin. Calculus forms in a calcospheric manner as the calcium salts derived from saliva are deposited within the organic matter. The glycoprotein matrix and the bacteria become mineralized if the oral environment maintains an alkaline pH. As the plaque mineralizes, it loses its ability to produce an acid environment. Calculus varies in composition and in hardness. Very hard calculus con-

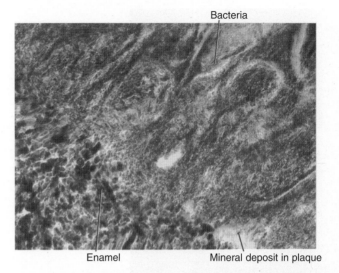

Fig. 18.**19** Electron micrograph of minute crystals on the surface of enamel denotes calculus formation. A calcified bacterial matrix is seen.

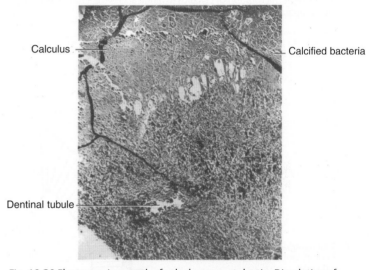

Fig. 18.**20** Electron micrograph of calculus on root dentin. Dissolution of mineral in dentinal tubule indicates reversal of caries process.

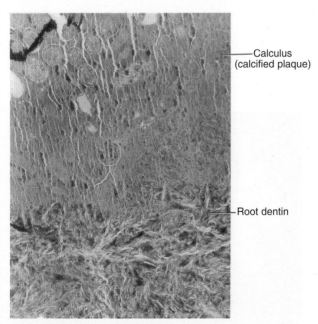

Fig. 18.**21** Electron micrograph of calculus on irregular surface of dentin after root scaling. Note the minute size of the crystals in the calculus compared with those in the dentin.

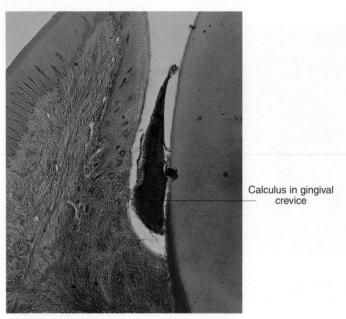

Fig. 18.**22** Light micrograph of calculus in gingival crevice. Enamel was lost in tissue preparation.

Calculus in gingival crevice

tains a higher percentage of inorganic salts. Softer calculus has a higher percentage of protein. Calculus is most often found near the opening of the parotid excretory ducts, on the buccal surfaces of the mandibular incisors, near the opening of the submandibular and sublingual gland ducts.

Calculus can be categorized clinically into two types: supragingival or *salivary*, appearing above the gingival crest, and subgingival or *serumal* within the gingival crevice. Subgingival calculus is much harder and forms more slowly than salivary calculus.

A typical picture of calculus appearing in a gingival crevice is shown in Figure 18.**22**. This deposit has caused gingival inflammation, and inflammatory cells can be seen in the lamina propria of the gingiva. Observe the location of the gingival attachment on the dark-staining cementum rather than on the enamel. Where there is calculus, inflammatory cells usually can be found in the underlying gingival epithelium.

The mouth is said to be a microuniverse of organisms. The acquired pellicle is an amorphous organic deposition on enamel, on which plaque may form. Plaque is derived from desquamated epithelial cells and is composed of mucin, dextrans, sugars, and bacteria. The composition of the plaque changes with the time, location, and extent of the disease process. The composition of supragingival and subgingival plaque varies, as does the bacterial composition in the periodontal pocket. These variables are expressed in Figure 18.**23**. If the pH of the saliva is alkaline, calculus may develop from mineralization of the plaque, and this may be salivary or serumnal.

Figure 18.**24** is an example of a mouth that requires extensive care and patience. This patient is dependent on your knowledge of oral hygiene.

A. Supragingival plaque
Predominantly Gram-positive rods and cocci
Very few Gram-negative rods and motile forms

B. Subgingival plaque
•Marginal plaque
Mostly Gram-positive rods and cocci
Some Gram-negative rods and motile forms

—Calculus

•Pocket plaque
Predominantly Gram-negative rods and motile forms

Fig. 18.**23** Summary of presence and identification of bacteria in supragingival, subgingival, and periodontal pocket.

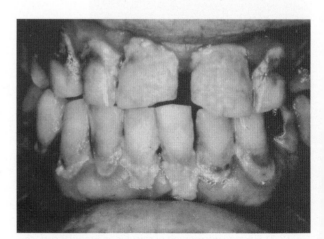

Fig. 18.**24** Plaque, calculus, and severe periodontal problems can be seen in this patient's mouth.

Clinical Application

Saliva bathes the tooth's surface and assists in the formation of the protective organic membrane, the pellicle. Micro-organisms collect in protected sites forming a deposit. Thus, saliva, which usually serves a protective function in bathing the tooth, then serves as a medium for the growth of organisms on the tooth.

Clinical Application

Cells of the saliva include, most commonly, epithelial cells shed from the mucosa, lymphocytes, and leukocytes. The two latter cells are termed salivary corpuscles and are prevalent when either of these sites of origin is infected. Lymphocytes arise from the tonsils and leukocytes from gingival crevices.

Summary

Figure 18.**25** is a diagram summarizing the activity occurring within plaque. This diagram illustrates the typical location of development of plaque at the interdental gingival margin. Above the gingiva the washing action of saliva is seen, which assures the self-cleansing of enamel areas. Plaque accumulates at the gingival margin, and the presence of sucrose gives rise to a synthesis of slimy extracellular oligosaccharides and glucose, which diffuse into the deeper layers of the plaque. There they may be fermented to lactic acid, which penetrates the enamel and causes mineral diffusion onto the plaque. The large polysaccharide molecules of starches do not diffuse into the plaque.

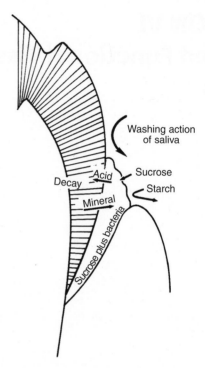

Fig. 18.**25** Summary of plaque activity and enamel dissolution.

Self-Evaluation Review

1. Name and characterize the outermost layer of enamel.
2. Describe the changes that occur in the plaque from 1 day to 3 weeks.
3. On what matrix does calculus form?
4. What changes occur in the pellicle underlying the plaque?
5. Describe some histologic characteriestics of the plaque.
6. Where does plaque usually form?
7. Describe the cells found in saliva and their origin.
8. Describe the composition of a pellicle.
9. Name the organisms found deep in the plaque supragingivallyand subgingivally.
10. How long does it take for an acquired pellicle to form?

Acknowledgements

Photomicrographs in Figures 18.**9A**, 18.**17**, 18.**18**, and 18.**19** were provided by Dr Robert Frank, Professor and Dean, and by Dr Mendel, Faculté de Chirurgie Dentaire, Strasbourg, France. Photomicrographs for Figures 18.**20** and 18.**21** were provided by Dr Knut Selvig, Professor and Head, Department of Dental Research, School of Dentistry, University of Bergen, Norway. Photographs for Figures 18.**13**, 18.**14**, and 18.**15** were provided by scientists at the National Institute of Dental Research, Bethesda, Maryland.
Data for Figure 18.**24** was provided by Dr Walter Loesche, University of Michigan School of Dentistry, Ann Arbor, Michigan.

Suggested Readings

Frank RM, Brendel A. Ultrastructure of the proximal plaque and the underlying normal and carious enamel. Arch. Oral Biol. 1996;11:888–912.
Hand AR. Salivary glands. In: Orban's Oral Histology and Embryology. 11th ed. Bhaskar SN, ed. St Louis Mo: CV Mosby; 1990.

SECTION VI
Related Functional Tissues of the Oral and Paraoral Areas

19 Histology of the Nasal Mucosa and Paranasal Sinuses

Geoffrey H. Sperber

Introduction

This chapter discusses the nasal cavity, the paranasal sinuses, and olfaction. The nasal cavity protrudes from the median pyriform fossa of the skull, whereas the paranasal sinuses are buried within the bones surrounding the nasopharynx. The nasal septum divides the cavity into two parts. The lateral walls contain projections that vastly increase the area exposed to respiratory air. The mucosa of the nasal cavity aids in humidification and warming or cooling of the air during respiration. Epithelium lining the nasal cavity is respiratory epithelium (ciliated pseudostratified columnar epithelium with goblet cells), and the lamina propria contains numerous glands and a rich venous sinusoidal network.

The paranasal sinuses are a group of air-containing spaces around the nasal cavity. In the adult, the frontal, sphenoid, and maxillary sinuses are large paired sinuses. There are numerous ethmoid sinuses in the superior parts of the nasal cavity. The mucosa of these sinuses is similar to that of the nasal cavity, but the epithelium and lamina propria are thinner.

Olfactory mucosa is found in the superior parts of the nasal cavity. Neuroreceptor cells for the sense of smell are located within the epithelium of this mucosa. The neuroreceptor cells are first-order neurons and are considered to be part of the central nervous system. These cells have the ability to regenerate and re-establish connections with the central nervous system.

Objectives

After reading this chapter, you will be familiar with the microscopic structure of the nasal tissues and paranasal sinuses. Included in this knowledge will be an understanding of the function of these tissues. You should be able to describe the histologic detail of the olfactory mucosa and the basic neuroanatomic connections for olfaction. Also, you should be able to discuss the regeneration capacity of the olfactory epithelium, and to describe the anatomic basis for the sense of smell (olfaction).

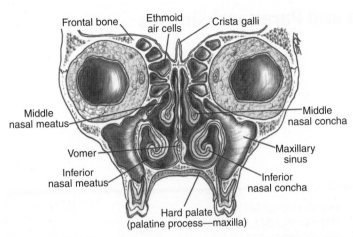

Fig. 19.**1** Diagram of relations of oral, nasal, and paranasal cavities: frontal view. Note the opening of the maxillary sinuses into the nasal cavity and the relations of its floor to the molar teeth.

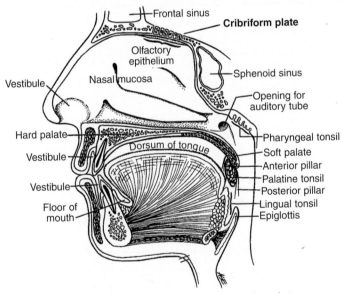

Fig. 19.**2** Diagram of relations of nasal and oral cavities: lateral view.

Nasal Cavity

In early embryonic development, the oral and nasal cavities are a single chamber—the stomodeum. The stomodeal chamber becomes horizontally divided into upper (nasal) and lower (oral) compartments by the elevation of palatine shelves (see palate development, Chapter 2). Coincidentally, the epithelia of the nasal and oral cavities specialize to accommodate the different needs of these areas—respiration for the nose and mastication for the mouth. The nasal cavity is divided into two halves separated by the nasal septum. The midline septum is composed of hyaline cartilage and of two bony parts: the vomer bone and the perpendicular plate of the ethmoid bone (Figs. 19.**1** and 19.**2**). The nasal septum is frequently deflected from the midline, impairing nasal breathing and resulting in mouth breathing with deleterious consequences. During fetal life (8 to 30 weeks postconception) a transient vomeronasal organ (Jacobson organ) develops in the nasal septum, which may serve as a temporary endocrine gland. It normally atrophies and disappears by birth, but may persist and possibly act as a pheromone detector.

At the entrance to the nostrils are nasal hairs that serve as a filter of inhaled particulate matter. The hairs are characterized by their constrained growth in length, in contrast to facial and scalp hairs, thus resembling eyelash hairs.

The inferior floor of the nasal cavity is much wider than the superior aspect. The lateral walls have bony, curved protuberances that project into the nasal cavity and are termed conchae or turbinates (Fig. 19.**1**). Usually, there are three conchae: superior, middle, and inferior. The superior and middle conchae are formed from the ethmoid bone. The inferior concha develops as a separate bone and is much larger than the other conchae. Beneath each concha is a channel called a meatus. These are the superior, middle, and inferior meatus. The bony surfaces and cartilage of the nasal cavities are covered by respiratory epithelium. This is a pseudostratified, ciliated, columnar epithelium and contains numerous goblet cells. The nasal cavity extends from the nares (nostrils) anteriorly to the two posterior nasal apertures (choanae), with the nasopharynx directly posteriorly (Fig. 19.**2**).

In the superior aspect of the nasal cavity, the olfactory epithelium underlies the cribriform plate of the ethmoid bone (Fig. 19.**2**). The cribriform plate is perforated by numerous foramina through which pass neural connections from the olfactory epithelium to the olfactory bulbs of the brain. This epithelium differs from the remainder of the nasal cavity in that it contains cells that are the receptors for smell (olfaction).

The nasal cavity ends posteriorly in the nasopharynx at the posterior border of the vomer bone. The respiratory epithelium continues into the nasopharynx. In areas of the nasopharynx, where the soft palate approximates the posterior wall of the nasopharynx in functional movements (speech and swallowing), the epithelium is stratified squamous.

Mucosa of Nasal Cavity

Nasal mucosa, like oral mucosa, is composed of overlying epithelium and subjacent connective tissue termed lamina propria. The respiratory epithelium of the nasal cavity is structurally different from the stratified squamous epithelium of the oral cavity. However, respiratory epithelium is not limited to the nasal cavity, similar epithelia are located in parts of the pharynx, trachea, bronchi, and bronchioles.

Respiratory epithelium is composed of basal, ciliated, and mucous cells. All of these cells rest on a prominent basement membrane. In a histologic section, the cell nuclei appear at different levels, giving the appearance of a stratified epithelium. The adjective "pseudostratified" is used to describe this epithelium. The cells that reach the lumen (ciliated and mucous) are columnar; therefore, the full description of this epithelium is "pseudostratified columnar epithelium."

Basal cells are the site of cell divisions. Daughter cells then continuously replace the mucous and ciliated cells. Mucous cells have a thin stem–like extension of the cell arising from the basement membrane, and the apical cytoplasm is filled with varying amounts of mucus. The nucleus is situated between these parts of the cell. When full of mucus, these cells look like goblet glasses; hence, the term "goblet cells" is commonly used to describe these mucous cells. A blanket of mucus coats the surface of the respiratory epithelium. The mucus is a product of the goblet cells and the seromucous glands in the lamina propria. This mucus traps dust and other particulate material, and the mucous coat is moved by action of cilia of the ciliated cells. The mucociliary system is responsible for clearing inhaled particles and pathogens from the airways.

Cilia arise from basal bodies found in the apical (luminal) end of the cell. They are round, finger–like processes numbering over 200 per cell, and project out into the lumen about 5 µm. Inside each cilium is an outer ring of nine paired microtubules and a central pair of microtubules. The cilia beat at 10 to 20 cycles/second with a fast whiplike forward stroke and a slower recovery stroke. These cilia beat in a local fluid environment (periciliary layer) that is less viscous than the blanket of mucus that coats the surface above the cilia. The periciliary fluid is thought to be secreted by the ciliated cells, and the mucous coat by the goblet cells and glands in the lamina propria. The coordinated movement of the cilia moves the mucous coat posteriorly to the nasopharynx where the mucus can be either swallowed or expectorated.

In the more exposed areas, such as the medial aspects of the conchae and the surfaces of nasal septum, where air is continuously being inspired and exhaled, the mucosa is thickest (up to several millimeters) (Figs. 19.**3** and 19.**4**). The basement membrane is prominent, and there are numerous goblet cells in the epithelium (Fig. 19.**3**). These areas are in contrast to the areas in the nasal meatus and floor of the nasal cavity, where the epithelium and basement membrane are much thinner and fewer goblet cells appear.

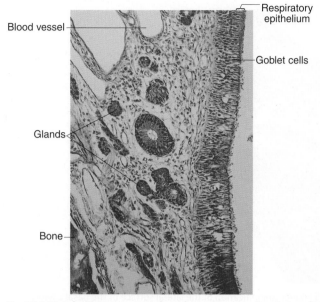

Fig. 19.**3** Histologic appearance of nasal sinus mucosa. Respiratory lining epithelium with goblet cells is on the right, and bone is on the left. Observe mixed glands and blood vessels in the lamina propria.

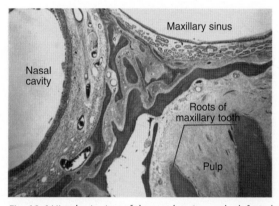

Fig. 19.**4** Histologic view of the nasal cavity on the left and the maxillary sinus on the upper right reveals the thickness of the respiratory epithelium. Note the numerous glands underlying the sinus mucosa. Molar tooth roots are on the lower right.

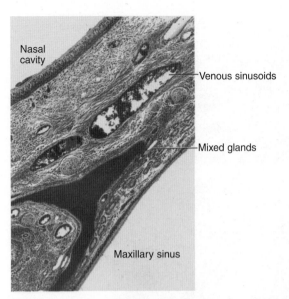

Fig. 19.**5** Higher magnification of the lateral surface of the nasal cavity (above) and maxillary sinus mucosa (below). Note the venous sinusoids underlying the mucosa and the mixed glands.

The medial surfaces of the conchae and septum are areas directly exposed to incoming drafts of air, and these areas have numerous mixed glands present in the lamina propria. The glands are very numerous (6 to 10 glands/mm^2), and the cells of the glands include serous, mucous, and mixed types. Serous demilunes are present in some of the glands. The lamina propria is also richly supplied with blood vessels that freely anastomose, and prominent venous sinusoids are present. This network of large veins is similar to erectile tissue (Figs. 19.**3**–19.**5**). Secretions of the goblet cells and the glands coat the surface of the epithelium and protect it from dehydration. The watery component of these secretions humidifies the inspired air, and the rich blood supply of the underlying lamina propria heats (or cools) this air. Many free nerve endings are found in the lamina propria and, when irritated, reflexly give rise to sneezing fits. Few encapsulated nerve endings are found here.

Allergic reactions and respiratory infections, such as the common cold, cause the venous sinusoids to become engorged with blood and the glands to produce abundant quantities of secretions. This accounts for the nasal discharge and "stuffed-up" feeling in the nasal cavity associated with these conditions. Medications to counteract the nasal symptoms of minor infections and allergies act on the vascular system causing vasoconstriction. These medications also affect the mucous glands by interfering with the secretomotor stimuli (mainly arising from the parasympathetic system). In the connective tissue of the lamina propria, many mast cells, eosinophils, lymphocytes, plasma cells, and even diffuse lymphatic tissue can be seen along with the regular or usual cellular constituents of the lamina propria.

Paranasal Sinuses

The paranasal sinuses are the frontal, maxillary, ethmoid, and sphenoid sinuses (Figs. 19.**6** and 19.**7**). The numerous ethmoid sinuses are located around the supe-

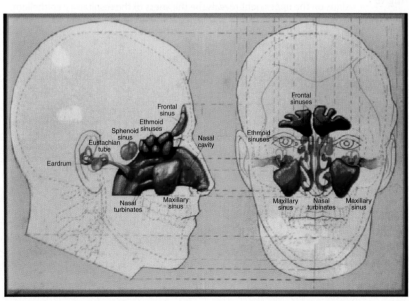

Fig. 19.**6** Lateral (left) and frontal (right) views of paranasal sinuses.

rior and superior-lateral parts of the nasal cavity and are connected via the nasopharynx and auditory (Eustachian) tube to the middle ear (Figs. 19.**7** and 19.**8**). All of the paranasal sinuses drain into the nasal cavity. Their openings are termed ostia. These openings represent the site of the original outpouching during the development of the sinuses.

The internal cavitation of the sinuses continuously and variably encroaches the surrounding bones, becoming larger and more complex with advancing age. The sinuses are often subdivided by septa, resulting in extremely intricate internal morphology, which complicates any endoscopic surgical intervention.

Maxillary Sinuses

The maxillary sinuses are the only sizable sinuses present at birth (Figs. 19.**1** and 19.**9A** and **B**). At birth, these sinuses are approximately the size of a small lima bean and are situated with their longer dimension directed anteriorly and posteriorly. The maxillary sinuses develop in the space existing between the oral cavity and the floor of the orbit (Fig. 19.**10**). They enlarge with facial growth to occupy the space between the posterior maxillary teeth and the floor of the orbits. Maxillary sinus

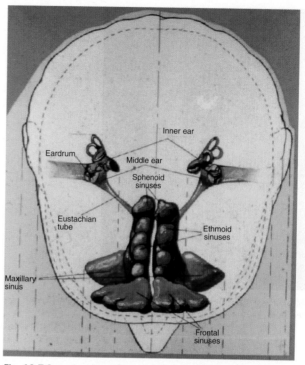

Fig. 19.**7** Superior view of paranasal sinuses and middle ear connections.

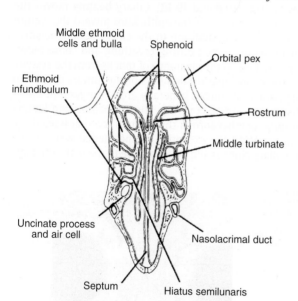

Fig. 19.**8** Detailed diagram of sphenoid and ethmoid sinuses: frontal section. (With permission.)

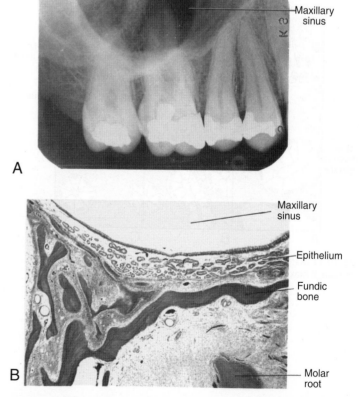

Fig. 19.**9 A** Radiograph of maxillary sinus (above) and adjacent molar roots. Radiographically, the roots appear to project into the sinus. Refer to Figure 19.1. **B** Histologic view of maxillary sinus from a section comparable with that in **(A)**. Molar fundic bone lines the socket below.

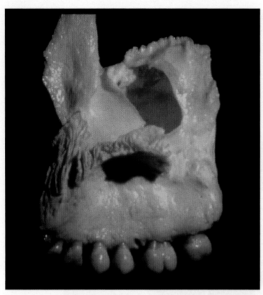

Fig. 19.**10** Maxillary sinus in the body of the maxilla above the palate in a disarticulated skull. Lingual aspect of palate shadowed.

growth slows down with the decline of facial growth during puberty, but continues throughout life. In the adult, a maxillary sinus is shaped like a pyramid, with its base against the lateral wall of the nasal cavity and its apex growing into the zygomatic bone (Fig. 19.**10**). Significantly, the maxillary ostium (opening) is located near the roof of the sinus, toward which the cilia beat to discharge secreted mucus.

The epithelium of the maxillary sinuses is similar to that of the nasal cavity (ciliated pseudostratified columnar), but has fewer goblet cells. The medial wall of the maxillary sinuses possesses a mucosa that is thicker and richer in seromucous glands than that of the lateral walls (Figs. 19.**4** and 19.**5**). The epithelium is thinner than in the nasal cavity, and the lamina propria is much thinner than in the nasal cavity (Fig. 19.**11**).

Frontal, Ethmoid, and Sphenoid Sinuses

These three sinuses have a thinner mucosa than the maxillary sinuses. They have only a moderate number of seromucous glands, and have a reduced number of goblet cells in their epithelium. The columnar epithelial cells lining their surfaces contain cilia. All of these sinuses have openings (ostia) to the lateral walls of the nasal cavity (Figs. 19.**8** and 19.**12**). Ciliary beating moves the mucous coating over the epithelium toward the ostium of each sinus. In addition to the ciliary action, negative air pressure created during breathing and "nose blowing" can help in the clearance of mucus from the system.

The connective-tissue fibers of the lamina propria in the paranasal sinuses generally are not organized into a distinct periosteal covering. The epithelium and lamina propria together form a thin membrane that lines these sinuses. With the exception of the medial walls of the maxillary sinuses and an area close to the ostia, the lam-

Goblet cells

A. Nasal mucosa
  • thicker basement membrane
  • thicker ephithelium with more goblet cells
  • thicker lamina propria than in maxillary sinus
B. Maxillary sinus, medial wall
C. Maxillary sinus, lateral wall
  • fewer glands
  • thinner lamina propria than in medial wall

Sero-
mucous
glands

A   B   C

Fig. 19.**11** Diagram of mucosa of the nasal and paranasal sinuses. **A** Nasal mucosa. **B** Maxillary sinus, medial wall. **C** Maxillary sinus, lateral wall.

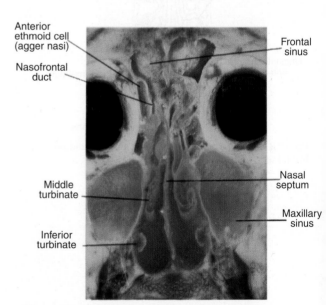

Anterior
ethmoid cell
(agger nasi)

Nasofrontal
duct

Frontal
sinus

Nasal
septum

Maxillary
sinus

Middle
turbinate

Inferior
turbinate

Fig. 19.**12** Coronal section of skull revealing frontal, ethmoid, and maxillary sinuses superior and lateral to the nasal fossae. (With permission.)

Clinical Application

Smoking seriously diminishes ciliary activity, accounting for increased predisposition to respiratory infections.

ina propria of the paranasal sinuses does not contain many seromucous glands.

The paranasal sinuses normally maintain their prenatal sterility throughout life, despite their proximity to the bacterially colonized nasal cavities. This sterility is the result of the production of bacteriostatic nitric oxide and immunoglobulins, as well as ciliary activity by the mucous membrane. Loss of sterility results in sinusitis infection.

Fluid resulting from infections of the mucosa (sinusitis) accumulates on the floor of the maxillary sinus, since the opening of the sinus (ostium) lies near the roof (Fig. 19.**13**). Drainage of this fluid may require an artificial opening (oroantral fistula) to be created surgically (Caldwell-Luc procedure).

Root tips from teeth broken during extraction can lodge in the maxillary sinus. The surgical approach (Caldwell-Luc) to this area is intraorally through the maxillary alveolar mucosa, high in the buccal vestibule and into the maxillary sinus. Also after extractions of maxillary teeth, bone between the sinus and tooth may be perforated and an oroantral fistula may result. Most of these fistulae will heal without treatment, although surgical intervention may be necessary.

Apices of maxillary posterior teeth can project into the maxillary sinus. Bone forming the floor of the sinus can also be the bone surrounding the apex of the tooth. Consequently, periapical infections of teeth can spread to the maxillary sinus, and the reverse can occur with maxillary sinus infections being perceived as originating from teeth. Pain from carious lesions or other insults to the dental pulp may be referred to the sinus. The maxillary sinus enlarges with age and may advance anteriorly as far as the canine root, so relations discussed previously cannot be limited to the posterior teeth. Nerves that supply the maxillary teeth are the same as those that supply the maxillary sinus, accounting for dental pain from healthy teeth arising from maxillary sinusitis.

It is usually difficult to place osseointegrated type implants into the posterior parts of the maxilla due to the lack of bone present and the proximity of the maxillary sinus. However, surgical procedures have been designed to place bone from the patient or bone substitutes into an enlarged space between the sinus mucosa and the bony floor. The purpose is to create newly organized osseous tissue to support the implant.

Orthognathic surgery for moving the maxillary arch sometimes requires the separation of the maxillary alveolar process and teeth as a block (Le Fort I ostectomy). Ostia of the nasolacrimal ducts should be superior to the surgical cuts that free the maxillary segment. Scarring or closure of the duct results in tears flowing over the face from the inner corners of the eye.

Patients with defects between the oral and nasal cavities (cleft palate or surgical defects) require a physical sepa-

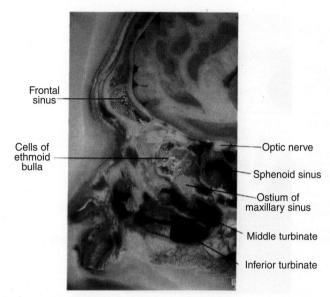

Fig. 19.**13** Sagittal section of skull revealing maxillary sinus ostium in nasal fossa. (With permission.)

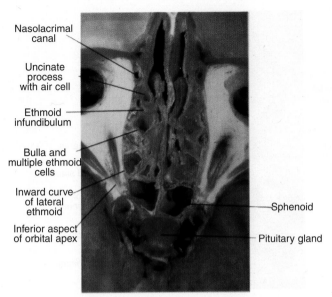

Fig. 19.**14** Horizontal section of skull revealing the nasal fossae and septum anteriorly and the sphenoid sinus and pituitary sella turcica posteriorly. (With permission.)

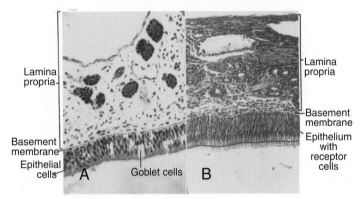

Fig. 19.**15 A** Respiratory mucosa. **B** Olfactory mucosa.

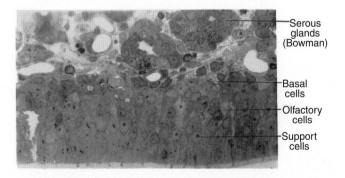

Fig. 19.**16** Olfactory mucosa with three layers of nucleated cells (bottom to top); superficial (light-stained) support cells; wide band of olfactory cell nuclei (dark nuclei); and basal cell nuclei at junction with basal lamina.

ration of these cavities so that breathing can occur when ingesting food or for normal-sounding speech to occur. An oral prosthesis (obturator) can be constructed to help close the defect.

Olfaction

Olfaction occurs as airborne substances contact cilia of sensory cells that are located in the superior region of the nasal mucosa. There are direct neural pathways between olfactory stimuli and the central nervous system. How the olfactory receptors sense and discriminate between various odors is not fully understood.

Olfactory Mucosa Structure

The zone of olfactory mucosa is located in the superior aspects of the nasal cavity. This area is above the superior nasal conchae and includes the roof of the nose and the upper part of the nasal septum (Figs. 19.**12** and 19.**14**). This area is out of the main air flow. Consequently, the receptors in this area are activated by eddy currents carrying the odorific substances to them. In histologic sections the junction between the olfactory mucosa and the nasal mucosae is abrupt. A comparison of the thickness of the nasal olfactory mucosa is seen in Figure 19.15. With increasing age the amount of olfactory mucosa diminishes, and there is an uneven border between the two types of mucosa. However, when viewed microscopically, the boundary is clearly seen, In some areas, islands of olfactory mucosa are surrounded by nasal mucosa.

The olfactory receptors arise embryologically from neuroblasts that differentiate directly from cells of the paired olfactory placodes. The placodes are thickenings in the superficial ectoderm of the face and they invaginate to form the olfactory pits. Primary receptor (sensory) cells develop from this ectoderm, and then form axons that join with the olfactory nerve that is part of the brain.

The olfactory mucosa consists of an epithelial cell layer and a lamina propria that is adjacent to the underlying bone (Fig. 19.**15**). In the lamina propria are serous glands (Bowman's) whose ducts drain into the surface of the epithelium. In Figure 19.**15**, the respiratory epithelium (A) and olfactory epithelium (B) can be seen side by side. However, there are several basic differences. Both are pseudostratified, columnar-type epithelium, but the olfactory epithelium (approximately 70 μm) is taller than the respiratory epithelium (45 μm). Both types of epithelium have cilia. The respiratory epithelium contains goblet cells, whereas the olfactory epithelium contains olfactory receptor cells. Both have basal cells. Respiratory epithelium has a distinct basement membrane visible with the light microscope; the olfactory epithelium has a basement membrane, but is less distinct and is best visualized at the ultrastructural level. Beneath the olfactory mucosa is the periosteum of the ethmoid bone (Fig. 19.**16**). There is no submucosa underlying the olfactory epithelium. In contrast, there is a significant submucosa found under respiratory epithelium; this submucosa contains numerous venous sinusoids and glands.

Olfactory epithelium consists primarily of three cell types: tall, ciliated, columnar receptor cells; supporting cells with microvillar cells; and basal cells that lie adjacent to the basement membrane. When olfactory epithelium is viewed with the electron microscope, distinct layers are seen (Fig. 19.**16**). The nuclei of supporting cells lie close to the surface of the epithelium. The nuclei of the neural cells form a band midway from the free surface to the deep-lying basal cells. On the free surface of the mucosa is a mucous layer some 10 to 40 μm thick. At higher magnification (Fig. 19.**17**), the cilia of the neural receptor cells and the microvilli of the supporting cells can be seen. The tall slender olfactory receptor cells end at the epithelial surface with a bulb-shaped olfactory vesicle from which the cilia extend onto the surface of this epithelium (Figs. 19.**17**–19.**19**). Cilia of the epithelial cells of nasal mucosa (respiratory epithelium) move or beat constantly whereas cilia of olfactory epithelium do not.

The olfactory receptor cell is a primary neuron. This slender, flask-shaped columnar cell with its cylindrical dendrite terminates as an olfactory vesicle at the epithelium–mucus interface (Fig. 19.**20**). This vesicle may appear flat or dome-shaped. It contains neurotubules indicating its neural function in olfaction, and contains the ciliary basal bodies of numerous cilia (10 to 60) per cell (Figs. 19.**19** and 19.**20**). The cilia vary in length from 50 to 200 μm and exhibit the usual pattern of "9 + 2" microtubules in each cilium. The cilia probably play a role in olfactory transduction. Adjacent to the olfactory vesicle is a constricted zone and junctional complex. This junctional complex has characteristic zonulae

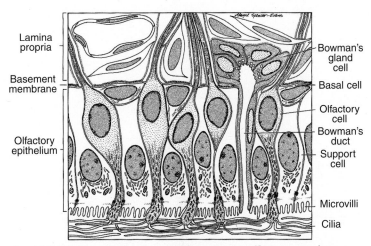

Fig. 19.**17** Diagram of olfactory epithelium denotes olfactory neural receptor and supporting cells. Serous glands underlie the olfactory epithelium.

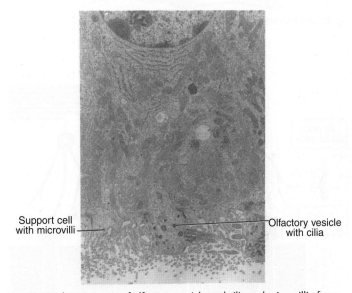

Fig. 19.**18** Ultrastructure of olfactory vesicle and cilia and microvilli of support cells.

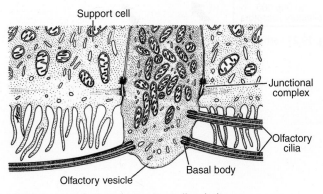

Fig. 19.**19** Diagram of olfactory receptor cell and cilia.

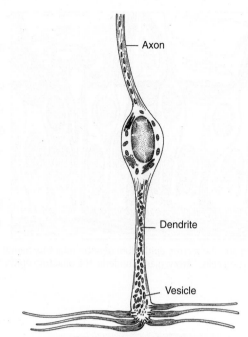

Fig. 19.**20** Diagram of olfactory cell and axon.

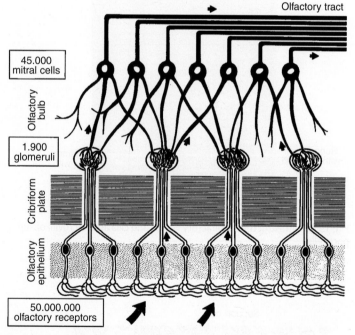

Fig. 19.**21** Pathway of how smell impulses pass to the brain.

occludens, zonulae adherens, and maculae adherens (desmosomes), with adjacent supporting cells. This junctional complex seals the intercellular space from the external environment. The receptor cells vary from 5 to 8 μm in diameter, with a nucleus almost as large. Most of the cell cytoplasm is thus at the distal pole, where it is continuous with the cylindrical dendrite (olfactory rod) (Fig. 19.**20**). Figure 19.**21** is a diagram of the pathway of smell impulses to the brain. The olfactory sensory cell is a first-order neuron. The process that extends from the proximal pole of the olfactory cell is actually an unmyelinated axon. This axon joins with other axons to form small Schwann cell-wrapped bundles. These bundles then join with other similar bundles and pass through the cribriform plate of the ethmoid bone to terminate in the glomeruli of the bilateral olfactory bulbs. The glomeruli are areas where axons of the olfactory sensory cells intermingle with dendrites of the mitral cells.

The basal cells shown in Figure 19.**17** are pyramid-shaped and in direct contact with the basement membrane. Basal cells are the site of numerous mitotic figures, and thus produce cells that replace the supporting and receptor cells (Fig. 19.**17**). New cells are required to replace the cells that normally turn over because of age, injury, or exposure to noxious chemicals. The new neural receptor cells re-establish their contact with the olfactory nerves of the brain and with adjacent cells. Olfactory neogenesis is unique in the body as neural cells are not normally replaced elsewhere and the process continues throughout life.

Observe the relationship of the adjacent olfactory support cells and basal cells seen in Figure 19.**19**. On their free surface, microvilli are seen extending from the support cells, and their cytoplasm is filled with secretory granules. In addition to the ciliated receptor cells, support cells, and basal cells, an additional support cell with microvilli may be a second type of receptor cell. Olfactory cells contain many neurotubules and mitochondria, and cilia protrude from the surface of the olfactory vesicle (Fig. 19.**19**). Underlying the olfactory epithelium in the lamina propria are the serous *glands of Bowman*. These glands are tubular alveolar glands with secretory cells penetrating the epithelial cell layer; their ducts open onto the surface (Fig. 19.**17**). Although these cells are classified as serous cells, they contain mucopolysaccharide-staining granules. These glands, as well as the supporting cells, contribute to the mucous layer overlying the olfactory epithelium.

Olfactory Receptor Nerve Supply

Although the first cranial nerve is responsible for olfaction, trigeminal nerve fibers (cranial nerve V) have been found in olfactory mucosa. These fibers, arising from terminal nasal branches, terminate among the olfactory cells. Their role in olfaction is unknown, but they may provide a role in sensory function.

Olfactory Receptor Function

What part the cilia provide in olfactory reception is not known, although cilia and microvilli considerably increase the surface of these receptors. Findings indicate that the secretion from Bowman's glands, along with the secretory products of the supporting cells, play a role in the diffusion of odor molecules over the epithelial surface. These secretions are renewed by production of new materials within these cells. Functionally, the olfactory receptor is thought to be an independent unit. Recent information on replacement of receptor cells and their close relation to adjacent cells by junctional complexes indicates that the differences in the basal and supportive cells may relate to stages of growth.

Figure 19.**21** illustrates a large number of receptor cilia in the olfactory mucosa. Considering the number of cilia per cell and the number of receptor cells in the olfactory mucosa, there are millions of these cilia. Cilia are at the luminal end of the cell, which is the dendritic end of this bipolar sensory neuron. At the opposite end is the axon of this cell. The axons from hundreds of receptor cells cluster, are wrapped by Schwann cells, and pass to the bilateral olfactory bulbs. At the bulbs, the axons synapse at sites called glomeruli, which are composed of the dendrites of mitral cells. The mitral cells are the second-order neurons. The dendrites of the mitral cells then carry olfactory impulses by their axons that form the olfactory tract. These axons proceed to centers in the brain. There are far fewer mitral cells (45 000) than sensory neurons (they number 50 million on one side), and there are even fewer (1900) glomeruli. Hence, large numbers of sensory axons synapse with each mitral cell. The axons of the mitral cells collectively form the olfactory tract, which travels to the higher brain centers. Not shown in Figure 19.**21** are the many interconnections between right and left olfactory bulbs.

A regional organization of the olfactory bulb corresponds to that of the olfactory mucosa; fibers from the anterior part of the mucosa extend to the anterior part of the bulb, and fibers from the posterior portion of the mucosa extend to the posterior part of the bulb. Smells can therefore be discriminated by both detailed signal pattern and area of signal origin. Attempts have been made to classify smells into a smaller number of groups, but have not proven successful. Of interest, the olfactory epithelium can become fatigued to one odor but not to others. Recent investigations into the mechanism of olfaction have suggested that the sensed odors affect the enzyme balance of the olfactory cell. The responses of olfactory receptor neurons are rarely specific to only one odor; the majority of cells respond to a broad range of substances. Arrays of neurons are activated in response to a specific odor, with overlapping sensory profiles.

Summary

The nasal passages function not only in conduction of air but in the warming (and cooling) of it by numerous blood vessels, and in adjusting the moisture content with secretions from the serous and mucous glands. Each bilateral nasal cavity contains three conchae that increase the surface area of the nasal cavities. These cavities are lined with pseudostratified, ciliated columnar epithelium situated on a prominent basement membrane. Beneath the basal lamina, mucous and serous glands appear in the lamina propria. The paranasal sinuses are located around the superior and lateral parts of the nasal cavity, and drain into the nasal cavity. Maxillary sinuses are the largest of the sinuses, and molar roots lie adjacent to or in the sinus floor. Therefore, maxillary sinusitis may cause painful teeth. The frontal, ethmoid, and sphenoid paranasal sinuses contain ciliated, stratified columnar epithelium, which is much thinner than the epithelium of the nasal cavity and contains no seromucous glands and few goblet cells.

Odors are transmitted to olfactory epithelium as airborne substances. At the epithelium odors combine with fluid-covered mucosa at the receptor site. Olfactory receptors are bipolar neurons that use cilia to detect odors, and then transmit the impulse via the olfactory nerve to the olfactory bulb and the brain. The cells of the olfactory epithelium are continuously being replaced, and the receptor neurons re-establish connections with the olfactory bulb (cranial nerve I).

Self-Evaluation Review

1. Indicate the mechanisms of air conditioning (heating, cooling, humidification) of respired air available in the nasosinusal complex.
2. Relate the major differences between the nasal and paranasal sinusal mucosae.
3. Indicate the origin, functions, and disposal of mucus.
4. Identify the ostial site of opening of the maxillary sinus and its clinical consequences.
5. What is the relationship of maxillary molar roots to the maxillary sinus and its surgical and pathologic significance?
6. Describe the mechanism of sterility of the sinuses versus the bacterial infectivity of the nasal and oral cavities.
7. What is the Caldwell-Luc procedure and for what purpose is it undertaken?
8. How is the sense of smell (olfaction) perceived and conducted to the brain?
9. What sinuses have their ostial openings into the middle meatus?
10. Identify the sensory nerves and the sensations they convey from the nasosinusal complex.

Acknowledgements

Permission to reproduce Figures 19.**16** and 19.**18** was granted by Professor PPC Graziadei, Florida State University. Appreciation is expressed to Dr Stephen P Becker and the Annals of Otology, Rhinology,and Laryngology for permission to reproduce Figures 19.**8**, 19.**12**, 19.**13**, and 19.**14**. Gratitude is expressed to Anne-Marie McLean for the word processing.

Suggested Readings

Anagnostopoulou S, Venieratos D, Spyropoulos N. Classification of human maxillary sinuses according to their geometric features. Anat. Anz. 1991;173(3):121-130.

Ariji Y, Kuroki T, Moriguchi S, Ariji E, Kanda S. Age changes in the volume of the human maxillary sinus: a study using computed tomography. Dento-Maxillo-Facial Radiology. 1994;23(3):163-168.

Baroody FM, Suh SH, Naclerio RM. Total IgE serum levels correlate with sinus mucosal thickness on computerized tomography scans. J. Allergy Clin. Immunol. 1997;100(4):563-568.

Beahm E, Teresi L, Lufkin R, Hanafee W. MR of the paranasal sinuses. Surg. Radiol. Anat. 1990;12(3):203-208.

Becker SP. Applied anatomy of the paranasal sinuses with emphasis on endoscopic surgery. Ann. Otol. Rhinol. Laryngol; 1994; Supp. 162,103(4), Part 2.

Bolger WE, Clement PAR, Hosemann W, et al. Paranasal sinuses: Anatomic terminology and nomenclature. Ann. Otol. Rhinol Laryngol. 1995;104(101):7-16.

Caliot P, Midy D, Plessis JL. The surgical anatomy of the middle nasal meatus. Surg. Radiol. Anat. 1990;12(2):97-101.

Corsten MJ, Bernard PA, Udjus K, Walker R. Nasal fossa dimensions in normal and nasally obstructed neonates and infants: preliminary study. Int. J. Pediatr. Otorhinolaryngol. 1996;36(1):23-30.

Davis WE, Templer J, Parsons DS. Anatomy of the paranasal sinuses. Otolaryngol. Clin. North Am. 1966;29(1):57-74.

Eberhardt JA, Torabinejad M, Christiansen EL. A computed tomographic study of the distances between the maxillary sinus floor and the apices of the maxillary posterior teeth. Oral Surg. Oral Med. Oral Pathol. 1992;73(3):345-346.

Graney DO. Anatomy of the paranasal sinuses. Immunology & Allergy Clinics of North America. 1994;14(1):1-15.

Hawke M, Bingham B, Calhoun KH. Surgical anatomy of the lateral nasal wall. Otolaryngol. Head Neck Surg. 1991;105(1):135.

Krennmair G, Ulm C, Lugmayr H. Maxillary sinus septa: Incidence, morphology and clinical implications. J. Craniomaxillofac. Surg. 1997;25(5):261-265.

Kubal WS. Sinonasal anatomy. Neuroimaging Clin. North Am. 1998;8(1):143-156.

Lundberg JON, Farkas-Szallasi T, Weitzberg E, et al. High nitric oxide production in human paranasal sinuses. Nat. Med. 1995;1(4):370-373.

McDonnell D, Esposito M, Todd ME. A teaching model to illustrate the variation in size and shape of the of the maxillary sinus. J. Anat. 1992;181(2):337-380.

Medina J, Hernandez H, Tom LW, Bilaniuk L. Development of the paranasal sinuses in children. Am. J. Rhinol. 1997;11(3):203-209.

Miller AJ, Amedee RG. Functional anatomy of the paranasal sinuses. [Review] [20 refs] Journal of the Louisiana State Medical Society. 1997;149(3):85-90.

Nakashima T, Tanaka M, Inamitsu M, Uemura T. Immunohistopathology of variations of human olfactory mucosa. Eur. Arch. Otorhinolaryngol. 1991;248(6):370-375.

Philippou M, Stenger GM, Goumas PD, Hillen B, Huizing EH. Cross-sectional anatomy of the nose and paranasal sinuses. A correlative study of computer tomographic images and cryosections. Rhinology. 1990;28(4):221-230.

Riederer A, Held B, Mayer B, Wörl J. Histochemical and immunocytochemical study of nitrergic innervation in human nasal mucosa. Ann. Otol. Rhinol. Laryngol. 1999;108:869.

Scuderi AJ, Harnsberger HR, Boyer RS. Pneumatization of the paranasal sinuses: normal features of importance to the accurate interpretation of CT scans and MR images. Am. J. Roent. 1993;160(5):1101-1104.

Smith T, Siegel MI, Mooney MP, Burdi A, Todhunter J. Vomeronasal organ growth and development in normal and cleft lip and palate human fetuses. Cleft Palate Craniofac. J. 1996;33(5):385-394.

Smith TD, Siegel MI, Mooney MP, Burrows AM, Todhunter JS. Formation and enlargement of the paranasal sinuses in normal and cleft lip and palate human fetuses. Cleft Palate Craniofac. J. 1997;34(6):483-489.

Stammberger H. History of rhinology: anatomy of the paranasal sinuses. Rhinology. 1989;27(3):197-210.

Stammberger HR, Kennedy DW. Paranasal sinuses: anatomic terminology and nomenclature. The Anatomic Terminology Group. Ann. Otol. Rhinol. Laryngol. Suppl. 1995;167:7-16.

Uchida Y, Goto M, Katsuki T, Akiyoshi T. A cadaveric study of maxillary sinus size as an aid in bone grafting of the maxillary sinus floor. J. Oral Maxillofac. Surg. 1998;56(10):1158-1163.

Vinter I, Krmpotic-Nemanic J, Hat J, Jalsovec D. The frontal sinus and the ethmoidal labyrinth. Surg. Radiol. Anat. 1997;19(5):295-298.

Watson L. Jacobson's organ and the remarkable sense of smell. London, UK: Allen Lane; 1999.

Weiglein A, Anderhuber W, Wolf G. Radiologic anatomy of the paranasal sinuses in the child. Surg. Radiol. Anat. 1992;14(4):335-339.

Zinreich SJ. Functional anatomy and computed tomography imaging of the paranasal sinuses. Am. J. Med. Sci. 1998;316(1):2-12.

20 Structure and Function of the Temporomandibular Joint

James K. Avery and Sol Bernick

Introduction

The temporomandibular joint (TMJ), the mandibular articulation, is a bilateral diarthrosis between the condyles of the mandible and the articular eminences of the temporal bone, arteriorly, and the mandibular fossae, posteriorly. The TMJ allows the mandible to move as a unit in both a hinge and a gliding movement.

The TMJ consists of: the condylar head of the mandible, the articulating surfaces of the temporal bone, the articulating disc, and the articulating capsule. The disc separates the head of the condyles from the temporal bone. Therefore, the disc divides the joint into two portions, an upper and a lower compartment. The disc is an oval plate of fibrous tissues whose periphery blends into the articulating capsule. In front, the disc is anchored to the tendon of the lateral pterygoid muscle. It is lightly attached to the condyle, so that it follows the jaw in sliding movements. There are two synovial membranes in the joint: one lines the capsule above the disc, and the other lines the capsule below the disc.

A loose articular capsule is attached to the articular tubercles, the squamotympanic fissure, and the margins of the mandibular fossa between these two attachments. Below, it is attached to the neck of the mandible, so that posteriorly a portion of the mandible is intracapsular (Fig. 20.**1**).

The lateral (temporomandibular) ligament is intimately related to the fibrous capsule. Above, it is attached to the zygoma, and below, it is attached to the lateral surfaces and posterior border of the neck of the mandible.

In addition, there are two accessory ligaments associated with the TMJ. The stylomandibular ligament attaches to the styloid process and to the posterior border of the ramus; the sphenomandibular ligament extends between the spine of the spenoid bone and the lingula of the mandible (Fig. 20.**1C**).

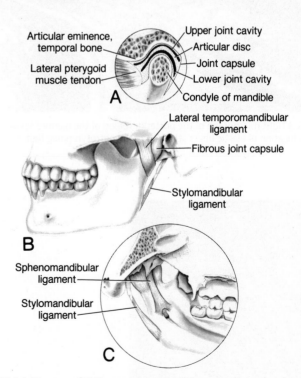

Fig. 20.**1 A** Diagram of TMJ compartments. **B** Diagram of lateral and posterior ligaments of the TMJ. **C** Diagram of medial ligaments of the TMJ.

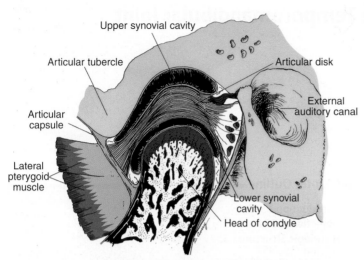

Fig. 20.**2** Diagram of the TMJ with articular disc, capsule, and relations to the lateral pterygoid muscle and external auditory canal.

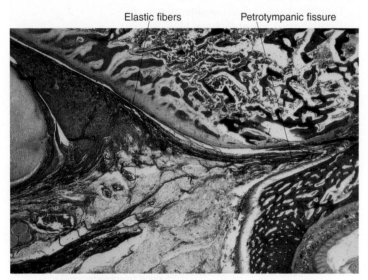

Fig. 20.**3** Light micrograph of the posterior region of the glenoid fossa shows location of elastic fibers attached to the petrotympanic fissure.

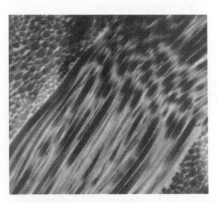

Fig. 20.**4** Ultrastructure of collagen fibers of the articular disc.

Objectives

After reading this chapter you should be able to describe the structure of the condyles, the temporal fossae, and the articulating disc and capsule. You should also be able to discuss the function of this joint and the relation of the muscles of mastication to its actions.

Histologic Structure

The microscopic structure of the TMJ reveals a fibrous capsule enclosing the joint, which is attached anteriorly to the articulating tubercle of the temporal bone above, and the neck of the condyle below (Fig. 20.**2**). Posteriorly, the capsule is attached to the temporal bone anterior to the external auditory canal above and the posterior aspects of the condyle below (Fig. 20.**2**). Suspended from the internal walls of the capsule between the condyles and the fossae is the fibrous disc, which is composed of collagen fibers (Fig. 20.**3**). This disc is seen to separate the superior and inferior joint cavities. In this diagram, the cartilage is in the condylar head underlying the fibrous perichondrium. The condition indicates that the mandible has not completed its growth, as cartilage has not been entirely replaced by bone. Growth occurs in the formation of new cells underlying the periochondrium of the condylar surface and also at the site of the transformation of cartilage to bone in the neck of the condyles. As long as there is cartilage in the condylar head, growth may occur. Observe the inclined plane of the anterior articulating surface of the condyle, the thin area of the articulating disc anteriorly and the thick zone posteriorly (Fig 20.**2**). Far posteriorly, a number of blood vessels appear, known as the *vascular triangle* (Fig. 20.**3**). Above the vascular triangle, the elastic fibers of the disc emanate from the borders of the petrotympanic fissure, as seen in Figure 20.**3**. The articular disc is composed of collagen fibers, as seen in Figure 20.**4**. Because the condylar head slides along the articular plane during function, the capsule is described as loose. It is supported by a medial ligament (sphenomandibular), a lateral ligament (temporomandibular), and a posterior ligament (stylomandibular). These relative positions are seen in Figures 20.**1B** and **C**.

Condyles

Condyles are ovoid in shape mediolaterally and consist of a smooth bony surface covered with a fibrous connective tissue (Fig. 20.**5B**). The condyles grow laterally during development, gaining the oval shape as they reach maturity at 6 years of age. For example, the porous appearance of the cartilage-covered condyle is apparent in Figure 20.**5A**. Histology of the condyle confirms in an early-teenaged individual that the condyle has thinned considerably, with further thinning occurring as the age of the individual nears 20 (Fig. 20.**6**). The condylar head and head of long bones differ in that long bones form secondary ossification sites (Fig 20.**7**). These secondary ossification sites produce epiphyseal lines where lengthening of the long bone occurs. Like the heads of long bones, the condylar heads grow by developing new chondroblasts, with growth of new cartilage matrix and replacement by bone. In long bones, however, the cartilage cells appear to be arranged in long rows adjacent to the cartilage bone junctions. In the mandibular joint cartilage the cells appear scattered, as seen in Figures 20.**6** and 20.**7**.

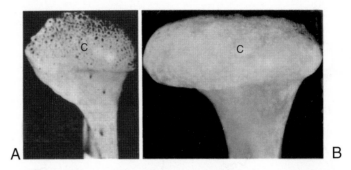

Fig. 20.**5** Comparison of a 6-year-old condyle (**A**) and adult condyle (**B**). Note the increase in the lateral dimension.

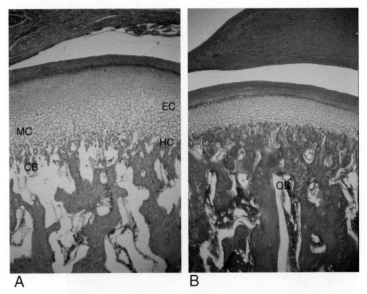

Fig. 20.**6 A** Histology of young postnatal codyle and disc. Reserve cartilage zone (EC), multiplication of cells (MC), cartilage zone, hypertrophy zone (HC), calcifying zone (CB). **B** Thin cartilage zone later postnatally, bone formation (OB).

Clinical Application

The most important formative time for the TMJ is from the 8th to 12th weeks of embryonic age. At that time the condylar heads differentiate and articulate with the temporal bone, which also appears at this time. The articular disc then forms, and the capsule, ligaments, and masticatory muscles begin to differentiate. Any factor that would affect growth and differentiation at that time would be likely to alter development of the TMJ.

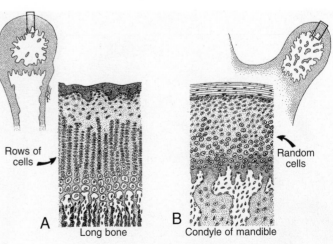

Fig. 20.**7** Diagrams of the cartilage of long bone (**A**) and condyle (**B**). Observe the lack of palisading and the thick perichondrium in the condyle.

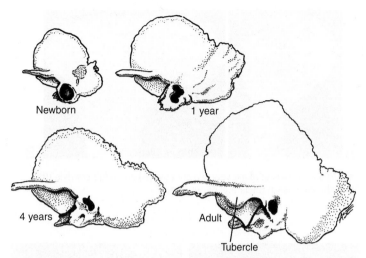

Fig. 20.**8** Development of the glenoid (temporomandibular) fossa from birth to maturity.

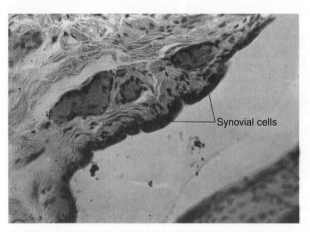

Fig. 20.**9** Light micrograph of synovial cells lining the TMJ.

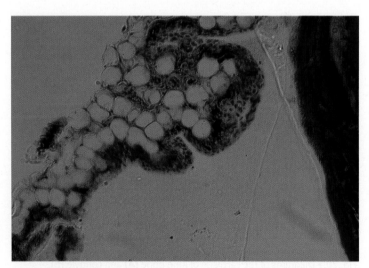

Fig. 20.**10** Light micrograph of sinovial and fat cells in the TMJ.

Temporomandibular Fossa (Glenoid Fossa)

The temporomandibular fossa is composed of an anterior zone in the form of an eminence (articular) and a posterior part, which is a depression or cavity on the inferior aspect of the temporal bone. This fossa is located at the posterior medial end of the zygomatic arch (Fig. 20.**8**). To compensate for the increase in lateral dimension of one condylar head, the glenoid fossa extends laterally as well (Fig. 20.**8**). By maturity, the articular eminence becomes prominent. The articular eminences are smooth with rounded ridges on whose posterior slope the condyles slide during articulation. On the posterior wall of the fossa, the petrotympanic fissure separates the anterior squamosa and the more posterior petrous parts of the temporal bone (Figs. 20.**3** and 20.**8**). It is the only location in the disc in which elastic fibers are found. Because of their location, these fibers may be a remnant of the anterior ligament of the malleus.

Synovial Membrane

A synovial membrane (stratum synoviale) lines the entire articular capsule of the joint—both the upper and the lower compartments. The synovial cells appear to be a continuous layer, but usually are intermingled with connective-tissue fibers and fat cells. Thus, the synovium is not a true membrane (Fig. 20.**9**). In this posterior region of the joint, synovial folds may be found on the free surfaces of the joint. Within these folds the cells may be piled up and may project into the cavity. Some folds may be nonvascular while others have associated connective tissue or contain adipose cells (Fig. 20.**10**). Ultrastructurally, it has been shown that there are two types of synovial cells, types A and B (light and dark). It has been suggested that type A secretes hyaluronic acid, whereas type B produces a protein-rich secretion. The matrix of the synovial membrane contains collagen fibrils, unbanded fibrils, and electron-dense amorphous material (Fig.20.**11**).

The synovial membrane is richly supplied with blood vessels. Capillary networks are found not only in the subsynovial tissues, but also adjacent to the synovial cells. Three types of synovial capillaries are found: continuous, fenestrated, and discontinuous. The fenestrated type is found in the matrix of the synovial membrane. Lymphatic vessels are observed a short distance from the synovial surface, draining into the capsular collecting lymphatic vessels.

Synovial fluid, with hyaluronic acid, is an infiltrate or distillate of the blood (as is tissue fluid). Here, hyaluronic acid has a high viscosity and provides the lubricating property of synovial fluid.

Vascular and Neural Supply

Vascular Supply

Blood is supplied to the TMJ through branches of the *superficial temporal, deep auricular, anterior tympanic,* and *ascending pharyngeal* arteries. These branches converge into the capsule of the joint (Fig. 20.**12**). Small arteries, arterioles, and capillaries pass into the peripheral third of the articular disc. Note the extensive vascularity in the peripheral region of the disc, taken from a section of peripheral third of the joint (Fig 20.**13**). On the other hand, a section of the central portion of the joint (Fig. 20.**14**) reveals that the thin portion of the disc is avascular. Note also the vascular channels within the articular vessels; they have been injected with latex and the connective tissue has been removed. The high vascularity of the peripheral disc is clearly seen in Figure

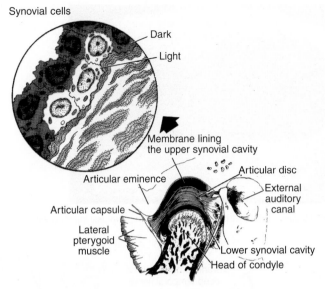

Fig. 20.**11** Diagram of light and dark synovial cells in the TMJ. Circled inset is the diagram of a magnified view of the upper synovial cavity.

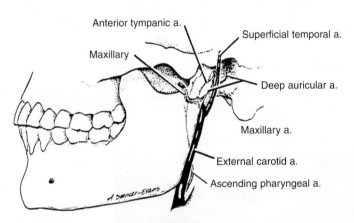

Fig. 20.**12** Diagram of the blood supply of the TMJ.

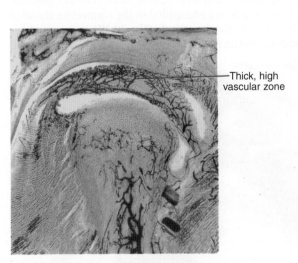

Fig. 20.**13** View of peripheral articular disc, with blood vessels illustrated. Specimen is injected with India ink.

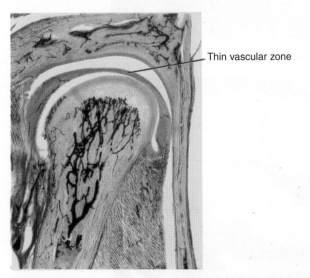

Fig. 20.**14** View of central zone of articular disc without blood vessels. Specimen is injected with India ink.

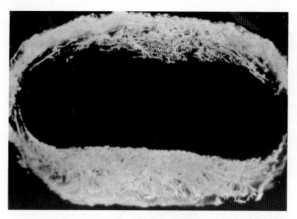

Fig. 20.**15** View of disc, with vascular network in periphery injected with latex.

20.**15**. Note that the disc is oval and that its lateral and medial extremities are right and left respectively; its anterior aspect is above, and its more highly vascularized posterior region is below. There are no vessels throughout the central portion of the disc.

Neural Supply

The nerve supply to the TMJ is through the mandibular division of the trigeminal nerve, the same nerve that supplies the muscles of mastication. The neural branches are the *auriculotemporal*, *masseteric*, and *deep temporal* nerves (Fig. 20.**16**). Nerves containing myelinated and nonmyelinated fibers enter the capsule and disc to sup-

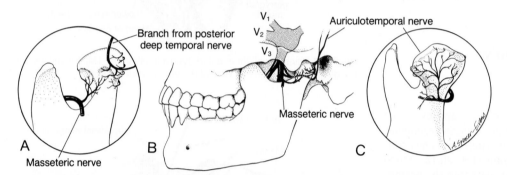

Fig. 20.**16** Diagram of nerve supply of the TMJ. Auriculotemporal masseteric and deep temporal branches of the fifth nerve supply the joint. **A** Anterior. **B** Lateral. **C** Posterior.

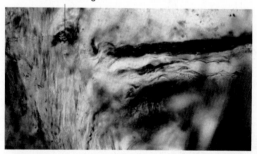

Fig. 20.**17** Nerve ending in disc.

ply the anterior, posterior, medial, and lateral regions of the joint (Fig. 20.**16**). Nerve endings as receptors for pain, as well as such specialized nerve endings as receptors for temperature, touch, and deep pressure, are found in, and pass from, the joint into the peripheral region of the articular disc and synovial folds (Figs. 20.**17** and 20.**18**). Only free nerve endings, as receptors for pain, have been found in the peripheral region of the disc (Fig. 20.**17**). The thin central portion of the disc is free of nerves. Both myelinated and nonmyelinated nerves are found in the connective-tissue core of the synovial folds (Fig. 20.**18**). Those nerves that terminate in various encapsulated structures appear to be coiled or globular in nature, and are embedded in the connective tissue of the articular disc or capsule (Fig. 20.**19**). In the condylar region, myelinated nerves are traced passing through

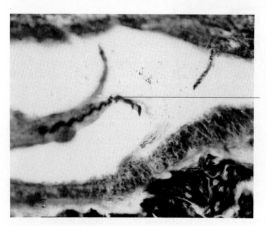

Fig. 20.**18** Nerve ending in the synovial fold.

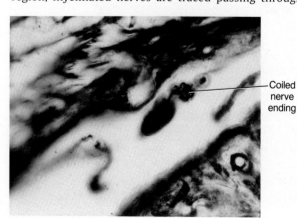

Fig. 20.**19** Coiled nerve ending in the TMJ.

the muscle to enter the capsular connective tissue. These nerves may end as nonmyelinated free nerve endings or specialized coiled endings, similar to Ruffini corpuscles (Fig. 20.**20**).

Muscles of Mastication

There are eight powerful muscles of mastication, four on each side. Each has a different location; therefore, the direction of fiber contraction results in a different functional relation. Three of the muscles on each side—the medial pterygoid, masseter, and temporalis—exert vertical forces in closing the jaws, whereas the function of the lateral pterygoid muscles is to protract the mandible and stabilize the joint. These muscles do not function alone but work as a group with the muscles of the tongue and the superhyoid muscles. *Free movements* of the mandible relate to the interplay of masticatory muscles and the morphology of the teeth in the absence of food. *Masticatory movement*, on the other hand, is the synergistic action of the three groups of muscles—the elevators, depressors, and protractors—that function together and at different times during mastication of food.

The *medial pterygoid* muscle arises from the medial surface of the lateral pterygoid plate and inserts in the inferior surface of the ramus and angle of the mandible. Blood supply is from the maxillary artery, and nerve supply from the mandibular division of the trigeminal. It functions to protract and elevate the mandible (Fig. 20.**21**). From this inferior view, the medial part is seen to run downward and backward, below and behind the angle of the mandible, to meet the externally located masseter in a tendinous raphe, and forming the pterygo-masseteric sling (Figs. 20.**21** and 20.**22**).

The *lateral pterygoid* muscle has two heads: the upper arising from the greater wing of the sphenoid and the lower from the lateral pterygoid plate. They insert into the front of the neck of the condyle and the capsule (Fig. 20.**22**). Blood supply is from the maxillary artery, and nerve supply is from the pterygoid branch of the mandibular nerve. The function of both heads of the muscle is to protrude the mandible and pull the articular disc forward (Figs. 20.**21** and 20.**22**).

The *temporalis* muscles fibers originate from the floor of the temporal fossa and temporal fascia and insert on the anterior borders of the coronoid process and ramus of

Clinical Application

The TMJ is a complex and precisely integrated bilateral joint with the functions of mastication and speech. By placing our fingers on the condylar heads and then opening and closing the jaw, it is possible to follow the downward and foreword path of their sliding action.

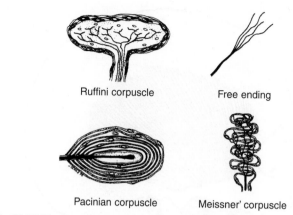

Ruffini corpuscle

Free ending

Pacinian corpuscle

Meissner' corpuscle

Fig. 20.**20** Diagram of types of nerve endings in the joint capsule and disc.

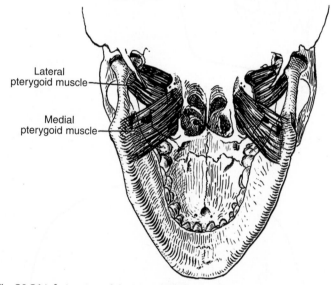

Lateral pterygoid muscle

Medial pterygoid muscle

Fig. 20.**21** Inferior view of the lateral and medial pterygoid muscles of mastication.

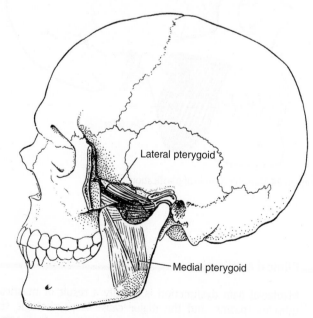

Lateral pterygoid

Medial pterygoid

Fig. 20.**22** Lateral view of the lateral and medial pterygoid muscles of mastication.

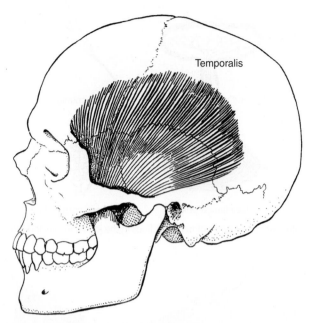

Fig. 20.**23** Temporalis muscle of mastication.

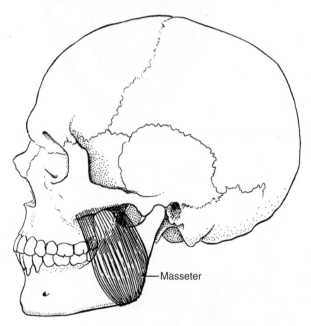

Fig. 20.**24** Masseter muscle of mastication.

▗ **Clinical Application** ▗▗▗▗▗▗▗▗▗▗▗

Myofacial pain dysfunction is usually a result of masticatory muscles spasms, and the major cause is psychologic stress. There are four cardinal symptoms: preauricular pain, muscle tenderness, limitation of mouth opening, and clicking.

the mandible (Fig. 20.**23**). Blood supply is from the superficial temporal and maxillary arteries, and nerve supply is from the deep temporal branches of the mandibular nerve. Functions of the temporalis muscle are elevation of the jaw, retraction of the mandible, and clenching of the teeth.

The *masseter* muscle has a deep part and superficial part. The superficial fibers originate from the anterior two-thirds of the lower border of the zygomatic arch, and the deep fibers form the medial surface of the same arch. The superficial fibers are at right angles to the occlusal plane of the posterior teeth, and the deep fibers are directed downward and slightly anteriorly. The masseter muscle inserts into the lateral surface of the coroniod process of the mandible, the upper half of the ramus, and the angle of the mandible. Blood supply is from the superficial temporal and maxillary arteries, and the nerve supply comes from the mandibular division of the trigeminal nerve. The functions of the masseter muscle are elevation of the jaw and clenching of the teeth (Fig. 20.**24**).

Functional and Clinical Considerations

The sensations of pain and pressure are important symptoms in temporomandibular disorders. The nature of the transmission of these sensations from this joint is still not fully understood. In view of the previously described innervation of the joint, pain and pressure may be explained by the following malfunctions: 1) Changes in occlusion, from various causes, may produce displacement of the condyle—disc to disc—fossa relation and irritate the peripheral disc areas and associated nerve receptors; 2) Inflammation and associated increases in synovial fluid would produce pressure effects and irritation of the specialized nerve endings in the synovial folds; 3) Muscle tensions may act on the nerves not only in muscle per se but also on the endings in the periosteal connective tissue.

Disturbances to the TMJ are, in part, no different from those in other joints. There are dissimilarities in the disorders of the TMJ, however, as a result of its specific anatomic and functional features. The TMJs are bilaterally coupled as a single unit by the mandible, which prevents unilateral motion. Its articular surfaces are covered by articular fibrous tissue rather than hyaline cartilage, and are found in other joints. There is a functional relation with the dentition, periodontal tissues, muscles of mastication, and the joint. Pathology in one component may affect another, which complicates diagnosis of a disease; therefore, the TMJ is exposed to functional changes seen in the oral cavity.

Developmental Disturbances

Although uncommon, developmental disturbances do occur. Condylar aplasia may occur either unilaterally or bilaterally. Usually, it is associated with other anatomically related defects, such as a defective or absent external ear. The intimate relation in the development of the external ear, mandible, and TMJ may clarify this association. Underdevelopment or defective formation of the mandibular condyle may be congenital or acquired as a result of toxic agents interfering with normal prenatal and postanatal development of the condyle. These defects may result from infection, dietary insufficiency, hormonal dysfunction, or trauma.

Dislocation

Dislocation, or luxation and subluxation of the TMJ, occurs when the head of the condyle is displaced anteriorly over the articular eminence and cannot be returned voluntarily to its normal position. It may occur after a condylar fracture or, more frequently, in overstretching, usually at the attachment point of the lateral pterygoid into the capsule. It is commonly characterized by sudden locking and immobilization of the jaws when the mouth is open, and it is accompanied by prolonged spasmodic contraction of the temporal, medial pterygoid, and masseter muscles with protrusion of the jaw. The normal position and relation of the muscles of mastication are shown in Figures 20.**21**–20.**24**.

Ankylosis

Ankylosis of the TMJ is a debilitating condition involving immobility of the jaw. The cause of ankylosis may be intra-articular or extra-articular. In intra-articular ankylosis, there is progressive destruction of the meniscus, flattening of the fossa, thickening of the condyle, and shrinkage of the capsule with partial or even complete abolition of the joint. Usually, the ankylosis is fibrous, although the fibrous type may ossify. After infection, extra-articular ankylosis leads to "splinting" of the joint by a fibrous or a bony mass external to the joint proper.

Injury to the Articular Disc

Inflammation and, more commonly, malocclusion may result in articular disc injury. The latter usually results from abnormal patterns of mandibular excursion carried out during mastication. During these excessive movements, the capsule is overstretched, which prevents too great an anterior condylar movement. The adaptation of the disc to the condyle is lost, and disc degeneration occurs.

After an acute traumatic injury to the jaw, a *condylar fracture* accompanied by pain, swelling, and limitation of motion over the involved area is not unusual. The condylar fragments usually are displaced anteriorly and medially into the infratemporal fossa because of the pull of the lateral pterygoid muscle.

Clinical Application

In no instance does the TMJ operate independently of the surrounding muscles. It is the action of these muscles of mastication to function in groups for elevation, protrusion, and lateral motion.

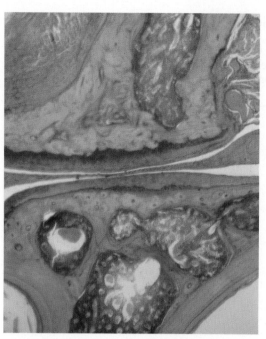

Fig. 20.**25** Flattened condyle in old age.

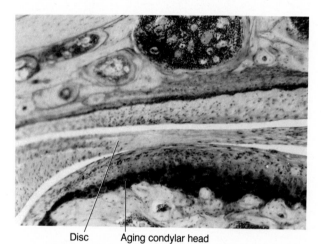

Disc   Aging condylar head

Fig. 20.**26** Aging condylar head.

Arthritis

Inflammation of the joints, or arthritis, also involves the TMJ. Three types of arthritis occur in the TMJ, the most common of which usually is caused by direct extension of infection into the joint. Such an extension may result from dental infection, infection of the parotid gland, or an ear infection. Rheumatoid arthritis in the TMJ is not common; more common is osteoarthritis. The changes in the articular cartilage consist of a loss of elasticity and surface erosion, with vertical cracks that may extend into the subchrondal bone. There is complete destruction of the chondrocytes. The disc may exhibit cracks and fissures and may be hyalinized or even mineralized. Sometimes, necrosis or destruction of the disc may occur.

Age Changes in the Temporomandibular Joint

With aging, the TMJ undergoes changes similar to those of other masticatory structures. The condyle appears flattened in outline (Fig. 20.**25**), and it is not unusual to find a remnant of condylar cartilage in aged joints. The fibrous covering of the condyle, which consists of dense collagen fiber bundles, is thicker in older specimens than in younger ones. In addition, it is not surprising to see chondroid changes. Osteoporosis of the underlying bone of the condyle is a common feature of the aging TMJ complex. The loss of bone has been reported to be more marked in women than in men over 60 years of age. The osteoporosis may become so advanced that the ramus and condyle of the mandible appear to be a thin shell of cortical bone.

The articular disc becomes thinner and exhibits hyalinization and chondroid changes similar to those described for the connective-tissue layer of the condyle (Fig. 20.**26**). In addition, there are small acellular areas where tears appear. Similar alterations are found in the connective-tissue capsule.

The synovial folds appear fibrotic, and a thick basement membrane develops that separates the synovial lining cells from the underlying stroma. The walls of the blood vessels are thickened. Nerves appear decreased in number in the capsule and peripheral portion of the disc.

These changes in the various components of the joint could lead to its dysfunction in older individuals. The changes in the connective-tissue elements in the capsule and disc could lead to a decrease in their extensibility and result in impaired motion. The chondroid changes to the collagenous elements of the articular tubercle, articular disc, and condyle may affect the degree of resiliency during masticatory function. The alterations found in the synovial folds may lead to a decrease in the formation of synovial fluid and decreased lubrication of the two compartments.

Summary

In the adult TMJ, the condyle consists of a fibrous articulating surface, a thin cartilaginous zone overlying the bone of the condyle. The articular disc is characterized by collagen fibers with a few fibroblasts. The central portion of the disc is very thin. The articulating surface of the glenoid fossa also is fibrous in nature. Synovial membranes and villi are found lining the capsule. The TMJ is well vascularized. A rich vascular plexus appears from the superficial temporal, anterior tympanic, and ascending pharyngeal arteries to terminate in the articular capsule. These arteries form a "crown" circumferentially around the central region of the disc. There are no blood vessels in this thin portion of the disc. Capillary networks are found in the capsular synovia and villi. The capillaries are adjacent to the synovial membrane, and their positions are important for the production of synovial fluid.

Nerves originating from the auriculotemporal, masseteric, and deep temporal areas can be traced into the capsule, disc, and synovial villi. Nerve fibers end in the capsule as free nerve endings and encapsulated endings. Only free nerve endings are observed in the peripheral portion of the disc. There are no nerves in the central portion of the disc. Specialized end bulbs of varying types are found in the synovial villi. These specialized end organs may be proprioceptive.

Changes to the TMJ caused by aging include chondroid changes to the articular surfaces of the glenoid fossa and condyle as well as to that of the disc. In addition, there is thinning or absence of the cartilaginous zone of the condyle. Finally, there are varying degrees of osteoporosis of the bony portion of the condyle, ramus of the mandible, and temporal bone.

Self-Evaluation Review

1. Describe the functions of the superior and inferior TMJ compartments.
2. Describe the function of the TMJ capsule and its supporting ligaments.
3. Describe and compare the action of the two heads of the lateral pterygoid muscle.
4. In what direction do the TMJ condyles grow during childhood?
5. Describe how the connective tissue of the condylar head perichondrium plays a role in the blood supply to the cartilage of the TMJ.
6. Describe the development of new cartilage and its replacement by bone in the condylar head.
7. What is meant by sling muscles? Do the separate muscles in the sling have the ability to work in synchrony?
8. Describe the nerve supply to the joint. Where do the nerve endings terminate in the joint?
9. Compare the condylar heads in a young adult and in an aging person.
10. Describe the blood supply to the TMJ.

Acknowledgements

Dr Donald Wright contributed Figures 20.**5A** and **B**. Dr CC Boyer contributed Figure 20.**15**, and Dr S Bernick, now deceased, contributed Figures 20.**6**, 20.**13**, 20.**14**, and 20.**17**–20.**19** as well as much of the written material of this chapter.

Suggested Readings

DuBrul EL. The craniomandibular articulation, In: Sicher's Oral Anatomy. 7th ed. St louis: CV Mosby Co; 1980:Chaps 4,16.

Dixon AD. Structure and functional significance of the intra-articular disc of the temporomandibular joint. Oral Surg. 1962;15:48.

Griffin CJ, Hawthorne R, Harris R. Anatomy and histology of the human temporomandibular joint. Monogr. Oral Sci. 1975;4:1.

Gugenheim B, Shipiro S. Oral Biology at the Turn of the Century. Basel: Karger; 1998.

Karakasis D, Tsakakis A. Aging changes in the articular disk of the temporomandibular disk in the guinea pig. J. Dent. Res. 1976;55:262.

Meikie MC. The role of the condyle in the postnatal growth of the mandible, Am. J. Orthop. 1973;64:50.

Sarnat BG, Laskin DM. Temporomandibular Joint: Biological Basis for Clinical Practice. Springfield Ill: Charles C Thomas; 1979.

Thilander B. Innervation of the temporomandibular disc in man. Acta. Odontol. Scand. 1964:22:151.

21 Histologic Changes during Tooth Movement

Carla A. Evans

Introduction

Adjustments in tooth position are possible throughout life because the components of the periodontium (periodontal ligament, alveolar bone, cementum, and gingiva) remodel continually. Some tooth movements occur spontaneously. Tooth buds may change position within the jaw before beginning to erupt. After active eruption to the occlusal level, teeth continue to erupt passively and migrate as they compensate for late growth changes and tooth wear.

Tooth movement also may occur in response to the sustained mechanical forces emanating from orthodontic appliances or other stimuli. This chapter focuses on the histologic features of mechanically induced tooth movement.

In most instances, the periodontal structures respond well to movements induced by the clinician because the alveolar bone and gingiva show a remarkable ability to be modified (Figs. 21.**1** and 21.**2**). Mechanical loads activate cells, and tissues remodel to resist stresses and strains. The sequence and timing of the remodeling process are known, but the biologic basis for orthodontic tooth movement is not well understood.

Objectives

After reading this chapter, you should be able to describe typical histologic changes in the periodontium that result from tipping, bodily movement, and intrusive, extrusive, and rotational force on the tooth root during clinical treatment. Also, you should be able to describe potential diverse changes resulting from orthodontic tooth movement.

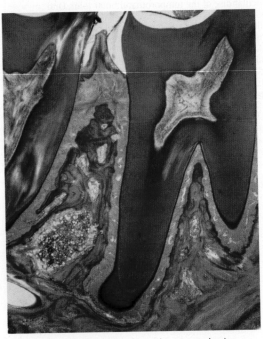

Fig. 21.**1** Normal periodontium (rhesus monkey).

Clinical Application

Dental implants and ankylosed teeth lack fibrous attachment to alveolar bone and do not move in response to orthodontic forces; investigators are exploring the potential uses of implants as anchor units in orthodontic treatment.

Fundamentals of Tooth Movement

Clinical tooth movement requires a periodontal ligament. Forces applied to teeth are mediated through the periodontal ligaments and result in remodeling of the periodontal tissues (Figs. 21.**1** and 21.**2**). When an appliance is attached to a tooth and the tooth is moved, as shown in Figure 21.**2**, the entire surface of the socket is affected. The pressure side of the tooth root compresses the periodontal ligament and alveolar bone, which results in bone resorption. On the opposite surface of the root, the movement stretches the ligament fibers, which causes tension. This situation is, of course, similar in the case of a single or multirooted tooth, although it is more complex in the latter (Fig. 21.**2**). Forces had only recently been applied to the tooth in Figure 21.**2**: consequently, the ligament is narrower on the compression side than on the tension side.

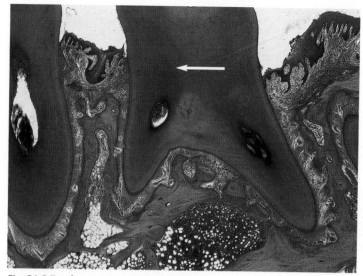

Fig. 21.**2** Tooth movement to the left (arrow).

Sites of Remodeling

On the compression side of the ligament, collagen fiber bundles initially are disorganized and compacted. Vascular flow decreases; cell death may occur and osteoclasts may appear along the bone front (Fig. 21.**3**). On the tension side of the ligament, the collagen fibers are stretched. The fibroblasts become more spindle-shaped and appear oriented with their long axis in the direction of the fiber bundles (Fig. 21.**4**). A two-rooted tooth, as shown in Figures 21.**2** and 21.**5**, has two or more zones of compression as well as two or more zones of tension. Note that the bifurcation zone has a region of tension toward the left root and a region of compression toward the right root. The apical areas demonstrate transition from tension to compression and are vulnerable locations during tooth movement

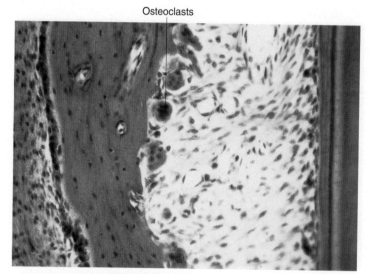

Fig. 21.**3** Compression zone (early).

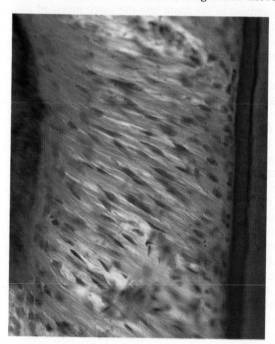

Fig. 21.**4** Tension zone (early).

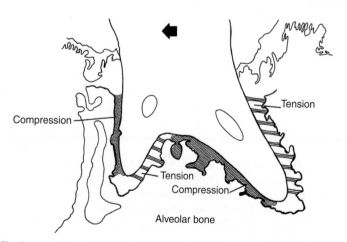

Fig. 21.**5** Zones of compression and tension in tooth movement.

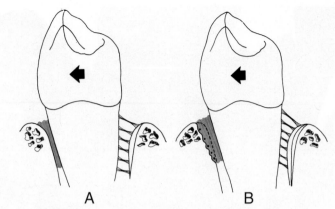

Fig. 21.**6** Results of tipping type of tooth movement. **A** Early. **B** Late.

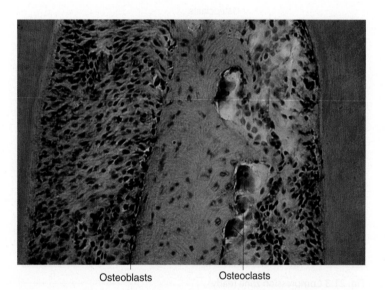

Osteoblasts   Osteoclasts

Fig. 21.**7** Osteoblasts and osteoclasts in the bifurcation zone. Left: tension zone. Right: compression zone.

Clinical Application

Clinically applicable advances related to tooth movement have come primarily from improvements in orthodontic materials and statistical observations on growth and development. Basic biologic research on the remodeling process and mechanisms of tooth movement is desirable to produce faster and more stable tooth movement.

because too much pressure could cause death of the pulp tissue by interfering with the tooth's vascular supply.

The initial response to physical force is displacement of the tooth; permanent structural changes follow. The histologic features accompanying the changes include a change in cell type and number, vascular changes, and changes in the extracellular matrix.

Transduction

The mechanism of transduction—that is, the conversion of physical force into biologic response—is not known, but numerous hypotheses have been introduced. Some of the mechanical and chemical signals proposed as initiators of metabolic changes are: altered blood and lymphatic flow; pressure and volume changes within the periodontal space; distortion of matrix molecules, cell membranes, and cell cytoskeleton; stress-generated bioelectric effects from alveolar bone bending; hormonal influences; and inflammatory phenomena and other nervous and immune cellular events. The explanations propose ways for local and systemic factors to influence alveolar bone, periodontal and gingival fiber bundles, cells (mesenchymal, vascular, neural, gingival epithelial), and tissue fluids. However, more investigation is needed to elucidate the cascade of changes involved in remodeling of the periodontium during tooth movement.

Force Variables

Time is an important variable in the response of alveolar bone to tooth movement. As might be expected, the histology of the compression and tension zones will change with time. Alveolar bone resorption allows for the gradual movement of the tooth into the space provided and begins on the compression front. On the tension side, bone formation compensates for tooth movement away from the bone under tension, as shown in Figures 21.**6A** and **B**. Figure 21.**6A** illustrates a tooth tipping to the left; on the left a compression zone is seen whereas on the right a tension zone is seen. Later (Fig. 21.**6B**), the zone of direct osteoclastic resorption is seen on the left, with bony deposition occurring in the tension zone on the right. Direct or frontal resorption is a desirable clinical goal because it is not a destructive process. Osteoclasts appear a few hours after tooth movement begins as they are recruited from monocytes arising from blood vessels. Both osteoclasts and osteoblasts stain with oxidative enzymes. Figure 21.**7** illustrates both osteoblasts (left) and osteoclasts (right) in the interradicular bone between the roots of a molar tooth. Compare the resorption sites that have large, multinucleated, black-stained osteoclasts (right) with the highly cellular, fibrous zone (left). In which direction is the tooth therefore moving? Fibroblasts proliferate and synthesize new matrix in tension sites and participate in the degradation of necrotic ligament in areas of compression along with osteoclasts and macrophages.

Histologic Changes

The tissue response to mechanical forces in tooth movement will vary with force magnitude (light, heavy), duration (continuous, itermittent), direction, and point of application. Should the force be too great in magnitude or the movement too rapid, hyalinization of the periodontal ligament may occur. Hyalinization results in the loss of cell activity and vascularity in the pressure zone of the ligament. This zone of the ligament may appear glass–like; hence, the origin of the term. A hyalinized ligament is shown in Figure 21.**8A**, where the tooth is in close apposition to bone. Viewed at higher magnification (Fig. 21.**8B**), a loss of the fibrillar nature of the collagen fibers can be seen. Loss of cells interrupts bone resorption and tooth movement stops temporarily.

Another feature of hyalinization is its association with undermining resorption. Because resorption cannot occur on the compressed surface of the alveolar bone, osteoclasts are activated in the marrow spaces opposite the compressed alveolar bone surface. When the osteoclasts finish removing the intervening bone, the tooth will move again. Note the osteoclasts in Figure 21.**8B** that are destroying the bone adjacent to the hyalinized zone. Some of the cells in the zone of compression do not recover. As they are destroyed and resorption relieves the compression, new cells from adjacent tissues rebuild the destroyed zone. It is not yet known why compression of the ligament and alveolar bone results in undermining resorption, but lack of blood supply and cell death in the hyalinized zone may contribute. Also, changes in bioelectric potential may signal the onset of resorption. In addition to delaying orthodontic treatment, undermining resorption of alveolar bone is potentially more damaging to the alveolar process than is direct resorption, as it may result in extensive bone loss and root resorption. What protects the root surface from damage during routine tooth movement is not known. Undermining resorption is not easily controlled and the extent of damage is unpredictable. Forces applied to the teeth can also cause distant changes, such as those in periosteum, endosteum, sutures, and possibly even mandibular condyles. A complete explanation of tooth movement must include mechanisms for bone remodeling alveolar bone marrow spaces, alteration of the gingiva, and transmission of forces to distant sites. Intermittent force and continuous force cause different histologic appearances. When the tissues are temporarily relieved of stress, circulation is partially restored, cell activity is restored, and repair takes place. Tooth mobility may be increased, however, which can become a problem.

A lower level of cellularity in the periodontal ligament is found in older individuals and may be related to an initial slower rate of response during tooth movement. Increased age, however, does not reduce the prospect of a successful clinical outcome.

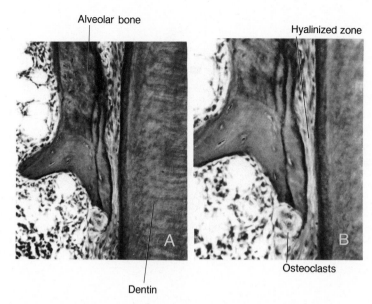

Fig. 21.**8 A** Compression and hyalinization of the periodontal ligament caused by excessive tooth movement. **B** Higher magnification of (**A**) shows undermining resorption adjacent to the hyalinized zone.

Clinical Application

The clinician must choose a force level and an appliance that are effective, efficient, and safe. Regular monitoring of the progress of treatment is extremely important so that forces and appliances can be altered as required.

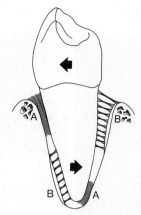

Fig. 21.**9** Tipping of tooth causing crown movement to the left and root movement to the right. Observe the zones of compression and tension.

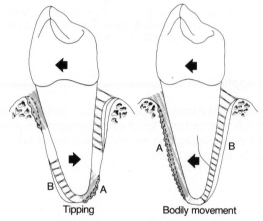

Tipping   Bodily movement

Fig. 21.**10** Tipping movement compared with bodily movement. In the latter, changes occur over the entire periodontium of the root surface.

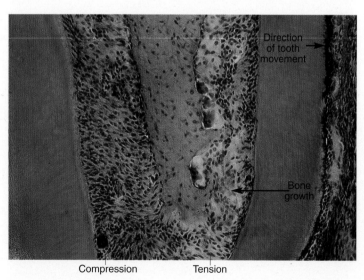

Direction of tooth movement

Bone growth

Compression   Tension

Fig. 21.**11** Bifurcation zone during late tooth movement. Left: active resorption. Right: bone formation.

Tipping and Bodily Movement

Tipping of a tooth (Fig. 21.**9**) results in nonuniform alteration of the sockets, whereas bodily movement affects the entire socket in a more constant fashion, as is illustrated in Figure 21.**10**. Compression, and possibly hyalinization, occur at points A, whereas tension and bone deposition occur at points B. When the crown tips to the left, the root apex moves to the right, producing zones of compression and tension on opposite sides of the tooth apex relative to the cervical region. Likewise, both bone resorption and deposition occur on the same side of a tooth as it is tipped (Fig. 21.**10**).

Figure 21.**11** shows a histologic section of the bifurcation zone of a molar tooth during the process of being tipped to the right. The direction of force is indicated by the small arrow in the upper right-hand corner. At the point of the large arrow, on the tension side of the tooth, new alveolar bone is being formed. The active bone-forming osteoblasts as well as osteocytes are seen stained black by a histochemical stain, which indicates vital functioning cells. Along the dentin (right), the cementoblasts are also stained, which indicates the formation of new cementum in response to tension on the perforating fibers. Resorption of bone and degenerative changes are occurring in the compression zone on the left of the alveolar bone. This is indicated by inactivity of the bone front. Most of the lacunae are unstained, which indicates the absence of vital cells. Spaces where bone loss has occurred indicate resorptive activity.

In Figure 21.**12**, the small circle on the roots indicates the center of resistance, or the fulcrum of rotation of each tooth. In the case of a short, incompletely developed root (Fig. 21.**12A**), tipping causes resorption at two sites and tension at the opposite two sites. The root apex of a young, completely formed tooth, as shown in Figure 21.**12B**, tips in a direction opposite to the crown. In the adult, as shown in Figure 21.12C, tipping is complicated by strong apical fibers that resist movement and a narrow ligament space. In this case, tipping causes less movement at the root apex, but causes resorption along most of the length of bone on the compressed side.

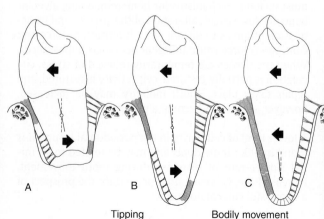

A   B   C

Tipping   Bodily movement

Fig. 21.**12** Change in point of rotation of tooth in young forming root (**A**), completed root (**B**), and mature periodontium (**C**).

A micrograph of the cemental surface reveals the activity of oxidative enzymes during tooth movement in the cementoblasts adjacent to the cementum (Fig. 21.**13**, center). Observe the bundles of collagen fibers projecting from the cementum. The stain indicates that the cementocytes, probably newly differentiated, have high functional activity. This is also true for the osteoblasts in the adjacent alveolar bone. New cementum will be deposited, and attachment fiber bundles will be formed in response to the tension.

Both the cementum and the alveolar bone may undergo resorption (Fig. 21.**14**). If compression is great and over a long period, both opposing surfaces will be affected. Note the osteoclasts along the bone and cementum. (Fig. 21.**14**).

Extrusive and Intrusive Movement

Figure 21.**15A** illustrates the orientation of principal fibers when extrusive forces are applied to the tooth. Note the direction of the arrows. This type of movement causes tension in all the ligament fibers with resultant bone deposition along the lamina dura, especially in the alveolar crest and fundic regions. Light extrusive forces are most effective at producing compensatory bone growth. Intrusive forces cause relaxation of the free and attached gingival fibers, as well bone loss at the alveolar crest and over the entire socket (Fig. 21.**15B**). Good results are less easily obtained with intrusive movements than with tipping. This mode of movement requires a light, persistent force proceeding at a slow rate.

The tooth shown in Figure 21.**16** is in the process of being intruded. The applied forces depicted by the arrow on the left of this micrograph, on the pulpal side of the root dentin, cause the principal fibers to appear oblique, except at the gingival area at the top of the field where they are collapsed. The bone in this area has been partially resorbed and will undergo further resorption, as will the compressed alveolar bone in the apical zone.

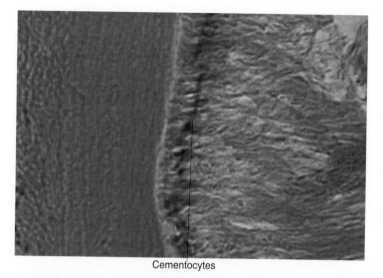

Cementocytes

Fig. 21.**13** Activation of cementocytes along the surface of the root.

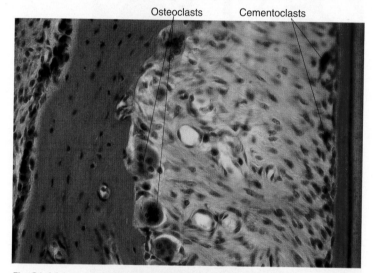

Osteoclasts   Cementoclasts

Fig. 21.**14** Activity in the compression zone (late). Observe the osteoclasts on bone and the resorption of the root surface.

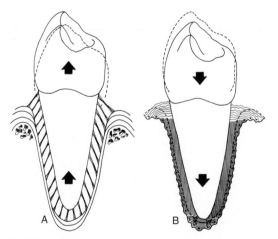

A   B

Fig. 21.**15 A** Extrusion of tooth, causing tension over the entire socket. **B** Intrusion of tooth, causing resorption over the entire surface of the alveolar bone proper.

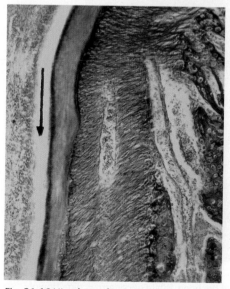

Fig. 21.**16** Histology of intrusive movement. Note the loss of bone and cementum.

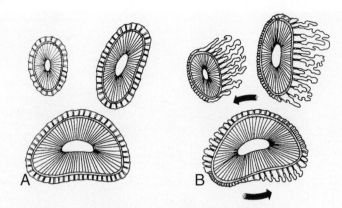

Fig. 21.**17 A** Normal periodontium around three-rooted tooth. **B** Rotation of three-rooted tooth, causing bone loss and deposition of new bone.

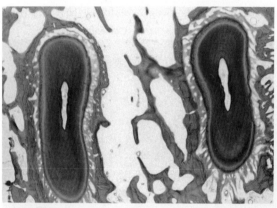

Fig. 21.**18** Histology of rotation of roots. Observe the direction of the periodontal fiber bundles.

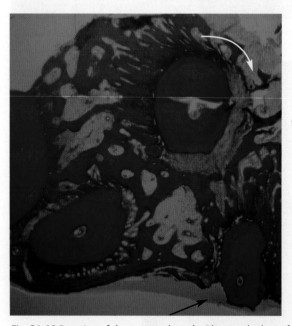

Fig. 21.**19** Rotation of three-rooted tooth. Observe the bone formation along the tension surfaces of the bone. White upper arrow: direction of rotation. Black lower arrow: perforation of cortical bone by root.

Rotation and Bodily Movement

Figure 21.**17** illustrates the consequence of rotational forces on a three-rooted molar tooth. At the left in these diagrams is the direction of the principal fibers before treatment. As the tooth is rotated, deposition will occur along the tension surface. The result after 4 months is shown in Figure 21.**17B**. Observe the distance each root has moved. Not all roots may move the same distance; for example, one root rotates in place whereas the others are moved around this axis. Restructuring of the socket in the alveolar bone during rotation therefore occurs by development of zones of tension and compression as shown in Figure 21.**17B**. The oval shape of the root also complicates resorptive patterns.

Figure 21.**18** shows two teeth in the early stages of clockwise rotation illustrated by the direction of the collagen fiber bundles of the periodontal ligament. Bone resorption and bone formation are minimal at this early time, although resorption of bone on the inferior aspect of the root on the right and some cemental loss along the root surface on the right are seen.

Figure 21.**19** illustrates the clockwise rotation of a three-rooted molar after 4 months. In this micrograph, the root on the left has rotated in position, which demonstrates the characteristic changes in socket shape that result from movement of an oval root. These are the same changes shown in Figure 21.**17**. The other two roots also show evidence of clockwise movement and more extensive remodeling of the socket. The pattern of bone deposition stimulated by tension placed on the periodontal ligament fibers can be seen on the left of the uppermost root. Observe that bone formation has occurred along the direction of the periodontal ligament fibers. This deposition pattern indicates the path of root movement. Excessive application of rotational force in the tooth has resulted in the undesired perforation of the cortical bone plate by the buccal root, which can be seen at the lower right of the micrograph (Fig. 21.**19**, black arrow). In Figure 21.**20**, the long horizontal trabeculae of bone can be seen deposited behind the moving tooth root. Incremental deposits of cementum also can be seen along the tension side of the root (Fig. 21.**20**). Cementum, like bone, will resorb or form in areas of pressure and tension. This figure demonstrates an extreme case of socket remodeling and shows the alveolar bone's potential for remodeling.

Figure 21.**21** demonstrates an extreme case of intrusion of a tooth in a socket. The molar tooth is in contact with the underlying bone. Observe the extent of bone loss on the left and right. Bony change is indicated by the dark-stained bone surrounding the root. Resorption has caused a thinning of the bone on the left of the root. Remodeling of the bony tooth socket and alteration of the periodontal ligament fibers are not only considerations in tooth movement. As shown in Figure 21.**22**, black-stained neural elements pass from the periodontal ligament (right) into the alveolar bone (left). These neural elements must adjust to positional changes of the tooth and bone. The vascular network within the periodontal ligament will be modified according to any changes caused by tooth movement and will adapt to maintain a normal vascular supply (Fig. 21.**23**). Lack of

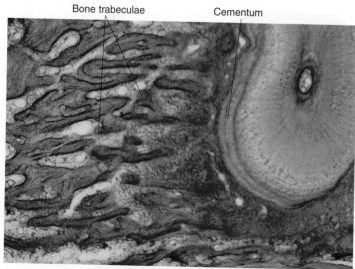

Fig. 21.**20** Bone trabeculae and cementum on the tension side of the root. This tooth is undergoing rotation.

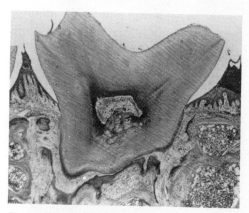

Fig. 21.**21** Intrusion of tooth (early). Observe the contact of the tooth and alveolar bone.

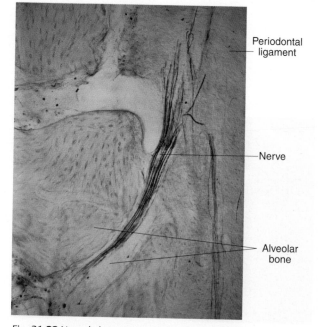

Fig. 21.**22** Neural elements enter the ligament from the alveolar bone.

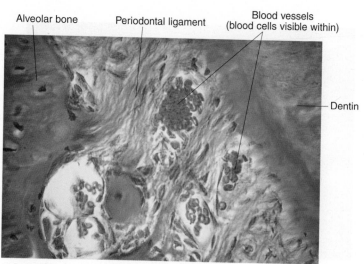

Fig. 21.**23** Normal vascularity of the periodontal ligament.

vascular supply to this area results in hyalinization, possibly with resultant undermining and surface resorption.

Root resorption is a potential complication of orthodontic tooth movement. Figures 21.**24A** and **B** show an unusual case of generalized extreme root resorption that occurred during orthodontic treatment.

Stability and Relapse

Teeth remain in position on a day-to-day basis because the forces acting on them from the tongue and cheeks and from chewing and swallowing are in equilibrium. Even in severe malocclusions (Fig. 21.**25**), the alignment of the teeth is stable. The clinician faces two challenges: first, to move the teeth and second, to find a second position of equilibrium so that the results of tooth movement with orthodontic appliances will be stable. Figure 21.**26** shows relapse of dental crowding after completion of comprehensive treatment, which included extraction of premolars, fixed orthodontic appliances, and a long period of retention with removeable retainers.

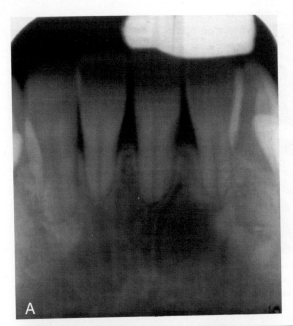

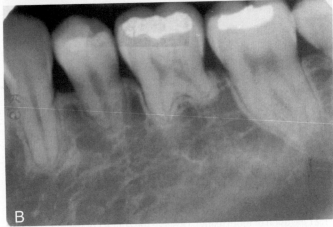

Fig. 21.**24 A**, **B** A rare case of generalized extreme root resorption.

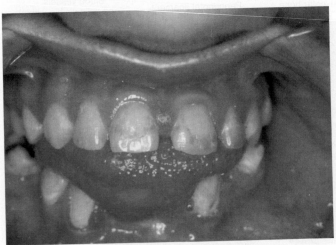

Fig. 21.**25** Tooth position is stable in this anterior open bite malocclusion associated with a lymphatic malformation.

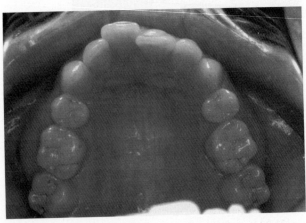

Fig. 21.**26** Orthodontic relapse

Summary

Changes in the periodontal structures during tooth movement depend on the magnitude, duration, direction, and point of application of the force, as well as health and age of the tissues. Changes on the tension side of tooth movement are characterized by an initial increase in periodontal ligament width with stretching of the periodontal ligament fibers. Later, bone deposition follows in the form of plates or spurs. On the compression side of the tooth, either direct bone resorption or hyalinization with undermining resorption ensues. Variations of these changes are demonstrated in Figure 21.**27**, which illustrates forces causing tipping (A), bodily movement (B), extrusive force (C), intrusive force (D), and rotational force (E). Determination of the center of resistance of the tooth is an important factor in planning treatment mechanics.

Most routine clinical tooth movement produces a successful, stable, nondestructive result. In some unusual instances, however, substantial permanent loss of bone or root structure may occur. Remodeling of the periodontium after tooth movement is necessary to maintain the correction. In contrast to the rapid reorganization seen in the alveolar bone, gingival fibers require a prolonged period of retention and may never fully remodel.

Self-Evaluation Review

1. Regarding tipping, what differences or changes in the periodontium would you expect of a young versus mature individual?
2. What changes are noted along the cemental surface at a tension site?
3. Describe hyalinization of the periodontal ligament. From what may it result?
4. What complications may arise from hyalinization of the periodontal ligament?
5. What adverse results would you expect when a tooth is moved too rapidly?
6. Compare the effects of intrusive and extrusive forces.
7. Describe undermining resorption. What complications may arise?
8. What role would vascularity play in bone resorption?
9. What tissue resorbs more rapidly, tooth or alveolar bone, and why?
10. Compare rotation with rotation plus bodily movement of a tooth.

Clinical Application

Although commonly associated with excessive force or long duration of treatment, root resorption may also arise surprisingly quickly during use of light forces; however, this is very rare.

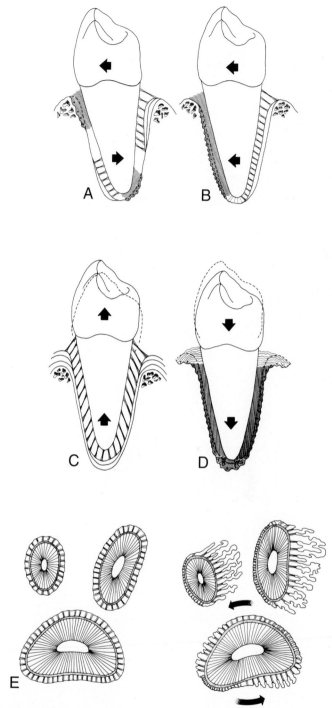

Fig. 21.**27** Summary diagrams of tipping **(A)**, bodily movement **(B)**, extrusion **(C)**, intrusion **(D)**, and rotation **(E)**.

Clinical Application

Stability of the orthodontic outcome depends on attaining equilibrium of forces and total remodeling of the periodontium. Gingival fibers in particular remodel very slowly and will cause rotations and spacing anomalies to recur. Gingival fiber resection and permanent fixed retention may be required to maintain the correction.

Suggested Readings

Atherton JD. The gingival response to orthodontic tooth movement. Am J Orthod. 1970;58:179.

Azuma M. Study on histologic changes of periodontal membrane incident to experimental tooth movement. Bull Tokyo Med Dent Univ. 1970;17:149.

Baumrind S, Buck DL. Rate changes in cell replication and protein synthesis in the periodontal ligament incident to tooth movement. Am J Orthod. 1970;57:109.

Beersten W, Everts V, Hoeben K, Niehof A. Microtubules in periodontal ligament cells in relation to tooth eruption and collagen degradation. J Periodont Res. 1984;19:489–500.

Davidovich Z. Tooth movement. Crit Rev Oral Biol Med. 1991;2:411–450.

Davidovich Z, Montgomery PC, Eckerdal O, Gustafson GT. Cellular localization of cyclic AMP in periodontal tissues during experimental tooth movement in cats. Calcif Tissue Res. 1976;19:317.

Edwards JG. A study of the periodontium during orthodontic rotation of teeth. Am J Orthod. 1968;54:441–459.

Kuam E. Organic tissue characteristics on the pressure side of human premolars following tooth movement. Angle Orthod. 1973;43:18–23.

Proffit WR. The biologic basis of orthodontic therapy. In: Rudolph P. Contemporary Orthodontics. St. Louis, MO: CV Mosby Co; 1993:266–288.

Roberts WE, Goodwin WC Jr, Heiner SR. Cellular response to orthodontic force. Dent Clin North Am. 1981;25:3–17.

Rygh P. Ultrastructural changes in pressure zones of human periodontium incident to orthodontic tooth movement. Acta Odontal Scand. 1973;31:109–122.

Rygh P. Orthodontic root resorption studied by electron microscopy. Angle Orthod. 1977;47:1–16.

Stenvick A, Mjor IA. Pulp and dentine reactions to experimental tooth intrusion. Am J Orthod. 1970;47:370–385.

Ten Cate AR, Deported DA, Freeman E. The role of fibroblasts in the remodeling of periodontal ligament during physiologic tooth movement. Am J Orthod. 1976;69:155.

Thilander B, Lindhe J, Okamato H. The effect of orthodontic tilting movements on the periodontal tissues of infected and non-infected dentitions in dogs. J Clin Periodontol. 1977;14:231.

22 Histology of Endosseous Implants

Robert B. O'Neal and Marion J. Edge

Introduction

The documented high survival rate of osseointegrated root from dental implants, since 1981, has lead to their acceptance as a realistic treatment alternative in modern dentistry to that of traditional prostheses. Branemark et al and Schroeder et al independently demonstrated a predictable tissue healing of dental implants that resulted in direct bone-implant contact. Successful osseointegration is predictable when specific criteria regarding choice of materials and clinical procedures are observed. The development of dynamic functioning interfaces of implants with epithelium, connective tissue, and bone is important for the long-term success of implant-supported dental prostheses (Fig. 22.**1**). The first implant-supported prostheses were limited to the completely edentulous patient. Four or five fixtures were placed so that they engaged both the superior and inferior cortical plates of the anterior mandible (Fig. 22.**2**). These fixtures were connected together by a rigid framework to which artificial teeth were attached. The patient went from

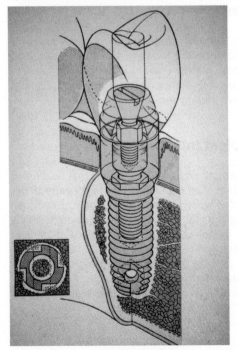

Fig. 22.**1** Schematic representation of a dental implant with components: fixture, abutment, and center screwed attached prostheses. The unique interfaces of the implant with epithelium, connective tissue, and bone will be discussed in this chapter.

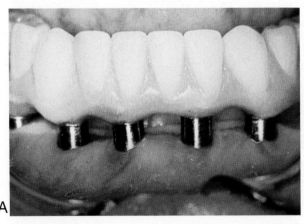

A

Fig. 22.**2 A** Patient with a mandibular prosthesis supported by five titanium dental implants.

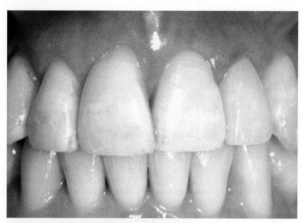

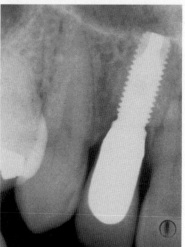

B

Fig. 22.**2 B** Maxillary single implant replacing the left lateral and radiograph of the final restoration.

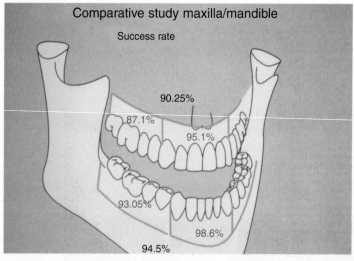

Fig. 22.**3** Schematic diagram of the success rates of implants.

wearing a loose-fitting lower denture to a prostheses that was as stable as their original teeth. Patients were able to eat and speak without having to concern themselves about the denture dislodging or food being trapped under their appliance. A functional and esthetic maxillary implant is seen in Figure 22.2**A** and a radiograph of this tooth in Figure 22.2**B**. Today, because of the results of long-term clinical trials and improvements in implant design, especially in the abutment connections, implants are approved for the replacement of a single tooth in both the maxillary and mandibular arch. The success rate over 5 years is slightly higher in the mandible (94%) than in the maxilla (90%). This difference in the success rate is mainly due to the difference in the quality of the bone between the arches and the location within each arch (Fig. 22.**3**). The approval by the Federal Drug Administration, and acceptance by the dental implant profession has lead to a major change in the replacement of missing teeth. This has been especially beneficial to patients with congenitally missing teeth and teeth lost to trauma, caries, and periodontal disease. The ability to replace a tooth or teeth without affecting the adjacent natural teeth has even been accepted by many insurance companies as an approved benefit. This approach has proven to be cost effective, in the long run, and preserves the adjacent natural dentition. Knowledge of basic histology and implant biocompatibility characteristics will not only enhance our ability to choose the right implant system, but will also increase implant integration capability and further ensure long-term implant success.

Objectives

After reading the information in this chapter, you should be able to describe the unique epithelium, connective tissue, and bone interface with the implant surface. You should also be able to describe peri-implant infections and supportive therapy for implant success.

Bone-implant Interfaces

In 1952 Branemark embarked on studies that resulted in the introduction of an implant design. In the early 1980s, after years of extensive study, the cylindrical threaded endosteal implants for tooth replacement were formally accepted by organized dentistry. A variety of implant models and surgical techniques have led to the development of our present concepts of fibro-osseous integration, osseointegration, and bio-integration. *Fibro-osseous integration* is defined as the connective-tissue-encapsulated implant within bone (Fig. 22.**4**). This type of integration was an early histologic finding in implant development. Fibro-osseous integration resulted from: 1) early types of implant materials; 2) lack of primary stability; 3) premature loading of the implant; and/or 4) a traumatic surgical procedure causing heat-induced bone necrosis. Long-term clinical studies have demonstrated a success rate of less than 50% over a 10-year period for this type of implant integration. Materials that stimulate this type of reaction are non-precious metals, acrylates, polymers, and vitreous carbon. These materials are no longer used. With the newer materials, fibro-osseous integration makes up a much smaller percentage of the interface to the implant, while osseointegration or bio-integration compromise the majority of the interface.

Branemark defined *osseointegration*, at the light microscope level, as a direct structural and functional connection between ordered living bone, and the surface of a load-carrying implant without soft-tissue intervention (Fig. 22.**5**).

In a more comprehensive way, osseointegration is characterized as "a direct structural and functional connection" between ordered living bone and the surface of a load-bearing implant. This type of integration has been shown to yield the most predictable success for long-term implant stability. Factors that enhance osseointegration include: 1) atraumatic surgical procedures with minimal heat generated, and 2) close fit of the implant fixture to the formed socket. Present implant surgical research indicates that the best result is achieved with a low drilling speed (under 1200 rpm) and abundant irrigation with chilled saline, which minimizes bone-tissue injury. The use of a precision drilling system increases the initial implant–bone contact. The implant materials, surface characteristics of the implant, and type of recipient bone are factors that help determine the final implant–tissue interface (Table 22.**1**). In addition, the appropriate timing of placing the implant in function supporting a prosthesis is an essential element in maintaining osseointegration. Procedurally, for most implants there is a waiting time of 3 to 6 months prior to placing the implants in function, depending on the quality of the bone.

Biointegration is a form of implant interface that is achieved with bioactive materials, such as hydroxyapatite (HA) or bioglass that bond directly to bone similar to ankylosis of natural teeth. The bone matrix is deposited on the HA layer as the result of a physiochemical interaction between the collagen of the bone and HA crystals of the implant. HA-coated implants appear to develop bone contact faster than non-coated implants. However, after a year there seems to be little difference in bone contact between coated and non-coated

Table 22.**1** Osseointegration factors

Sterile environment
Precision drilling system
Low-speed cutting
Chilled saline irrigation
Surface characterization of implant
Timing when placed in function

Clinical Application

Because of their comfort, stability, esthetics, and longevity, implant placement has increased 20-fold in the last 20 years. Today, implants are considered an acceptable alternative to conventional prostheses. They are also approved for the replacement of even a single tooth in either the maxillary and mandibular arch.

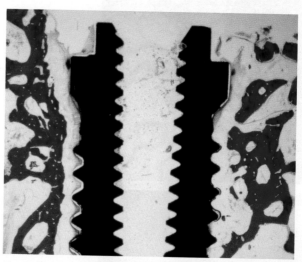

Fig. 22.**4** Light micrograph of fibrous-tissue encapsulation around titanium implant in a human. The fibers run parallel to the implant surface rather than inserting into the titanium.

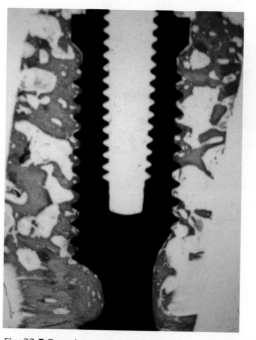

Fig. 22.**5** Osseointegration: a direct structural and functional connection between ordered living bone and the surface of a load-bearing implant. Photomicrograph showing both cortical and cancellous bone in direct contact with a titanium implant.

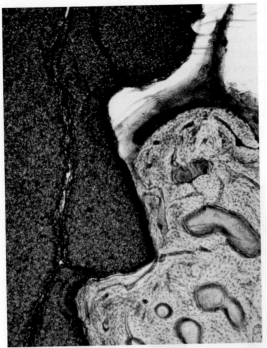

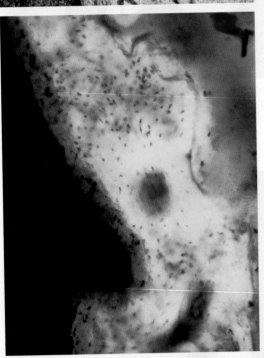

Fig. 22.**6** Bio-integration: **A** Light micrograph of bone contact with aluminum-oxide ceramic implant in a primate. **B** HA-coated implant in contact with the cortical bone in a rabbit tibia.

implants. The HA-coated implants continue to be improved in their purity and manufacturing processes (Figs. 22.**6A** and **B**).

Dental implants differ significantly from natural teeth in their interface with the alveolar bone and connective-tissue fibers. The sulcular and junctional epithelium, however, appears to have the same interface characteristics with implants as with natural teeth (Fig. 22.**7**). Because implants do not have a cemental surface for the insertion of the periodontal ligament and gingival connective-tissue fibers, successful implants depend on direct contact with the alveolar bone. The connective-tissue and epithelial adhesion coronal to the alveolar housing are the primary barriers to bacterial invasion. A successful implant at the light microscopic level would be defined as having 35 to 90% direct bone contact, a connective-tissue adhesion above the bone, and an intact non-inflamed junctional epithelium. Clinically, the implant should be non-mobile and free of discomfort in function. An implant is considered successful if: 1) Mucosal health is substantiated by clinical parameters such as lack of redness, bleeding or suppuration on probing. Soft-tissue inflammation, when present, should be amenable to treatment. 2) There is no significant or progressive loss of supporting bone. 3) There is no persistent infection. 4) The implant functions in the absence of discomfort. 5) There is no increasing mobility of the implant when evaluated on removal of the prosthesis. 6) The implant is prosthetically useful.

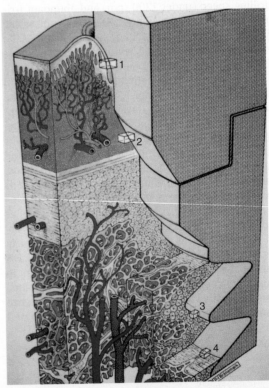

Fig. 22.**7** Three-dimensional diagram of tissue–titanium interrelation showing an overall view of the intact interface zone around osseointegrated implants. Numbers 1 to 4 indicate specific sites discussed in this chapter: [1] sulcular epithelium, [2] junctional epithelium, [3] connective tissue, [4] bone.

Bone is a specialized, calcified connective tissue. The alveolar bone is a combination of both cortical and cancellous bone. Both forms of bone have been shown to osseointegrate with the implant surface. In addition, blood vessels within the bone have been shown to proliferate in contact with the implant surface. To date, the implant materials that have demonstrated the most rapid ability to integrate are the calcium phosphate material (HA) and titanium (commercially pure and alloy). Attempts to improve the bone implant contact with titanium have used several methods to increase the surface area to accomplish this goal. The first method, in the early 1980's, was spraying titanium particles on the surface of the titanium implant (Fig 22.**8**). Other methods have included sand and grit blasting, titanium oxide (TiO_2) blasting, acid etching, or a combination of these. The roughened surface implants have become increasingly popular in implant dentistry. Further improvements in surface configuration are expected to emerge.

The biologically active surface on titanium is a dense protective oxide (TiO_2) layer 15 to 50 μm thick. This TiO_2 layer forms quickly after processing and is relatively resistant to further corrosion by proteolytic enzymes or chemical attack. Titanium plasma spraying of the implant increases the surface area for osseointegration almost six-fold. The other methods increase the surface area to a lesser degree, but it is felt to be easier to maintain than the plasma-sprayed surface in case of exposure to the oral environment. The HA-coated implants appear to osseointegrate more rapidly and have a higher percentage of bone contact than titanium. However, within a year's time the difference does not appear to be clinically significant. The HA coating is manufactured with a commercially pure material that has been proven to be non-toxic and has a resemblance to the inorganic phase of the human skeleton. The healing of bone—implant interface with a stable implant is the same as that of a direct fractured bone healing and follows an orderly sequence of events (Table 22.**2**). Without initial stability, which is determined by the design of the implant and the precise drilling of the implant site, the implant may become fibro-osseous encapsulated. The percentage of cortical bone in contact with implants increases over the first year, because of the remodeling of the bone associated with functional adaptation. Once activated, osseointegration follows a common, biologically determined program of healing that is subdivided into three stages:

1. Incorporation by woven bone.
2. Adaptation of bone mass to load (lamellar and parallel-fiber bone deposition).
3. Adaptation of bone structure to load (bone remodeling).

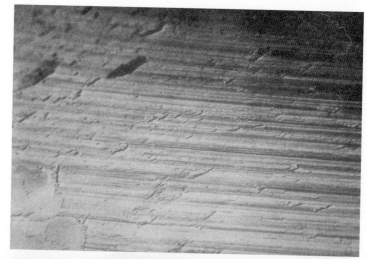

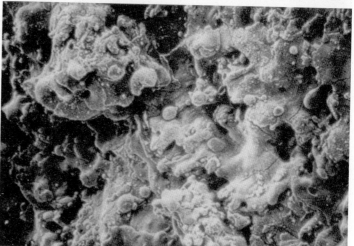

Fig. 22.**8** Comparison of machined titanium (**A**) and plasma sprayed (**B**).

Table 22.**2** Healing stages of the bone—implant interface

Initial healing of the bone—implant interface with gap of less than 0.5 mm
1. Primary stability—appropriate implant design and precise drilling
2. Clot formation between bone and implant
3. Replacement of the blood clot by blood vessels and osteo-progenitor cells
4. Proliferation and differentiation into osteoblast
5. Deposition of bone on the surface of the implant
Healing after implant is placed in function
1. Incorporation by woven bone
2. Adaptation of bone mass to load (lamellar and parallel fiber bone deposition)
3. Adaptation of bone structure to load (bone remodeling)

Clinical Application

HA-coated implants appear to achieve integration faster than other types of implant where there is minimal cortical bone available. These implants are favored by many, especially in areas of poor bone quality. The major disadvantage of the HA-coating is that it can dissolve in the presence of inflammation.

Clinical Application

Titanium implants have an exceptionally high success rate (98%) in the area of the anterior edentulous mandible, where there is a high ratio of cortical to cancellous bone. The changes in the surface characteristics have allowed titanium implants to be used in areas of poor bone quality with a good success rate (87%).

Epithelium Tissue Interface

The interface of epithelium to an implant is similar to that found with the natural tooth. The sulcus and the junctional epithelium are both in contact with the implant. The healthy sulcus consists of a 5 to 15-cell layer of non-keratinized epithelium with wide intercellular spaces. The junctional epithelium is approximately 2 mm in length and two to five cell layers thick, with basal and suprabasal cells in direct contact with the implant surface. These cells are attached to the implant surface by a basal lamina and hemidesmosomes (Figs. 22.**9A–C**). The epithelial interface is similar to the natu-

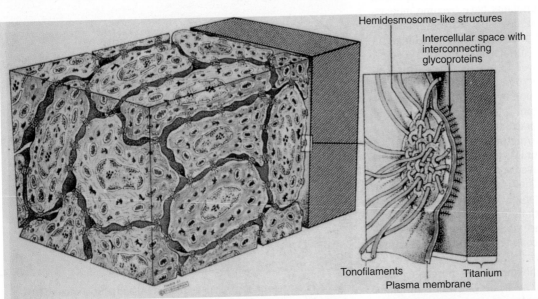

Hemidesmosome-like structures

Intercellular space with interconnecting glycoproteins

Tonofilaments

Plasma membrane

Titanium

A

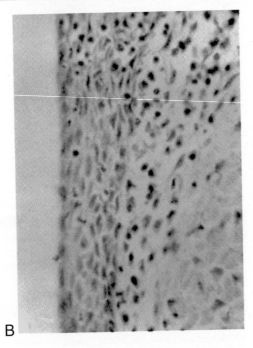

B

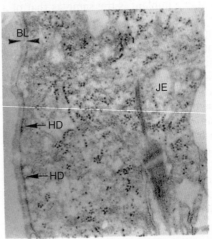

BL

JE

HD

HD

C

Fig. 22.**9 A** Enlarged schematic of gingiva–titanium-oxide contact zone. Inset demonstrates a hemidesmosomes–like structure anchoring the epithelial cells to the implant surface. **B** Light micrograph of the two to five-cell-layer thickness of the junctional epithelium at the interface of a titanium screw in a miniature pig. **C** Transmission electron micrograph of hemidesmosomes at an epoxy resin implant in a monkey. BL: basal lamina. HD: hemidesmosomes. JE: junctional epithelium cell.

ral tooth, whereas the connective-tissue interface is significantly different. In health the junctional epithelium cells migrate from the basal cells of the junctional epithelium toward the base of the sulcus with a turnover rate of 5 to 7 days. Probing around an implant is usually done with plastic probes to avoid scratching the metal surface of the abutment or fixture. The probe usually penetrates close to the base of the junctional epithelium when using light pressure (Figs. 22.**10A–D**). With increased levels of inflammation, the probe may penetrate to the crest of bone. Probing only disrupts the attachment momentarily and has no detrimental effect on the health of the implant. It is usually more difficult to probe around a restored dental implant because the crown is usually larger in diameter than the fixture. The clinician must probe around the height of contour of the crown causing the probe to be at a acute angle to the fixture.

Connective-Tissue Interface

The connective tissue that is attached to a tooth above the crestal bone is normally arranged into three different fiber groups: 1) dentogingival fibers extending from their insertion into cementum to the marginal connective tissue; 2) dentoperiosteal fibers extending from the cementum to the alveolar bone crest; 3) circular fibers present in the connective tissue of the marginal gingiva and supra-alveolar connective tissue. All these fiber groups are functionally oriented (perpendicular) to the tooth. The initial success of dental implants is determined by the ability of the implant material to integrate with the alveolar bone. With the placement of the implant abutment through the oral mucosa, the long-

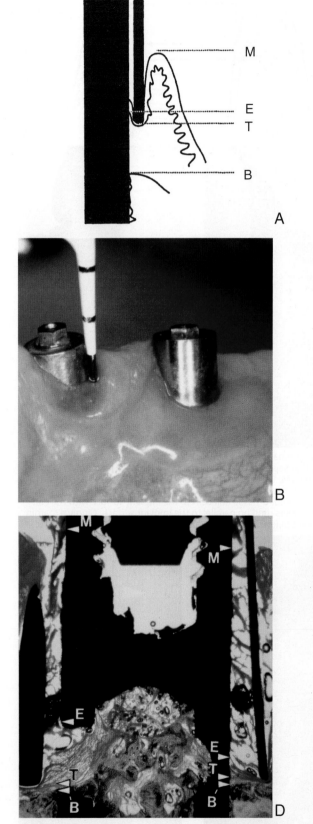

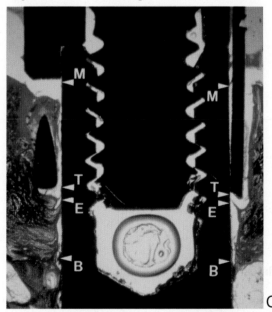

Fig. 22.**10** Probing around a dental implant. **A** Probing in health around an implant stops close to the base of the junctional epithelium. **B** Plastic probes avoid scratching the implant surface. **C** Micrograph of probe stopping in the base of the junctional epithelium in health. **D** Micrograph of probe stopping in the connective tissue with inflammation. Gingival margin (M); apical point of junctional epithelium (E); tip of probe (T); alveolar bone crest (B).

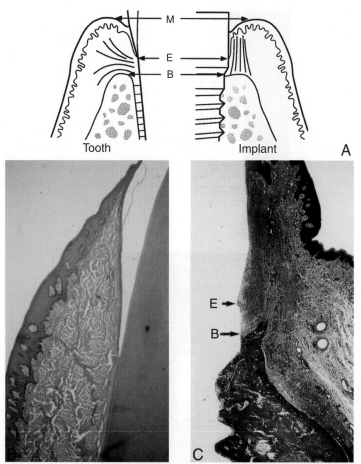

Fig. 22.**11 A** Schematic drawing demonstrating the landmarks on the tooth and implant that separate the area of the sulcus and the junctional epithelium, the connective tissue, and the alveolar bone. **B** The tissue adjacent to a tooth: The junctional epithelium is thin and the distinct collagen fiber groups are well demarcated. **C** Tissue adjacent to the implant surface with the connective-tissue fibers running parallel to the implant surface. Gingival margin (M); apical point of junctional epithelium (E); alveolar bone crest (B).

Fig. 22.**12 A** Light microscopic view of an implant demonstrating the parallel arrangement of the connective-tissue fibers. These fibers extend from the apical termination of the junctional epithelium to the marginal bone crest. **B** Higher magnification of **(A)** showing that the connective-tissue fibers (arrows) run predominantly parallel to the implant surface.

term success is dependent on the "transmucosal seal" that forms between the implant abutment's polished or machined surface and the mucosa's connective tissue and epithelium. In the peri-implant tissue, the vast majority of large collagen fiber bundles are attached to the marginal alveolar bone and insert into the marginal gingiva, not onto the titanium (Figs. 22.**11A–C**). These fiber bundles are highly organized and are oriented parallel to the surface of the machined titanium surface (Fig. 22.**12**). The collagen fiber bundles are consistently separated from the surface of the titanium-dioxide layer by a 20-nm-wide proteoglycan layer.

The width of supracrestal connective tissue around the neck of a healthy implant is approximately 1 to 1.5 mm. This width may vary, being based on either the initial thickness of the mucosa or the degree of adaptation of the mucosa at the time the transmucosal abutment is placed. If the direct bone implant contact is broken, connective tissue will fill the space between the alveolar bone and implant. The connective-tissue fiber bundles run parallel and circular to the implant surface. With adequate home care, both the connective-tissue and epithelial interfaces have been proven to provide adequate resistance to oral function and marginal irritation.

Clinical Application

Ideally, implants should be placed 3 to 4 mm apart, external surface to external surface, to provide adequate space for the development of a soft-tissue interface with each implant. This distance allows room for adequate oral hygiene around each implant.

Peri-implant Infection

The term *peri-implant mucositis* (gingivitis) has been proposed for reversible inflammation of the soft tissues surrounding implants in function. *Peri-implantitis* is defined as an inflammatory process affecting the tissues around osseointegrated implants in function, resulting in loss of supporting bone (First European Workshop on Periodontology, 1994).

Peri-implant health can normally be maintained with a good oral hygiene program. Although plaque accumulation and marginal inflammation are generally low, severe inflammation of the peri-implant tissue occurs in some cases. Clinical inflammatory reactions, as studied in animals, are characterized by an increased number of inflammatory cells infiltrating the connective tissue. Microflora associated with implants in both healthy and slightly inflamed tissues are similar to those of teeth with healthy gingiva. The histologic picture of *early gingivitis* is similar for both the tooth and the implant (Fig. 22.**13**). Early gingivitis consists of an inflammatory cell infiltrate in the connective tissue, lateral to the sulcular epithelium. With *long-standing gingivitis*, the inflammatory cell infiltrate around an implant has a more apical

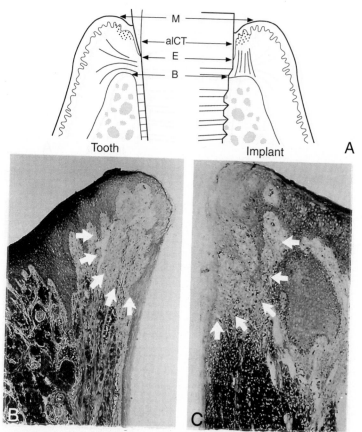

Tooth   Implant   A

Fig. 22.**13 A** Schematic demonstrating the early inflammation with a tooth and implant. **B** With the tooth, infiltrate (arrows) is still above the base of the junctional epithelium. **C** With the implant, the infiltrate (arrows) is still above the base of the junctional epithelium, but occupying a larger area.
Gingival margin (M); area of inflammation in the connective tissue (alCT); apical point of junctional epithelium (E); alveolar bone crest (B). Arrows: outline the borders of inflammation in the connective tissue.

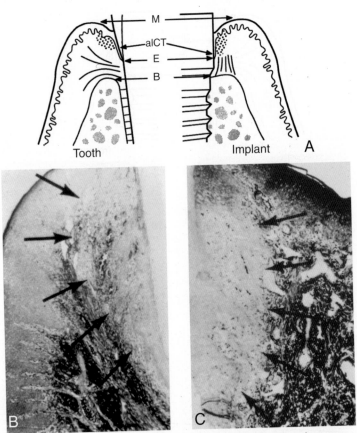

Fig 22.**14 A** Schematic drawing of 3 months of plaque formation, demonstrating the area of inflammatory connective-tissue infiltrate. **B** This inflammation with the tooth extends from the gingival margin to just short of the apical termination of the junctional epithelium (arrows). **C** With the implant, the inflammation extends from the gingival margin to the apical termination of the junctional epithelium.
Gingival margin (M); area of inflammation in the connective tissue (aICT); apical point of junctional epithelium (E).

extension than a corresponding lesion in gingival tissue, and the sulcular epithelium has the appearance of an ulcerated pocket epithelium (Figs. 22.**14A–C**).

The microbiota associated with implants and teeth affected by *marginal bone* loss are more complex and consist primarily of Gram-negative anaerobic rods. *Bone loss around teeth* begins with bone around blood vessels (perivascularly). Despite this perivascular bone resorption, a layer of collagen-rich connective tissue inserted in cementum separates the inflammatory-cell-infiltrated connective tissue from the crestal bone adjacent to the tooth. Inflammatory cells are rarely seen in the periodontal ligament space. The inflammatory infiltrate causing resorption of *bone around an implant* is usually more pronounced than around a tooth, and the inflammatory zone extends directly to the implant and has a more apical extension than a corresponding lesion in gingival tissue. The junctional epithelium cells are turning over more rapidly, and they are less organized with larger spaces between the hemidesmosomes. The inflammatory infiltrate causing resorption of bone around an implant is usually more pronounced than around a tooth, and the inflammatory zone extends directly to the crestal bone (Figs. 22.**15A–C**). The difference can be explained by the parallel orientation of the connective tissue adjacent to the implant, which is less resistant than collagen fibers inserting at right angles into a cemental surface of a tooth. The parallel arrangement of connective tissue and the resulting pathway for bone resorption explains the typical saucerization (circumferential cratering) associated with bone loss around implants, as observed on radiographs (Figs. 22.**16A–C**).

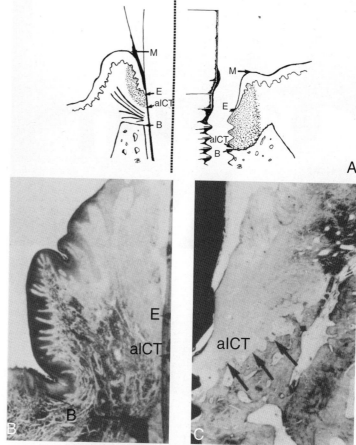

Fig. 22.**15 A** Schematic drawing of destructive periodontitis demonstrating the area of inflammatory connective-tissue infiltrate. **B** This inflammation with the tooth extends to the apical termination of the junctional epithelium. **C** Cross-section of implant and peri-implant tissues with inflammation consistent with peri-implantitis. Arrows indicate the close relation between the inflamed connective tissue and the bone. The bone margin is cupped out, demonstrating active bone resorption.
Gingival margin (M); apical point of junctional epithelium (E); area of inflammation in the connective tissue (aICT); alveolar bone crest (B).

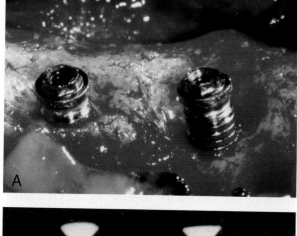

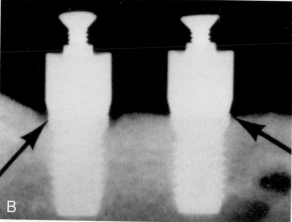

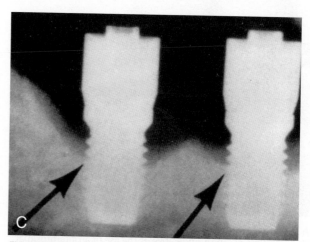

Fig. 22.**16 A** Implants with established peri-implantitis. With the soft tissues removed, the classic circumferential bony defect (saucerization) is apparent. **B** Radiograph consistent with health. **C** Radiograph with bone loss exposing three to four threads of the implant. Arrows: alveolar bone crest.

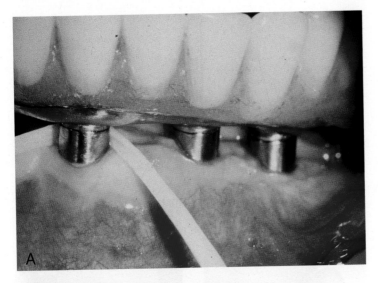

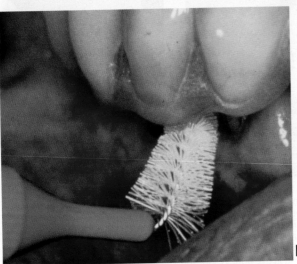

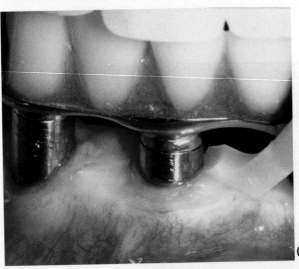

Fig. 22.**17 A** To maintain a high level of plaque and calculus control, daily oral hygiene with dental floss or tape is imperative. **B** The use of an interproximal brush with plastic coating of the metal stem is an excellent method of personal oral hygiene, especially in areas difficult to reach with an ordinary toothbrush. **C** Scaler made of soft material that will not damage the surface of the fixture or abutment.

Supportive Therapy for Peri-implant Mucositis

Patients receiving dental implants have made a significant financial investment in tooth replacement therapy. Although the rate of implant failure is very low, it is significant to those that experience the loss of an implant and possibly the entire restoration. Patients must be given detailed instruction and required to demonstrate their ability to perform proper daily oral hygiene procedures for their dental implants. Implants are a different shape from natural teeth and cleaning around them takes practice. In many cases, specially designed dental aids are needed so that the patient can maintain proper plaque control around their implants. Patients should be instructed to use materials that are not abrasive or that will not scratch the implant surfaces (Fig. 22.**17A**). Interproximal brushes are now manufactured with a coating of nylon over the wire center to prevent damage to the implant surface (Fig. 22.**17B**).

Patients should be in a systematic dental supportive maintenance program with both their restorative and surgical dentist. The repeated assessment should include the following parameters around each implant: The presence of plaque; the bleeding tendency of the implant tissues; the presence of suppuration; the probing depths; relative attachment levels; and the occlusal status of the restoration. To date, there is no evidence that probing around a dental implant is detrimental to the soft-tissue interface with the implant; although some clinicians are concerned about this procedure. Radiographic evidence of bone change over time should be recorded. The goal of a daily home care and a systematic recall program is to intercept peri-implant tissue destruction as early as possible and prevent loss of osseointegration. All instruments that are used in the supportive therapy session should be made of materials that do not damage the surface of the fixture or abutment. There are many commercial companies that manufacture scalers and curettes made of soft materials, which do not damage the implant (Fig. 22.**17C**). Many clinicians have patients using daily rinses of anti-microbial agents and will irrigate with these agents as part of the supportive therapy. In most cases, patients that perform adequate daily home care and stay in a supportive therapy program never progress beyond a peri-mucositis around their implants.

Therapy for Peri-implantitis

Persistant or acute peri-mucositis can lead to peri-implantitis with a state of inflammation that cannot be controlled with adequate daily home care and supportive implant therapy. Some clinicians will place patients on antibiotic therapy. Antibiotics alone do not seem to be a definitive method of treating peri-implantitis. The removal of bacterial bio-film and endotoxins from the implant surface are the major goal in treating peri-implantitis. The best method to decontaminate an implant surface has yet to be determined. If the use of plastic scalers is not sufficient to arrest the inflammation, most clinicians will perform access flap procedures and use either tetracycline or citric acid to remove the bacterial bio-film and endotoxins that contaminate the implant surface. Some clinicians have also used air abrasive materials to clean the implant surface. With peri-implantitis the surface of the implant may become exposed to the oral environment. These implants can be maintained as long as the occlusal forces are directed along the long axis of the fixture and the peri-implant tissues are maintained in a state of health.

The use of air abrasive material and citric acid along with guided bone regeneration (GBR) principles (the exclusion of connective tissue and epithelium with an exclusive membrane material) has been shown to allow 100% of bone height to be restored, although only a minimal amount of this new height is new osseointegration (Fig. 22.**18**). As the techniques of decontamination and GBR are better understood, re-osseointegration may become a predictable procedure for implants with bone loss.

Clinical Considerations

Osseointegration requires an implant composed of a biocompatible material. It must be placed in bone atraumatically and must be placed in function at the appropriate time. After an implant is integrated, the main goal is to maintain good oral hygiene and gingival health around the implant. If oral hygiene is neglected, bacterial plaque forms, resulting in gingivitis, which can progress into peri-implantitis. In the latter condition, bone resorption occurs and dental implants can be lost. Because of the unique pattern (saucerization) of bone resorption around implants, every effort should be made in the design of the implant restoration to allow for optimal hygiene by the patient. The shape and texture of the implant surface that interfaces with the dentogingival complex are important. A geometrically simple, polished, conical, tooth-shaped design is ideal to minimize the deposition of bacterial plaque and calculus. The design of oral implants must consider the possibility of bone resorption and gingival recession, which would expose more of the implant to the oral cavity. Close professional supervision of the implant patient must include continual reassessment of the occlusal forces placed on the implant and the integrity of the prosthetic components. Clinical assessment of the peri-implant soft-tissue interface and radiographic evaluation of the bone-implant interface must be carefully evaluated. Clinical parameters of mobility, tissue color and tone, probing and attachment levels, and bleeding upon probing must be recorded and compared over time. Standardized reproducible radiographs must be compared to evaluate bone height and quality of osseointegration. Any deviation from normal should be corrected to ensure the long-term success of the dental implant.

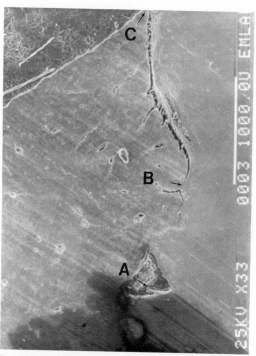

Fig. 22.**18** Scanning electron micrograph of bone contact to a titanium implant with connective-tissue interface, which occurred with a regenerative procedure using guided tissue regeneration (GTR). New bone extends from (A), the most concave point below the second thread, to (B), the most coronal point of reosseointegration. (C) is the most coronal height of new bone (original magnification x 33).

Clinical Application

Titanium implant abutments are easily marred or scratched by metallic instruments and abrasive oral cleaning materials. Implants and their prosthetic components must be designed so that adequate oral hygiene procedures may be performed. Home care products should be non-abrasive and non-metallic. Dental probes, scalers, and curettes made of plastic should be used in cleaning dental implants.

Table 22.**3** Comparison of natural tooth and implant

	Natural tooth	**Implant**
Structure	PDL, cementum	No
Tissue interface	Junctional epithelium	Biologic seal
Fiber orientation	Perpendicular	Most parallel
Inflammation	Plaque induced	Plaque induced

Table 22.**4** Integration call

Fibro-osseous integration	Least successful
Bio-osseous integration	Gold result
Osseointegration	Best result

Summary

The interfaces of oral tissues with an endosseous implant have been discussed and compared with the natural tooth (Table 22.**3**). Direct bone contact in the form of *osseointegration* or *biointegration* is the best choices of attachment (Table 22.**4**). The epithelial soft-tissue interface to endosseous oral implants is similar to the interface with natural teeth and is formed by a junctional epithelium and sulcus. The supracrestal collagen fibers run parallel to an implant's surface, whereas on natural teeth they are functionally oriented (perpendicular) and insert into cementum. The portion of the oral implant in contact with oral environment, epithelium, and connective tissue should have a geometrically simple, polished, conical, tooth-shaped design to minimize plaque accumulation and facilitate oral-hygiene procedures. The microbiota around dental implants and natural teeth are similar. Progression of inflammation directly from the connective tissue to the alveolar crest and into the marrow spaces is a unique pathway of inflammation seen around infected dental implants. This pattern of bone loss may be explained by the connective-tissue interface to the dental implant. The interface appears to be protective as long as an adequate level of oral hygiene is maintained.

Self-Evaluation Review

1. Define an oral implant.
2. What are the three possible types of hard-tissue interfaces that can be formed between endosseous oral implants and alveolar bone?
3. What are the most preferred hard-tissue interfaces for endosseous oral implants?
4. What does the term "osseointegration" mean?
5. What materials can produce a bioactive chemical and mechanical interface with bone?
6. Why is a soft-tissue interface around an endosseous oral implant not desirable by most implantologists?
7. What is "saucerization"?
8. What is the most important condition for healthy tissue around endosseous oral implants?
9. What is the difference between the interface of connective tissue to a tooth and an implant?
10. Adherence to what five factors will ensure the greatest probability of achieving osseointegration of implants?
11. What are the major differences between probing a tooth and a dental implant?

Acknowledgements

We thank: Dr MA Listgarten of Philadelphia, Pennsylvania, for use of Figure 22.**9B**; Drs BE Gysi and JR Strub of Freiburg, Germany, for use of Figure 22.**9C**; Dr PI Branemark and Dr T Albrektsson of Göteburg, Sweden, and the Quintessence Publishing Co. Inc., Chicago, Illinois, for use of Figures 22.**1**, 22.**7**, and 22.**9A**; Dr MA Listgarten and Munksgaard International Publishers Ltd for use of Figures 22.**12A** and **B**; Dr T Berglundh and Munksgaard International Publishers Ltd for use of Figures 22.**11A** and B, 22.**13A–C**, and 22.**14A–C**; Dr I Ericsson and Munksgaard International Publishers Ltd for use of Figures 22.**14A–C**; Dr J Lindhe and Munksgaard International Publishers Ltd for use Figures 22.**15A–C** and 22.**16B** and C; and Drs RV McKinney and RA James and Mosby Year Book Inc for use of Figure 22.**8**.

Suggested Readings

Adell R, Lekkholm U, Rockler B, Branemark PI. Marginal tissue reactions at osseointegrated titanium fixtures. Int. J. Oral Maxilliofac. Surg. 1986;15:39–52.

Berglundh T, Lindhe J, Ericsson I, Marinello CP, Liljenberg B, Thompson P. The soft tissue barrier at implants and teeth. Clin. Oral Imp. Res. 1991;2:81–90.

Berglundh T, Lindhe J, Ericsson I, Marinello CP, Ericsson I, Liljenberg B. Soft tissue reaction to de novo plaque formation on implants and teeth. An experimental study in the dog. Clin. Oral Impl. Res. 1992;3:1–8.

Buser D, Warrer K, Karring T. Formation of a periodontal ligament around titanium implants. J. Periodontol. 1990;61:597–601.

Ellingsen JE. Surface configurations of dental implants. Periodontology 2000. 1998;17:36–46.

Ericsson I, Berglundh T, Marinello C, Liljenberg B, Lindhe J. Long standing plaque and gingivitis at implants and teeth in the dog. Clin. Oral Impl. Res. 1992;3:99–103.

Hickey JS, O'Neal RB, Scheidt MJ, Strong SL, Turgeon D, Van Dyke TE. Microbiologic characterization of ligature-induced peri-implantitis in the microswine model. J. Periodontol. 1991;62:548–553.

Lindhe J, Berglundh T. The interface between the mucosa and the implant. Periodontology 2000. 1998;17:47–54.

Lindhe J, Berglundh T, Ericsson I, Liljenberg B, Marinello C. Experimental breakdown of peri-implant and periodontal tissues: A study in the beagle dog. Clin. Oral Impl. Res. 1992:3:9–16.

Listgarten MA, Lang NP, Schroeder HE, Schroeder A. Periodontal tissues and their counterparts around endosseous implants. Clin. Oral Impl. Res. 1991;2:1–19.

Listgarten MA, Buser D, Steinemann SG, Donath K, Lang NP, Weber HP. Light and transmission electron microscopy of the intact interfaces between non-submerged titanium-coated epoxy resin implants and bone or gingiva. J. Dent. Res. 1992;71:364–371.

McCollum J, O'Neal RB, Brennan WA, Van Dyke TE, Horner JA. The effect of titanium implant surface roughness on plaque accumulation. J. Periodontol. 1992; 63:802–805.

McKinney RV, Steflik DE, Koth DL. The epithelium-dental implant interface. J. Oral Implant. 1988;13:622–641.

Ten Cate AR. The Gingival Junction. In: Branemark PI, Zarb GA, Albrektsson T, eds. Tissue Integrated Prostheses. Chicago, IL: Quintessence; 1985:145–153.

Thomsen P, Ericson LE. Light and transmission electron microscopy used to study the tissue morphology close to implants. Biomaterials. 1985;6:421–424.

Schenk RK, Buser D. Osseointegration: a reality. Periodontology 2000. 1998;17:21–35.

Steinemann SG. Titanium—the material of choice. Periodontology 2000. 1998;17:7–20.

23 Wound Healing

Francisco Rivera-Hidalgo

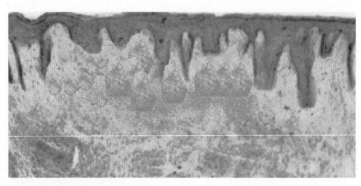

Fig. 23.**1** Gingival mucosa

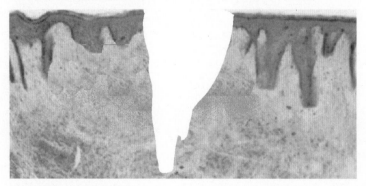

Fig. 23.**2** Incisional wound

Introduction

Healing is the process by which tissues are restored to an anatomic and physiologic arrangement after they have been injured. Figure 23.**1** illustrates the normal arrangement of the gingival mucosa and Figure 23.**2** diagrams an incision through this tissue. The normal cellular environment is composed of extracellular matrix (ECM) and extracellular fluid. This environment is also referred to as ground substance, connective-tissue matrix, or intercellular matrix. Cells communicate with their environment and become aware of their surroundings through contact with other cells, with ECM, and with extracellular fluid. Cells achieve this awareness through specific cell-surface receptors and communicate by releasing factors and chemical mediators. These factors and mediators are usually released to induce a local effect but some may have distant effects. The ECM may contain inactive factors or precursors that await a signal to become active. Injury represents a disturbance in the normal cell environment.

Whether injury results unintentionally from accidental trauma, or intentionally from the blade of the surgeon or the removal of a tooth, events are triggered that will eventually restore it to its normal state. Injury is cell and ECM damage that may result in cell death, damage to capillaries with disruption of their blood flow, and alteration of the normal structure and function of the area. When injury occurs, blood or plasma leak into the injured area, bringing cells and chemical substances that start a complex series of events. These events are: 1) clotting; 2) inflammation; 3) mobilization of cells; 4) formation of granulation tissue; 5) repair and remodeling. In this chapter, we will review these events as they relate to an incisional wound of the gingival tissues. Our incision cuts through and damages epithelium, connective-tissue cells, ECM, and capillaries of the area.

Objectives

After reading this chapter, you should be able to present the events that follow injury and the histologic changes associated with the repair process, as well as a fundamental knowledge of wound healing and some of the biochemical and immunologic events associated with it. You should also understand the special healing cases associated with healing adjacent to a tooth surface, with guided tissue regeneration, and with the extraction wound.

Events Associated with Healing

Early Events Leading to Clotting and Promoting Inflammation

The first changes resulting from injury are believed to occur at the vascular level. A transient episode of vasoconstriction (lasting a few seconds) is followed by prolonged vasodilation, which results in increased vascular permeability. Albumin and other blood constituents are spilled into the wound space, which changes hydrostatic pressure and leads to fluid accumulation (edema) and swelling. The resultant increase in extravascular pressure is sufficient to collapse adjacent capillaries and veins, and in this way to contribute to controlling the bleeding.

Extravasation of blood spills cells, platelets, and other blood substances into the wound site (Fig. 23.**3**). Prothrombin, plasma fibronectin, fibrinogen, plasminogen, kininogens, clotting factors, complement, and immunoglobulins are among the blood substances spilled.

Platelets reach the wound as a result of the hemorrhage from damage to capillaries. They become activated by the exposed collagen from injured capillaries (collagen types IV and V are found in association with small blood vessels). Activated platelets become sticky and change their shape, projecting pseudopods to aid in the aggregation of other platelets. Platelets attach themselves to the exposed collagen through a glycoprotein receptor on their surface, which in turn attaches to a protein (known as the "von Willebrand factor") released by platelets and endothelial cells in response to the injury (Fig. 23.**4**). The platelets reshape themselves to achieve broad contact with the exposed subendothelial structures, then release their granules, which contain important mediators (including adenosine diphosphate, fibronectin, platelet-derived growth factor [PDGF], platelet-activating factor [PAF], serotonin (5-hydroxytryptamine I5HT]), clotting factor V, insulin–like growth factor 1 (IGF-1), and synthesize thromboxane, a potent mediator of inflammation.

Most platelets aggregate through the action of calcium ions, adenosine diphosphate, and thromboxane. This platelet aggregation and plug formation occurs within 3 minutes after injury (Fig. 23.**5**). The platelet plug that forms aids in the temporary sealing of the damaged blood vessel. Thromboxane activates the blood-clotting cascade that leads to the formation of fibrin. Clotting factor V binds to the activated platelets, and together with clotting factor X, activates thrombin, which in turn leads to platelet activation and fibrin formation.

Clotting proceeds in the area of the platelet plug. Hemostasis, the process of clot formation, proceeds via intrinsic and extrinsic pathways that cascade to form a clot. Prothrombin is first converted to thrombin. In the presence of thrombin, fibrinogen is converted to fibrin monomer, which polymerizes, forming fibrin strands. Cross linkage is established between the fibrin strands,

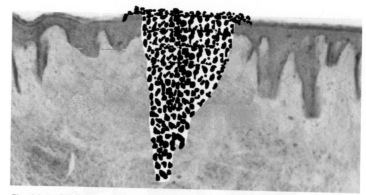

Fig. 23.3 Blood fills the wound gap.

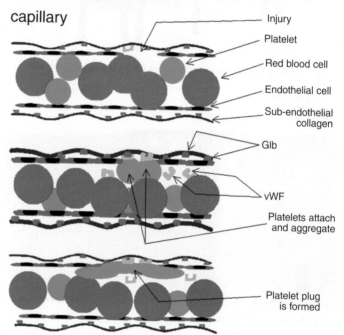

Fig. 23.**4** Platelet plug formation.

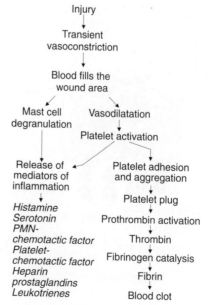

Fig. 23.**5** Early events following injury.

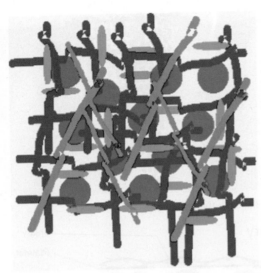

Fig. 23.**6** The clot is formed by a meshwork of fibers, red blood cells, and platelets.

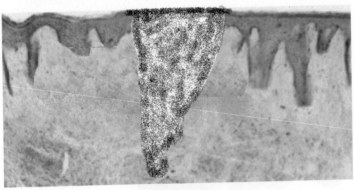

Fig. 23.**7** The blood clot fills the wound space.

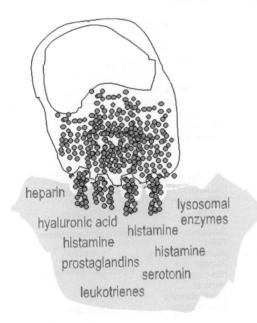

heparin
hyaluronic acid
lysosomal enzymes
histamine
histamine
histamine
prostaglandins
serotonin
leukotrienes

Fig. 23.**8** Mast-cell degranulation.

and a dense, tight clot is formed within 5 to 10 minutes after injury (Fig. 23.**6**). A matrix of fibrin, blood constituents, and cellular debris fills the wound defect and provides protection (Fig. 23.**7**). In skin, the surface of the clot dehydrates, forming a scab. In the oral cavity, the scab is soft and appears white because pigment has been washed away.

Plasma fibronectin is abundant in the wound. Found in plasma and in ECM, fibronectin comprises a group of glycoproteins that are secreted by fibroblasts, platelets, and endothelial and epithelial cells. In the wound, fibronectin accumulates to help in the removal of bacteria and to help in cell adhesion to the ECM.

As a result of injury, local mast cells and other mast cells that migrate to the wound area synthesize mediators and degranulate to release many bioactive substances, including lysosomal enzymes, hyaluronic acid, heparin, prostaglandins, chemotactic mediators for leukocytes, PAF, and histamine (Fig. 23.**8**). Histamine, a vasoactive amine, is responsible for vasodilation and increased vascular permeability during the first few minutes after wounding.

Damage to the cell membrane activates phospholipase A2, an enzyme that cleaves phospholipids normally found with cholesterol and triglycerides in the cell membrane. This enzyme will break down arachidonic acid, producing mediators known as eicosanoids (Fig. 23.**9**). Eicosanoids are compounds that have a cyclopentane ring, contain 20 carbon atoms, and consist of prostanoids and leukotrienes (Table 23.**1**). Prostanoids are converted via the cyclooxygenase pathway into thromboxane A2 (vasoconstrictor), prostacyclin (vasodilator), prostaglandin E2 (vasodilator), and prostaglandin F2α (vasoconstrictor and chemotactic). The leukotrienes are converted via the lipoxygenase pathway into leukotriene B4 (chemotactic) and leukotriene C4, known as slow-reacting substance, which induces smooth muscle contraction.

The Hageman factor or clotting factor XII is one of several blood-clotting factors spilled as a result of injury. This factor is activated by exposed collagen of damaged tissue and blood vessels. Its activation results in the

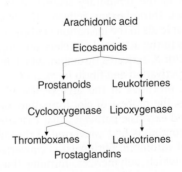

Arachidonic acid
↓
Eicosanoids
↓
Prostanoids   Leukotrienes
↓   ↓
Cyclooxygenase Lipoxygenase
↓
Thromboxanes   Leukotrienes
Prostaglandins

Fig. 23.**9** Inflammatory mediators from arachidonic acid.

establishment and amplification of an inflammatory response. Once activated, the Hageman factor activates directly or indirectly four important systems: 1) the clotting system; 2) the anticlotting (plasmin) system; 3) the kinin system; and 4) the complement system (Fig. 23.**10**).

Plasminogen, bound to tissues and present in blood, is activated by the Hageman factor and converted into plasmin, which activates the anticlotting system. Mast-cell-derived tryptase can activate plasminogen activator, which in turn can convert plasminogen to plasmin. Plasmin can degrade extracellular membrane components including fibrin, fibronectin, laminin, and proteoglycans; in effect inactivating the thrombin mediated clotting activity. Plasmin prevents the clotting process from spreading throughout the blood vessels (intravascular coagulation) and helps in the eventual dissolution of the fibrin clot.

Kininogens are the product of the interaction between kallikrein and Hageman factor. Kininogens are subsequently transformed into kinins, which exhibit potent biologic effects similar to those of histamine (Table 23.**1**). The kinins cause contraction of visceral smooth muscle and dilation of vascular smooth muscle. They increase capillary permeability, attract white blood cells, and are responsible for inducing pain. Once released, the kinins and the prostaglandins remain active longer than histamine (which is just a few minutes), and in that way lengthen the vasoactive changes. The kinins are considered responsible for prolonging the inflammatory state.

Complement is a group of 20 or more proteins that, when activated, generate mediators of the acute inflammatory response and damage or kill foreign cells (Table 23.**1**). These products of the activation induce the release of histamine from mast cells and platelets and attract granulocytic leukocytes. They also help in the elimination of foreign substance (antigen [Ag]) such as bacteria, viruses, and their products, and help in the mediation of the inflammatory process. Complement is classically activated by antibody-antigen complexes (Fig. 23.**11**). Activation of the complement cascade via an alternative pathway that bypasses the need for antibody is possible. This alternative pathway, dependent on the presence of thrombin, plasmin, and other factors present in tissue, may play an important role in defending the body against invaders during the initial phase of the inflammatory response, when antibody to a particular antigen may not be available.

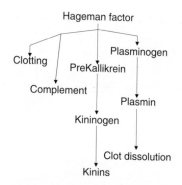

Fig. 23.**10** The Hageman factor activates four systems.

Table 23.1 Mediators of inflammation

Histamine/serotonin	Vasodilation
	Increased vascular permeability
	Smooth muscle contraction
Kinins	Vasodilation
	Increased vascular permeability
	Smooth muscle contraction
	Pain
Prostaglandins	Vasodilation
	Increased vascular permeability
	Pain
Leukotrienes	Vasodilation
	Increased vascular permeability
	Smooth muscle contraction
	PMN chemotaxis
Complement products	Vasodilation
	Increased vascular permeability
	Smooth muscle contraction
	PMN chemotaxis
	MΦ chemotaxis
	Mast-cell degranulation

PMN, polymorphonuclear neutrophils; MΦ, macrophage

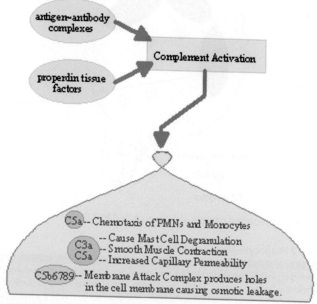

Fig. 23.**11** Complement activation and products.

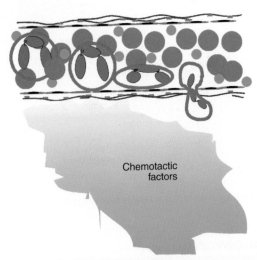

Fig. 23.**12** Polymorphonuclear neutrophils start to adhere to the endothelial cells in postcapillary venules (pavementing) and migrate through gaps between endothelial cells (diapedesis) following a chemotactic gradient.

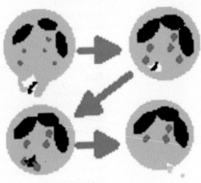

Fig. 23.**13** Steps involved in phagocytosis: engulfing, phagosome, phagolysosome digestion and excretion.

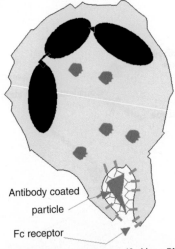

Fig. 23.**14** An opsonized particle or Ag is engulfed by a PMN.

Table 23.**2** Phagocyte-killing mechanisms

Oxygen-dependent killing within the phagosome oxygen is converted into superoxide, which becomes singlet oxygen, hydrogen peroxide, and hydroxyl radicals. These reactive oxygen intermediates can kill bacteria. Lysosomal granules contain enzymes such as myeloperoxidase, lysozyme, and lactoferrin that can kill bacteria.

Cellular Events and Establishment of Acute Inflammation

The granulocytes (polymorphonuclear neutrophils [PMNs], basophils, and eosinophils) are important to the defense of wound areas. Blood flow in the capillaries and arterioles of the wound area is slowed in responding to the action of chemical mediators. Changes in the cell's surface are responsible for the PMN accumulation (adhesion) next to the area of injury followed by a flattening or pavementing against the endothelial cells within a postcapillary venule (Fig. 23.**12**). Cell-adhesion molecules control this process. Lymphocyte functional antigen (LFA-1) is an adhesion molecule found on the surface of the PMN that attaches to another adhesion molecule, intracellular adhesion molecule (ICAM-1), on the endothelial cell. As PMNs begin to pass between endothelial cells, they release some of their granules containing enzymes that may aid in this passage. The process of migration of PMNs between endothelial cells and through the basement membrane is called diapedesis. Chemical substances such as complement product C5a guide their subsequent directional movement toward the injury site. This movement toward higher concentration of the mediator is known as chemotaxis.

During the first day the number of PMNs in the wound increases rapidly and their accumulation at the wound site is considered to be a histologic sign of acute inflammation. Clinical signs of inflammation, known as the classic signs of inflammation, are: pain (dolor), heat (calor), redness (rubor), swelling (tumor), and loss of function (functio laesa). These are signs of changes that allow increased blood flow to the area (heat and redness), release of mediators such as kinins (pain), and accumulation of fluid resulting in edema (swelling and loss of function).

Polymorphonuclear neutrophils function by engulfing (phagocytosis) and digesting foreign material and wound debris (Fig. 23.**13**). PMNs carry on their cell surface complement receptor one (CR1), a receptor for antibody fragment c (Fc), and nonspecific receptors for bacterial carbohydrate. Opsonization is when bacteria and debris are coated with antibody or complement products, facilitating their uptake by phagocytes (Fig. 23.**14**). The PMN binds to particles through these receptors, extends pseudopodia around the particles, and internalizes them into a phagocytic vacuole. The lysosomes merge with it (forming a phagolysosomal vacuole), and the PMN killing mechanisms are activated (Table 23.**2**). Eventually, the vacuole is opened to the cell exterior and the breakdown products of particles that were engulfed, as well as active or unused enzymes, are released. The enzymes released can digest debris or healthy tissue that is exposed to them. These unused enzymes can aid in the wound-cleansing process or may damage healthy tissue.

Polymorphonuclear neutrophils constitute the first line of defense and are the first phagocytic cell to arrive at the wound site. Their numbers reach a maximum during the first day and start to decrease during the third day after wounding, partially because their life span is limited to 2 days. PMNs release their enzymes toward the end of their life cycle or sometimes right after phagocytosis uses up all of their energy reserve (glycogen). The wound fluid that contains dead PMNs, wound debris, and other factors is known as pus.

Basophils and eosinophils are the other two granulocytes besides the PMNs. Basophils are found in blood vessels and are similar to mast cells in tissue. They can migrate into the tissue and function like a mast cell. Basophils are long-lived and can multiply in tissues.

Eosinophils are phagocytic cells with a bilobed nucleus and eosinophilic granules. They respond to chemotactic factors, especially those released by the mast cells. They have receptors for antibodies of the E class (IgE) and play a role in protection against parasitic infection. They release their granules by exocytosis to kill parasites too large to engulf. They may play a role in modulating the reactions mediated by mast cells. Later in the healing process, eosinophils produce an important growth factor known as transforming growth factor α (TGF-α) (Fig. 23.**15**).

Growth factors are proteins or peptides that induce cells to initiate DNA synthesis and to divide. Some growth factors can also be chemotactic. PAF, TGF-α, TGF-β, tumor necrosis factor (TNF-α or TNF-β), and PDGF are some of the factors involved in wound healing. Some of these factors are also considered cytokines.

Cytokines are a group of nonantibody molecules produced by white blood cells and tissue cells and that influence or signal other cells. They are involved in regulating the activity of cells. Lymphokines are cytokines produced by lymphocytes, whereas monokines are cytokines produced by monocytes. Cytokines include four main groups: colony-stimulating factors (CSF), interferons (IFN), interleukins (IL), and TNF. Another cytokine produced by keratinocytes is nitric oxide (NO). A short-lived mediator of inflammation, it is a gas that functions as a biologic messenger and induces vasodilation.

Monocytes in circulation are mobilized at the same time as PMNs. They are attracted into the area by chemotaxis induced by C5a and preferentially by TGF-β (probably from platelets), to which they are especially sensitive. As monocytes migrate into the wound site, they are activated by high concentrations of TGF-β or bacterial products and are transformed into tissue macrophages (MΦ). The phagocytic function of the macrophage is similar to the function of the PMN, but MΦs have a longer lifespan than PMNs and have the ability to synthesize enzymes at the wound site. The phagocytic role of the PMN as a barrier to bacterial infection is different from the role of the MΦ, which is one of cleaning up the wound site in preparation for repair.

Macrophages release prostaglandins and leukotrienes to influence the inflammatory response, collagenase, which is required to degrade the collagen in the connective tissue, interleukin-1 (IL-1), interleukin-6 (IL-6), TNF,

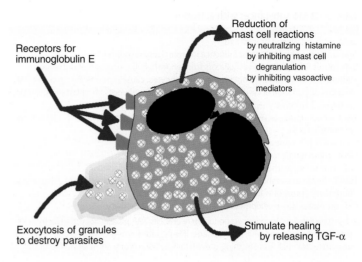

Fig. 23.15 Eosinophils contribute to the enhancement of inflammation and later to the healing process.

Table 23.**3** MΦ substances with activities

Collagenase: collagen breakdown.

Arachidonic acid metabolites: influence inflammatory response.

IL-1: causes fever; releases vasodilators from endothelium; increases endothelial adhesiveness to PMNs, monocytes, and lymphcytes; causes endothelial release of PAF; induces degradation of cartilage and bone resorption; enhances fibroblast proliferation, activates T lymphocytes; and co-regulates B-cell antibody production.

TNF (or cachectin): same activities as IL-1 plus induction of production of IL-1 by MΦ and endothelial cells.

IL-6 (or IFN-β₂): same activities as IL-1.

PDGF: chemotactic for fibroblasts and PMNs.

TGF-α: promote epithelial growth, keratinization, and angiogenesis.

TGF-β: chemoattractant for monocytes, stimulates fibroblast production of collagen and fibronectin, promotes formation of granulation tissue.

CSF: promotes the development of leukocytes and PMN activity.

IL-1: interleukin-1; PMN, polymorphonuclear neurophils; PAF, platelet-activating factor; TNF, tumor necrosis factor; MΦ, macrophage; IFN-β₂, interferon-β₂; PDGF, platelet-derived growth factor; TGF, transforming growth factor; CSF, colony-stimulating factor.

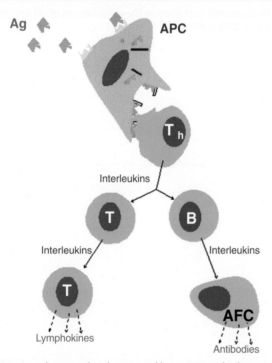

Fig. 23.**16** Ag is endocytosed and processed by an APC and subsequently presented to a T helper cell. In turn, the T helper cell presents the Ag to a B lymphocyte and releases interleukins that influence other T and B lymphocytes ultimately to produce antibodies and lymphokines.

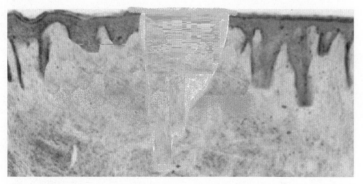

Fig. 23.**17** On the outside, the wound is covered and protected by the blood clot, whereas on the inside the inflammatory mechanisms are actively establishing an acute inflammation.

PDGF, CSF, TGF, adhesion molecules, and other mediators of inflammation. Growth and chemotactic factors leading up to the proliferation and migration into the wound of fibroblasts and endothelium are released by the MΦ (Table 23.**3**).

In the wound, MΦ numbers reach a maximum during the second day and decrease after the fourth day. The presence of MΦs at the wound site is histologically associated with late, acute inflammation or with chronic inflammation.

Macrophages aid the specific immune response by preparing antigens for lymphocyte recognition and by producing soluble mediators required for T-lymphocyte activation. A somewhat similar role has been attributed to the Langerhans' epithelial cells. Both of these cells function as immunologic accessory cells. Cells that support the activities of other cells are called accessory cells; those that carry out the activities are called effector cells. An immunologic accessory cell is a lymphoid cell capable of presenting antigens to B and T lymphocytes. Accessory cells are also called antigen-presenting cells (APCs). MΦs can function as APCs (Fig. 23.**16**).

Lymphocytes are not normally associated with acute inflammation, but they are found at the wound site. Their role is mediation of the specific immune response. Accessory cells help T lymphocytes (helper) in the recognition of antigen. These activated cells in turn induce effector T lymphocytes to produce lymphokines that mediate delayed hypersensitivity (cell-mediated) reactions. After antigen recognition and help from helper T lymphocytes, B lymphocytes are transformed into plasma cells. These cells produce and release specific antibodies (Fig. 23.**16**). These antibodies react with available antigens to form the complexes that activate complement through the classic pathway. These antibodies will opsonize antigens and prepare them for phagocytosis.

As the inflammatory response continues, the acidity of the wound site increases, in some cases reaching a pH of 6.8. Complement activation produces more chemotactic factors for attracting PMNs and monocytes. These cells phagocytize wound debris and release their enzymes, enhancing the inflammatory state (Fig. 23.**17**). Fluid continues to accumulate as a result of the combined effects of increased blood-vessel permeability, the action of enzymes, and increased protein concentration in the extravascular space. As the inflammatory events peak, the degree of hypoxia (low oxygen content) in the wound microenvironment increases (Fig. 23.**18**).

The lymphatic circulation contributes an important role in the inflammatory process. The lymphatic endothelial cells and vessels next to the wound contract rhythmically, moving fluids, cells, large molecules, and debris along the lymphatic vessels and away from the wound toward regional lymph nodes. This activity aids in resolution of the inflammatory state. Antigens, debris, and particulate are brought to the regional lymph nodes, where cells remove them by phagocytosis and where they are processed by APCs. In the nodes, APCs and lymphocytes interact and mount an immunologic response. The inflammatory response is an essential step that prepares the wound site for the repair that follows.

Events Leading to Repair of the Wound

Once acute inflammation peaks, numerous other activities begin to shift the wound environment from one where inflammation is being constantly amplified and enhanced to one where reparative processes are amplified and enhanced. At a cellular level, there is a decrease in inflammatory mediators coupled with an increase in growth mediators. The wound microenvironment itself may trigger some of these changes. Once the initial clot and fibrin network is established, mast-cell-derived mediators are released to attract endothelial cells and fibroblasts to the area. In addition, factors that stimulate mitosis (mitogenic factors) of endothelial cells and fibroblasts are also released.

Epithelial–Related Events

In their normal state the epithelial cells at the basal layer are occupied with the production of keratin as their principal activity, and thus are called keratinocytes. Keratin is a family of 20 proteins that constitute the intermediate filaments, also known as tonofilaments of the epithelial cell. Some of these filaments are connected to the hemidesmosomes and the desmosomes that attach the epithelial cells to each other. Epithelial cells express different keratins at different layers, mainly expressing keratin 5 and 14 at the basal layer and 1 and 10 at the upper layers.

Upon wounding, the basal cells at the wound margin undergo significant changes. During the initial 12 hours after injury, epithelial cells at the margin of the wound

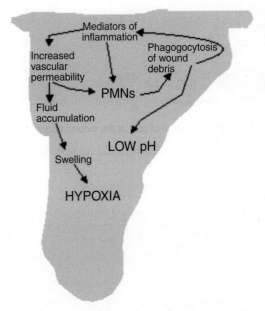

Fig. 23.**18** Inflammation induces changes that lead to a low pH and hypoxia of the wound.

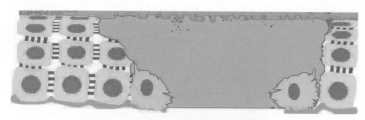

Fig. 23.**19** Dedifferentiation of cells at the wound edges leads to motile and phagocytic activity.

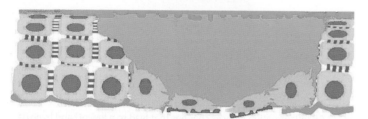

Fig. 23.**20** Cells migrate over the clot's dense fibrillar matrix, digesting debris and at the same time forming the new basement membrane.

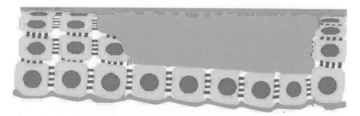

Fig. 23.**21** When contact between cells is established (contact inhibition) cells differentiate, become more mature, increase the production of keratins, and eventually form the original epithelial architecture.

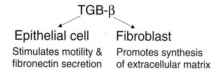

TGB-β

Epithelial cell   Fibroblast

Stimulates motility &   Promotes synthesis
fibronectin secretion   of extracellular matrix

Fig. 23.**22** Cell activities induced by TGF-β.

undergo a dedifferentiation process (i.e., they become more primitive) (Fig. 23.**19**). This results in a number of cellular modifications: cells acquire the potential for ameboid movement; they undergo organelle reduction; their membranes exhibit ruffled borders; they have fewer cell junctions (desmosomes); they have a higher metabolic rate; their surface expresses receptors that interact with the wound environment; and they become phagocytic. The modified epithelial cells increase the number of gap junctions (for better cell-to-cell communication), flatten out toward the wound, and use the clot as a scaffold. Modified epithelial cells move into the wound by ameboid movement, phagocytizing fibrin and debris as they dissect their way (with the help of collagenase and plasminogen activator) as a one or two cell thick layer between the clot and the base of the wound (Fig. 23.**20** and Fig. 23.**21**).

As they move, the cells rest on a dense fibrillar matrix principally composed of fibrin and fibronectin. Fibronectin promotes keratinocyte motility and phagocytosis. TGF-β promotes motility and secretion of fibronectin by the epithelial cell (Fig. 23.**22**). The movement of epithelial cells along fibrin has been termed "contact guidance." Hyaluronic acid, a component of the ECM, interacts with fibrin and aids in the establishment of a scaffold for epithelial-cell migration. A cell receptor that attaches the cell to fibronectin (known as the fibronectin receptor) mediates this attachment. This receptor is probably an integrin transmembrane link protein, one of a family of cell-surface molecules also known as adhesion molecules.

Cells attach to the ECM through the adhesion complex (or hemidesmosome), which is a multiprotein complex. The adhesion complexes are cell surface receptors made of three classes of proteins: the extracellular protein that attaches to the ECM portion of the basement membrane; the transmembrane protein that connects the extracellular protein with the cell interior; and the cytoplasmic plaque protein where the cell's cytoskeletal fibers (tonofilaments) are anchored. Besides anchoring, adhesion complexes have other functions. Integrins (one of several families of adhesion complexes) are composed of α and β chains; these serve to transduce signals that can affect cell function and cell phenotype. In this way, signals from the extracellular environment can alter the organization of the cytoskeleton, cell proliferation, cell differentiation and apoptosis (programmed cell death).

Basement-membrane epithelial cells do not routinely express (produce) matrix metalloproteinases (MMPs) on their surface. MMPs are a family of enzymes responsible for the degradation of collagen and other ECM components. However, as epithelial cells prepare to migrate, stromelysin–1 (MMP-3) is expressed, and while they are migrating they express collagenase-1 (MMP-1) and stromelysin-2 (MMP-10). It is believed that the activity of these MMPs is required for cell migration and the formation of new epithelium over the wound.

As they move, the epithelial cells have to reform the missing basement membrane. Epithelial cells produce fibronectin, collagens type IV and V, and laminin to form an immature basement membrane. The basement membrane (a structure seen with light microscopy) attaches the basal epithelial cells to the underlying ECM. Ultrastructurally, the basement membrane consists of: an electron-lucent layer (lamina lucida), made of laminin (glycoprotein) and heparan sulfate (polysaccharide); an electron-dense layer (basal lamina) or lamina densa, containing type IV collagen; and an electron-lucent layer, (the fibroreticular lamina), containing anchoring fibrils (type VII collagen) extending from the basal lamina into the ECM (Fig. 23.**23**). The fibroreticular lamina merges with the ECM. In cases where the basement membrane remains intact after wounding, the epithelial-cell movement is facilitated, resulting in faster repair of the wound.

It is mostly accepted that the epithelial cell at the wound margin moves toward the wound while the cell next to it divides to fill the space. This sequence is repeated until the wound is covered. However, there is some evidence to suggest that once the marginal epithelia cell has moved it stays put and the cell immediately behind "leapfrogs" to become the leading cell.

Epithelial-cell movement as a layer stops when cellular contact is re-established (contact inhibition) (Fig. 23.**21**). When contact is re-established, these cells differentiate (i.e., they become more specialized) and begin to multiply, eventually returning to their usual stratified arrangement (Fig. 23.**24**). Internal rearrangement of the cell occurs again to produce keratins as the main activity. Recent studies suggest that epithelial growth and differentiation is enhanced by the release of TGF-∝ by the eosinophils in the wound area. The chemical structure of TGF-∝ is partially similar to epithelial growth factor (EGF), a factor produced by the salivary glands that promotes epithelial growth and differentiation.

Connective-Tissue and Vascular Events

At the center of the repair-process events are the MΦs, which have the capacity to accomplish many functions. Actions mediated by MΦs include: debridement of the repair site; release of mediators of inflammation and enzymes; release of mediators of bone resorption; release of angiogenic factors, and release of factors that promote proliferation of endothelial cells and fibroblasts. Among the many products of macrophages, MMPs play an important role in degrading all components of the ECM. MMPs are a family of 15 enzymes that appear in the fluid recovered from wounds and play a proinflammatory role early in wound healing. Furthermore, MΦs monitor the wound environment and react to changes in it. This role could be compared to that of a project director who supervises and controls several activities, making adjustments as the microenvironment dictates. MΦ-released factors induce the transition from inflammation to repair.

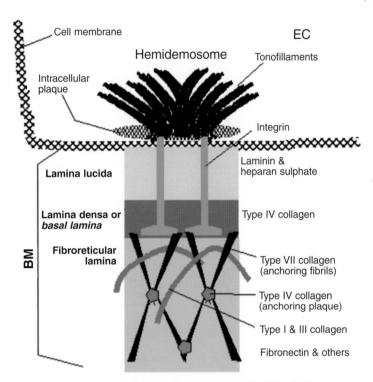

Fig. 23.**23** Basement membrane is formed as the epithelial cell migrates across the wound.

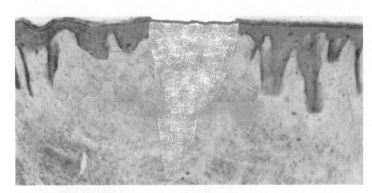

Fig. 23.**24** The epithelium covers the wound.

The role of the MΦ as director of events is mediated by factors within the wound microenvironment. The MΦ, a producer of large amounts of lactate, reacts to the lactate in the same way it reacts to the hypoxia of the area: by inducing the formation of new blood vessels through the release of angiogenic factor and chemoattractants for endothelium. Fibroblasts also react to the hypoxic environment, to TGF-β, and to PDGF by migrating into the area and producing ECM (Fig. 23.**25**).

The MΦ releases TGF-β, collagenase, IL-1, insulin–like growth factor-1, and large amounts of lactate into the wound. A high concentration of lactate in the wound causes the MΦ to release angiogenic factor and chemoattractants for endothelium, which is also induced by hypoxia. The hypoxic stimulus decreases as new capillaries form and the level of oxygenation of the wound increases.

In response to PDGF and TGF-β, the fibroblasts deep within the wound begin to multiply rapidly and then migrate into the wound, reaching maximum numbers during the sixth day. The role of the fibroblast is to produce the substances that will constitute the new connective tissue, participate in wound contraction, and continue the remodeling of the wound. The fibroblasts are the factory where the constituents of the matrix are produced.

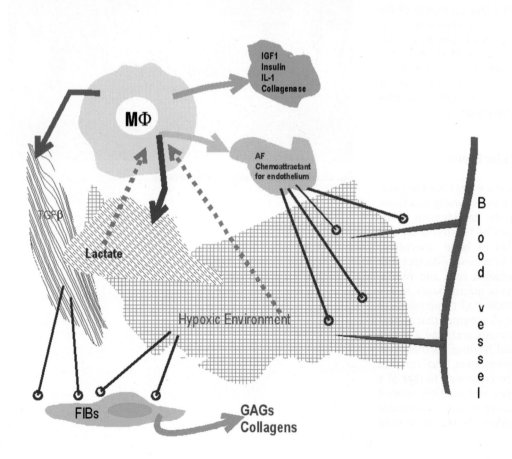

Formation of Granulation Tissue

In response to stimuli from mediators, capillaries in adjacent connective tissue develop bud–like structures that ramify and form loops; these loops penetrate the wound site in a process known as angiogenesis. Heparin released from basophils and mast cells stimulates the migration of capillary endothelium into the clot. Heparin also binds some of the growth factors needed for the formation of new vessels. As capillary branches meet they form a tissue rich in blood vessels, fibroblasts, and fibroblast products. This replacement tissue that gradually displaces the clot is known as granulation tissue (Figs. 23.**26** and 23.**27**). The name is derived from the "granulated" appearance of the tissue resulting from the new capillary loops. This tissue is rich in collagens and fibronectins. Fibronectins play a role in the organization of the granulation tissue and in the synthesis of the new connective-tissue (extracellular) matrix.

The fibroblasts in the granulation tissue produce the major constituents of the ECM: fibrillar proteins and GAGs (Table 23.**4**). The ECM is a hydrophilic gel composed of fibrillar and nonfibrillar proteins in close association with glycosaminoglycans or GAGs (large polysaccharides with high molecular weights). The GAGs have the property of retaining water and positive ions. GAGs can become covalently attached to proteins forming proteoglycans (protein polysaccharides) that can hold large amounts of water. The proteoglycans are a subclass of glycoproteins. Matrix proteoglycans are: chondroitin sulfate (dermatan sulfate), heparan sulfate (and heparin), hyaluronic acid, and keratan sulfate. Besides binding water, the GAGs function to facilitate diffusion of molecules and in the attachment of cells.

Collagen (mostly a fibrillar protein with the exception of type IV) forms the fibers that provide the tissue with its tensile strength (Table 23.**5**). Collagen constitutes 60% of total tissue protein in gingiva. Approximately 13 types of collagen have been identified, based on the content of collagen monomer. The collagen monomer is formed from three genetically distinct polypeptide chains. Each monomer differs in the amino-acid sequence of the chains. The collagen monomers aggregate to form the collagen fibers. Ultrastructurally, type III collagen fibers are fine, short, thin, and striated (sometimes called reticulin fibers) whereas type I collagen fibers are formed in dense, large, striated bundles.

Normal gingival tissue contains type I and type III collagens at a ratio of 5:1, which account for 99% of the collagen; type IV, which is associated with the basal lamina and produced by the epithelial cell, accounts for 1%. In granulation tissue, type III collagen predominates initially and, as it matures, decreases gradually to approximately 20% of the total collagen. The ratio of type V to type I collagen is increased at extraction sites in the early healing stages and gradually diminishes to usual levels, as does the ratio of type III to type I. The increase is probably related to angiogenesis, in which type V collagen may facilitate the migration of endothelial cells. The tensile strength of the wound augments as the content of

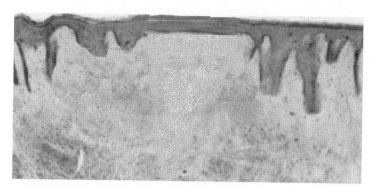

Fig. 23.**26** Granulation tissue fills the wound.

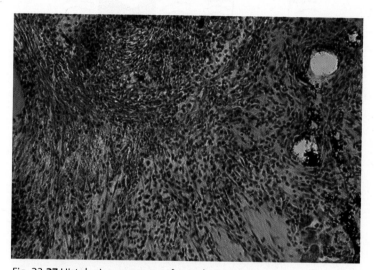

Fig. 23.**27** Histologic appearance of granulation tissue.

Table 23.**4** Connective-tissue matrix components

Fibrillar proteins
Collagen
Elastin
Fibronectin
Proteoglycans
Chondroitin sulfate
Dermatan sulfate
Heparan sulfate
Heparin
Hyaluronic acid
Keratan sulfate

Table. 23.**5** Collagens

Type	Form	Location	Cell
I	Fiber	Gingiva, skin	Fibroblast
I	Fiber	Bone	Osteoblast
II	Fibril	Cartilage	Chondroblast
III	Fibril	Gingiva, skin	Fibroblast
IV	Meshlike	Basal lamina	Keratinocyte
V	Fibrils	Placenta, skin	Fibroblast
VI	Microfibrils	Ubiquitous	Fibroblast
VII	Short fibrils	Basement membrane	Fibroblast

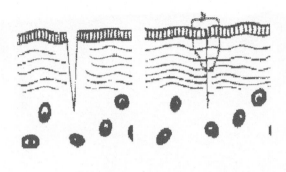

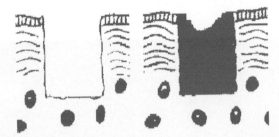

Fig. 23.**28** Primary and secondary intention healing is a function of the width of the wound.

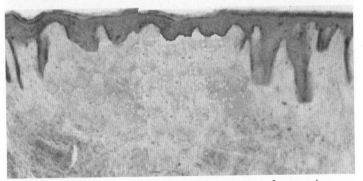

Fig. 23.**29** The wound is healed but remodeling continues for several months. It may take 6 months or more for the tissue to achieve its usual tensile strength.

type I collagen increases. Through the healing process, collagen is formed, broken down, and reformed.

The assembly of collagen type I and type III occurs extracellularly within the tissue matrix. This matrix has a high content of water (70% in the periodontal ligament).

Maturation of the Wound—Repair and Remodeling

As healing progresses, vascularization diminishes as granulation tissue is replaced by young, new connective tissue. This tissue is different from normal connective tissue in that it is more cellular and has many immature collagen fibers. Many of the blood vessels disappear as a result of apoptosis. Early in the maturation process, wound contraction begins. Wound contraction results from the contraction of connective tissue, which starts around the fourth day and continues for several weeks. It involves the movement of the wound edge, both the epithelium and the connective tissue, as a whole.

Interspersed throughout the wound are myofibroblasts, highly differentiated fibroblasts that have contractile microfilaments and properties associated with smooth muscle cells. Their intracellular proteins (vinculin and actin) join extracellular material composed of fibronectin and collagen types I and III to interconnect to other myofibroblasts. These connected myofibroblasts apply the forces necessary to achieve contraction. It appears that the force is generated uniformly throughout the wound. These cells increase early in the repair process and diminish gradually, eventually disappearing from the site. In wounds where the edges are far apart and large volumes of tissue are to be replaced, there is more contraction. When the wound edges are closely approximated, there is less contraction.

The width of the clot formed between the edges of a wound determines whether the wound will heal by primary intention (narrow clot) or by secondary intention (wide defect) (Fig. 23.**28**). The net result of contraction is a scar area that is significantly smaller than the wound. A scar is a mark left in the tissue after a wound heals. Histologically, a scar represents an area that has a slightly higher than normal ratio of collagen fibers to cells. In an incision made to reflect a mucosal flap (mucosa that has been partially detached), the wound edges are closely approximated (coapted), which makes the intervening clot and area to be repaired very narrow: thus, the resultant scar is small (Fig. 23.**29**) The gingival tissues will heal with practically no scar formation, whereas the alveolar mucosa will form scar tissue. Contraction is observed in the alveolar mucosa but practically not observed in the attached gingiva; the reason for this is not clearly understood.

Remodeling is a process that results in the rearrangement of the collagen fibers and proteoglycans. It starts around the third week and continues for several months. A certain level of remodeling always occurs as part of the maintenance of normal tissue. Remodeling is the result of the breaking down of collagen that was deposited in excess, increasing collagen cross-linking and decreasing the proteoglycan content. Once formed, collagen fibers continue to undergo chemical changes that decrease their solubility and increase their tensile strength for several months. Because of its capacity to simultaneously degrade and synthesize collagen, the fibroblast plays an important role in this process.

Wounds Associated with Teeth

Tissue–Tooth Interface

How a wound edge heals against a tooth represents a special case of healing that will be explored in this section. The normal tissue–tooth interface (Fig. 23.**30**) is a complex structure that includes a multitude of tissues: junctional epithelium, ECM, periodontal ligament, cementum, and bone (Fig. 23.**30**). Whenever a surgical separation occurs, most of these tissues are involved in the healing process that follows. When this interface has been modified, as with periodontal disease and treatment, the local morphology may dictate how the healing will occur.

In the case of a simple incision through the soft tissue, the previous description of how an incisional wound heals applies (Fig. 23.**30A**). In other cases, as with an intrasulcular incision, additional activity must occur to reestablish the tissue–tooth interface (Fig. 23.**30B**). This activity will result in either regeneration (healing by reestablishing lost tissues and normal architecture) or repair (healing that does not re-establish lost tissues or normal architecture). Regeneration is the most desired result of surgical interventions of this area. However, the result most frequently obtained is repair.

In many instances when the tooth surface has been exposed to the oral environments as the result of periodontal disease, repair by an abnormally long junctional epithelium is obtained. This modified interface may occur because of the different rates at which tissues can fill the wound (Fig. 23.**31**).

Guided Tissue Regeneration

The rate at which the epithelial cells can move exceeds the rate at which other tissues in the wound can move to fill the wound. The migration rate for epithelium is between 0.1 and 1 mm per day. Epithelium will migrate down a root surface toward the tooth apex until it encounters the ECM. It is at this point that the apical termination of the epithelial attachment to the tooth will be established. An extracellular matrix zone follows immediately apical. This zone of 1 to 2 mm of extracellular-matrix attachment to the root is always present, and is sometimes referred to as the biologic width. Apical to this zone bone, periodontal ligament, and cementum are reformed. When the root surface is

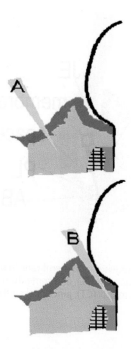

Fig. 23.**30** Normal tissue–tooth interface with simple incision in **A** and an intrasulcular incision in **B**.

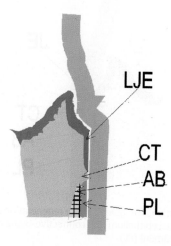

Fig. 23.**31** Healing with an abnormally long junctional epithelium (LJE) is a modified tissue–tooth interface. Connective-tissue matrix (CT); periodontal ligament (PL); bone (AB).

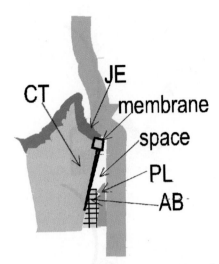

Fig. 23.**32** Guided tissue regeneration membrane in place allows cells from bone (AB), periodontal ligament (PL), and cementum to repopulate the space. Connective-tissue matrix (CT); junctional epithelium (JE).

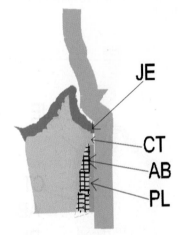

Fig. 23.**33** Regeneration after guided tissue regeneration and removal of the membrane. Junctional epithelium (JE); connective-tissue matrix (CT); bone (AB); periodontal ligament (PL).

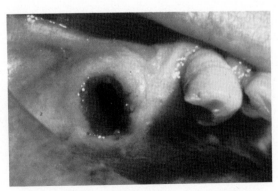

Fig. 23.**34** Tooth socket immediately after extraction.

exposed by periodontal disease-induced changes in the attachment, the most commonly observed healing is by formation of an abnormally long junctional epithelium (Fig. 23.**31**).

If the epithelial cell movement down the root could be slowed or prevented, a virtual empty space would be created to allow growth of slower-moving tissues and there would be an opportunity for regeneration (Fig. 23.**32**). This is the principle behind guided tissue regeneration. In guided tissue regeneration, an inert membrane is placed in the wound to satisfy these requirements.

In guided tissue regeneration, the membrane is a two-part, semipermeable structure of polytetrafluoroethylene (similar to Teflon). The part forming the collar of the membrane is a multilayer structure that when implanted looks like ECM to the epithelial cells. The main portion of the membrane has a cell-occlusive structure. The membrane is placed on top of the bone and the collar is tightly sutured to the tooth to prevent apical migration of the epithelial cells and to exclude the ECM. After being implanted for 4 to 6 weeks, the membrane has to be surgically removed. The tissue that forms under the membrane will eventually mature to become normal tissue (Fig. 23.**33**). Newer, resorbable, membranes do not have to be removed because they are broken down and assimilated by the body. Membranes are also used in conjunction with endosseous implants.

The Extraction Wound

After the removal of a tooth, the wound that remains represents a special case of healing. An extraction wound, with injury extending to the alveolar bone, heals by secondary intention.

At the precise instant of extraction, the tooth socket can be visualized as an area in which junctional epithelium, gingival fibers, periodontal ligament fibers, blood vessels, and nerve fibers have been torn or severed, and bone may have been fractured.

Figure 23.**34** is the clinical picture of a site immediately after an extraction. No blood clot can be seen in this photograph. In Figure 23.**35**, however, bleeding has occurred and a clot can be seen forming.

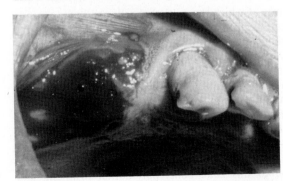

Fig. 23.**35** Bleeding shortly after extraction with a clot forming.

The lining bone of a socket after a wound would be covered by periodontal ligament fibers that anchor in the bone and by blood vessels that pierce its surface as they traverse into the supporting bone (Fig. 23.**36**). The lining bone, being somewhat more dense than spongy bone but less dense than cortical bone, is recognized radiographically as a radiopaque line paralleling the root (the lamina dura [Fig. 23.**37**]). The dynamic events secondary to tooth extraction lead to the formation of a clot that fills the socket (Fig. 23.**35**). During the first 3 days, changes occur at the base and periphery of the clot as fibroblasts migrate into the clot and up toward the converging epithelial cells.

At 4 days, a vascular network within the clot is evident (Fig. 23.**38**). Bone resorption begins to take place at the adjacent areas of the socket, at the alveolar crest, and in the interradicular area. Figure 23.**38** shows fibroblasts migrating into the clot and the periodontal-ligament area being remodeled. Thus, at the end of the first week, the clot has become organized into granulation tissue and bone formation has begun.

During the second week, collagen bundles can be seen running through the area (Fig. 23.**39**). The oral epithelium grows in an attempt to cover the surface of the wound. The wound area appears to be well vascularized, and there is continued bone formation.

By the third week, the epithelium has migrated under the remaining clot that covers the granulation tissue, and new bone is evident at the base of the socket (Fig.

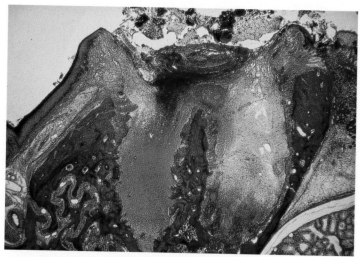

Fig. 23.**36** Histology of the extraction site after 24 hours.

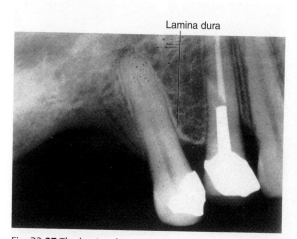

Fig. 23.**37** The lamina dura is a radiographic structure depicting the bone that lines the socket.

Clot, zone of lysis

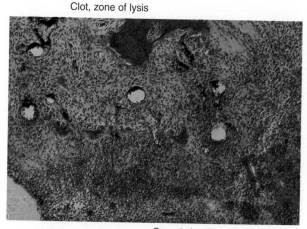

Granulation tissue in socket

Fig. 23.**38** Histology of extraction site at 4 days.

Oral epithelium

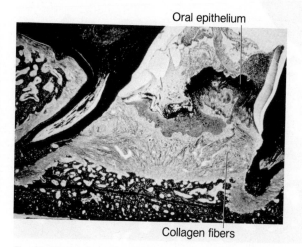

Collagen fibers

Fig. 23.**39** Histology of extraction site at 14 days.

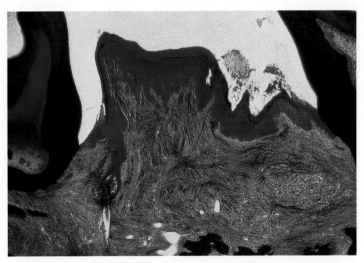

Fig. 23.**40** Histology of extraction site at 3 weeks.

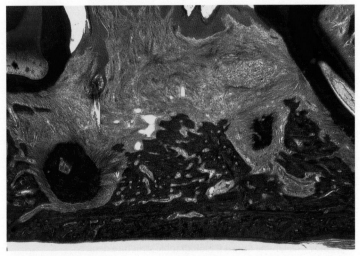

Fig. 23.**41** Histology of extraction site at 4 weeks.

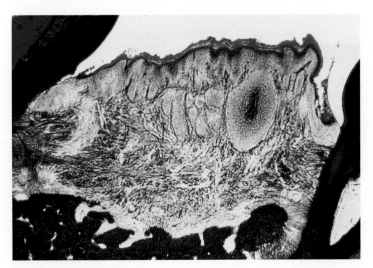

Fig. 23.**42** Histology of extraction site at 12 weeks.

23.**40**). The granulation tissue is maturing into ECM.

The fourth week is characterized by the presence of collagen bundles and new bone. This new bone fills a large portion of the socket (Fig. 23.**41**).

By the eighth week, the keratinized oral mucosa overlying the socket is well differentiated, as is the lamina propria (ECM, blood vessels, and other components adjacent to the epithelium). The base of the socket has been filled with bone to a new height below the preextraction level (Fig. 23.**41**). The height of the lingual plate is usually higher than that of the buccal plate. During this period, the bone is remodeled by alternating resorption and deposition. The process of remodeling continues throughout the life of the individual.

After 12 weeks, the extraction site cannot be distinguished from the normal adjacent tissues (Fig. 23.**42**). Approximately 85% of individuals who have undergone extractions exhibit a residual ridge whose density is greater than that of the trabecular bone forming the inner portion of the alveolar bone, but is less than that of the cortical bone of the buccal and lingual plates.

Healing of the Osseous Wound

Healing of alveolar bone (whether it is in direct contact with the tooth or not) after an extraction or surgery is carried out in an attempt to restore normal morphology (form and structure) and function. The original bone found in these areas is known as lamellar bone on account of its thin sheets and regular, parallel collagen-fiber arrangement. However, the initial new bone that forms in the wound area has a random organization of collagen fibers and is known as woven bone. Gradually, this bone matures into lamellar bone (Figure 23.**43**). In most cases, total regeneration of the lost bone after surgery is not achieved.

Bone contains a series of compounds that, when demineralized and implanted subcutaneously or in muscle, can induce bone formation (osteoinduction). It is these compounds, released at the time of surgery, that start and modulate the bone regeneration. These compounds are known as bone morphogenetic proteins or BMPs (a morphogen is a substance that instructs and controls three-dimensional architecture of developing tissue by controlling gene expression). At least 15 BMPs have been identified; all are members of the cytokine TGF-β superfamily, except for BMP-1 that is a protease.

BMPs, mainly BMP 2, 4, and 7, can induce the differentiation of stem cells into preosteoblasts and the terminal differentiation of other mesenchymal cells including preosteoblasts. Once released from bone matrix, BMPs attach to cell surface receptors on osteoblasts to signal the cell to initiate intracellular responses. BMPs can initiate the cascade for bone formation eventually ending with the mineralizing osteoblasts.

Since these compounds hold the key to new bone formation, their commercial production as human recombinant bone morphogenetic proteins could open the door for their routine use in clinical treatment. (Figs. 23.**43** and 23.**44**).

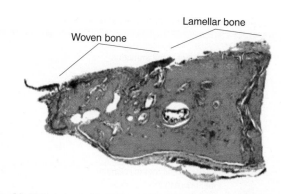

Fig. 23.**43** New bone formation in the calvaria of a rat. H&E section.

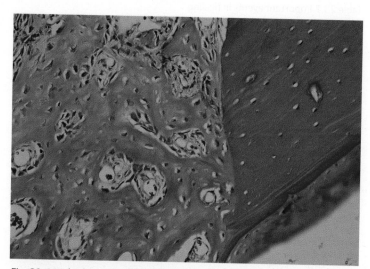

Fig. 23.**44** A higher magnification of Figure 23.43 shows empty lacunae in the lamellar bone next to the new woven bone produced by the trauma of creating the incision.

Table 23.6 Healing phases with approximate start and duration

0-2 d
  Establishment of inflammation
2 d to 1 wk
  Clean-up of the wound
1–2 wk
  Proliferation and production
    Epithelial migration starts 12 h
    Collagen synthesis starts 2–3 d
    GAGs synthesis starts 4–5 d
  Orientation and organization
    Functional changes in collagen
    Fiber orientation
    Wound contraction
1–6 mo
  Maturation and Remodeling
    Increase in tensile strength

Table 23.7 Important events in healing

Injury
↓
Formation of platelet plug
Activation of clotting system
Release of chemoattractants
Release of inflammation mediators
↓
Blood clot
↓
Mast-cell degranulation
Production of eicosanoids
Activation of plasmin, kinin, and complement systems
Infiltration by granulocytes, especially PMNs
↓
Inflammation
↓
Opsonization and phagocytosis
Production of cytokincs
Infiltration by macrophages
Production of growth factors
Angiogenesis
Infiltration by fibroblasts
Epithelial cell migration
Formation of basement membrane
Epithelial differentiation
↓
Granulation tissue
↓
Production of proteoglycans
Production of collagens organization of cell products
Establishment of young connective tissue
Maturation of new tissues
Maturation of matrix components
Increase in myofibroblast activity
↓
Wound contraction
↓
Rearrangement of collagen
Rearrangement of proteoglycans
Formation of scar
Increased wound strength
Increased collagen strength
Decreased collagen solubility
Decreased vascularity
↓
Remodeling

Summary

Although the events reviewed in this chapter are depicted as independent events, wound healing is a continuous process. Many of these events occur concurrently, and their activities may overlap each other. In a large wound, many microenvironments may exist with variations in the duration of healing events. Based on estimated duration of events from animal and human studies, the healing process could be divided into five phases, as summarized in Table 23.6.

Factors not directly associated with the wound may affect the healing process and its duration. Some of these factors are related to the location of the wound, the blood circulation of the area, the nutritional or hormonal status of the patient, and the existence of infection at the site. Wounds that are located in an area where trauma can reinjure the wound or where infection occurs will heal more slowly. In areas where the blood supply is compromised by either the wound trauma itself or secondary to another factor such as radiation therapy, the capacity of the tissues to heal properly will be affected. Healing in malnourished individuals is altered or defective. Hormonal problems such as those in uncontrolled diabetes may lead to an impaired inflammatory response, which in turn could lead to diminished formation of connective-tissue elements.

Healing will be faster in children and younger individuals than in older individuals. How aging affects healing is not completely understood. Overall, the available information suggests that in older individuals the start of the healing process is slightly delayed, whereas changes that add strength to the wound stop earlier than in a younger individual.

Smoking can also affect healing. Several clinical studies have implicated smoking as a factor leading to the postsurgical loss of bone or implants. Other clinical studies have found the development of postextraction pain to be associated to smoking immediately after tooth extraction. Smoking can induce vasoconstriction and affect oxygenation of the tissues.

A summary of the major events of the wound-healing process is presented in Table 23.7. Without the capacity to heal, we could not survive.

Self-Evaluation Review

1. Describe the events that lead to the formation of a blood clot.

2. Describe the contribution of PMNs to the establishment of acute inflammation.

3. Describe the role of the Hageman factor in inflammation.

4. Describe the role of eosinophils in inflammation and healing.

5. Why is the monocyte-macrophage cell considered to play such an important role in wound healing?

6. Describe the composition of the basement membrane.

7. What is the role of hypoxia and lactate in wound healing?

8. What is granulation tissue?

9. Describe the major components of connective tissue.

10. Define long junctional epithelium, guided tissue regeneration, and lamina dura.

Acknowledgements

Leo Korchin, DDS, MS and Sol Bernick, PhD contributed some of the histologic material.

Suggested Readings

Croteau S, Rauch F, Silvestry A, Hamdy RC. Bone morphogenetic proteins in orthopedics: from basic science to clinical practice. Orthopedics. 1999;22(7):686–695.

Gutmann JL, Harrison JW. Surgical wound healing. In: Surgical Endodontics. Boston: Blackwell Scientific Publications Inc; 1991;300–337.

Hill MW. The influence of aging on skin and oral mucosa. Gerodontology. 1984;3:35–45.

Janeway CA. How the immune system recognizes invaders. Sci. Am. 1993;269:73–79.

Jones JK, Triplett RG. The relationship of cigarette smoking to impaired intraoral wound healing: a review of evidence and implications for patient care. J. Oral Maxillofac. Surg. 1992;50:237–239.

Keene DR, Sakai LY, Lunstrum GP, Morris NP, Burgeson RE. Type VII collagen forms an extended network of anchoring fibrils. J. Cell Biol. 1987;104:611–621.

Pelissier A, Ouhayoun, JP, Sawaf MH, Forest N. Changes in cytokeratin expression during the development of the human oral mucosa. J. Periodont. Res. 1992;27:588–598.

Ross R. Wound healing. Sci. Am. 1969;220:40–50.

Rothe MJ, Nowak M, Kerdel FA. The mast cell in health and disease. J. Am. Acad. Dermatol. 1990;23:615–624.

Singer AJ, Clark RAF. Cutaneous wound healing. N. Engl. J. Med. 1999;341(10):738–746.

Todd R, Donoff BR, Chiang T, et al. The eosinophil as a cellular source of transforming growth factor alpha in healing cutaneous wounds. Am. J. Pathol. 1991;138:1307–1313.

Whalen GF, Zetter BR. Angiogenesis. In: Cohen IK, Diegelmann RF, Lindblad WJ. Wound Healing: Biochemical and Clinical Aspects. Philadelphia Pa: WB Saunders; 1992:77–95.

Glossary

Accessory canals. Canals leading from the radicular pulp laterally through the root dentin to the periodontal tissue. They are particularly numerous in the apical third of the root.

Accessory root canal. Subordinate chamber of the dental pulp lying within the root portion of the tooth.

Acellular cementum. That part of the cementum covering one-third to one-half of the root of a tooth adjacent to the cemento-enamel junction. It usually is opposed by a layer of cellular cementum. It consists of collagenous fibers and a uniform ground substance, but has no cellular components.

Acid hydrolases. The content of lysosomes, the enzymes specialized for intracellular degradation.

Acini. The secretory end pieces comprising acinar cells that produce the primary saliva in the major and minor salivary glands. The end pieces may be serous, mucous, or seromucous (mixed) type.

Acquired cuticle. Acellular organic film that is deposited on the surface of teeth after eruption. Microscopically, it is made up of several layers.

Adrenergic. Nerve fibers that secrete norepinephrine at a synapse usually associated with sympathetic nerve fibers.

Agonist. A substance that produces an effect similar to the naturally occurring substance.

Allantois. Fetal tubular diverticulum developing from the hindgut. In humans it is vestigal and contributes to the formation of the umbilical cord and placenta.

Alloplastic material. Material suitable for implantation that is not from the human body, such as metal, plastic, or mineral.

Alveolar bone. The ridge of bone on the surface of the body of the maxilla and mandible. This term is applied to the tooth-bearing part of the mandible and maxilla, as it contains the tooth sockets.

Alveolar bone proper. A thin lamina of bone that surrounds and supports the roots of the teeth and gives attachment to principal fibers of the periodontal ligament.

Alveolar crest fibers. Those principal fibers of the periodontal ligament extending between the crest of the alveolar bone and the neck of the tooth.

Alveolar fundus. Bottom or base of the alveolar bone proper, lining the tooth socket.

Ameloblast. One of the cells of the inner layer lining the cap of the enamel organ. These cells give rise to the enamel of the teeth.

Amelogenesis. The process of production and development of enamel.

Amelogenin. A hydrophobic proline-rich protein found in newly deposited enamel matrix. Its molecular weight is about 25 000 daltons. Amelogenins are lost during maturation of enamel.

Amylase. Enzyme that catalyzes the hydrolysis of starch into smaller, water-soluble carbohydrates. In mammals, there are two forms: 1) Pancreatic amylase, found in the pancreatic juice, and 2) salivary amylase (ptyalin), found in the saliva.

Anastomosis. A communication or union between two structures.

Anatomic crown. That portion of the tooth covered by enamel; the true crown.

Angiogenesis. The process by which capillaries develop bud–like structures that will form new capillary branches.

Ankyloglossia. Restricted movement of the tongue, which results in speech difficulty.

Ankylosed. Stiffened; bound by adhesions; fused; denoting a joint in a state of ankylosis; rigid fixation of a tooth to the surrounding bony alveolus as a result of periodontal membrane ossification.

Annexins. A group of calcium-binding proteins that interact with acidic phospholipids in membranes. They are also known by other names (e.g., lipocortins, endonexins).

Antibody. An immunoglobulin molecule that reacts with or binds to the substance (antigen) that induced its synthesis. These proteins are produced by plasma cells.

Antigen. A substance that is recognized as foreign by the body.

Aortic arches. A series of arterial channels encircling the embryonic pharynx in the mesenchyme of the branchial arches.

Apical cementum. Cementum deposited on the apical region of the tooth root.

Apical foramen. Opening at the apex of the root of a tooth that gives passage to the nerves and blood vessels.

Apocrine. Sweat gland; a large tubular exocrine gland that accumulates secretion in its cell apices and ruptures the surface membrane during the secretory activity.

Apoptosis. Cell death programmed as part of development or induced during cell interactions.

Appositional growth. Growth by layered incremental deposition at surfaces.

Aquaporin (AQP). A family of homologous integral membrane water channel proteins expressed in fluid-transporting epithelia. Aquaporins modulate the osmolarity of fluids in the salivary glands and epithelia of other organs such as the lung, kidney, brain, eye, and lacrimal gland. These proteins are conserved from bacteria to mammals and even plants and are highly selective.

Arches, aortic. See *Aortic arches.*

Arches, pharyngeal. See *pharyngeal arches.*

Articular disc. Of the temporomandibular joint; the fibrous disc that separates the joint into upper and lower cavities.

Attached gingiva. That part of the oral mucosa which is firmly bound to the tooth and alveolar process.

Attached pulp stones. Mineralized tissues that are partly fused with the dentin of the coronal or root pulp.

Basal lamina. Structural scaffolding composed of glycosaminoglycans, glycoproteins, and collagen; synthesized by epithelial cells throughout the body. Probably plays an important role in developing systems and in homeostasis of adult epithelia. Thickening of the basal laminae to the body occurs in diabetes mellitus and other pathologic conditions.

Bell stage. Tooth development stage characterized by the differentiation of inner enamel epithelial cells into ameloblasts and the formation of the crown outline by these cells.

Bifid tongue. Split or cleft; separating the tongue into two parts.

Biocompatibility. The ability of a material to perform with an appropriate host response in a specific situation. The material may be required to trigger or elicit a biologic response from the body, such as bone formation of protein adhesion, without being harmful to the tissues.

Biologic age. The maturational age; not the chronologic age, but the dental/skeletal age.

Birbeck's granule. A specific granule located in Langerhan's cells.

Birth. Passage of the child from the uterus to the outside world; the act of being born.

Blastocyst. The postmorula stage of development; a blastula with a fluid-filled cavity.

Bodily movement of a tooth. When force is applied through the center of resistance the tooth moves in a bodily fashion. All parts move the same amount and in the same direction.

Bone. Mineralized animal tissue consisting of an organic matrix of cells and fibers of collagen impregnated with mineral matter, chiefly calcium phosphate and calcium carbonate.

Bone morphogenetic protiens (BMPs). A class of proteins belonging to the transforming growth factor beta family having cartilage or bone-inducing potential.

Bradykinin. A kinin composed of nine amino acids secreted in response to the action of trypsin on a globulin of blood plasma.

Branchial. Bar–like; resembling the gills of a fish.

Buccinator muscle. Muscle forming the principal substance of the cheek.

Bud stage. Initial stage of tooth development; the enamel organ develops from this structure. The dental papilla and the dental sac enclose the bud.

Bundle bone. Specialized bone lining the tooth socket into which the fibers of the periodontal ligament penetrate; synonymous with the radiographic term "lamina dura."

Calciotraumatic line. An incremental line in dentin found at the junction of secondary and reparative dentin.

Calculus. An abnormal concretion within the body, usually formed of inorganic matter and often deposited around a minute fragment of inorganic material, the nucleus.

Calculus, dental. Hard stone–like concretion formed on the teeth or prosthesis. It varies in color from creamy yellow to black and is mostly composed of calcium phosphate.

Calvaria. Skullcap; the superior, dome–like portion of the cranium.

Canaliculi. Small microscopic spaces that contain cellular projections of osteocytes and cementocytes. In dentin, the spaces occupied by branches from the main dentinal tubule.

Cap stage. Tooth development, an early stage in enamel organ formation; follows the bud stage.

Caries, dental. Localized, progressively destructive disease of the teeth that starts at the external surface (enamel) with the apparent dissolution of the inorganic components by organic acids.

Cartilage. Connective tissue characterized by its non-vascularity and firm consistency. There are three kinds: hyaline cartilage, fibrocartilage, and elastic cartilage.

Catecholamines. One of a group of similar compounds that have a sympathomimetic action.

Cell differentiation. An increase in morphologic or chemical heterogenicity.

Cell proliferation. The developmental process in which cells pass through the cell cycle, with parent cells dividing to form two daughter cells and thereby increasing the number of cells in the tissue or organ.

Cell rests (Malassez). The epithelial remnants of the root sheaths found in the periodontal ligament.

Cell-free zone. Relatively cell-free layer adjacent to odontoblasts, overlying the cell-rich zone of the dental pulp, and composed of delicate fibrils embedded in the ground substance.

Cell-rich zone. Layer of the dental pulp situated between the pulp core and the cell-free zone, which is richly supplied with cellular elements, blood vessels, and nerves.

Cellular cementum. That part of the cementum covering the apical one-half to two-thirds of the root of a tooth. It is usually opposed by a layer of acellular cementum. It contains cemetocytes embedded in the calcified matrix.

Cementicles. Calcified spherical bodies composed of cementum either lying free within the periodontal ligament, attached to the cementum, or embedded in it.

Cementoblast. Connective-tissue cell type responsible for the formation of cementum.

Cementocyte. A cell found in the lacuma of cellular cementum, from 8 μm to more than 15 μm in diameter, with a wide variety of shapes from round to oval to flattened. Numerous cytoplasmic processes extend from its free surface.

Cementum. Bone–like connective tissue that covers the tooth from the cementoenamel junction to and surrounding the apical foremen.

Cementoenamel junction. Represents the boundary between enamel and cementum that lies at the cervix of the tooth. These two tissues may overlap or be sightly separated.

Cervical loop. Growing free border of the enamel organ. The outer and inner enamel epithelial layers are continuous and reflected into one another.

Cervix. The portion of the tooth that lies at the border of the anatomic crown and root of the tooth. It is often at the cementoenamel junction.

Chemotaxis. The movement of cells following a concentration gradient (moving toward higher concentration) of a chemical substance.

Choanae. Paired openings between the nasal cavity and nasopharynx.

Cholinergic nerves. Nerve fibers that secrete acetycholine at a synapse primarily associated with postganglionic parasympathetic fibers.

Chorda tympani. A branch of the facial nerve that joins the lingual nerve for parasympathetic supply to the sublingual and submandibular glands.

Chondrocranium. Cartilaginous skull; the embryonic skull before ossification.

Chronologic age. Record of time elapsed since birth.

Circumpulpal dentin. Inner portion of the dentin located near the pulp organ of the tooth.

Circumvallate papilla. Papilla vallata; one of eight or 10 projections from the dorsum of the tongue that form a V-shaped row anterior to the sulcus terminalis. Each is surrounded by a circular trench having a slightly raised outer wall.

Cis **Golgi network.** This is a specialized tubular region of the Golgi apparatus. It receives incoming transport vesicles that bud off from the transitional elements of the rough endoplasmic reticulum (RER) and fuse with the cis-face of the Golgi.

Clathrin. A protein that assembles into a basket–like cage, facilitating formation of a coated pit by, in turn, facilitating the pulling of the membrane bilayer into the basket. The coated pit buds off to form a clathrin-coated vesicle. Clathrin-coated vesicles were first identified in the endocytic pathway involving internalization of receptor-ligand complexes from the plasma membrane. Clathrin-coated vesicles, however, are also involved in vesicular transport between the TGN of the Golgi apparatus and the plasma membrane during exocytosis.

Cleft lip. A congenital defect of the lip, usually the upper lip. Failure of the median nasal and maxillary process to fuse.

Cleft palate. Palatum fissum; a congenital fissure in the median line of the palate or lateral to the premaxillary process, or both. It usually is associated with cleft lip.

Clinical crown. That portion of the crown exposed above the gingiva and visible in the oral cavity.

Clinical eruption. Emergence of the crown of a tooth, that portion of which can be observed clinically.

Cocci. Bacteria with a round, spheroid, or ovoid form, including *Microcossus*, gonococcus, meningococcus, *Staphylococcus*, *Streptococcus*, and pneumococcus.

Col. Valley–like depression in the facial lingual plane of the interdental gingiva. It conforms to the shape of the interproximal contact area.

Collagen. White fibers of the corium of the skin, tendon, and other connective tissue. The fiber is composed of fibrils bound together with interfibrillar cement; the fibrils are, in turn, formed from ultramicroscopic filaments. An albumoid found in connective tissue, bone, and cartilage and notable for its high content of the amino acids glycine, proline, and hydroxyproline.

Collagen fiber. High-molecular-weight protein composed of a number of structural types that vary in diameter from less than 1 μm to about 12 μm and are usually arranged in bundles.

Compact bone. Hard, external, more highly calcified than cancellous (spongy) portion of bone.

Competence. The ability of a tissue or cell to respond to inducing factors.

Complement. A group of proteins that react with the antibody antigen complex producing mediators of inflammation and causing death of foreign cells.

Concha. A shell–like or scroll–like bone. Anatomically it relates to the turbinate bones projecting into the nasal cavity.

Connective-tissue adhesion. Protein adhesion of connective tissue to other substances such as teeth or alloplastic materials.

Connective-tissue stroma of salivary glands. Capsule and septa formed from mesenchyme and the blood vessels.

Constitutive secretion. Secretion occurring continuously with molecules transported in vesicles from the Golgi apparatus to the plasma membrane in the presence or absence of secretagogue. Some transport vesicles may bud from the secretory vesicles, shuttling proteins to the plasma membrane.

Cord growth of salivary glands. Solid cord of epithelial cells that characterizes an early stage of development of salivary glands.

Corpus luteum. Yellow endocrine body, 1 to 1.5 cm in diameter, formed in the ovary in the site of a ruptured ovarian follicle.

Cranial. Pertaining to the bones covering the brain on the superior end of the body in humans.

Cranial base. Lower portion of the skull constituting the floor of the cranial cavity.

Cribriform. Bone containing perforations or numerous foramina.

Crypts. Pit–like depressions or tubular recesses.

Cuticle, developmental. Skin of the teeth consisting of an extremely thin layer of organic material covering the enamel of recently erupted teeth.

Cuticle, primary. A thin film on the enamel of an unerupted tooth. A product of the degenerating ameloblasts.

Cyclic AMP (cAMP). Adenosine 3':5'-cyclic phosphate; the second or intracellular messenger of target cells. Hormones or pharmacologic agents interact and bind to a membrane-bound receptor associated with an adenyl cyclase enzyme system. Adenyl cyclase catalyzes the conversion of ATP to AMP.

Cystic fibrosis (CF). Lethal genetic disease characterized by a generalized dysfunction of the exocrine glands of the body and therefore resulting in digestive and pulmonary problems. CF is caused by mutations in the gene that encodes for the cystic fibrosis transmembrane conductance regulator (CFTR) protein.

Cystic fibrosis transmembrane conductance regulator (CFTR). A cyclic AMP-regulated chloride channel that is essential for chloride and bicarbonate secretion and regulates other ion channels in salivary and other epithelia.

Cytodifferentiation. The process by which an undifferentiated cell attains a more differentiated phenotype.

Cytokines. A group of non-antibody molecules produced by cells that function to influence and signal other cells. The principal function is the induction of cell division and the regulation of differentiation.

Dead tracts. Empty tubules left after the odontoblastic processes degenerate.

Deciduous dentition. Primary teeth or first-formed set of teeth that undergo exfoliation to provide space for the permanent teeth.

Degenerating lamina. Lysis and disappearance of the dental lamina, characteristic of teeth in the bell stage of development.

Demilune (serious demilune). Half-moon or crescent-shaped serous cells of a mixed-type acinus that form a cap over the ends of the mucous acinar cells.

Dental lamina. Horseshoe-shaped epithelial bands that traverse the upper and lower jaws and give rise to the ectodermal portions of the teeth.

Dental papilla. Formative organ of the dentin and primordium of the pulp.

Dental plaque. Organic deposit on the surface of teeth. Site of growth of bacteria or nucleus for formation of dental calculus.

Dental pulp (endodontia). Soft tissue contained within the pulp cavity, consisting of connective tissue and containing blood vessels, nerves, and lymphatics.

Dental sac (follicle). Area surrounding the developing tooth that produces the alveolar bone, cementum, and periodontal ligament and consists of (ecto)mesenchymal cells and fibers that surround the dental papilla and the enamel organ.

Denticles. A calcified structure found in the pulp of a tooth.

Dentin. Body of the tooth; surrounds the pulp and underlies the enamel of the crown and the cementum on the roots of the teeth. About 20% is organic matrix, mostly collagen, and 10% is water. The inorganic fraction (70%) is mainly hydroxyapatite, with some carbonate, magnesium, and fluoride. It is yellowish in color.

Dentin phosphoprotein (DPP). A highly phosphorylated protein found in the dentinal matrix, also referred to as phosphophoryn. A component of a larger protein, dentin sialophosphoprotein (DSPP).

Dentin, reactionary. Dentin that is formed by primary odontoblasts in response to an external stimulus. It has irregular tubules and was formerly known as irritation dentin or irregular secondary dentin.

Dentin, reparative. Dentin that is formed following the death of primary odontoblasts. Its structure is tubular and dystrophic. This dentin is deposited by a new generation of odontoblasts.

Dentin sialophosphoprotein (DSPP). A phosphorylated, highly glycosylated protein containing high amounts of sialic acid. Expressed exclusively by ameloblasts (transiently) and odontoblasts. Genetic evidence indicates that DPP and DSP are transcribed as parts DSPP.

Dentin sialoprotein (DSP). A phosphorylated, highly glycosylated protein containing high amounts of sialic acid.

Dentinal tubule. The space in dentin that contains, or at one time contained, an odontoblastic process.

Dentinoenamel junction. Interface of the enamel and dentin of the crown of a tooth.

Dentinogenesis. Process of dentin formation in the development of teeth.

Desmosome. Macula adherens; site of adhesion between two cells, consisting of a dense plate near the cell surface, separated from a similar structure in the adjacent cell by thin layers of extracellular materials believed to have adhesive properties. Intercellular tonofilaments are associated with this structure.

Diapedesis. The migration of cells like neutrophils through gaps between endothelial cells.

Differentiation. Growth associated with or having a distinguishing character or function from the surrounding structures or from the original type; specialization.

Diphyodont. Having two sets of teeth, as in humans and most mammals.

Displacement. Change in position of a bone due to growth at its border or movement of an adjacent bone. Change in attachment when one element, radical, or molecule is removed and is replaced by another.

Drift. The change in position of a bone due to remodeling (apposition on one side and resorption on the other). Movement of a tooth to a position of greater stability.

Drug. Any substance used as a medicine in the treatment of disease; to give medicine; to narcotize.

Duct. Tube with well-defined walls for passage of excretions or secretions.

Duct, intercalated. The smallest-diameter intralobular duct of salivary glands that conducts saliva from the acinar cells to the striated ducts. These ducts modify salivary secretions.

Duct, interlobular. Channels located outside lobes of the salivary glands.

Duct, intralobular. Channels located within lobes of the salivary glands.

Duct, striated. A type of intralobular duct of the salivary glands that is composed of columnar cells with centrally placed nuclei and striations at the basal ends of cells. These cells modify salivary secretions.

Dystrophy. Any disorder arising from defective or faulty nutrition.

Eccentric growth. Process whereby one part of the developing tooth germ remains stationary, while the remainder continues to grow. This leads to a shift in its center.

Ectoderm. Outer layer of cells of the three primary germ layers; forms nervous system epidermis and derivatives.

Ectomesenchyme. Neural crest cells, mesectoderm. This term is used to describe cells derived from the neural crest and found in the mesodermal tissues. Functions in induction. Forms spinal ganglia, much of the face, and pharyngeal arches.

Edema. The swelling that results from fluid accumulation within the tissue following a spill of blood constituents.

Edentulous. Without teeth, having lost the natural teeth.

Eicosanoids. A group of compounds that are converted to biologically active substances that act as mediators of inflammation.

Embedded pulp stones (denticles). Small calcified masses of dentin appearing as a function of age or trauma. They may protrude from the existing dentin wall into the pulp tissue.

Enamel cord. A structure connecting the enamel knot to the enamel navel.

Enamel crystals. Hydroxyapatite crystals found in enamel rods. They are deposited during tooth mineralization.

Enamel knot (primary knot and secondary knots). A collection of epithelial cells associated with the inner enamel epithelium of the enamel organ of a developing tooth near the developing cusp tips. It is a transient structure responsible for the production of signaling molecules that control the development of both the enamel epithelium and papilla.

Enamel lamellae. Thin, leaf–like structures that extend from the enamel surface toward the dentinoenamel junction. They represent defects or spaces filled entirely or partly with organic material.

Enamel navel. A collection of epithelial cells connected to the outer enamel epithelium during the early stages of tooth development.

Enamel organ. Originates from the stratified epithelium lining the primitive oral cavity organ; consists of four distinct layers: outer enamel epithelium, stellate reticulum, stratum intermedium, and inner enamel epithelium. The latter becomes the ameloblastic layer.

Enamel pearls. Enameloma, a developmental anomaly in which a small nodule of enamel is formed near the cemetoenamel junction, usually at the bifurcation zone of molar teeth.

Enamel rod. One of the structural units of enamel, extending from the dentinoenamel junction to the surface of the tooth, averaging about 5 μm in width and 9 μm in height, and normally having a translucent crystalline appearance.

Enamel spindles. Tubular spaces in enamel found at the dentinoenamel junction in which a terminal extension of the odontoblast processes may be found.

Enamel tuft. Narrow, ribbon–like structure whose inner end arises at the dentinoenamel junction, extends one-third of the distance to the enamel surface, and consists of hypocalcified enamel rods; may be filled with organic substance and extend at near right angles to the dentinoenamel junction.

Enamelin. An acidic glycosylated phosphoprotein of mature enamel. It has a molecular weight of about 55,000 daltons.

Ectochondral. Relating to the type of formation of bone formed within cartilage and replacing it.

Endocrine. Refers to glands of internal secretion that release their secretory product(s) (hormones) directly into the bloodstream rather than through a duct system.

Endocytosis. The process by which material enters the cell by invagination of the plasma membrane to form a membrane-bound pit, which eventually buds off to form a membrane-bound vesicle. Calthrin is the coating material of pits and vesicles in the endocytic pathway.

Endosseous implants. Implants that are embedded in bone and fixed throughout the entire length of the implant. The various implant types are screw, blade, and cylinder.

Enhancer. Regulatory sequences in DNA that influence the rate of transcription (e.g., enhancing the action of the promoter). They are recognized by gene regulatory factors (transcription factors) and function irrespective of : 1) Their orientation relative to the transcribed DNA (e.g., they may be many thousands of base pairs away from the transcribed gene); and 2) their sequence polarity.

Entactin. An extracellular matrix glycoprotein associated with the basal lamina.

Epidermal growth factor (EGF). A small peptide (molecular weight = 6045) originally isolated from the male mouse submandibular gland and now known to have a very wide distribution in the body. EGF stimulates cell proliferation and/or differentiation in various organs and tissues through EGF receptors that activate tyrosine-specific proteins kinases.

Epimers. Dorsal form of a myotome that forms muscles innervated by the dorsal ramus of the spinal nerve.

Epiphyseal plate of condylar head. Cartilage of the head of the mandibular condyle, a growth site.

Epithelial attachment. Dentogingival junction attachment of the gingival epithelium with the tooth's surface. The basal lamina of the epithelium is attached by means of hemidesmosomes.

Epithelial cell rests. Remains of (Hertwig's) root sheath. The epithelial cells that cover the roots during root development. Later, they are located in the periodontal ligament near the surface of the cementum as groups of cells called "rests." There are three types: proliferating, resting, and degenerating. Occasionally, they develop into the dental cysts.

Epithelial diaphragm. Formed by the root sheath at the beginning of root development; important in formation of the root. It finally serves to narrow the width of the cervical opening of the root.

Epithelial pearls. Discrete, rounded, or ovoid groups of epithelial cells, frequently keratinized, found in the lamina propria. The cells are arranged in a whorled or concentrically laminated pattern, with polygonal cells centrally flattened and with more mature cells found peripherally. They are most often found in the midline of the palate and are remnants of epithelium in the line of fusion.

Epithelium. Cellular, avascular layer covering all the free surfaces of the body internal and external and the lining of vessels. Consists of cells and a small amount of intercellular substance. Includes the glands and other structures derived therefrom.

Epithelium, inner enamel. The cells that line the concavity of the enamel organ in the cap and early bell stages of tooth development and differentiate into ameloblasts.

Epithelium, outer enamel. Cuboid peripheral cells of the cap or the bell stage of tooth development that line the convexity of the cap.

Eruption, teeth. Appearance of teeth in the oral cavity; a stage coordinated with root growth and maturation of tissues surrounding the tooth.

Esterase. The enzyme responsible for catalyzing the hydrolosis of an ester into an alcohol and acid.

Excretory duct. Pertaining to excretion; is an interlobular duct draining the intralobular ducts, possessing a pseudostratified or stratified columnar epithelium, and believed to be involved in ionic transport.

Exfoliate. To shed or eliminate something, such as scales from the surface of the body, or loss of teeth from the jaws.

Exocrine. Denotes glands that release their secretory product(s) into a duct system.

Exocytosis. Discharges of secretory products(s) from the cell, preserving the cell membrane through fusion of the secretory vesicle with the cell membrane.

Exon. The coding sequence of a eukaryotic gene. The exon encodes the sequence of nucleotides in messenger RNA (mRNA) that represents the amino acids in a protein.

Extracellular matrix. Macromolecular products of mesenchymal and epithelial (basement membrane components) cells that provide a role in cellular adhesion. These substrate adhesion molecules are important in induction of epithelia and regulation of cellular migration.

Extravasate. Fluid that extrudes or escapes from a vessel into the tissues.

Fenestrated. Perforated with one or more openings.

Fertilization. Rendering gametes fertile; contact and fusion of spermatozoa and ovum and formation and merging male and female pronuclei and development of zygote.

Fibroblasts. Elongated, ovoid, spindle-shaped, or flattened cells found in connective tissue that form the connective-tissue fibers.

Fibronectin. An adhesive V-shaped glycoprotien present in the basement membrane that has collagen-binding domain. There is also a heparin-binding domain and a fibrin-binding site on the molecule. Fibronectin binds to integrins called fibronectin receptors on cells. One cell-binding site contains a tripeptide sequence known as the RGD sequence. (Arg-GY-Ash).

Fibrous capsule. Capsule composed chiefly of fibrous elements.

Filamentous bacteria. Long, pleomorphic, branched, rod-shaped microorganisms.

Filiform papillae. The most numerous type of papillae of the dorsum of the tongue. They are thread–like papillae pointing toward the throat.

Fissure sealant. Composite resin "bonded" directly to the enamel surface that functions to seal out bacteria that cause caries.

Fontanelles. One of several membranous intervals at the angles of the cranial bones in the infant. Normally there are six, corresponding to the pterion and asterion, on either side, and to the bregma and lambda, in the midline.

Fordyce's spots (granules). Ectopic sebaceous glands, located at the angles of the mouth.

Free gingiva. That portion of the gingiva that surrounds the tooth and is not directly attached to the tooth surface; the outer wall of the gingival sulcus.

Free pulp stones (denticles). Small calcified masses of dentin that appear as a function of aging or trauma. They develop in the connective tissue of the pulp without obvious relationship to the secondary dentin of the tooth.

Frontonasal. Region of the upper anterior face between the eyes. Nasal placodes arise here.

Fungiform papillae. One of numerous minute elevations of the dorsum, tip, and sides of the tongue, of a mushroom shape, with the tip being broader than the base.

Furcation. An atomic area of a multirooted tooth where the roots divide.

G protein. Guanosine 5'-triphosphate-binding regulatory protein that alters an intracellular messenger (e.g., cyclic nucleotides or Ca^{++}).

Gap junctions. Specialized intercellular junctions between cells, with pores permeable to ions and small molecules.

Genetic. Relating to genetics or ontogenesis.

Gingiva. The soft tissue surrounding the necks of erupted teeth. It is composed of two parts: the masticatory mucosa facing the oral cavity and the sulcular (crevicula) epithelium and epithelial attachment facing the tooth. The gingiva consists of fibrous tissue, enveloped by mucous membrane, which covers the alveolar process of the upper and lower jaws.

Gingival sulcus. The shallow V-shaped trench around each tooth, bounded by the tooth surface on one surface and the epithelial-lined free margin on the other.

Glycosaminoglycan (GAG). Noncollagenous macromolecule previously referred to as mucopolysaccharide.

Gnarled enamel. The enamel located at the tips of the cusps, in which the rods or groups of rods are twisted, bent, and intertwined.

Gonial angle. Angle between the lower border and posterior ramus of the mandible.

Granular layer of Tomes. A thin layer of defective dentin adjacent to the cementum, which appears granular and located along the root surface.

Granulation tissue. The tissue that replaces the blood clot and is formed by new connective tissue and new capillaries.

Granulocytes. Blood cells that have granules in their cytoplasm. These include neutrophils, eosinophils, and basophils.

Granuloma. A nodule of granulation tissue containing growing fibroblasts and capillaries in response to chronic inflammation.

Growth factors. Chemical substances that induce cells to initiate DNA synthesis.

Guanosine triphosphatases (GTPases). Controls molcular switching processes within the cell. There are two types: trimeric G proteins, which are involved in signal transduction (e.g., G_s, G_q), and monomeric GTPases (e.g., Ras, Rab, and Rho).

Gubernacular cord. Fibrous cord connecting two structures; a connective-tissue band uniting the tooth sac with the alveolar mucosa.

Hageman factor. The clotting factor XII that becomes activated following injury, and in turn activates the clotting complement kinin and plasmin systems.

Hard palate. Anterior part of the palate, consisting of the bony palate covered above by the respiratory mucosa of the floor of the nose and below by the keratinized stratified squamous oral mucosa of the roof of the mouth. The hard palate contains palatine vessels and nerves, adipose tissue, and mucous glands.

Haversian bone. Compact bone containing tubular channels with blood vessels, nerves, and bone cells with concentrically located lacunae that are termed the Haversion system or osteon.

Hemidesmosomes. Similar to a desmosome but represents only half of it. Located on the surface of some epithelial cells and forming at the site of attachment between the epithelial cell and the basal lamina. Consists of single attachment plaque, the adjacent plasma membrane, and a related extracellular structure that attaches the epithelium to the connective tissue.

Hemostasis. The process leading to stoppage of bleeding.

Heparan sulfate. A glycosaminoglycan consisting of N-acetyl-glucosamine alternating with D-glucuronic acid of D-iduronic acid. When covalently linked to protein, heparan sulfate proteoglycan is formed.

Heterotypic contacts. During development, these represent the close approximation of epithelium and mesenchyme without an intervening basal lamina.

Histamine. A vasoactive amine that induces vasodilation and increases vascular permeability.

Histodifferentiation. The acquisition of discrete functional layers of cells within the enamel organ and dental papilla during tooth development.

Homeobox. A conserved DNA sequence of 180 base pairs that codes for a 60 amino-acid-long DNA-binding motif; this is important in pattern formation during development, including morphogenesis, organogenesis, and cell differentiation. Homeoboxes are found in the genomes of lower animals and vertebrates. The homeobox codes for a protein domain that is involved in binding to DNA.

Homeodomain. The 60 amino acid DNA-binding region (motif) that is encoded in the homeobox sequence. Homeodomain-containing proteins are transcription regulators controlling the coordinate expression of genes involved in development and differentiation.

Homeotic gene. Gene containing the homeobox sequence. Expression is set during embryogenisis in response to positional cues that direct the later formation of site appropriate tissues.

Hormone. Chemical substance formed in one organ or part of the body and carried by the blood to another part where it stimulates or depresses functional activity.

Howship lacunae. Tiny depressions, pits, or irregular grooves on the surfaces of bones, the result of resorption by osteoclasts.

Hox genes. Conserved across phyla and specifying regional differences along the anteroposterior axis of the vertebrate embryo.

Hunter-Schreger bands. Alternating dark and light bands in enamel. Resulting from absorption and reflection of light caused by differences in orientation of adjacent groups of enamel rods originating at the dentinoenamel junction and extending to near the outer enamel surface.

Hyalinization. A result of compression of the periodontal ligament in which all vascularity and most cells are lost from the zone of compression, creating a glass–like appearance. As a result, tooth movement will cease.

Hyaluronidase. Enzyme catalyzing the hydrolosis of hyaluronic acid that forms the backbone of proteoglycan molecules in connective tissue.

Hydrodynamic. Branch of physics that deals with factors determining the flow of liquids. In dentistry, it refers to a theory of pain conduction through dentin.

Hypertrophic zone. Endochondral cartilage zone characterized by enlargement of existing cells.

Hydroxyapatite. The inorganic matrix of bone, enamel, cementum, dentin, and cartilage having the chemical formula $Ca_{10}(PO_4)6(OH)_2$.

Hypomere. Portion of the myotome that extends ventrolaterally to form body wall muscle and is innervated by the primary ventral ramus of a spinal nerve.

Hypoxia. Refers to low oxygen content of tissues.

Iatrogenic. An adverse condition resulting from the activities of a health professional.

IgA (secretory immunoglobulins). One of the classes of immunoglobulins; the principal immunoglobulin found in exocrine secretions—milk, intestinal and respiratory mucin, saliva, and tears. Antigens entering the oral cavity stimulate IgA synthesis and secretion in the salivary glands to protect the oral mucosa from pathogenic microbes.

Immunoglobulins. Serum proteins that function as antibodies and are responsible for humoral immunity. There are five classes of immunoglobulins: IgG, IgA, IgM, IgD, and IgE.

Impaction. Position of a tooth in the alveolus so that it is incapable of eruption into the oral cavity. Impaction may be due to crowding of teeth that results in a lack of available space for eruption. Teeth being driven into the alveolar process or surrounding tissues as a result of trauma.

Increment. The amount by which a given quantity is increased. A measurable amount.

Incremental deposition. Deposition of material in discrete amounts, rather than constant deposition. Rhythmic recurrent deposition of enamel, bone, dentin, or cementum.

Induction, embryonic. The act or process of causing the occurrence of a specific morphogenic effect in the developing embryo through the influence of organizers.

Innervation. Presence and distribution of nerves in a part, or the supply of nerve stimulation of a part.

Instructive influence. The ability of an embryonic tissue to change the fate of the responding tissue.

Instructive interaction. An embryonic interaction between two tissues in which the responding tissue differentiates by receiving specific signals (instructions) from the inducing tissue. The fate of the responding tissue is determined by the tissue with which it interacts.

Integrins. A class of transmembrane cell adhesion molecules. The fibronectin receptor (FN-R) and lamin receptors (L-R) are the best characterized members of this family. FN-R links the intracellular actin network with the extracellular matrix. LN-R promotes binding of epithelial cells to the basal lamina.

Intercalated duct. Intralobular-type salivary-gland duct draining the acinus. Intercalated duct cells are cuboidal and contain secretory granules and rough endoplasmic reticulum (RER). They are the smallest ducts within the salivary gland.

Interdental septa. Bony partitions that project into the alveoli between the teeth; interalveolar.

Interglobular dentin. A zone of a globular, rather than linear, formed dentin in the crowns of teeth, underlying enamel specifically in the zone separating the mantle and circumpulpal dentin. Characterized by interglobular spaces that are unmineralized or hypomineralized dentin between normal calcified dentinal layers.

Interlobualr ducts. Ducts of the salivary glands that traverse in connective-tissue septa between lobules; also termed excretory ducts.

Intertubular dentin. The dentin between zones of peritubular dentin that immediately surrounds the tubules.

Intratubular duct. Located within the lobules of the salivary glands. There are two types: intercalated, lined by low cuboidal epithelium, and striated, lined by tall cuboidal to columnar epithelium.

Intramembranous bone. Bone formation within or between connective-tissue membranes. It does not replace cartilage, as does endochondral bone.

Intratubular dentin. The hypermineralized layer of dentin that lies between the sheath of Neuman and the dentinal tubule.

Intron. A noncoding segment of DNA which is transcribed into the primary transcript of RNA, but is excised by RNA splicing to obtain the messenger RNAs. Introns are located adjacent to exons.

Junctional complex. Specialized region of contact between adjacent cells; it consists of three regions (moving in order from the apical region of the cell): zonula occludens, zonula adherens, and desmosome.

Junctional epithelium. Epithelial attachment. That epithelium adhering to the tooth or implant surface at the base of the gingival crevice and consisting of one or several layers of non-keratinizing cells.

Keratinized. Having developed a horny layer of flattened cells containing keratin.

Keratinized mucosa. Stratified surface of cornified epithelial cells that lack a nucleus and whose cytoplasm is replaced by large amounts of keratoyalin protein. Keratinized oral epithelium has four cells layers: basal, spinous, granular, and cornified.

Keratinocyte. Epithelial cells of the mucosa and skin whose main activity is the production of keratin.

Korff's fibers. First-formed argyrophilic dental fibers associated with glycosaminoglycans. They extend between odontoblasts from the dental pulp. Their existence is controversial.

Lamella. Thin leaf or plate, as of bone.

Lamella enamel. Imperfectly calcified, thin, leaf-shaped areas of enamel extending from the outer surface toward the dentin.

Lamina dura. Radiographic term describing the hard compact bone layer lining the dental alveoli.

Lamina propria. Layer of connective tissue underlying the epithelium of skin or a mucous membrane.

Lamin. A glycoprotein found in the basal lamina. Binds to type IV collagen; cells, particularly epithelial cells; and neurons through a laminin receptor (integrin) on the cell membrane, and glycosaminoglycans. It is believed to play a role in extracellular matrix regulation of cell migration and differentiation.

Langerhans' cells. Clear or dendritic cells found in both superficial and deep layers of the epidermis and oral epithelium. They contain no desmosomes or tonofilaments. Probably arising from bone marrow, they may have immunologic function in recognizing antigenic material.

Lateral lamina. Band of cells believed to be functionally and structurally similar to the parent dental lamina. Lateral lamina connects the developing tooth germs to the dental lamina.

Leukoplakia. Dysfunction of the keratinization process of stratified squamous epithelium resulting in a white appearance of the surface cells.

Lingual tonsil. Collection of lymphoid follicles on the base, posterior, or pharyngeal portion of the dorsum of the tongue.

Lining mucosa. Non-keratinized oral mucosa covering the cheeks, lips, soft palate, floor of the mouth, and ventral surface of the tongue.

Lobe. Subdivision of an organ bounded by structural demarcations such as connective-tissue septa or fissures.

Lobules. Small lobes or subdivisions of a lobe that are separated by thin partitions of connective tissue.

Long-range signals. Interactions involving diffusion of molecules far from their site of production.

Lymphokines. Cytokines produced by lymphocytes.

Macroglossia. Enlargement of the tongue, usually due to local lymphangiectasia or to muscular hypertrophy; megaloglossia.

Macrophage. Term generally used as a designation for the large mononuclear phagocytes that are found in various tissues and organs of the body, where they are called histocytes, "wandering cells," or other terms. They are found in conspicuous numbers in the sinusoids of the spleen, lymph nodes, liver, lungs, and bone marrow. In the brain and spinal cord, they are designated microglia.

Major salivary glands. The paired parotid, submandibular (submaxillary), and sublingual salivary glands that are responsible for the production of enzyme amylase, mucins, secretory immunoglobulin A (IgA), and other constituents of saliva.

Mallassez' epithelial rests. Epithelial remnants of Hertwig's sheath in the periodontal ligament. These groups of epithelial cells appear near the surface of the cementum; occasionally they develop into dental cysts.

Mandible. Horseshoe-shaped bone forming the lower jaw and articulating, by its upturned extremities, the condyles, with the temporal bone on either side. The mandible is composed of the body and the ramus that is located posteriorly. The body includes the alveolar process that contains the teeth.

Mannose-6-phophate (M6P). A marker on lysosomal hydrolases added only to the N-linked oligosaccharides in the cis-Golgi. M6P binds to M6P receptors that form on the clathrin-coated vesicles and provides the intracellular target signal to direct these enzymes into the lysosomal pathway.

Mantle dentin. The initially deposited portions of the dentin formed immediately beneath enamel.

Marginal leakage. Seepage of microorganisms, fluids, and debris along the interface between a dental restoration and the walls of a cavity preparation.

Mastication. Process of chewing food in preparation for swallowing and digestion.

Masticatory mucosa. The mucosa that functions in mastication. It tends to be bound to bone and is therefore immovable. It bears forces generated when food is chewed. The mucosa of the hard palate and gingiva.

Matrix vesicles. Membrane-bounded vesicles that arise by budding and lie free in the extracellular matrix. These vesicles may represent the initial sites of calcification in dentin, bone, and cartilage.

Maturation stage. The stage of enamel development following postsecretory transition in which the enamel gains mineral and loses water and organic matrix.

Maturation zone. Zone of cartilage characterized by chondrocyte enlargement.

Maxilla. Upper jaw bone; an irregularly shaped bone articulating with the nasal, lacriminal, zygomatic, palatine, ethmoid, sphenoid, and frontal bones of the face and containing teeth.

Maxillary sinus. Paired sinus cavities occupying the space beneath the floor of the orbit and above the roots of the posterior maxillary teeth.

Meatus. An opening, passageway, or channel.

Meckel's cartilage. The initial skeletal component of the first pharyngeal arch. It is the supporting cartilage of the mandibular arch in the embryo.

Melanocyte. A cell that forms melanin pigment found in the skin and mucous membranes.

Membrane performativum. Basement membrane separating the enamel organ and the dental papilla preceding dentin formation.

Merocrine. Type of glandular secretion in which the secreting cells remain intact during formation and release of the secretory products.

Mesenchyme. Loose, undifferentiated embryonic type of connective tissue that is usually of mesodermal origin but is a mixture of mesodermal and neural-crest derivatives in the head and neck region. See *Ectomesenchyme.*

Mesial drift. Gradual movement of a tooth or teeth anteriorly toward the midline.

Mesoderm. Mesoblast; the third primary germ layer of the embryo to differentiate. It is positioned between the ectogerm and endoderm.

Microglossia. Smallness of the tongue.

Mid-range. Interactions involving the diffusion of signaling molecules to responding cells in the immediate vicinity.

Mineralization front. The junction between mineralized and unmineralized tissue—for example, between predentin and dentin, osteoid and bone, or cementoid and cementum.

Minor salivary glands. The numerous glands located throughout the oral cavity in the lips (labial), cheeks (buccal), hard and soft palate (palatine), tongue (lingual; e.g., von Ebner's gland), and glossopalatine.

Mixed dentition. The state of possessing primary and secondary teeth simultaneously.

Modulation. A reversible change in form and function.

Monokines. Cytokines produced by moncytes.

Morphodifferentiation. The process occuring during tooth formation that is responsible for determining the space of the tooth's crown.

Morphogenesis. The development process that creates the shape and form of an organ. The branching process that occurs during salivary-gland development is an example of morphogenesis.

Morphogens. Signaling molecules that influence growth and development of a tissue or tissues.

Morula. Mass of blastomeres resulting from the early cleavage divisions of the zygote.

Mucoceles. Retention cysts of the minor salivary-gland ducts, which contain mucous secretion. Usually the result of rupture of the excretory duct of a minor-salivary gland, causing pooling of saliva in the tissues. The resulting versicular elevation is a mucocele.

Mucoperiosteum. A periosteum with a mucous surface. Close combination of mucous membrane (epithelium and lamina propria) with the periosteum of bone to form an apparent single layer.

Mucous acinus. Minute, sac–like secretory portion of a mucous gland. This is the functional unit of the gland.

Mucous glands. Glands that secrete viscous proteinaceous secretions, such as the sublingual gland; glands of the hard palate.

Mumps, parotitis. Enlargement of the parotid gland. An acute, contagious viral infection marked by bilateral or unilateral inflammation and swelling and manifested by chills, fevers, and headache.

Myoepithelial cells. Spindle-shaped cells with a stellate body and processes containing darkly staining fibrils found in all the glands of the oral cavity. Located in the epithelium of the terminal portion of the salivary gland acini, they are believed to have contractile ability that facilitates movement of the glandular secretion into the ducts.

Myofibrils. Fine longitudinal fibrils (parallel with long axis) occurring in a muscle fiber. They are composed of myofilaments.

NSF, N-ethylmaleimide sensitive factor. NSF is a cytosolic factor required for binding of vesicles to target membranes. NSF requires **s**oluble **N**SF **a**ttachment **p**rotein**s** (SNAPs) as cofactors to mediate its binding to membranes.

Naris. One of the orifices of the nasal cavity; nostril. May be the anterior internal or posterior naris.

Nasal region. Relating to the area of the nose, subdivided into internal naris, olfactory region, and nasopharynx.

Neonatal line. Accentuated incremental line or hesitation line seen in hard tissue such as bone, dentin, and deposited enamel. Probably due to metabolic changes occurring at or near the time of birth.

Neovascularize. To form new blood vessels after an injury.

Nerves. Whitish cords composed of fibers arranged in bundles (fascicles) and held together by a connective-tissue sheath. Nerves transmit stimuli from the central nervous system to the periphery or from the periphery to the central nervous system.

Neural crest. Ganglionic crest; a band of ectodermal cells that appear along either side of the line of closure of the embryonic neural groove. With the closure of the neural groove to form the neural tube, these bands then lie between the developing spinal cord and the superficial ectoderm. They later separate into cell groups that constitute the primordia of the ganglia of cranial and spinal nerves. Other derivatives migrate ventrally to induce formation of various other tissues.

Neurocranium. That part of the skull enclosing the brain, as distinguished from the bones of the face.

Nociception. The process of responding to pain.

Non-keratinocytes. Cells not producing keratin. Clear or dendritic cells found in oral epithelium, such as pigment cells (melanocytes). Langerhans' cells, Merkel's cells, and inflammatory cells such as lymphocytes.

Non-keratinized mucosa. Lining mucosa in which the stratified squamous epithelial cells retain their nuclei and cytoplasm. They contain no keratohyalin protein. Lining mucosa is found on the lips, cheeks, soft palate, vestibular fornix, alveolar mucosa, floor of the mouth, and undersurface of the tongue.

Occlusion. Relation of the maxillary and mandibular teeth when in functional contact during activity of the mandible.

Odontoblast. Layer of columnar cells with processes in the dentinal tubules, lining the peripheral pulp of a tooth. These cells function to form dentin.

Odontoblastic process. Slender protoplasmic process in dentinal tubule. It is a cytoplasmic extension of the cell bodies of the odontoblasts in the dental pulp. They extend from the cell possibly as far as the dentinoenamel junction and the cementoenamel junction.

Odontogenesis. The entire process of tooth formation, which includes amelogenesis, dentinogenisis, and cementogenesis.

Olfactory mucosa. Site of most of the receptors for the sense of smell. It occupies the superior aspect of the nasal cavity between the superior nasal conchae, roof of the the nose, and upper part of the septum and is composed of three cell types: receptor, supporting, and basal.

Oral vestibule. When the mouth is closed and the teeth are in occlusion, it is the space between the teeth and lips or cheeks.

Organic matrix. Formative portion of a tooth, as opposed to mineralized hydroxyapatite.

Oropharyngeal membrane. The embryonic transient membrane portion separating the oral and pharyngeal cavities. It ruptures and disappears during the fourth prenatal week. This membrane is located central to the pharynx and extends from the level of the palate to the vestibule of the larynx.

Osmiophilic. Tissue components stained easily with osmium or osmic acid.

Osseointegration. A direct structural and functional connection at the light microscope level between living bone and at the surface of a load-carrying implant.

Osteoblasts. Bone-forming cells derived from mesenchyme. They form the osseous matrix in which they may become enclosed to become osteocytes.

Osteoclasts. Larger multinucleated cells derived from monocytes with abundant acidophilic cytoplasm, formed in bone marrow and functioning in the absorption and removal of osseous tissue.

Osteocytes. Cells of the bone located in lacunae, which function in maintenance and vitality of bone.

Osteodentin. A form of reparative dentin in which cells become trapped in the matrix, giving it a bone–like appearance.

Oxytalan fibers. Type of connective-tissue fiber histochemically distinct from collagen or elastic fibers and found in the periodontal ligament and gingiva. May function in support of blood vessels and principal fibers of the ligament.

Palatine rugae. Transverse ridges located in the mucous membrane of the anterior part of the hard palate. They extend laterally from the incisive papilla. They have a core of dense connective tissue.

Palate, primary. That part of the palate formed from the median nasal process. The first palate to form, which is anterior to the secondary palate.

Palate, secondary. The palate proper, formed by fusion of the lateral palatine processes of the maxilla.

Palatine tonsils. Faucial; a large oval mass of lymphoid tissue embedded in the lateral wall of the oropharynx bilaterally located between the pillars of the fauces.

Parakeratinized. Superficial epithelial cells that have retained their pyknotic nuclei and show some signs of keratinization; the stratum granulosum generally is absent, however.

Parenchyma. Functional elements of glandular tissue rather than the supporting framework (strome) of the gland.

Parotid. The parotid salivary gland located anterior to the ear. It is encapsulated and produces 26% of the secretions of the major salivary glands.

Pellicle. Thin skin or film as on the surface of the teeth.

Perforating fibers (Sharpey's fibers). Penetrating connective-tissue fibers by which the tooth's surface is attached to the adjacent alveolar bone. These bundles of collagen fibers penetrate both the cementum and the alveolar bone.

Perikymata. Wave–like grooves, believed to be the manifestations of Retzius' striae, on the surface of enamel. They appear transverse to the long axis of the tooth.

Periodontal ligament. Connective-tissue structure attaching the tooth to the alveolus. It consists of collagenous fibers arranged in bundles, between which are loose connective tissue, blood vessels, and nerves.

Peritubular dentin. The zone of dentin forming the wall of the dentinal tubules. This dentin has a 9% higher mineral content than the remainder of intertubular dentin.

Perivascular. Located around a blood vessel.

Permissive interaction. An embryonic interaction between two tissues in which the responding tissue differentiates along a predetermined path. Only the presence of inducing tissue is necessary for differentiation.

Phagocytosis. The engulfing and digesting of cells, debris, and other substances by cells.

Pharyngeal-arch cartilages. One of the cartilages formed in a pharyngeal arch of the embryo.

Pharyngeal arches. One of a series of mesodermal thickenings between the pharyngeal clefts, appearing in higher forms only vestigially. During embryonic stages they contribute to the formation of the face, jaws, and neck.

Pharyngeal tonsil. Third (Luschka's) tonsil. A collection of more of less closely aggregated lymphoid cells located superficially in the posterior wall of the nasopharanx, the hypertrophy of which constitutes the condition called adenoids.

Phosphoinositide cycle. A signal transduction pathway in which binding to a cell surface receptor activates a G protein that subsequently activates phospholipase C. This enzyme forms two important intermediates from phosphatidyl-inositol-bisphosphate: inosital triphosphate (IP3) and diacylglycerol (DAG). IP3 releases Ca^{++} from intracellular compartments, while DAG activates protein kinase C leading to pholphorylation within the cell.

Phosphoproteins. A conjugated protein in which phosphoric acid is esterified with hydroxyamino acid, usually serine.

Placode. A plate–like thickening or layer of ectoderm appearing in the embryo.

Plaque, dental. Deposit of material on the surface of a tooth, which may also serve as a medium for growth of bacteria. May serve as a site for formation of dental calculus.

Plasma cells. Cells derived from B lymphocytes, which actively synthesize and secrete antibody (Ig) from an extensive rough endoplasmic reticulum (RER). Under appropriate conditions, antigen stimulation induces proliferation and morphologic alterations in B lymphocytes to form plasma cells.

Polarized cell. Exhibits apical and/or basal specializations and an asymmetric distribution of intercellular organelles.

Postsecretory transition. The stage of amelogenisis in which the enamel organ is in transition from the secretory to the maturation stage of development.

Predentin. Organic fibrillar matrix of the circumpulpal dentinal matrix before its calcification into dentin.

Preeruptive phase. Developmental stage preparatory to eruption of teeth and characterized by movements of the growing teeth within the alveolar process.

Primary curvatures of the dentinal tubule. These are the two curvatures of the dentinal tubule in the crown of the tooth that give the tubule its S shape.

Primary enamel cuticle. The epithelial attachment or the organic matrix responsible for binding the epithelium to the tooth. It is essentially the basal-lamina material formed by the epithelium.

Primary intention healing. The healing that occurs when wound edges can be sutured together, thereby minimizing scar formation.

Proliferative cell zone. Zone in endochondral bone formation characterized by the presence of dividing chondrocytes.

Proliferative period. Time during which cells grow and increase in number by cell division.

Proline. Naturally occurring non-essential heterocylic amino acid.

Promoter. A core promoter sequence of DNA specifies the exact point of transcription, that is, RNA chain elongation and positioning of the RNA polymerase. These sequences are recognized by gene regulatory factors (i.e., transcription factors) and are located very close to the transcribed gene. Promoter sequences are often enriched in adenine and thymidine bases (TATA box) and cytosine, adenine, and thymidine bases (CAAT box).

Prostiglandins. A group of hormones or hormone–like substances found in semen or menstrual fluid.

Proteoglycan. A glycoprotein with a very high carbohydrate content. These proteins are produced by odontoblasts and fibroblasts, are usually found in younger pulps or during active dentinogenesis, and are found reduced in older pulps.

Protein kinase A. Cyclic AMP-dependent protein kinase that is the intracellular effector molecule activated by cyclic AMP.

Proximate tissue interactions. Another term for secondary induction, referring specifically to the requirement that the epithelium and mesenchyme be in close proximity to one another.

Pulp bifurcation. Zone of branching of the pulp organ, as found in multirooted teeth.

Pulp organ. Soft tissue within the tooth, consisting of connective tissue, blood vessels, nerves, and lymphatics.

Pulpal blood vessels. Characteristic capillary thin-walled blood vessels of the dental pulp. Large vessels in central pulp with loops among odontoblasts.

Pulpal stones (denticles). Calcified mass of dentin–like substance located within the pulp or projected into it from its attachment in the dentin wall. (See *Attached, Embedded,* and *Free pulp stones.*)

Pulp chamber. The space surrounded by dentin in which the pulp organ resides.

Pus. A wound fluid mainly composed of dead neutrophils and their products.

Pyknotic. A reduction in size, condensation. Usually refers to a cell or nucleus of a degenerating cell in which the chromatin condenses to a structureless mass.

Rab. A monomeric G-protein required for vesicle transport and docking within the cell.

Radiation. Transmission of rays: light rays, short radiowaves, ultraviolet rays, or X rays. The latter are used for treatment or diagnosis.

Radicular. Concerning a root.

Ramus. General term to designate a smaller structure given off a larger one or into which a larger structure divides.

Ramus of mandible. Quadrilateral process projecting superiorly and posteriorly from the body of the mandible.

Rathke's pouch. Rathke's diverticulum; the pituitary diverticulum. A sac–like opening extending from the roof of the stomodeum toward the base of the brain.

Red blood cell (corpuscle, erythrocyte). A non-nucleated, biconcave cell bearing hemoglobin and responsible for transport of oxygen to tissues via the circulatory system.

Reduced enamel epithelium. The several layers of the epithelial enamel organ remaining on the surface of the enamel after enamel formation is complete.

Regulated secretion. Secretion in a direct response to the binding of a secretagogue to a cell surface receptor, leading to stimulation of a signal transduction pathway (e.g., cyclic AMP-G or protein or phosphoinositide cycle-calcium) causing secretion. Typically, the secretion product is stored in secretory vesicles and released in response to a secretagogue. There is no secretion in the absence of the secretagogue.

Remodeling. Altering of the structure by reconstruction. The continuous process of turnover of bone carried out by osteoblasts and osteoclasts.

Reparative dentin. The deposition of new dentin by newly differentiated odontoblasts at the site of pulpal trauma. A defensive reaction whereby hard-tissue formation walls off the pulp from the site of the injury.

Reserve cell zone. Site in endochondral bone characterized by the presence of resting cells, termed prechondroblasts. This zone lies adjacent to the perichondrium.

Respiratory mucosa. Lining of the respiratory system consisting of pseudostratified columnar epithelium containing numerous goblet cells and bearing true cilia in the apical region of the cell.

Retrovirus. A large class of RNA-containing viruses that reverse the classic pattern of DNA→RNA→protein by using RNA as a template to form a double-stranded DNA intermediate. Reverse transcriptase is found within retroviruses and uses RNA as a template to make DNA.

Retzius' striae. Lines reflecting successive incremental deposition of mineralized tissue (enamel).

Reversal lines. Lines separating layers of bone or cementum deposited in a resorption site from the scalloped outline of Howship's lacunae. The latter is obliterated by action of osteoblasts or cementoblasts. Deposition of new hard tissue leaving a visible line where the reversal of resorption took place.

Rod sheaths or arcades. Hypomineralized area in enamel representing the outline of the distal portion of Tomes' process. It lies at the intersection between rod and interrod enamel.

Root canal. Space containing pulp tissue of the tooth's root.

Root resorption. Dissolution of the root of a tooth by addition of osteoclasts. May occur anywhere along the surface of the tooth root in response to caries, trauma, or the loss of a primary tooth.

Root sheath cells (Hertwig's). Merged outer and inner epithelial layers of the enamel organ, extending beyond the region of the crown to invest the developing root. The cells induce dentinogenesis of the root and atrophy as the root is formed, but when the cells persist, they are called (Malassez') epithelial rests.

Root trunk. That part of the tooth immediately below the crown neck, covered by cementum and fixed in the alveolus.

Sagittal plane. Median plane in the anteroposterior direction.

Saliva. Clear, sightly alkaline, somewhat viscid mixture of secretions of the salivary glands and gingival fluid exudate. It functions to moisten the mucous membranes and food, facilitating speech and mastication. Contains water and 0.58% solids.

Salivary calculi. Calcium phosphate concretions (salivary stones) found within a salivary gland or duct, most commonly in the main excretory duct of the submandibular gland (Wharton's duct); the pathologic state known as sialolithiasis.

Salivary corpuscle. One of the leukocytes or lymphocytes found in saliva.

Salivary gland. Exocrine glands whose secretions flow into the oral cavity.

Sclerotic dentin. Dentin in which tubules are occluded with mineral. This dentin then is non-tubular and is termed transparent. Occurs mostly in elderly people, especially in the roots of teeth.

Sealant, dental. Agent that protects this enamel surface against the access of saliva. A resin capable of bonding to the surface of a tooth and offering protection against outside chemical or physical agents.

Secondary curvatures of the dentinal tubule. These are microscopic undulations of the dentinal tubule formed during deposition and mineralization of the dentinal matrix.

Secondary dentin deposition. Deposition of dentin circumpulpally formed after tooth eruption.

Secondary enamel cuticle. The epithelial covering of reduced enamel epithelium that is lost soon after eruption due to abrasion. It is the same as Nasmyth's membrane.

Secondary induction. Embryonic induction other than the primary neural induction, which involves the interaction of epithelium and mesenchyme occurring in the teeth and salivary glands. In induction one cell population (A) responds to a second group of cells (B), which causes a change in phenotype of the first population (A) to form a new cell type (C). The newly differentiated cells (C) will only form if the inducer (B) is present. After differentiation, these cells may serve as inducers when they are proximate to other cells.

Secondary intention healing. The healing that occurs when wound edges cannot be approximated, which causes healing with significant scar formation.

Secretagogue. Signal in extracellular environment that stimulates the release of secretory product within the regulated pathway. ß-Adrenergic and muscarinic drugs are secretagogues for salivary-gland acinar cells.

Secretory canaliculus (secretory capillary). Canaliculus found between acinar cells. Spaces provide communication between the serous acinar cells and the lumen. They rarely are found between mucous cells.

Secretory granules. A prominent feature of the secretory cell accumulating in its apical cytoplasm. Granules are about 1 μm in diameter and have a distinct, limiting membrane and a dense homogenous content.

Senescence. The state of growing old; beginning in old age.

Seratonin. A vasoconstrictor found in serum and body tissues that has the ability to modify neuronal function.

Serous. Relating to, containing, or producing a serious substance with a watery consistency.

Serous demilumes. Half-moon or crescent-shaped serous cells associated with the terminal external surface of mucous alveoli.

Serous glands of tongue (von Ebner). Serous glands opening in the bottom of the trough surrounding the circumvillate papillae and functioning in cleansing action.

Sheath of Neuman. Boundary between the intratubular and peritubular dentin. It represents the initial boundary of the dentinal tubule prior to intratubular dentin deposition.

Short-range matrix-mediated interaction. An embryonic interaction that is mediated by inductive molecules within the extracellular matrix, the matrix itself, or paracrine factors liberated in the immediate area.

Sialoadenitis. Inflammation of the salivary glands.

Sialography. Diagnostic X-ray technique visualizing salivary-gland ducts by injection of a radiopaque substance into the main excretory duct.

Sialolithiasis. Salivary calculi or stones which most often obstruct the main excretory duct of the parotid, submandibular, or sublingual glands (see also *Salivary calculi*).

Signal hypothesis. The hypothesis proposed by Dr. Gunther Blobel, Nobel prize winner, to explain the translocation of nascent peptides (destined for export) into the cisternal space of the rough endoplasmic reticulum (RER). The signal peptide for translocation in the RER is an N-terminal sequence of about 20 amino acids which directs newly synthesized transmembrane and secretory peptides to the lumen of the RER. The signal hypothesis, in general, explains the targeting of all proteins within the cell.

Signal recognition particle. The signal recognition particle binds to a newly synthesized peptide resulting in temporary arrest of protein synthesis and binding to a signal recognition particle receptor on the cytoplasmic face of the RER membrane. The signal recognition particle is recycled and protein synthesis subsequently continues.

Sinusoid. Resembles a sinus, a cavity. A form of terminal blood channel.

Sjögren's syndrome. Disease often associated with rheumatoid arthritis and believed to be an autoimmune disorder. Lymphoid infiltration of the parotid, submandibular, labial, and palatine glands leads to atrophy of gland parenchyma, which results in exocrine gland dysfunction.

Smear or smear layer. Debris formed by instrumentation of the tooth. The debris or smear particles form a layer that occludes dentinal tubules.

SNAPs. This abbreviation is short for **s**oluble NSF **a**ttachment **p**roteins. SNAPs form a complex with NSF. The NSF-SNAP complex binds to specific receptors called **SNAP re**ceptors **(SNAREs)**.

SNARE hypothesis. The hypothesis which explains vesicle docking in subcellular compartments along the secretory pathway. **NSF** and **SNAP** form a complex that binds to **SNAREs**. The Rab family of guanosine-triphosphatases (GTPases) is also present on the vesicle membrane and required for docking.

SNAREs. These are the SNAP receptors which bind NSF-SNAP complexes. There are two classifications of SNAREs: v-SNARE, which is located on the vesicle membrane, and t-SNARE found on the target membrane.

Soft Palate. The posterior muscular portion of the palate, forming an incomplete septum between the nasopharanx and the oral cavity.

Somatic growth. The growth pattern of the body in general.

Specialized mucosa. Mucosa found on the dorsum of the tongue that consists of four types of papillae: filiform, fungiform, circumvillate, and foliate.

Squamosal. Relating to the flat squama, as of the temporal bone.

Squamous epithelium. Composed of a single layer of flat scale–like cells, as in the lining of the pulmonary alveoli; oral epithelium.

Stapedial artery. Artery that supplies the region of the middle ear (stapes). Important in prenatal facial development.

Stellate reticulum. A network of star-shaped cells in the center of the enamel organ between the outer and inner enamel epithelium.

Stomedeum. The future oral cavity of the embryo; an invagination lined by ectoderm.

Stratified epithelium. A type of epithelium composed of a series of layers. The cells of each may vary in size and shape, as seen in skin and some mucous membranes.

Stratum germination. The inner layers of the epidermis resting on the corium; consists of several layers of polygonal cells (stratum spinosum) and a basal layer.

Stratum intermedium. The epithelial cell layer of the enamel organ that lies external and adjacent to the inner enamel epithelium and is attached to it by desmosones. Stratum intermedium also refers to the intermediate layer of non-keratinizing epithelia.

Striated duct. An intralobular salivary-gland duct involved in ionic transport, located between the intercalated and interlobular ducts. It is named for the basal striations created by infoldings of the basal membrane that produce compartments containing numerous mitochondria.

Stroma. Supporting framework of a gland, such as the capsule and trabeculae, rather than the functional parenchyma.

Sublingual. Area beneath the tongue, subglossal.

Sublingual gland. The smallest of the three pairs of major salivary glands. A pure mucous gland located in the anterior floor to the mouth.

Submandibular. Area beneath the lower jaw.

Submandibular gland. Largest of the three paired major salivary glands contributing 65% of the saliva. These two bilateral glands are a mixed seromucous type.

Submucosa. Layer of tissues that lies beneath the lamina propria underlying the mucous membrane of the lip, cheek, palate, and floor of the mouth.

Successional lamina. Portion of the dental lamina lingual to the developing deciduous teeth. It gives rise to the enamel organs that differentiate into permanent teeth.

Supporting bone. Bone tissue functionally related to the roots of the teeth. It surrounds, protects, and supports the tooth roots through the alveolar bone proper.

Sympathomimetrics. Imitating the effects of postganglionic adrenergic nerves.

Synarthrosis. A suture between two bones, with the uniting medium being a fibrous membrane continuous with the periosteum.

Synchondrosis. A type of cartilaginous joint that usually is temporary. The intervening hyaline cartilage ordinarily converts to bone before the person reaches adult life.

Syndesmosis. A type of fibrous joint in which opposing surfaces are united by fibrous connective tissue, as in the union between most of the facial bones.

Synovial cells. Cells that secrete synovial fluid. These are of two types: A and B. Type A is thought to secrete hyaluronic acid, while type B produces a protein-rich secretion.

Synovial membranes. Membranes that line joint cavities and function to secrete a small amount of clear, transparent, alkaline fluid in the articular spaces. Synovial fluid acts as a lubricant and nutrient for the avascular tissue covering (i.e., the condyle and articular tubercle of the temporomandibular joint). Also called synovial fluid.

Taste bud. Receptor of taste in the oropharanx. One of a number of goblet-shaped cells oriented at right angles to the surface by the epithelium. They consist of supporting cells and gustatory cells.

Temporomandibular joint. Joint formed between the condyle of the mandible and the mandibular fossa (concavity of the temporal bone).

Temporomandibular ligaments. Four ligaments: on the medial surface, the sphenomandibular; on the posterior surface, the stylomandibular; on the lateral surface, the temporomandibular and capsular.

Tenascin. An extracellular matrix molecule, transiently expressed during development, that slightly resembles fibronectin. It interacts with fibronectin in the extracellular matrix to regulate cell adhesiveness, and important environmental factor in cell migration and tissue remodeling during development.

Teratogen. Agent or factor that causes the production of physical defects in the developing embryo.

Terminal bar apparatus. That part of the ameloblast separating Tomes' process from the cell proper; localized condensations of cytoplasmic substance associated with the cell membrane.

Tic douloureux. Trigeminal neuralgia, repeated contraction, spasm, or twitching of the masticatory muscles usually resulting in extreme pain.

Tight junction. Fusions of the outer portions of adjacent cell membranes believed to provide a seal and communication between cells.

Tomes' granular layer. A granular-appearing layer in the dentin of the root adjacent to the cementum.

Tomes' process. Specialized apical zone of the ameloblasts. The apical Tomes' process is conical and interdigitates with the forming enamel rods.

Tonofibrils. Systems of fibers found in the cytoplasm of epithelial cells, which function with the desmosomal plaque to hold adjacent cells together.

Tooth crypt. Space filled by the dental follicle and developing tooth in the alveolar process.

Traction bands of the palate. Bundles of collagen that firmly attach the oral mucosa to the underlying bone of the hard palate.

Trans-Golgi network (TGN). The TGN is a meshwork of tubules and vesicles, which is the export (trans) face of the Golgi. It is the site of sorting to the plasma membrane and endosomes through vesicular transport of vesicles emanating from it surface.

Transcription. The process in eukaryotic cells by which the DNA sequence is converted into an RNA sequence by the action of RNA polymerase. It is the first step in the synthesis of proteins, which is followed by translation of the message (mRNA) on ribosomes.

Transduction. Conversion of physical force into biologic response. Theory proposing that odontoblasts are sensory receptors for pain stimuli transmitted through the dentin.

Translation. This process occurs on ribosomes and involves the conversion of the messenger RNA code, in the form of a nucleotide sequence, into specific amino acid incorporation into a nascent peptide.

Transport vesicles. Vehicles for the transport of materials from the intracellular compartment to another compartment (e.g., from the rough endoplasmic reticulum [RER] to the Golgli apparatus).

Trimer. A molecule composed of three identical simpler molecules.

Tufts. Clump or cluster of organic filled spaces in enamel that extends from the dentinoenamel junction for one-third of the thickness of enamel. Results in a defect in mineralization.

Turnover. Quantity of a material metabolized or processed in the body or a tissue within a given length of time.

Types I and III collagen. Two of the fibrillar collagens that form collagen fibrils after secretion into the extracellular milieu. Type I collagen is the most prominent form, accounting for about 90% of the collagen in the body. It is found in bone, tendon, and skin. Type III collagen is found in loose connective tissue, blood vessels, and in hematopoietic and lymphoid tissues, and is associated with the connective tissue side of the basement membrane.

Type IV collagen. The type of collagen associated with the basement membrane.

Vasculature. Reference to the blood vessels and circulating blood system.

Vermilion zone of the lip. Transitional zone between the skin of the lip and the mucous membrane of the lip, known as the red zone. Color due to thin epithelium, the presence of eleiden in the cells, and superficial blood vessels apparent in humans.

Vestibular lamina. Lip furrow band labial and buccal to the dental lamina; forms the oral vestibule between the alveolar portions of the jaws and the lips and cheeks.

Vicerocranial. Those parts of the facial cranial skeleton that are of pharyngeal-arch origin.

Vomer. Flat, unpaired bone located in the midline of the face, shaped like a trapezoid, and forming the inferior and posterior portion of the nasal septum. It articulates with the spheroid, ethmoid, two maxillary, and two palatine bones.

Waldeyer's ring. Group or ring of tonsilar tissue at the oropharyngeal–nasal junction.

Xerostomia. Dry mouth caused by lack of salivary secretion. Causes for xerostomia include pharmacologic agents such as antihistamines, radiation of head and neck tumors, and Sjögren's syndrome.

Zona pellucida. Translucent zone, non-cellular secreted layer, surrounding an ovum. It has a striated appearance due to the numerous fine canals with which it is pierced.

Zonula adherens (intermediate junction). Part of the junctional complex of columnar epithelial cells located deep to the zonula occludens where the plasma membranes of two adjacent cells divert to form a 15 to 20-nm-wide space.

Zonula occludens (tight junction). Part of the junctional complex immediately beneath the free surface and continuing all around the perimeter of the cell. There is no intercellular space, and the zonula occludens provides a permeability barrier to luminal material.

Zymogen. An inactive precursor that is activated to an enzyme by the action of an acid and an enzyme. Granules in serous cells of enzyme-secreting glands, such as the salivary glands and the pancreas.

Index

Note: page numbers in italics refer to figures and tables